Edited by

CHARLES F. FERGUSON, M.D., F.A.C.S.

Senior Otolaryngologist,
The Children's Hospital Medical Center;
Clinical Instructor in Otolaryngology,
Harvard Medical School,
Boston, Massachusetts

EDWIN L. KENDIG, JR., M.D., Sc.D. (Hon.)

Professor of Pediatrics, Medical College of Virginia,
Health Sciences Division,
Virginia Commonwealth University, Richmond, Virginia;
Director, Child Chest Clinic,
Medical College of Virginia Hospitals;
Director of Medical Education, St. Mary's Hospital,
Richmond, Virginia

PEDIATRIC OTOLARYNGOLOGY

Volume II

of

Disorders of the Respiratory Tract in Children

1972

W. B. SAUNDERS COMPANY

Philadelphia • London • Toronto

W. B. Saunders Company: West Washington Square
Philadelphia, Pa. 19105

12 Dyott Street
London, WC1A 1DB

833 Oxford Street
Toronto 18, Ontario

PEDIATRIC OTOLARYNGOLOGY

Volume 2 of Disorders of the Respiratory Tract in Children ISBN 0-7216-3615-2

 Made in the United States of America. Press of W. B. Saunders Company. Library of Congress catalog card number 70-173337.

Print No.: 9 8 7 6 5 4 3 2 1

To my dear wife, Elsa K. Ferguson,
for her patient understanding,
long-suffering forbearance and constant encouragement.

CONTRIBUTORS

GAYLE G. ARNOLD, M.D.

Associate Clinical Professor of Pediatrics, Health Sciences Division, Medical College of Virginia, Virginia Commonwealth University; Staff Physician, St. Mary's Hospital and Richmond Memorial Hospital, Richmond, Virginia

JOSEPH P. ATKINS, M.D.

Professor of Bronchoesophagology and Laryngeal Surgery, University of Pennsylvania Hospital; Attending Physician, Graduate Hospital; Surgeon, Children's Hospital, Philadelphia; Attending Physician, Bryn Mawr Hospital, Bryn Mawr, Pennsylvania

JOSEPH P. ATKINS, JR., M.D.

Resident, Johns Hopkins University School of Medicine, Division of Otolaryngology, Baltimore; Staff Otolaryngologist, U.S. Naval Hospital, National Naval Medical Center, Bethesda, Maryland

DANIEL C. BAKER, JR., M.D.

Professor and Chairman, Department of Otolaryngology, Columbia University College of Physicians; Director of Otolaryngology Service, Columbia Presbyterian Medical Center, New York, New York

DAVID ROZIER BEAM, M.D., D.D.S.

Chief Resident, Tampa General Hospital, Tampa, Florida

LESLIE BERNSTEIN, M.D., D.D.S.

Professor of Otolaryngology and Maxillofacial Surgery, University of Iowa College of Medicine, Iowa City, Iowa

MARIE A. CAPITANIO, M.D.

Associate Professor of Radiology, Temple University School of Medicine; Associate Radiologist, St. Christopher's Hospital for Children, Philadelphia, Pennsylvania

HENRY G. CRAMBLETT, M.D., F.A.A.P.

Professor and Chairman, Department of Medical Microbiology, Professor, Department of Pediatrics, College of Medicine, The Ohio State University; Attending Staff, Children's Hospital and University Hospitals, Columbus, Ohio

JOHN F. DALY, M.D.

Professor and Chairman, Department of Otolaryngology, New York University School of Medicine; Director of Otolaryngology, Bellevue and University Hospitals, New York, New York

RICHARD T. FARRIOR, M.D.

Clinical Professor, Department of Otolaryngology, College of Medicine, University of Florida, Gainesville; Senior Attending Physician, Plastic Surgery and Otolaryngology and Maxillo-Facial Surgery, Tampa General Hospital, Tampa, Florida

BLAIR FEARON, M.D., F.R.C.S. (C), F.A.C.S.

Assistant Professor, Otolaryngology and Broncho-Esophagology, University of Toronto; Senior Surgeon, Department of Otolaryngology and Broncho-Esophagology, Hospital for Sick Children, Toronto; Chief, North York General Hospital, Toronto; Consultant, Women's College Hospital, Toronto; Toronto and Oakville-Trafalgar

Memorial Hospital, Oakville, Ontario, Canada

CHARLES F. FERGUSON, M.D., F.A.C.S.

Senior Otolaryngologist, The Children's Hospital Medical Center; Clinical Instructor in Otolaryngology, Harvard Medical School, Boston, Massachusetts

JOHN P. FRAZER, M.D.

Professor of Otolaryngology, University of Rochester School of Medicine; Chief of Otolaryngology, Strong Memorial Hospital, Rochester, New York

PARK SPEARIN GERALD, M.D.

Professor of Pediatrics, Harvard Medical School; Chief, Clinical Genetics Division, Children's Hospital Medical Center, Boston, Massachusetts

GEORGE H. GIFFORD, Jr., M.D.

Assistant Clinical Professor of Surgery, Harvard Medical School; Associate in Surgery, Division of Plastic Surgery, Children's Hospital Medical Center; Staff Physician, New England Deaconess Hospital; Visiting Plastic Surgeon, Boston City Hospital, Boston; Senior Visiting Surgeon, Consultant Staff, Division of Plastic Surgery, Cambridge Hospital, Cambridge; Plastic Surgeon, Active Staff, Faulkner Hospital, Jamaica Plain; Visiting Staff Surgeon, Division of Surgery, Cardinal Cushing General Hospital, Brockton, Massachusetts

ALLAN C. GOODMAN, Ph.D.

Assistant Professor of Otology (Audiology), Assistant Professor of Rehabilitation Medicine, Tufts University School of Medicine; Director of Audiology, New England Medical Center Hospital, Boston, Massachusetts

JOHN M. HODGES, M.D.

Assistant Professor, Department of Otolaryngology and Maxillofacial Surgery, University of Tennessee College of Medicine; Head, Division of Facial Plastic and Reconstructive Surgery, City of Memphis Hospital, Memphis, Tennessee

PAUL H. HOLINGER, M.D.

Professor of Bronchoesophagology, Department of Otolaryngology, Abraham Lincoln School of Medicine, University of Illinois; Attending Bronchoesophagologist, Presbyterian-St. Luke's Hospital, The Children's Memorial Hospital, University of Illinois Hospital, and Eye & Ear Infirmary of University of Illinois, Chicago, Illinois

EDGAR M. HOLMES, M.D.

Senior Consulting Surgeon, Massachusetts Eye and Ear Infirmary; Consultant, Robert B. Brigham Hospital; Consultant, Free Hospital for Women; Consultant, Massachusetts Hospital for Crippled Children, Boston; Senior Consulting Surgeon, Newton-Wellesley Hospital, Newton Lower Falls; Consultant, Waltham Hospital, Waltham, Massachusetts

WILLIAM ALLEN HOWARD, M.D.

Clinical Professor of Pediatrics, George Washington University School of Medicine; Chief, Allergy Section, Children's Hospital, and Children's Hospital Research Foundation, Washington, D.C.

ROBERT M. HUI, M.D.

Professor of Clinical Otolaryngology, Columbia University College of Physicians and Surgeons; Attending Otolaryngologist and Chief of Ear-Nose-Throat Out-Patient Clinics, Columbia Presbyterian Medical Center, New York, New York

BURTON F. JAFFE, M.D.

Assistant Professor of Otolaryngology, Harvard Medical School; Chief, Department of Otolaryngology, Children's Hospital Medical Center; Chief, Department of Otolaryngology, Beth Israel Hospital; Associate Staff Member, Massachusetts Eye and Ear Infirmary, Boston, Massachusetts

JOHN A. KIRKPATRICK, M.D.

Professor of Radiology, Temple University School of Medicine; Radiologist, St. Christopher's Hospital for Children, Philadelphia, Pennsylvania

FRANK D. LATHROP, M.D.

Associate Clinical Professor of Otolaryngology (Emeritus), University of Vermont Medical School, Burlington; Attending Otolaryngologist, Medical Center Hospital of Vermont; Courtesy Staff, Otolaryngology, Rutland Hospital, Rutland, Vermont

WILLIAM E. LAUPUS, M.D.

Professor and Chairman of Pediatrics, Medical College of Virginia, Health Sciences Division, Virginia Commonwealth University; Director of Pediatrics, Medical College of Virginia Hospitals, Richmond, Virginia

DONALD W. MacCOLLUM, M.D.

Assistant Clinical Professor in Surgery, Harvard Medical School; Senior Associate in Surgery, Children's Hospital Medical Center, Division of Plastic Surgery, Boston, Massachusetts

HARRY LOUIS MUELLER, M.D.

Associate Clinical Professor of Pediatrics, Harvard Medical School; Chief, Division of Allergy, Department of Medicine, Children's Hospital Medical Center, Boston, Massachusetts

ARTHUR M. OLSEN, M.D., F.A.C.P.

Professor of Internal Medicine, Mayo Graduate School of Medicine, University of Minnesota; Consultant, Division of Thoracic and Internal Medicine, Mayo Clinic, Rochester, Minnesota

PETER N. PASTORE, M.D.

Professor and Chairman, Departments of Otorhinolaryngology, Facial-Maxillary Surgery, and Biocommunications. Audiology, and Speech Pathology, Medical College of Virginia, Health Sciences Division of Virginia Commonwealth University; McGuire Veterans Hospital; Crippled Children's Hospital; Richmond Ear-Nose-Throat Hospital, Richmond, Virginia

ROBERT J. RUBEN, M.D.

Professor and Chairman, Department of Otorhinolaryngology, Albert Einstein College of Medicine; Attending Physician and Chairman, Department of Otorhinolaryngology, Hospital of Albert Einstein College of Medicine, Bronx Municipal Hospital, and Lincoln Hospital; Attending Physician, Montefiore Hospital and Medical Center; Consultant, Department of Surgery, Misericordia Hospital; Senior Medical Consultant for Otorhinolaryngology, Department of Health; Consultant, U.S. Public Health Service Hospital, Staten Island, New York, New York

JOYCE A. SCHILD, M.D.

Clinical Assistant Professor of Otolaryngology, Abraham Lincoln School of Medicine, University of Illinois; Assistant Attending Otolaryngologist, Presbyterian-St. Luke's Hospital; Associate Attending Bronchologist, The Children's Memorial Hospital, Chicago, Illinois

HARVEY D. SILBERMAN, M.D.

Clinical Assistant Professor, Temple University School of Medicine; Albert Einstein Medical Center, Northern Division, Philadelphia, Pennsylvania

LEROY SMITH, M.D.

Clinical Professor of Surgery and Acting Chairman, Division of Plastic Surgery, Medical College of Virginia; Chief, Plastic Surgery, Crippled Children's Hospital; Attending Surgeon, Richmond Memorial Hospital; Attending Surgeon, St. Mary's Hospital; Attending Surgeon, Retreat for the Sick Hospital; Attending Surgeon, St. Elizabeth's Hospital, Richmond, Virginia

ROBERT M. SMITH, M.D.

Associate Clinical Professor of Anesthesia, Harvard Medical School; Director of Anesthesia, Children's Hospital Medical Center, Boston, Massachusetts

GABRIEL F. TUCKER, M.D.

Clinical Professor of Laryngology and Bronchoesophagology, Temple University School of Medicine; Professional Associate, Chevalier Jackson Clinic, Temple University Hospital; Chief, Department of Bronchoesophagology, St. Christopher's Hospital for Children, Philadelphia, Pennsylvania

JOHN A. TUCKER, M.D.

Professor of Surgery and Director, Division of Otolaryngology, Hahnemann School of Medicine; Department of Otolaryngology, Hahnemann Hospital, Philadelphia, Pennsylvania

MYLES G. TURTZ, M.D.

Associate Professor, Bronchoesophagology, Temple University School of Medicine; Chief, Department of Otorhinology, Laryngology, and Bronchoesophagology, St. Christopher's Hospital for Children, Philadelphia, Pennsylvania

J. LATANE WARE, M.D.

Assistant Clinical Professor of Surgery, Medical College of Virginia; Attending Surgeon, Medical College of Virginia, Crippled Children's Hospital, Richmond

Memorial Hospital, St. Mary's Hospital, and Retreat for the Sick Hospital, Richmond, Virginia

ROBERT HOWARD WILKINSON, M.D.

Assistant Professor of Radiology, Harvard Medical School; Radiologist and Associate in Medicine, Children's Hospital Medical Center, Boston, Massachusetts

NORMAN M. WOLDORF, M.D.

Instructor, Department of Otorhinolaryngology, Facial-Maxillary Surgery, and Biocommunications, Audiology, and Speech Pathology, Medical College of Virginia, Health Sciences Division of Virginia Commonwealth University, Richmond, Virginia

ARNOLD A. ZIMMERMANN, DR. ÈS SC.

Professor Emeritus of Anatomy, University of Illinois, Chicago, Illinois, and Baylor College of Medicine, Houston, Texas

PREFACE to Volume II

For many years it has been apparent that a textbook dealing with otolaryngological problems oriented to the very young patient is necessary for more adequate preliminary education of the medical student as well as for advanced training for the hospital resident. As pediatrics during the past 40 years has evolved into a most important and very broad specialty, so has increasing interest in its various sub-specialties proportionately expanded. Problems in otolaryngology now play a major role in the everyday practice of all busy pediatricians.

It is the intent of the editors and publishers that this work be geared especially to medical students, residents in pediatrics as well as in otolaryngology, to practicing pediatricians and to otolaryngologists who may only infrequently see young patients. Thus, the approach herein employed, along with the contents of the presented material, will differ from that found in the standard, general otolaryngological text.

Attempts to define the proper scope of such a text, however, have posed many difficult problems. The first edition of *Disorders of the Respiratory Tract in Children* contained several small chapters dealing with otolaryngology. The success of that edition clearly indicated to the publishers that a second edition should be undertaken. A logical sequence of that decision was to expand it into two volumes—the bulk of the original material to be covered in *Pulmonary Disorders,* and a new second book, *Pediatric Otolaryngology,* containing revision of some of the original material, but for the most part a new and more expanded text.

Although advances in pediatric otolaryngology during the past two decades have stimulated much greater interest in the field, it has been necessary for the student interested in otolaryngological problems to cull most of his information from lectures, original material in the literature, and from the annual Transactions of the various specialty societies. We have attempted to collect a good deal of this scattered material into a single volume and have been most fortunate in obtaining as authors those who are universally recognized as specialists in a particular area of the broad field of general otolaryngology. Obviously, in order to keep the volume down to a practical size and scope, much material had to be omitted.

This volume, therefore, cannot be considered as a complete reference work, but bibliographies found at the ends of chapters will prove a most useful reference source. Numerous excellent standard texts on otolaryngology also are available in all libraries and should be employed as supplements for descriptions of many basic problems.

Considering the many contributing authors, each one of whom is an authority in his own field and, therefore, must be given *carte blanche* in the expression of his own ideas, the editors have realized that there is inevitably some overlapping of material as well as divergent and occasionally even contradictory opinions on the same subject. This, however, should prove to be an advantage, since different approaches to the same problem always are of more value than are the thoughts of a single man.

The editors and publishers wish to express gratitude to the contributors, all busy practitioners as well as specialists in their particular field of interest, for giving generously of their time and talents to this undertaking. Any value or success which has been attained is obviously due to their wholehearted cooperation, suggestions and continued assistance. Many of the authors contributed to the first edition of *Disorders of the Respiratory Tract in Children* and have now revised or expanded their material. We cordially "welcome them aboard" once again. To those who are new on the project, we also extend a most sincere welcome in joining us—and our deepest appreciation to both groups.

Special thanks are due also to my secretary, Mrs. Evelyn DeLuca, who has typed and retyped countless pages of manuscripts, read proofs, and efficiently carried on much involved correspondence in mailing and re-mailing of manuscripts, prints and galley proofs as well as a myriad of other tasks well beyond the line of duty.

Mr. Robert B. Rowan, Vice President of W. B. Saunders Company, to whose strong powers of persuasion I finally succumbed in accepting this editorship, has been of tremendous assistance in planning and organizing countless details of production and has served as a constant and much-needed source of inspiration. To Mr. Richard Lampert and Mr. John Hanley, of W. B. Saunders, also goes much credit for their strong moral support, especially during the discouraging days when it seemed as if the final manuscripts would never arrive!

Grateful acknowledgment is also due the family of the late Lyman G. Richards, M.D., a revered mentor and fond associate with whom I shared offices early in my career, for their kind permission to reproduce several of the excellent line drawings from his 1939 textbook *Otolaryngology for the General Practitioner.*

CHARLES F. FERGUSON

PREFACE to Volume I

With this volume the second edition of *Disorders of the Respiratory Tract in Children* makes its appearance. The objective of the second edition is the same as that of its predecessor: To provide an answer to almost any question about respiratory diseases in children raised by the practitioner, resident or intern in pediatrics, the chest physician, the roentgenologist, the medical student or general practitioner. To better accomplish this aim, this edition has been expanded to include a second volume.

Pulmonary Disorders in Children, Volume I, is limited to disorders of the lower respiratory tract. New chapters are The Lung as an Organ of Metabolism, Intensive Care of Respiratory Disorders, Bronchopulmonary Dysplasia, The Wilson-Mikity Syndrome, Desquamative Interstitial Pneumonitis, and Fatal Granulomatous Disease. Two other chapters have been rewritten by new authors, and all material has been revised and brought up to date.

Volume II, edited by Dr. Charles F. Ferguson and myself, deals more with disorders of the upper respiratory tract and is entitled *Pediatric Otolaryngology.*

I should like to express my appreciation to the contributors who have made this book possible. For their dedicated zeal, willingness and expert attention to their assignment I am most grateful.

Gratitude is also due to Dr. John Chapman, Dr. Rosa Lee Nemir, Dr. Louis Siltzbach, and Dr. Sami Said for generously reading and criticizing specific chapters of the book. Dr. William Laupus and Dr. Donald Brummer have been particularly helpful in reading some portions of the manuscript, and both have contributed valuable advice.

Mrs. Nellie Gentry and Mrs. Joy Dobinson have assisted in the collection of case material for several of the chapters, and Mrs. Judith Gauldin has assisted in the proofreading and typing of the manuscripts.

I should like to acknowledge gratefully the cooperation and assistance of the staff of the W. B. Saunders Company.

EDWIN L. KENDIG, JR.

CONTENTS

VOLUME I

SECTION X DISORDERS OF THE RESPIRATORY TRACT DUE TO TRAUMA

VOLUME II

SECTION XI GENERAL CHAPTERS

SECTION XIII NOSE AND ACCESSORY SINUSES

SECTION XI

GENERAL CHAPTERS

Chapter Sixty-Two

ANESTHESIA FOR PEDIATRIC OTOLARYNGOLOGY

ROBERT M. SMITH, M.D.

GENERAL PRINCIPLES OF PEDIATRIC ANESTHESIA

Both anesthetist and surgeon must be aware of several underlying differences between children and adults as subjects for operation. The child's emotional reactions are more extreme and sometimes uncontrolled. This means that preoperative preparation is more critical, and local anesthesia is considerably less practical.

In relation to size, this has tremendous importance in airway maintenance, for encroachment upon the airway, whether by secretions, blood, an instrument or a kinked endotracheal tube, will cause disproportionately greater obstruction in smaller subjects.

As is well known, children have more marked physiologic responses, and will readily develop a fever of 104° F., a heart rate of 200 beats per minute, or respirations over 100 per minute; such signs in adults are observed rarely and are cause for greater concern.

There has been a great deal of speculation as to whether the child is as good an anesthetic risk as an adult. Unfortunately, this particular question has arisen in numerous communities in an attempt to explain why a child died during a "simple" tonsillectomy. Although there has been higher mortality in newborn infants during and after operation, this has been due chiefly to related defects, such as prematurity or congenital heart disease. A normal, healthy child facing tonsillectomy, or similar procedures, should be the best possible anesthetic risk, and morbidity and mortality that occur in such instances must be attributed to other causes. All operations involving the nose or throat threaten the airway, and complications are usually caused by the innumerable combinations of pathologic lesions, spasm, ventilatory depression, and anesthetic and surgical manipulation. Probably the main reason underlying many anesthetic deaths in children undergoing tonsillectomy is that this procedure has long been regarded as one that could be done in small hospitals by surgeons and anesthetists (sometimes pediatricians) who rarely did other types of pediatric surgery or anesthesia. Seasoned anesthesiologists regard tonsillectomy with respect, and consider the dangers associated with its complications second to none.

In our experience, considerably greater risk is involved when children undergo procedures involving instrumentation of the trachea, larynx and bronchi. However, if skilled personnel are charged with management of these patients, and if there is equipment on hand to care for serious emergencies, mortality can be held near zero.

Preparation of Children for Operation

Prior to anesthesia, every patient should have a thorough examination that includes history, physical examination, hemoglobin or hematocrit determination and urinalysis, these laboratory tests being performed within 48 hours of the intended operation. The anesthesiologist should visit the patient prior to induction to be able to judge for himself the overall picture and what special problems might be involved. Such individual assessment is especially important when any lesion encroaches upon the airway.

Preanesthetic Sedation

When respiration is obstructed or depressed, sedation may be contraindicated, but in most situations a child's fears are quieted by a mildly hypnotic agent, after which a vagolytic drug is added. Innumerable combinations have been advocated with rather similar results. Pentobarbital and atropine have been satisfactory, and seldom show undesirable side effects. To avoid unnecessary injections, pentobarbital may be given by rectal suppository, 2 to 2.5 mg./lb. of body weight, in children up to 8 years, or by mouth, 1.5 to 2 mg./lb. of body weight, an hour before operation. Atropine, 0.1 mg. per 10 lbs. of body weight, has proverbially been administered subcutaneously 45 to 60 minutes before anesthesia. In this situation the child suffers a needle puncture and a dry mouth, but the vagolytic effect is largely gone before anesthesia is started. It is more reasonable to withhold atropine until anesthesia has begun, and then give it intramuscularly or, if possible, intravenously.

Agents and Techniques

Methods employed for pediatric anesthesia are chosen to suit the patient and the intended operation. Procedures about the ear, nose and throat call for complete airway control and a moderate degree of analgesia. Although gag reflex and laryngeal spasm must be prevented, relatively little general muscular relaxation is needed. Apparatus has been simplified considerably, and two variations satisfy most needs. For children under 25 lbs., a light-weight, nonrebreathing apparatus proves practical and safe; a standard circle-type technique may be used for larger patients.

Ether still has the useful advantage of providing good tracheal relaxation while respiration remains active. Nevertheless, the related irritation, nausea and potential explosive hazard have virtually eliminated its use. Halothane, although dogged by the shadow of occasional fatal liver "sensitization,"[1,2] is technically ideal for nose and throat procedures because it is free from irritation or reflex stimulation.[3] Methoxyflurane, another fluorinated hydrocarbon of relatively recent origin, was gaining popularity for procedures requiring relaxation, but its probable role in causing renal failure has led to reasonable limitation of its use.[4,5] Nitrous oxide with relaxants and intravenous narcotics and sedatives has been employed extensively in adults, and is being used for younger patients, especially for more prolonged procedures, such as tympanoplasty. Endotracheal intubation is now considered mandatory for the majority of nose and throat procedures, and should involve very few disadvantages.

The greatest improvement in anesthesia has not been related to agent or to apparatus, but to standards of monitoring and supporting children during operation. This is evident in the general use of a precordial stethoscope, plus blood pressure apparatus made in suitably small sizes, and accurate temperature recording to prevent unnoticed development of hypothermia or hyperthermia, either of which may prove fatal.

Anesthesia for Operations about the Ear

Emergency myringotomy for an acute bulging ear drum in a child with a high fever is indicated less frequently at present because of antibiotic drugs. Food should be withheld for four hours before anesthesia, which can then be given as a mixture of nitrous oxide, oxygen and halothane with maximum safety. Since pain before and after this procedure is slight, preanesthetic sedation often may be omitted; frequently the best sedative is to have the child's mother stay with him just while he goes to sleep, then withdraw.

If the child's temperature is over 102° F., it may be preferable to provide moderate pain relief with morphine, and avoid the use of general anesthesia.

Mastoidectomy and Tympanoplasty

Longer operations are now commonly required for mastoidectomy or tympanoplasty, either of which may be an emergency or an elective procedure. General anesthesia and endotracheal intubation will be required under any circumstance, with careful monitoring plus intravenous hydration. In an emergency procedure, it is still safest to delay the procedure for two to three hours after any oral intake, and then to use careful inhalation anesthesia with halothane, avoiding rapid intravenous induction. The major safeguard against aspiration of vomitus is passing an endotracheal tube and making sure that it is not removed until the child is actually awake after operation.

Elective tympanoplasty may involve several hours. Here a light plane of anesthesia and minimal postoperative vomiting may be provided by intravenous combinations of thiopental or Innovar with supplemental nitrous oxide and oxygen. Monitoring and supportive therapy are of increased importance with longer operations. Continuous measurement of the temperature is mandatory in such procedures. The complete draping of the entire body and head of the patient renders him less easily observed and places him in greater danger of heat retention and hyperthermia. A thermistor may be placed in the nose, esophagus, axilla or rectum for such procedures.

For supportive therapy, blood replacement is seldom necessary, but fluid, calories and electrolytes are needed to maintain daily requirements. Here, 5 per cent dextrose in lactated Ringer's solution, given at a rate of 5 ml. per kilogram of body weight per hour is a practical measure.

Anesthesia for Operations About the Nose

Reduction of Fractured Nose. A very brief period of analgesia with a minimum of relaxation usually is required for reduction of a fractured nose. This can be accomplished using nitrous oxide and halothane, or other agents, but Ketamine and intravenous barbiturates are better avoided because of extreme stimulation of respiratory reflexes. The chief problems will be in patients who have eaten or have swallowed blood. In such patients, it is preferable to postpone anesthesia several hours, and then use endotracheal intubation with general anesthesia. At this time the pharynx may be packed to prevent the passage of more blood into the hypopharynx.

Plastic Operations on the Nose. For plastic procedures on the nose, light general anesthesia with oral endotracheal intubation is sufficient. Several different anesthetic agents may be employed. Halothane is nearly always most easily administered, but intravenous combinations are also valuable, and may be indicated when the patient's reaction to previous halothane anesthesia is questionable or unknown. Innovar is satisfactory, as well as combinations of nitrous oxide, a relaxant and morphine. Local anesthesia is employed by many plastic surgeons for rather extensive operations about the face, but it seems a poor method for children unless they are sedated to a point approaching general anesthesia. Blood replacement may be necessary and an intravenous line should be kept available.

Polypectomy. Removal of multiple nasal polyps may be required in children with cystic fibrosis. This may be an extensive procedure with considerable blood loss in relatively poor-risk patients. Use of nitrous oxide with oxygen and curare with oral intubation has been advantageous here, avoiding problems of further liver toxicity and allowing the surgeon to use epinephrine and electrocautery to facilitate his work.

Choanal Atresia. Choanal atresia is a rare but interesting anomaly consisting of occlusion of the posterior nares or choanae. Nasal breathing is impossible, and ventilation is considerably embarrassed. A halothane-oxygen induction with only atropine for premedication furnishes the safest approach here, and oral intubation will be mandatory. Following operation, these children may still encounter respiratory difficulty, and must be attended by personnel skilled in managing airway problems.

Operations Involving the Pharynx, Larynx, Trachea and Esophagus

TONSILLECTOMY. Tonsillectomy must be considered a potentially hazardous operation if complications are to be avoided. At present, this operation is generally performed under general endotracheal anesthesia upon children who have been prepared and sedated as for any major surgical procedure. The fact that some continue to operate without intubation shows that it can be done by skilled personnel; however, enlarged tonsils always reduce the airway, and ventilation often is obstructed. An endotracheal tube insures a continuous airway, largely prevents the passage of blood down the trachea and also prevents the passage of gas and anesthetic into the stomach, thereby reducing postoperative problems. Halothane is admirably suited for tonsillectomy. The use of succinylcholine for intubation is mostly a matter of choice. It facilitates intubation, and speeds it slightly, but initiation of spontaneous respiration may involve a short period of instability, which is avoided if relaxants are not used. With surgeons who perform tonsillectomy in less than 20 minutes, it is of even greater advantage to avoid succinylcholine.

Since the surgeon must work around the endotracheal tube, he will need all available room. The anesthesiologist can help by choosing a tube one size smaller than would be used for other procedures. If the tube is long enough to keep all adapters out of the surgeon's way, this will be of additional assistance. The type of mouth gag has been of tremendous importance. The Ring adaptation of the Brown-Davis gag, in which the tongue blade is grooved to fit over the endotracheal tube, is excellent in its control of tube position (see Figure 1). With the surgeon sitting above the head of the child, and the anesthesiologist beside the child, the monitoring of respiration and circulation is relatively easy. The point of greatest concern must be the airway. One must pay strict attention to the position and patency of the endotracheal tube at all times, since it may be obstructed or dislodged by surgical manipulation, or may become jammed or kinked in its relationship to the mouth gag. Continuous stethoscopic monitoring

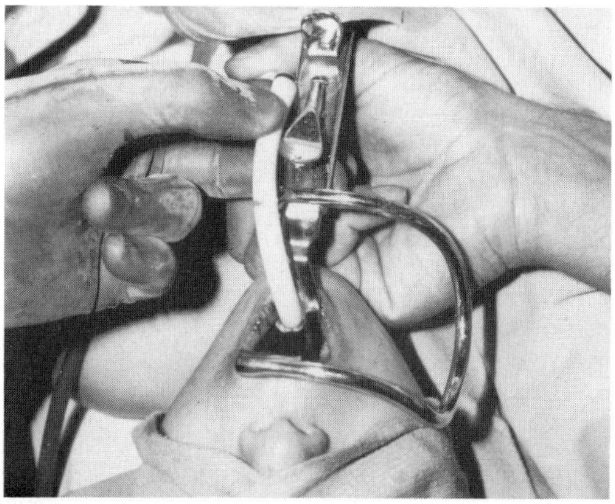

Figure 1. Tonsillectomy with endotracheal tube retracted by Ring tongue blade.

of breath sounds is helpful in all pediatric anesthesia, but it is mandatory for tonsillectomy.

Cardiac arrhythmias occur relatively often during tonsillectomy under halothane. These may be in the form of supraventricular arrhythmias, ventricular extrasystoles and bigeminy, and are seldom of serious consequence. It does not seem mandatory to use an electrocardiogram on all tonsillectomy procedures, but one should watch for any irregularities, and upon their appearance make certain that ventilation and oxygenation are excellent, and that blood pressure is unaffected. Should any of these conditions be abnormal, electrocardiographic diagnosis and elimination of halothane would be indicated.

Two characteristic complications may occur following tonsillectomy under halothane. Extubation may be followed by glottic spasm. This may be greatly reduced if extubation is performed while the child is still relatively deeply anesthetized. It is also helpful to use topical anesthesia, either by spray or by anesthetic jelly (4 per cent lidocaine), as an endotracheal tube lubricant. The second complication is a marked excitement stage during recovery, in which children are noisy and irrational prior to regaining consciousness. Although they do not remember it themselves, it can be disturbing to others, and may be prevented by adding a narcotic to the premedication, although some prefer to administer it intraoperatively and still others favor waiting until it is indicated, so that it will not cause unnecessary respiratory depression. Morphine or demerol may be used intramuscularly or intravenously. Morphine should be given 0.7 mg. per year of age intramuscularly or 0.3 mg. per year intravenously. Demerol should be given 1 mg./kg. of body weight intramuscularly or 0.5 mg./kg. intravenously.

Post-Tonsillectomy Bleeding. The proper handling of the "tonsil bleeder" is one of the major problems of pediatric anesthesia.[6] Assessment of the blood loss is an approximation at best, since an unknown amount of blood may have been swallowed, and emptying the stomach is too traumatic and unreliable to be indicated. Blood pressure, pulse rate, conjunctival color and hematocrit help evaluation, plus observation of stained bedclothes. Blood is cross-matched and intravenous infusion begun as primary acts. Atropine should be repeated. If signs are stable, general anesthesia may be induced with halothane and oxygen, observing all the safeguards used in patients with a full stomach, namely several suction tips of varied sizes, tongue blades, bite blocks, and succinylcholine drawn up in the syringe in case of uncontrollable spasm. The same sized endotracheal tube as previously used should be passed under halothane and oxygen anesthesia, without use of succinylcholine. The surgeon will then go ahead with hemostatic measures, after which the child is allowed to awaken with the endotracheal tube in place, to avoid regurgitation and aspiration.

Removal of Laryngeal Polyps. Polypoid growths (usually papilloma) occasionally are seen in children, and often recur many times, causing an appreciable emotional problem in addition to the vexing airway involvement. Unless there is definite obstruction, some sedation is helpful, after which halothane again provides gentle, nonirritating induction and adequate depth for endotracheal intubation without severe respiratory depression. A relatively small endotracheal tube is used, positioned posteriorly, allowing room for the surgeon to explore and remove the lesions while the airway is safely maintained.

Tracheostomy. Emergency tracheostomy is no longer performed on cyanotic, obstructed children, but more reasonably is undertaken only after an airway has been established by passage of an endotracheal tube or perhaps a bronchoscope. If the child is critically ill or hypoxic, no anesthesia may be required for the entire procedure. In others, local infiltration may suffice, but more often in

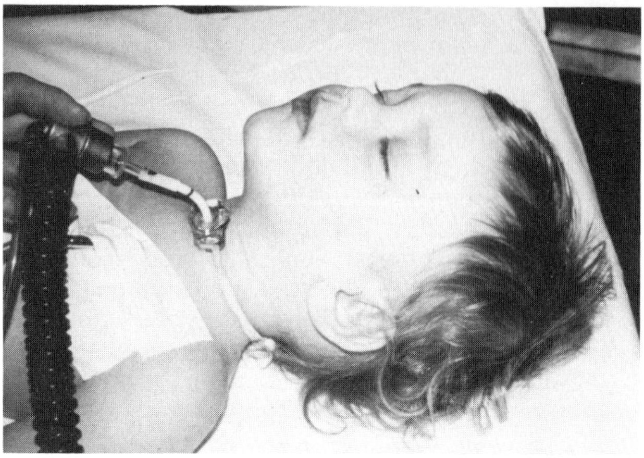

Figure 2. Anesthesia or supportive ventilation may be administered directly through tracheostomy.

prophylactic tracheostomy, general halothane-oxygen anesthesia is induced, the trachea is intubated, and controlled general anesthesia is administered, allowing the surgeon a safe, quiet field and ample time to perform this crucial procedure. To facilitate the operation, the shoulders are propped well up, with the head extended. When the trachea is opened, the anesthesiologist retracts the endotracheal tube just enough to clear the path for the tracheostomy tube, but it is not withdrawn above the vocal cords until satisfactory functioning of the tracheostomy is insured. If the child's ventilation is depressed, respiration should be assisted by adapting the anesthesia apparatus to the tracheostomy tube (see Fig. 2).

Removal of Foreign Bodies from the Esophagus

Foreign bodies that lodge in the esophagus are seldom a serious problem unless they are sharp or have become buried in the esophageal wall. Mild sedation plus halothane, nitrous oxide induction and endotracheal intubation should give the endoscopist reasonable opportunity to reach the offending object. Additional assistance can be furnished by the use of an endotracheal tube of minimal feasible bore but with adequate length to keep adapters out of the field.

Removal of Foreign Bodies from Trachea and Bronchi

Much greater difficulty (and danger) is met when some object finds its way into a child's trachea. Since children put everything imaginable into their mouths, pediatric endoscopists find currency of all nations, bones of mammals and fishes, pins, nuts, bolts, small parts of metal and plastic toys, and many other items. Some objects cause instant emergencies, but others go unsuspected for days or weeks.

Anesthesia for recovering aspirated foreign bodies first requires a quiet induction, which means light sedation supplemented by adroit handling. Intravenous agents are contraindicated because of the resultant exaggerated response to respiratory stimuli. Halothane is excellent here, since it is nonirritant and moderately rapid, and can be used without nitrous oxide when patients are hypoxic.

Anesthesia is induced evenly, with light inspiratory assistance. As soon as the patient can tolerate it, topical anesthesia of the glottis, trachea and carina is applied by spray, using 4 per cent lidocaine, up to 4 mg./kg. of body weight. Halothane is continued to provide even, moderately deep anesthesia, and an infusion is started. When the pupils are fixed and small, the patient is well relaxed and ventilation is quiet, the endoscopist is given an opportunity to pass the bronchoscope, to which the anesthetist should be able to attach his anesthesia apparatus, and thereby continue to deliver halothane and oxygen, the child breathing with quiet spontaneous respiration. The endoscopist can find and grasp the object without haste.

It is this moment that proves most critical, for as the endoscopist withdraws the bronchoscope, with forceps grasping the foreign body, the anesthesia often has become light enough to cause some adduction of vocal cords. If any edges of the foreign body project beyond the edge of the bronchoscope, the constricting vocal cords do not allow its passage. It falls from the grasp of the forceps and remains in the trachea, which may become completely occluded.

A most valuable maneuver to avoid this catastrophe is for the anesthetist to wait until the endoscopist grasps the foreign body, and then inject an intravenous dose of succinylcholine (2 mg./kg. of body weight), which promptly causes apnea and complete relaxation of vocal cords. The cords fall apart and allow maximum room for delivery of bronchoscope, forceps and foreign body.

Since the patient is still apneic at this point, the anesthetist must pass an endotracheal tube and ventilate the child until adequate spontaneous respiration returns. The endotracheal tube may then be removed and the endoscopist given an opportunity to re-examine the tracheobronchial tree.

Anesthesia for Diagnostic Procedures

LARYNGOSCOPY. Many small infants require laryngoscopy for diagnosis of stridor, and older children occasionally are seen with hoarseness and similar problems. Adequate examination frequently can be made using topical anesthesia, but general anesthesia with halothane plus topical anesthesia will give more satisfactory conditions, especially if a tracheogram is to be made. In larger children, a relatively small endotracheal tube can be introduced to maintain airway control during examination, but this should rarely be necessary.

BRONCHOSCOPY AND BRONCHOGRAPHY. In children, these procedures have always been a real test of skill and cooperation among endoscopist, anesthetist and radiologist, calling for the best in each. For bronchoscopy, the anesthetist prepares the child and manages induction of anesthesia, as was just described for removal of a foreign body, with halothane as the chief inhalation agent, supplemented when possible by nitrous oxide, and always by careful spraying of glottis, trachea and carina with topical anesthetic such as 4 per cent lidocaine (maximum safe dose, 1 ml. [40 mg.] per 10 lbs. of body weight).

When the child is relaxed, his respiration depressed, and his pupils fixed and contracted, the endoscopist passes the bronchoscope. The anesthetist continues to administer anesthesia by attaching the anesthesia apparatus to an outlet on the bronchoscope. Cardiac and respiratory action must be continuously and assiduously monitored throughout the procedure. Either stimulation of abnormal reflexes or airway obstruction may be produced by many factors. When room lights are dimmed, the anesthetist can use his laryngoscope as a flashlight to check signs.

Usually there will be a moderately large leak around the bronchoscope. If the patient needs assisted ventilation, this can be provided by running high gas flows and by having the endoscopist close the end of the bronchoscope with the glass end-plate or with his finger, or by using a ventilating bronchoscope.

When bronchography is undertaken following bronchoscopy, the bronchoscope is removed and an endotracheal tube passed. To facilitate passage of radiopaque material into the trachea, we employ a curved metal adapter (Rovenstine adapter) with a side arm, to which we fit a perforated rubber tip. The dye-containing catheter can be passed through this, and an air-tight system can be maintained, so that if apnea is required, artificial ventilation can be provided by compression of the breathing bag. Apnea can easily be produced by small intermittent intravenous doses of succinylcholine. Again, monitoring must be carried out with great care. When possible, two anesthetists should join in the management of these procedures, since filling the airway with sticky dye, then turning the child in many positions, in the dark, all combine to produce a potentially hazardous condition. At its conclusion, the child may be in a precarious condition, and one must clear his airway and promote adequate oxygenation before moving him from the examination table.

REFERENCES

1. Popper, H., Rubin, E., Gardiol, D., Schaffner, F., and Paronetto, F.: Drug-induced liver disease. *Arch. Intern. Med.,* 115:128, 1965.
2. Davidson, C. S., Babior, B., and Popper, H.: Concerning hepatotoxicity of halothane. *New Eng. J. Med.,* 275:1497, 1966.
3. Pittinger, C. B.: Halothane—its usefulness in otolaryngological procedures. *West. J. Surg. Obstet. Gyn.,* 69:189, 1961.
4. Crandell, W. B., and MacDonald, A.: Nephropathy associated with methoxyflurane anesthesia. *J.A.M.A.,* 205:798, 1968.
5. Frascino, J. A., Venemee, P., and Rosen, P. P.: Renal oxalasis and azotemia after methoxyflurane anesthesia. *New Eng. J. Med.,* 283:676, 1970.
6. Smith, R. M.: *Anesthesia for Infants and Children,* 3rd ed. St. Louis, C. V. Mosby, 1968.

Chapter Sixty-Three

GENETICS AND CHROMOSOMAL ABNORMALITIES

PARK S. GERALD, M.D.

Although the precise percentage of otolaryngologic disorders that may be assigned a genetic cause is unknown, it is undoubtedly of significant size. A recent tabulation of the varieties of hereditary deafness, for example, included over 70 different conditions (McKusick, 1971).

The various genetically determined disorders of otolaryngologic interest may be classified into three major groups: (1) those inherited in a simple dominant or recessive fashion, (2) those due to a demonstrable chromosome abnormality and (3) those that belong to neither of the two preceding groups but that nevertheless occur within certain families with a frequency greater than that observed in the general population. These three categories are discussed separately.

DISORDERS INHERITED IN A DOMINANT OR RECESSIVE FASHION

These conditions are representative of the group of diseases conventionally considered to be inherited. Since the individual inherited defects are considered at length in the separate chapters discussing the various organs and systems, the material of this section will be confined to a discussion of general principles.

The normal individual has 23 pairs of chromosomes (Fig. 1), including one pair of sex chromosomes (an X and a Y in the male and two X's in the female) and 22 pairs of nonsex chromosomes (the au-

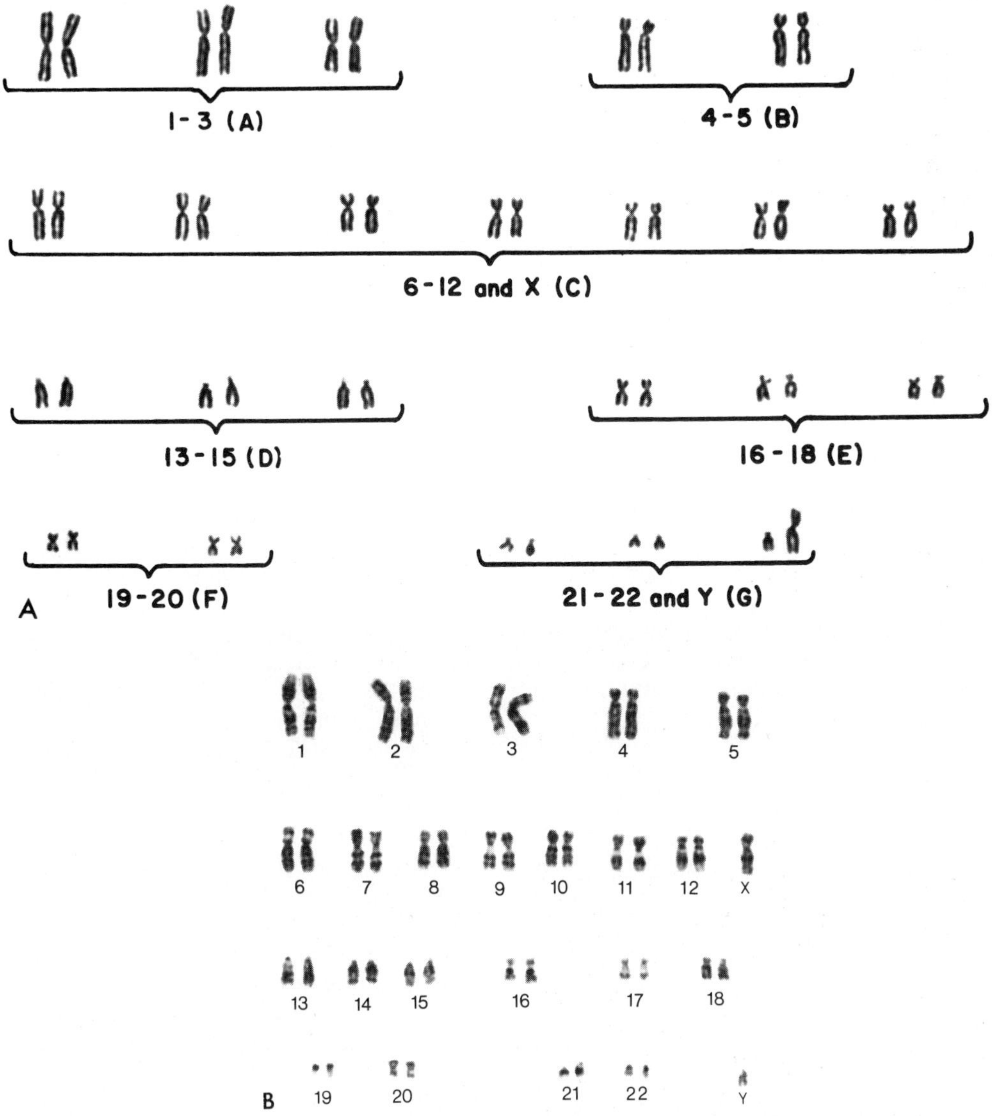

Figure 1. *A,* The standard (Denver) karyotype prepared with the conventional Giemsa staining technique. Classification is based upon chromosome size and relative length of chromosome arms. Only the individual pairs of group A (chromosomes 1, 2, and 3) and chromosome 16 may be identified by this means. By use of autoradiography (tritiated thymidine incorporation), further distinctions may be made (in groups B, D and E), but only with great labor and technical skill. *B,* Karyotype prepared with a "modified Giemsa stain" (Sumner et al., 1971) that distinguishes every pair of chromosomes. This karyotype may be adopted as the standard in the near future. Other special staining procedures, such as fluorescent staining, give comparable results. (Photograph provided by Drs. A. T. Sumner and H. J. Evans.)

tosomes). Each member of a pair is usually identical to its partner in its appearance and in the genes it contains. (The X and Y sex chromosomes in the male constitute a unique exception to this rule.) For this reason, the members of a pair are said to be homologous. Homologous chromosomes have comparable genes located at identical points along their length. The point at which a gene may be found in a particular chromosome (or in its homologue) is known as its locus. Loci, and the genes they contain, thus occur in pairs, and a pair of loci are referred to as homologous loci.

A given kind of gene, including any of its mutant forms, will always be found at its specific locus. Alternative forms of a gene that can occur together, each at one member of a pair of homologous loci, are said to be alleles, and they necessarily govern the same function. On the other hand, genes located at different, nonhomologous loci are apparently never identical, although they may govern related (but not identical) functions.

Ova and sperm normally possess only one member of each chromosome pair. Hence, each parent contributes one member of each pair of genes to any child. This behavior of genes explains the distribution in families of dominantly and recessively inherited conditions. If only one of a pair of genes need be altered for the disease or condition it controls to be expressed, then the condition will be dominantly inherited. On the average, half of the gametes formed by the individual who has a dominantly inherited condition will contain the altered gene. Hence, about half of his offspring will inherit the condition.

If both members of a pair of genes must be altered for a condition to be expressed, then the condition is recessively inherited. All of the gametes formed by an individual with a recessively inherited condition will contain one (and only one) altered gene. Hence, an individual with a recessively inherited condition cannot pass on both his altered genes to his children. An individual with a recessively inherited condition necessarily has inherited one altered gene from each of his parents. In most instances, each parent will have only a single altered gene and therefore will not express the condition themselves.

The foregoing strictly applies only to autosomal genes. Genes located on the X chromosome (X-linked genes) follow a different inheritance pattern, since a male has only one X chromosome and the Y contains at most only a few loci homologous to those on the X. Recessively inherited conditions determined by X-linked genes are therefore expressed in the male, even though he has only one altered gene. (For a more complete account of X-linked inheritance, the reader should consult a clinical genetics textbook such as those by McKusick [1969] and Porter [1968].)

A major feature of our present understanding of inherited disease is the recognition that a multiplicity of genetic defects may produce the same clinical picture (phenotype). A number of loci participate, for example, in the formation of the structures required for normal hearing. Defective genes at any one of these loci may produce deafness. Furthermore, at any one of these loci a number of allelic, mutant genes can exist, each of which may cause deafness. It is predictable, therefore, that inherited deafness will be genetically heterogeneous, and the present list of over 70 different types (McKusick, 1971) will probably be made even larger in the future.

It is generally true that a group of patients with apparently the same phenotype is often found, upon more intensive study, to be classifiable into clinically distinct subgroups, each resulting from a different genetic cause. Within a single family, however, no more than one or two relevant, abnormal genes will be found. For this reason, the clinical courses of affected members within an individual family are usually far more similar to one another than they are to the clinical picture in other families (or to the textbook description of the disease!).

A complete listing of the diseases that exhibit dominant and recessive inheritance, including the known inherited otolaryngologic defects, has recently been published by McKusick (1971). Descriptions of the clinical appearance associated with many of these disorders have also been compiled (Goodman et al., 1970; Gorlin et al., 1964; Smith, 1970).

DISORDERS RESULTING FROM CHROMOSOME ABNORMALITIES

A chromosome abnormality is found in about one out of every 200 newborn infants. Approximately half of these involve the sex chromosomes; the remainder are disorders of the autosomes (Table 1). Only the autosomal disorders are of concern here, since gross otolaryngologic abnormalities are rare in patients with sex chromosome disorders.

The autosomal disorders listed in Table 1 consist of the three relatively common trisomies, in which an extra but otherwise normal chromosome is present in the karyotype, and of a group of disorders known as chromosome rearrangements. The term rearrangement is used to describe an altered structure in a chromosome. These alterations in general result from multiple chromosome breaks and reunion of the chromosome fragments in an abnormal order. The rearrangement may be confined to a single chromosome or may involve transfer of genetic material between two chromosomes.

TABLE 1. OCCURRENCE OF CHROMOSOME ABNORMALITIES IN 4400 CONSECUTIVELY BORN INFANTS*

Sex chromosome abnormalities	11
Autosomal abnormalities	
Trisomy 13	1
Trisomy 18	1
Trisomy 21	3
Rearrangements†	6
Total (1/200)	22

*From Lubs, H., and Ruddle, F. H.: Applications of quantitative karyotypy to chromosome variation in 4400 consecutive newborns. In Jacobs, P. A., Price, W. H., and Law, P.: *Human Population Cytogenics.* Baltimore, Williams & Wilkins Co., 1970.

†All of these infants had a normal phenotype and the rearrangements were thought to be "balanced" translocations.

Chromosome abnormalities produce congenital malformations when they result in an excess or a deficiency of genes, or both. It is not yet known why such a genetic imbalance is deleterious. The disturbance is apparently a specific process, since each particular type of imbalance generally produces a relatively consistent phenotype. There are now a number of syndromes known to be due to chromosome abnormalities (Table 2). A comprehensive tabulation of the clinical findings associated with most reported chromosome disorders is now available (Levine, 1971).

Trisomy results from abnormal cell division, during which a chromosome is included in the wrong daughter cell. The process is generally termed nondisjunction and may occur during either meiosis (gametogenesis) or mitosis. (The term nondisjunction emphasizes that the extra chromosome arises from failure of the normal process of separation or disjoining of chromosomes during cell division. The extra chromosome is normal in its structure and gene content; it is merely out of place.) Nondisjunction is almost never familial, and the parents of a trisomic child have normal chromosomes. Nondisjunction of chromosomes 21, 18, and 13 occurs with increased frequency in older women (Levine, 1971), but the reason for this is still unknown.

Experience with conventional means of chromosome analysis (the staining procedure of Figure 1*A*) has demonstrated that among congenitally malformed children who lack any of the well-characterized phenotypes of Table 2, about 5 per cent will have a chromosome abnormality as the cause of their congenital malformations (Gerald, unpublished data). In almost every instance, the chromosome abnormality will be of the rearrangement type, with

TABLE 2. OTOLARYNGOLOGIC MANIFESTATIONS OF SOME CHROMOSOME ABNORMALITIES WITH CLEARLY DELINEATED PHENOTYPES*

Chromosome Abnormality	Otolaryngologic Abnormalities	Other Abnormalities
Trisomy 21	Poorly developed external ear	Severe mental retardation; typical facies; short, incurved fifth finger
Trisomy 18	Abnormal middle ear; low-set external ear; micrognathia	Severe mental retardation; failure to thrive; flexed fingers
Trisomy 13	Cleft palate with or without cleft lip; deafness; absent olfactory tracts	Severe mental retardation; ocular coloboma; polydactyly; arhinencephaly
Cat cry syndrome (deletion of short arm of 5)	Low-set external ears; laryngomalacia	Severe mental retardation; microcephaly
Deletion of long arm of 18	Atresia or stenosis of external ear; hearing defect	Severe mental retardation; characteristic facies; vertical talus
Cat eye syndrome (extra, small acrocentric chromosome, of undetermined origin	Preauricular tags or fistulae	Moderate mental retardation; imperforate anus; ocular coloboma; congenital heart disease

*The associated congenital malformations are usually numerous (Levine, 1971); only the most characteristic are listed here.

only small chromosome segments extra or missing.

It is believed that autosomal monosomies (absence of an entire autosome) or trisomies, other than those listed in Table 1, are lethal *in utero,* since they occur in abortuses but not in liveborn children (Carr, 1967). For most chromosomes, only small segments can be extra or missing if the fetus is to survive intrauterine life and be born as a congenitally malformed child. Even so, a seemingly endless variety of congenital malformation syndromes is possible—the precise phenotype in each instance will depend upon the specific combination of extra and missing chromosome segments. Even when relatively small chromosome segments are involved, the phenotype will consist of multiple congenital malformations rather than a single major malformation.

In view of the very large number of potential rearrangements, which individually will be quite rare, it is practical only to consider the general characteristics of rearrangements. The two commonest types of rearrangement of clinical significance are the deletions and the reciprocal translocations. Deletions are caused by the loss of a segment from an individual chromosome. (Deletions may be thought of as partial monosomies.) Two common deletion syndromes are now recognized (Table 2), and other, rarer types have been described. Deletions are nearly always sporadic and the other family members are free of chromosome defects.

A reciprocal translocation is a more complex type of rearrangement since two, usually nonhomologous, chromosomes are involved. If a break occurs simultaneously in each of two chromosomes and the segments separated from the centromeres in the process reattach, but to the wrong chromosome, a reciprocal exchange or translocation occurs (Fig. 2). When the process is reciprocal, no gain or loss of genetic material occurs, and the patient has a normal phenotype. The translocation in this case is said to be balanced. Mitosis is not affected by the presence of a balanced translocation, and the daughter cells produced by this type of cell division also contain the balanced translocation. When a cell with a balanced translocation enters meiosis, however, the adverse consequences of a balanced translocation may become evident (Fig. 2). This is illustrated by the following ex-

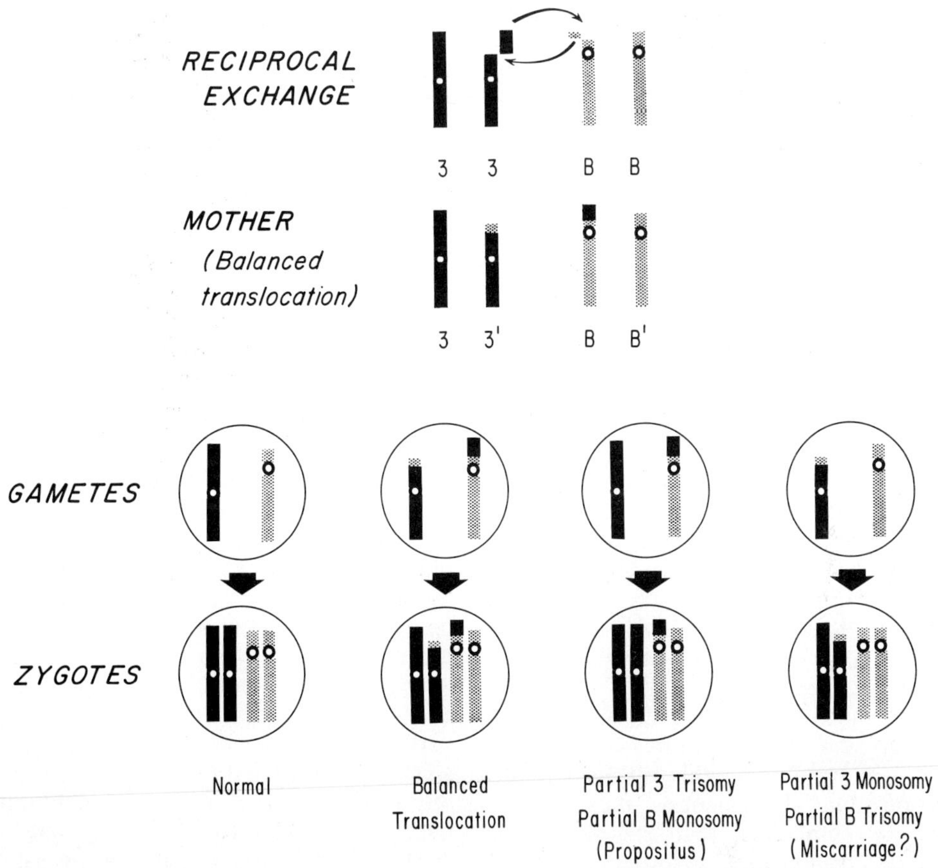

Figure 2. Schematic representation of a reciprocal translocation involving chromosome 3 and a B chromosome (Walzer et al., 1966). The four types of gametes and progeny (zygotes) expected for this translocation are shown.

ample from the author's experience (Walzer et al., 1966).

The propositus (Pedigree #2270) was born with bilateral cleft lip and complete cleft palate, a small mandible and low-set ears. A number of additional malformations were present, including iridial coloboma, bifid thumb, protuberant eye (secondary to a small orbit) and congenital malformations of the heart and great vessels. The patient developed congestive heart failure and died on the nineteenth day of life.

The family history initially obtained did not include other infants with congenital malformations. The propositus was found to have a chromosome abnormality, with one of his "B" chromosomes being increased in length. This was apparently the result of a reciprocal translocation, since his mother, who had no congenital defects, had a related chromosome abnormality. She had one abnormal "B" chromosome, identical to that in the propositus, as well as one #3 chromosome that was decreased in length. The increase in length of the abnormal "B" chromosome was equal to the decrease in length of the abnormal #3, suggesting that a reciprocal exchange of chromosomal segments had occurred (Fig. 2).

The reciprocal translocation could finally be traced to the great-grandfather and to five of his nieces and nephews. The descendants of these latter translocation carriers included five congenitally malformed infants (all were third cousins of the propositus) whose existence had not been previously known by the parents of the propositus. Of these congenitally malformed infants, three had cleft palate and the remaining two had both cleft lip and cleft palate, in addition to other defects resembling those noted in the propositus.

As Figure 2 indicates, two types of chromosome imbalance could be produced by the translocation in this family. The consistency in the phenotype of the affected infants suggests that only one of these occurred among the liveborn offspring. Presumably fetuses with the second type of imbalance could not survive intrauterine life and appeared only as miscarriages.

In slightly more than half of the families studied, the parents of individuals suffering from an unbalanced translocation have no chromosome abnormality (Gerald, unpublished data). In the remainder, one parent is a translocation carrier, with the balanced translocation occurring in every cell. In these families, the translocation can usually be traced through several generations.

Before concluding this discussion of chromosome abnormalities, it is necessary to emphasize that the study of human chromosome disorders is currently undergoing rapid development. The ability to identify every chromosome pair was not achieved until late in 1970 (Caspersson et al., 1970), and the simplified method of identification illustrated in Figure 1*B* was only developed in 1971 (Sumner et al., 1971). This visualization of internal detail will increase the probability of detecting subtle changes in chromosome structure and is certain to reveal chromosome rearrangements that were previously undetectable.

FAMILIAL DISORDERS WITHOUT SIMPLE GENETIC EXPLANATION

A number of morbid states that do not exhibit typical dominant or recessive inheritance and do not have an underlying chromosome abnormality may nonetheless occur among the members of certain families far more frequently than their occurrence in the general population would lead one to expect. Conditions with this characteristic are as diverse as cancer, pyloric stenosis and cleft lip–cleft palate. The familial concentration could result from either environmental or genetic factors or from some combination of the two. To date, only a few environmental factors have been shown to be relevant.

Diseases inherited in the typical dominant or recessive fashion are assumed to be determined by a pair of genes (at a pair of homologous loci), one or both of which are abnormal. This concentration upon a single locus ignores the vast number of other loci present in the human genetic complement. When the phenotype cannot be attributed primarily to the effect of a single locus, a more complicated genetic model, such as polygenic inheritance, must be considered. The polygenic model for inherited disease assumes that mutant genes at various loci individually have only a slight effect, but that these effects are additive, In that case, a disease might not be clinically manifest until, say, half a dozen or more mutant genes (at perhaps as many different loci) are present together in an individual. The number of loci involved, each of which may be inherited independently of the others, would preclude the transmission of polygenically determined disease in a simple dominant or recessive fashion.

The complexity of the polygenic model makes it difficult to test, although there is fairly general acceptance that pyloric stenosis is inherited in this fashion (Carter, 1970). It is possible that a number of otolaryngologic disorders, including certain types of cleft lip (Carter, 1970), may fit the polygenic model, but there is very little direct evidence to verify this.

REFERENCES

Carr, D. H.: Chromosome anomalies as a cause of spontaneous abortion. *Amer. J. Obstet. Gynec.*, 97:283, 1967.

Carter, C. O.: Multifactorial genetic disease. *Hosp. Prac.*, 5:45, 1970.

Caspersson, T., Zech, L., and Johansson, C.:

Analysis of human metaphase chromosome set by aid of DNA-binding fluorescent agents. *Exp. Cell Res.*, 62:490, 1970.
Goodman, R. M., and Gorlin, R. J.: *The Face in Genetic Disorders.* St. Louis, C. V. Mosby Co., 1970.
Gorlin, R. J., and Pindborg, J. J.: *Syndromes of the Head and Neck.* New York, McGraw-Hill Book Co., 1964.
Levine, H.: *Clinical Cytogenetics.* Boston, Little, Brown & Co., 1971.
Lubs, H., and Ruddle, F. H.: Applications of quantitative karyotypy to chromosome variation in 4400 consecutive newborns. In Jacobs, P. A., Price, W. H., and Law, P.: *Human Population Cytogenetics.* Baltimore, Williams & Wilkins Co., 1970.
McKusick, V. A.: *Human Genetics,* 2nd Ed. Englewood Cliffs, New Jersey, Prentice-Hall Co., 1969.
McKusick, V. A.: *Mendelian Inheritance in Man,* 3rd Ed. Baltimore, John Hopkins Press, 1971.
Porter, I. H.: *Heredity and Disease.* New York, McGraw-Hill Book Co., 1968.
Smith, D. W.: *Recognizable Patterns of Human Malformation: Genetic, Embryologic and Clinical Aspects.* Philadelphia, W. B. Saunders Co., 1970.
Sumner, A. T., Evans, H. J., and Buckland, R. A.: New technique for distinguishing between human chromosomes. *Nature,* 232:31, 1971.
Walzer, S., Favara, B., Ming, P. M. L., and Gerald, P. S.: A new translocation syndrome (3/B). *New Eng. J. Med.,* 275:290, 1966.

Chapter Sixty-Four

OTOLARYNGOLOGIC RADIOLOGY IN CHILDREN

ROBERT H. WILKINSON, M.D.

GENERAL PRINCIPLES

The goal of the radiologist is to obtain the maximum amount of information with the least possible radiation to the patient. For this reason, it is essential that experienced radiologists and radiographers use optimal equipment with proper tube filtration and beam collimation. High quality plain film should precede positive contrast examinations; all too frequently the latter are performed unnecessarily because standard films were technically unsatisfactory.

Fluoroscopy is especially valuable in children as an adjunct to preliminary films, since dynamic structures are being examined. Modern image amplification and minimal field size are essential to avoid excessive radiation. Positive contrast material should be used only under fluoroscopic control. If a volume of more than a few milliliters is to be used, one of the bronchographic agents rather than the more irritating water-soluble compounds should be selected, since aspiration into the tracheobronchial tree may well occur. Spot films, cinefluorography and video-tape are vital in recording anatomic changes and dynamics of function. Follow-up overhead films will frequently provide superior anatomic detail and should be used in conjunction with films exposed during the fluoroscopic examination.

Stereoscopic filming can be exceedingly helpful in skull, facial bone and chest problems, but the child must be cooperative or properly sedated for this method.

Laminograms (tomograms or body-section roentgenograms) are also useful diagnostic adjuncts. Since patient motion is unacceptable, this method has some limitations. Linear tomograms are satisfactory for many problems, but fine bony detail such as that required in the examination of the middle ear and the internal auditory canal is more clearly defined by a device capable of a more complex motion, such as a hypocycloidal tomographic unit.

THE NOSE

The most common nasal examination is for trauma, and two views are usually required. Right and left lateral projections and a Water's projection will usually suffice to permit evaluation of any displacement. Since a child's nose is small relative to the frontal bone, vertical beam views are generally not as satisfactory. The prominent nasofrontal and nasomaxillary sutures of children should not be mistaken for fractures.

Congenital anomalies such as absence of the nose, nasal encephaloceles and choanal atresia can be well defined radiographically. Bilateral choanal atresia may appear as a semi-emergent condition, since an infant experiences considerable distress during feeding when suffering from nasal obstruction. A presumptive diagnosis can be made if it is impossible to pass a small catheter through the nose. Preliminary removal of secretions by gentle suction is helpful, as is the instillation of a few drops of 0.25 per cent Neo-synephrine nose drops. Then the instillation of a small volume of oily Dionosil, preferably under fluoroscopic control, will demonstrate the obstruction (Fig. 1). It is desirable to allow

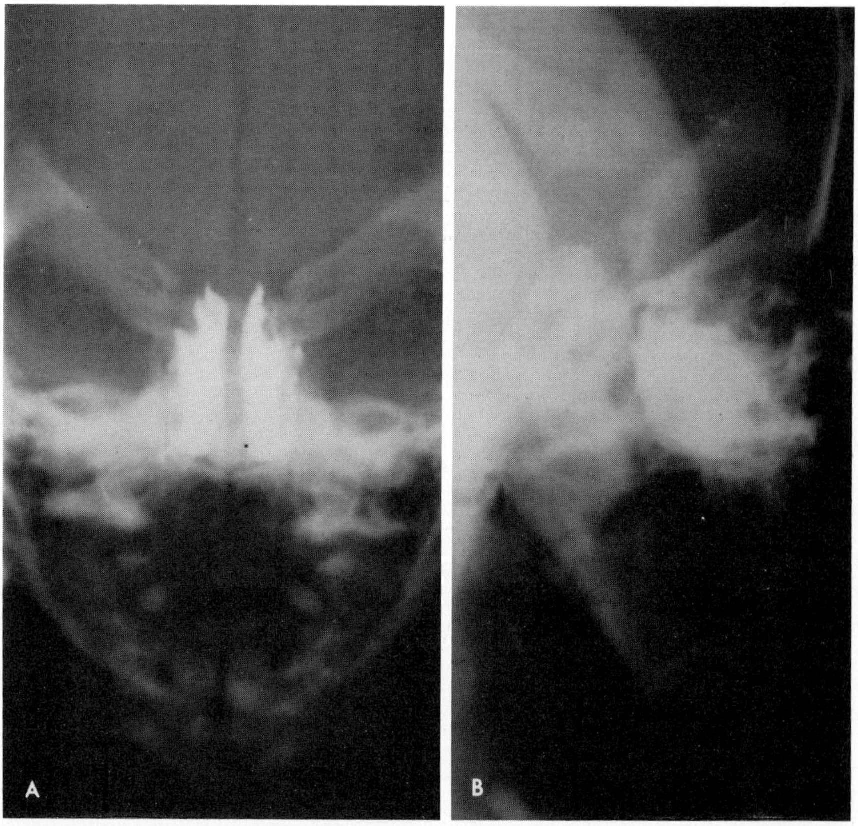

Figure 1. Dionosil has been instilled into both nares. It does not pass posteriorly because of the obstruction in this infant with choanal atresia. Frontal (*A*) and lateral (*B*) projections show the symmetrical obstruction.

the contrast agent to drain from the first side before examining the second, although using a base projection makes such a delay unnecessary. It may be necessary to introduce contrast material behind the obstruction to delineate its thickness.

Direct inspection may disclose the presence of polyps, but large polyps occasionally cause bone changes that can best be demonstrated radiographically with frontal, Water's and lateral projections.

EARS

Abnormalities of the middle and inner ears may require laminography for optimal demonstration. This is particularly true of the auditory ossicles. For preliminary evaluation, however, frontal, Towne, and oblique lateral projections such as Stenver's and Law projections should be obtained. These will permit definition of the middle ear, internal auditory canal and mastoids.

Eustachian Tubes

Wittenborg and Neuhauser (1963) have described a method for opacification of the eustachian tubes that occasionally is helpful in demonstrating obstruction of these structures by adenoid masses or neoplasms. This method also provides an additional means of examining the roof of the nasopharynx using oily Dionosil instilled under fluoroscopic control (Fig. 2).

MASTOIDS AND PARANASAL SINUSES

Pneumatization of the mastoids and paranasal sinuses occurs at varying ages. Caffey (1967) showed the usual sequence and rate of development. Infection may retard the development of

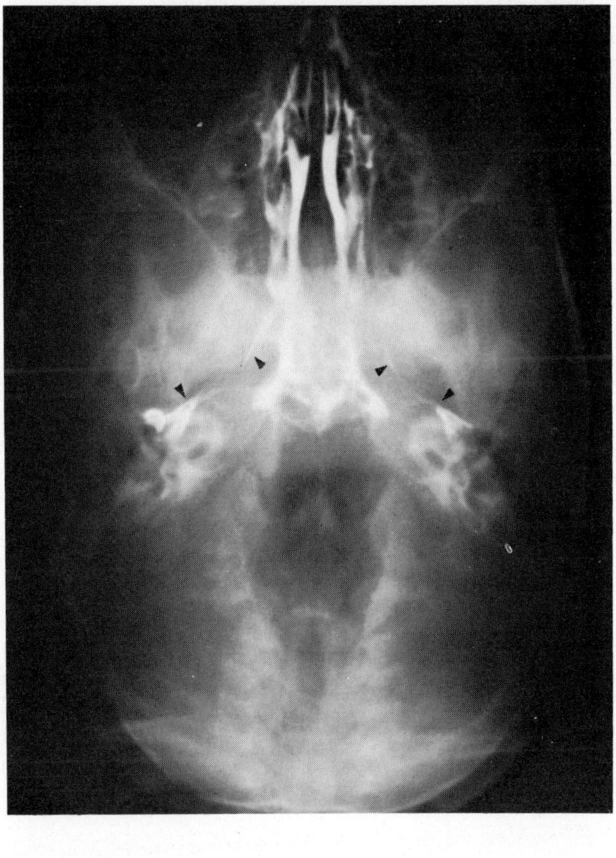

Figure 2. A submento-vertical projection shows patency of both eustachian tubes (arrows) in this normal child. The tubes open during swallowing but are closed in their medial two-thirds in their relaxed state.

these air spaces; this is particularly true of the mastoids. In infancy, the mastoids and sinuses are so small that roentgenologic definition may be very difficult. Since development varies so widely among individuals, it is unwise to assume that these structures will not be visible, even at an early age.

The normal mastoids and maxillary antra are quite symmetrical in size and shape. The frontal, ethmoid and sphenoid sinuses are usually asymmetrical even in the normal child, but this may be accentuated by inflammatory disease or by a more remote influence, such as asymmetric brain growth. Inflammatory disease of the sinuses and mastoids begins with thickening of the mucous membrane overlying the bony walls. This thickening cannot be differentiated radiographically from allergic edema. The presence of free fluid suggests inflammatory disease, and sclerosis of the bony walls, retarded growth and cyst formation within the mucous membranes indicate some chronicity. Destruction of the bony cell wall is seen with osteomyelitis and neoplasm. Since the normal sinus contains air, it is more lucent radiographically than the surrounding bone. Increased radiodensity of the sinus indicates less air and more soft tissue or fluid within it.

Radiographic evaluation of the mastoids should include at least a Towne's projection and oblique lateral views. Mayer and Shüller projections are more difficult to perform in children, but may add valuable information. It is helpful to compare both sides with radiographs symmetrically exposed.

The paranasal sinuses should be viewed in at least three projections: Water's, frontal or Caldwell, and lateral. If free fluid is to be demonstrated, a horizontal beam must be employed (an upright view).

Laminograms are particularly helpful in evaluation of the integrity of the bony margins of facial bones and paranasal sinuses. Fractures, especially of facial bones (e.g., blow-out fractures of the orbit), can be well demonstrated by laminograms.

THE PHARYNX

True lateral radiographs of the nasopharynx show the palate and adenoids to good advantage. In patients suspected of having agammaglobulinemia, this view is very important (Figs. 3 and 4). In addition, considerable information regarding palatal function can be obtained by exposing the lateral view during phonation by the patient who has a cleft palate or other speech defect. The palate should make contact with the posterior pharyngeal wall while making "s," "ba," "ka" and "pa" sounds and while hissing, blowing and speaking. Observation during these exercises permits evaluation of the child's ability to close off the nasopharynx to the passage of air from below. Properly timed lateral films will demonstrate this function (Figs. 5 and 6). A cine-examination shows this in a more dynamic fashion and also provides a good method of comparison and evaluation of results following palatal surgery.

Occasionally it is helpful to observe the patient swallowing opaque material to identify nasopharyngeal regurgitation on an anatomical or neuromuscular basis. This examination should be initiated with the child in the lateral position so that aspiration at any level can be recognized most readily. Subsequently, the child can be examined supine; some observers find the submento-vertex projection helpful in observing abnormalities of deglutition and of the pharyngeal anatomy.

Swallowing takes place so rapidly as to be difficult to record by spot films of the young child who will not swallow on command. A fasting child usually does not have to be urged to swallow and this facilitates examination. Video tape recording, rapid-sequence 70 or 90 mm. spot films, or cine-fluorography film will help record the pharyngeal function.

Evaluation of the soft tissue contours of the posterior pharyngeal wall requires that the neck be well extended and truly lateral. This is especially important in infants, since flexion and expiration will cause spurious thickening of the prever-

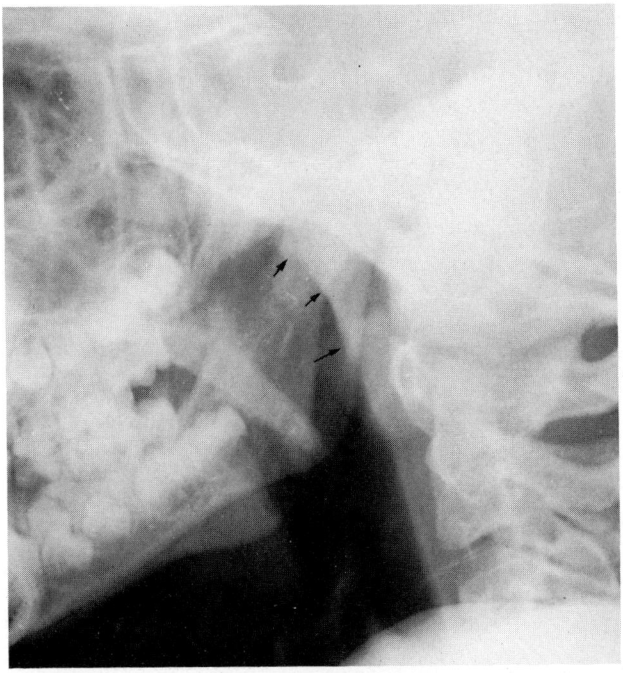

Figure 3. This 6-year-old boy with agammaglobulinemia has no adenoid mass in the nasopharynx. Even after surgical removal of hypertrophic adenoids, a small amount of tissue should be visible in the area of the upper arrow. A normal infant will not have a demonstrable adenoid mass prior to 9 or 10 months of age.

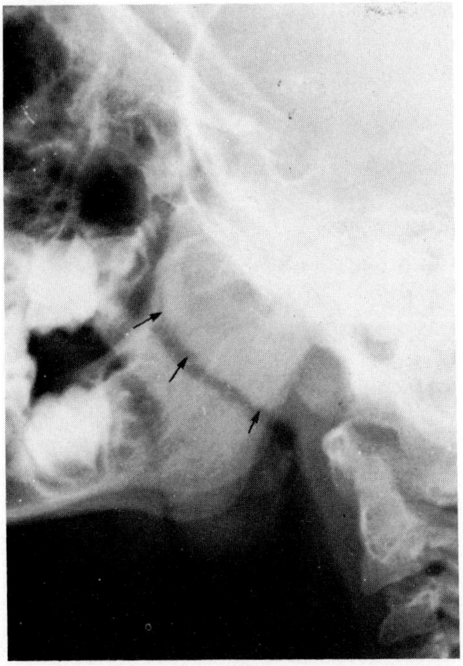

Figure 4. Hypertrophied adenoids (arrows) encroach upon the air passage in the nasopharynx and may obstruct it, causing mouth breathing. Chronic obstruction may lead to cor pulmonale. The false appearance of a uvular mass is caused by continuity of hypertropic tonsils and the soft palate.

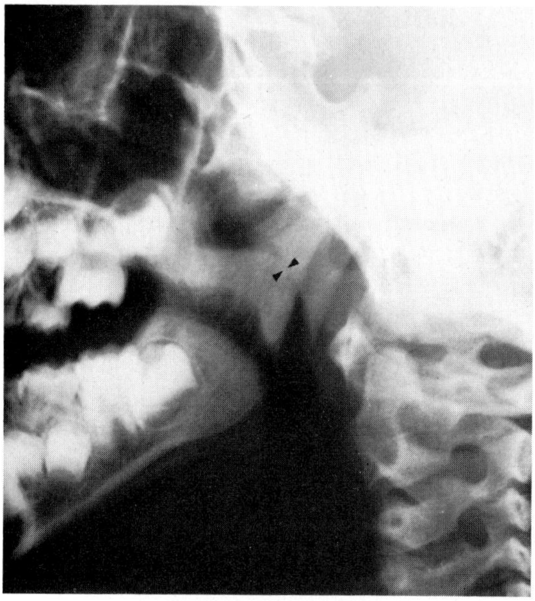

Figure 5. Normal palatal elevation during phonation shows apposition of soft tissue and closure of the airway so that air passes through the mouth rather than through the nose. The child was making an "ess" sound and was recorded on a spot film.

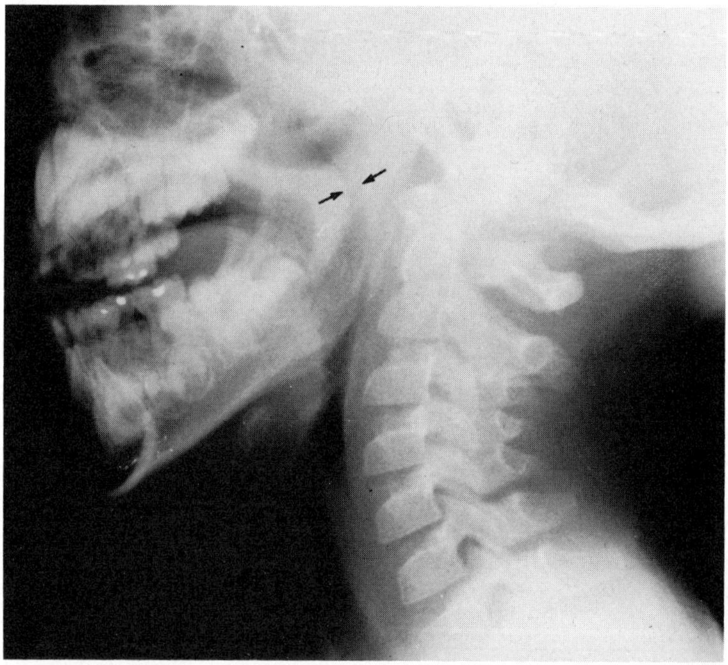

Figure 6. Palatal incompetence is demonstrated by the interval between the arrows. Such incomplete closure results in nasal speech. The interval illustrated is small, and should be surgically correctible.

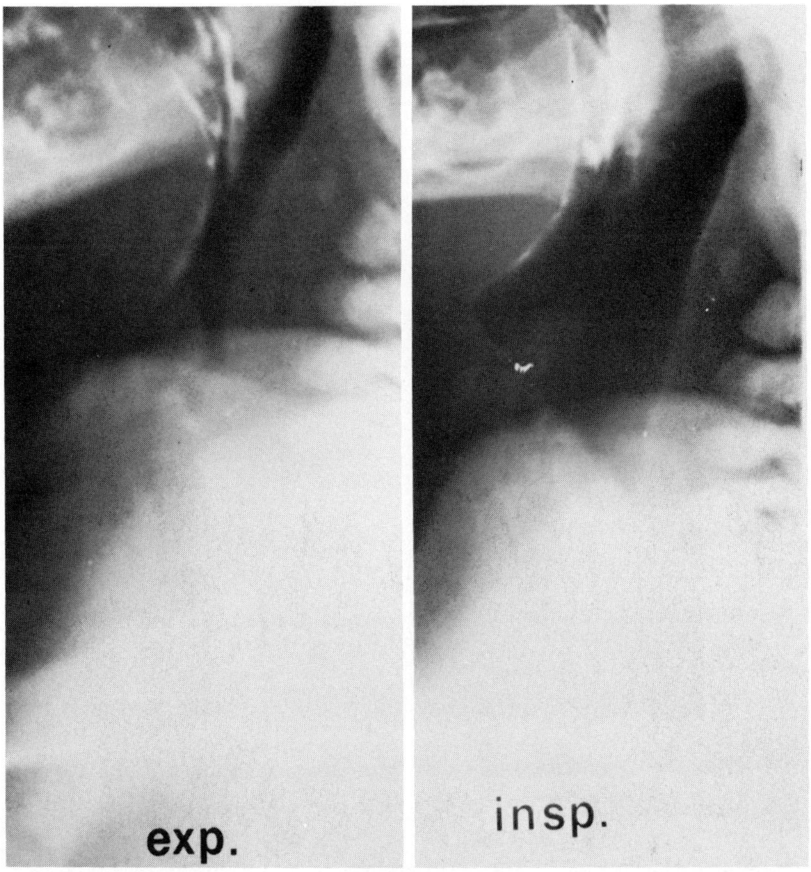

Figure 7. Lateral projections of the airway of a normal infant show the variation of caliber between expiration and inspiration. Note also the change in thickness of the prevertebral soft tissue. This tissue will also increase and decrease with flexion and extension of the neck.

tebral soft tissues (Fig. 7). Such apparent thickening may erroneously suggest myxedema, neoplasm or inflammatory disease.

LARYNX AND TRACHEA

Most examinations of this area are prompted by cough, stridor, dysphonia or dysphagia. Usually frontal and lateral radiographs of the neck will show sufficient anatomic detail for diagnosis using only air as the contrast medium (Fig. 8). The trachea in infancy is mobile in its midportion and relatively long. Even in the normal infant the trachea may buckle anteriorly and to the right, especially during expiration and with flexion of the neck. Deviation of the trachea to the left is less common and may indicate a right aortic arch (Fig. 9). Recognition of true displacement requires careful positioning of the head and neck.

Epiglottitis and croup (laryngotracheobronchitis) are two potentially dangerous conditions that warrant radiographic examination with as little manipulation as possible. The child with epiglottitis may be so severely embarrassed as to be unable to lie down; a lateral upright radiograph of the neck will be diagnostic (Fig. 10). The child with croup will usually be recognized with a frontal film of the chest if the trachea and larynx are included (Fig. 11). The lateral view will also show the characteristic subglottic edema.

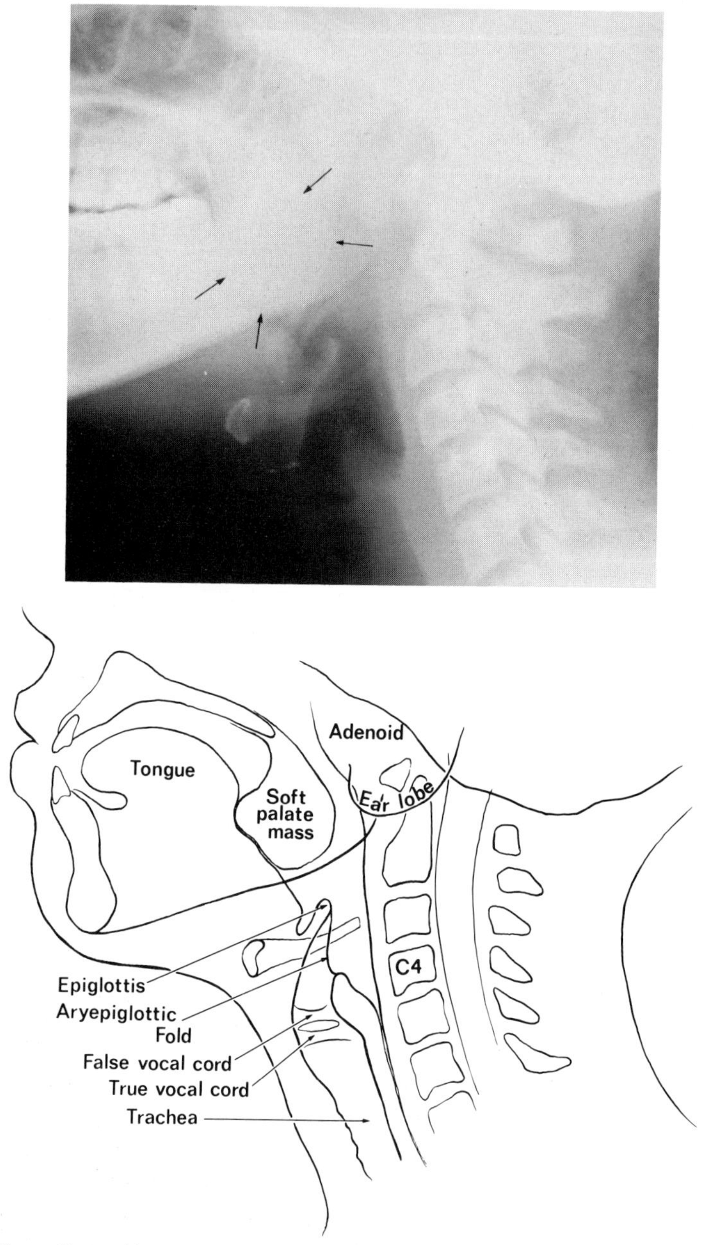

Figure 8. The radiographic anatomy of the upper airway is well visualized in this lateral projection of the neck. The ear lobe should not be mistaken for a pharyngeal mass; it continues beyond the limit of the posterior pharyngeal wall. The palatal mass is caused by cellulitis of the soft palate and uvula.

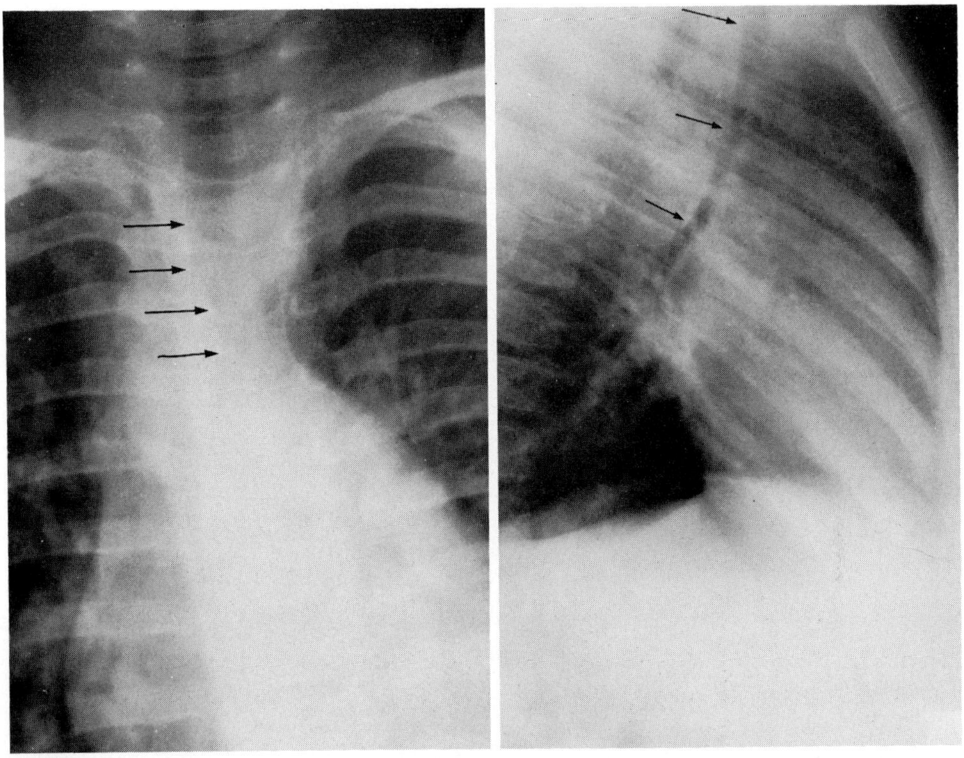

Figure 9. Frontal and lateral chest radiographs show abnormal tracheal displacement by a right aortic arch in a 3-year-old boy with recurrent stridor. A vascular ring was present in the form of a double aortic arch. The smaller vessel was on the left and was divided surgically with relief of the stridor.

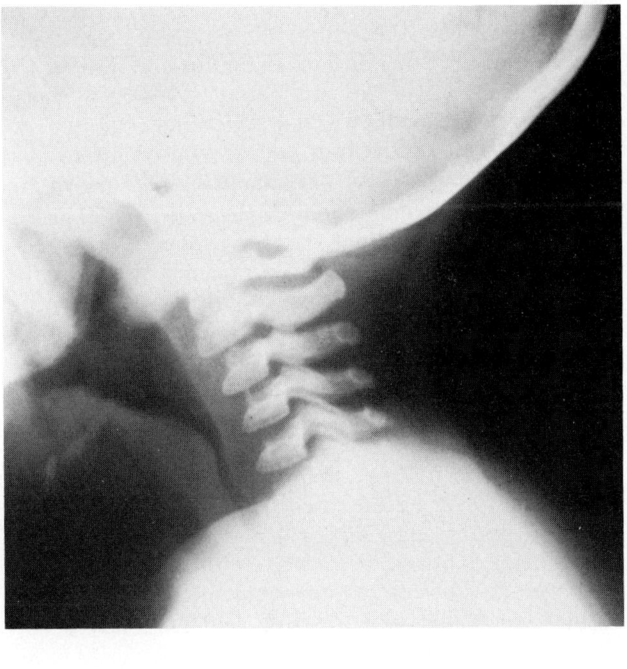

Figure 10. Edema of the epiglottis and aryepiglottic folds is present in epiglottitis. Note the straightened cervical spine and the air in the cervical esophagus as the child strains to get air past the obstructing edema.

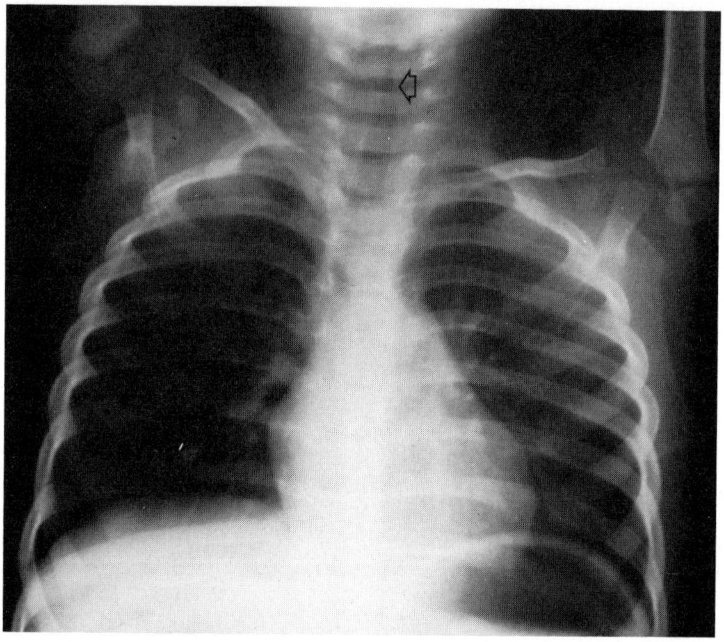

Figure 11. Croup can be diagnosed by the narrowed conus elasticus (arrow). Since this obstruction is inspiratory, the lungs are usually underinflated.

In the older child, standard radiographs of the larynx during phonation show laryngeal detail and motion well. Fluoroscopy with spot films, video tape or cine film are generally required in the infant.

The next step in evaluation of this portion of the airway is to opacify the esophagus and observe deglutition, since these two structures are so intimately associated both in location and in function. Again, fluoroscopic observation combined with some sort of permanent film documentation is employed. Some radiologists prefer to deliver barium to the esophagus via a catheter passed through the nose. This method is especially helpful in searching for fistulae, but it is unphysiologic and can probably be reserved for the uncooperative child or to differentiate aspiration at the laryngeal level from aspiration through an esophageal fistula.

Usually, lowering the child's head by tilting the fluoroscopic table can accentuate esophageal opacification and produce a retrograde flow of barium, even in a normal esophagus, which is sufficient to opacify a tracheoesophageal fistula in the absence of atresia.

Positive contrast examination of the larynx and trachea is occasionally required. In the older child, local anesthesia can be used; younger children require general anesthesia (Fig. 12). Some promising results have been obtained using powdered tantalum as the contrast agent, but good detail can be obtained with oily Dionosil. Generally there is no ill effect to the child from aspiration of a small amount of barium.

Tracheal dimensions normally increase during inspiration and decrease during expiration. Inspiratory collapse may occur at the cervicothoracic junction and is seen in laryngeal obstruction. Expiratory collapse is more common, occurring late in the expiratory phase and involving the intrathoracic portion of the trachea in children with obstruction of the peripheral airway, such as bronchiolitis and asthma. True segmental collapse of the trachea as an intrinsic tracheal abnormality must be extremely rare. Collapse is more commonly due to extrinsic compression.

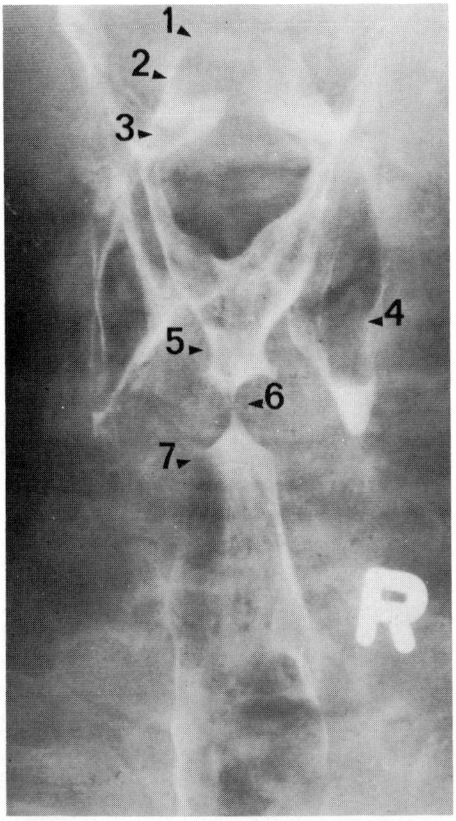

Figure 12. A Dionosil laryngotracheogram clearly demonstrates the normal landmarks: epiglottis (1), aryepiglottic folds (2), valleculae (3), pyriform sinus (4), false vocal cord (5), true vocal cord (6), and conus elasticus (7). (Courtesy of Dr. Jordon Greenfield, Boston Floating Hospital.)

Caution should be used in interpreting a single static film of the lumen of the airway, for it is such a dynamic structure (Fig. 13).

THE SALIVARY GLANDS

Radiographic examination of the salivary glands is most helpful in recognition of calculi, which usually are radiopaque. Tangential and oblique views are most helpful; the calculus must be projected free of the normal bony structures of the head and neck.

Identification of ectasia or stenosis of ducts, or demonstration of nonopaque calculi requires the gentle instillation of the proper amount of positive contrast material. Fluoroscopic control is helpful to avoid overfilling. General anesthesia is required for the infant but older children can be examined successfully after premedication with Demerol compound.

Inflammatory involvement may occasionally be recognized by demonstrating the edema of the overlying subcutaneous fat. Differentiation of inflammatory disease from neoplasia is best done with sialography.

Neoplasms generally cause extrinsic alveolar and ductal displacement. The normal gland, not excessively filled, will spontaneously expel the contrast material within 15 minutes. For this reason,

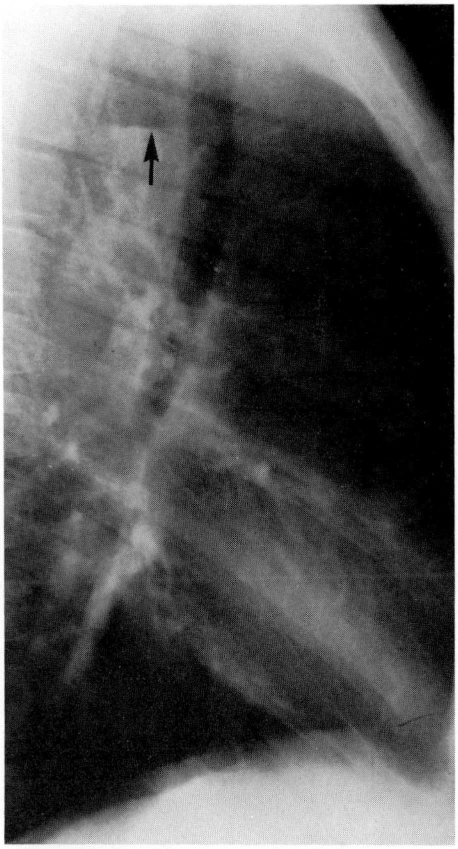

Figure 13. A dilated esophagus can displace the trachea anteriorly. This boy with achalasia has an air-fluid level in his chronically obstructed esophagus. This disease may be a cause of chronic aspiration pneumonia even in infants, but older children and adults are more commonly affected.

delayed radiographs should be obtained to demonstrate small areas of abnormal alveoli and ducts.

REFERENCES

1. Caffey, J.: *Pediatric X-ray Diagnosis,* 5th Ed. Chicago, Year Book Medical Publisher, Inc., 1967, pp. 95–113.
2. Capitanio, M. A., Kirkpatrick, J. A., Jr.: Upper respiratory tract obstruction in infants and children. *Rad. Clin. N. Amer., 6*:265, 1968.
3. Chang, L. W. M., Lee, F. A., and Gwinn, J. L.: Normal lateral deviation of the trachea in infants and children. *Amer. J. Roent., 109*:247, 1970.
4. Dunbar, J. S.: Upper respiratory tract obstruction in infants and children. *Amer. J. Roent., 109*:227, 1970.
5. Etter, L. E.: Opacification studies of normal and abnormal paranasal sinuses. *Amer. J. Roent., 89*:1137, 1963.
6. Etter, L. E.: Roentgen technique and anatomy of the temporal bone. *Semin. Radiol., 4*:104, 1969.
7. Gyepes, M. T., and Desilets, D. T.: Submentovertical projection: A new approach to the study of laryngeal and pharyngeal function in infants. *Radiology, 92*:758, 1969.
8. Hinchcliffe, W. A., et al.: Roentgenographic study of the human trachea with powdered tantalum. *Radiology, 97*:327, 1970.
9. Levy, A. M., Tabakin, B. S., Hanson, J. S., and Narkewicz, R. M.: Hypertrophied adenoids causing pulmonary hypertension and severe congestive heart failure. *New Eng. J. Med., 227*:506, 1967.
10. Luke, M. J., Mehrizi, A., Folger, G. M., Jr., and Rowe, R. D.: Chronic nasopharyngeal obstruction as a cause of cardiomegaly, cor pulmonale, and pulmonary edema. *Pediatrics, 37*:762, 1966.
11. Maine, F. J., and Woldshin, H. J.: Radiologic diagnosis of salivary gland tumors. *Rad. Clin. N. Amer., 8*:475, 1970.
12. O'Hara, A. E.: Roentgen evaluation of patients with cleft palate. *Rad. Clin. N. Amer., 1*:1, 1963.
13. Owsley, W. C.: Palate and pharynx: Roentgenographic evaluation in the management of cleft palate and related deformities. *Amer. J. Roent., 87*:811, 1962.
14. Samuel, E.: Inflammatory disease of the nose and paranasal sinuses. *Semin. Roent., 3*:148, 1968.
15. Seaman, W. B.: Examination of the pharynx. In Margulis, A. R., and Burhenne, H. J. (Eds.): *Alimentary Tract Roentgenology.* St. Louis, C. V. Mosby Co., 1967, pp. 247–252.
16. Valvassori, G. E.: Laminography of the ear: Normal roentgenographic anatomy. *Amer. J. Roent. 89*:1155, 1963.
17. Valvassori, G. E., and Pierce, R. H.: The normal internal auditory canal. *Amer. J. Roent., 92*:1232, 1964.
18. Wittenborg, M. H., Gyepes, M. T., and Crocker, D.: Tracheal dynamics in infants with respiratory distress, stridor, and collapsing trachea. *Radiology, 88*:653, 1967.
19. Wittenborg, M. H., and Neuhauser, E. B. D.: Simple roentgenographic demonstration of eustachian tubes and abnormalities. *Amer. J. Roent., 89*:1194, 1963.

SECTION XII

THE EAR AND MASTOID

Chapter Sixty-Five

EMBRYOLOGY, APPLIED ANATOMY AND PHYSIOLOGY

GAYLE G. ARNOLD, M.D.

The ear is an organ of hearing and equilibrium. It is divisible into the external ear, the middle ear and the inner ear. Embryologically, all three germ-layers contribute to the formation of the ear.

The ectoderm, lining the early first branchial groove and bounded by the first and second branchial arches, forms the covering of the auricle, lines the external auditory canal and contributes to the outer (epidermal) covering of the tympanic membrane. In addition, the ectoderm above the first branchial groove invaginates to form the otocyst (auditory vesicle), which eventually contributes the epithelium-lined membranous labyrinth of the inner ear, developing into the otic duct and sac, the cochlear duct, three semicircular ducts, the utricle and the saccule.

The entoderm lines the first pharyngeal pouch, and developmental expansion of this pouch contributes the eustachian tube, the tympanic cavity, the epitympanic recess, the mastoid antrum and the mastoid air cells. The entodermal layer of the pouch becomes the epithelium of the mucous membrane of the middle ear and also contributes the mucosal inner layer of the tympanic membrane.

Mesoderm contributes the cartilaginous capsule, the osseous labyrinth, the otic capsule, the ligaments and muscles of the middle ear ossicles, and the intermediate (fibrous) layers of the tympanic membrane (radial and circular fibers).

The external ear is formed by the auricle and the external auditory canal. The auricle is supported by the ear cartilage, and there are some seven intrinsic and extrinsic muscles to the cartilage, variably developed.

The auricle develops around the first branchial groove from six knoblike evaginations that coalesce at about the third month.

The external auditory canal has a lateral cartilaginous structure lined with skin that contains strong hairs (tragi) and wax glands. The medial portion is bony and belongs to the temporal bone, but is lined with skin. The medial boundary of the canal is the tympanic membrane. This membrane is located in a groove (sulcus) of the temporal bone, and the marginal connective tissue ossifies at about the third month, forming the supportive annulus. Superiorly, the annulus is deficient at the incisura and the membrane is looser (pars flaccida), having a small elevation caused by the lateral process of the malleus. The fixed portion of the drum (pars tensa) is concave, drawn inward by the tip of the handle of the malleus, the attachment of which is called the umbo.

The middle ear is formed by the tympanic cavity, the ossicles and the auditory (eustachian) tube. The tympanic cavity, lying in the temporal bone, has a lateral boundary, the tympanic membrane. The medial wall consists of the oval or vestibular window, closed by the footplate of the stapes, the promontory, and the cochlear or round window. The inferior wall is bone, with small pneumatic cells, and the superior wall is thin bone, above which is the middle cranial fossa.

The anterior wall is thin bone, also

with pneumatic cells, the upper part occupied by the orifice of the auditory (eustachian) tube. The posterior wall penetrates cranially as the epitympanic space, with the tympanic antrum joining it to the mastoid air cells posterolaterally.

The ossicles begin laterally with the malleus, touching the tympanic membrane and articulating with the incus, which in turn articulates with the head of the stapes, the base of which almost fills the oval window. These ossicles are derived from the branchial arch system, and undergo marked alterations to adapt for hearing. All this growth occurs during the first half of intrauterine life, and they increase to about five times their early dimensions.

The inner ear has three main parts, the otic labyrinth, derived from ectoderm, the periotic labyrinth, and the otic capsule, derived from mesoderm. The otic labyrinth is surrounded by the periotic labyrinth and its supporting connective tissue, and both lie within the bony capsule. Components of the otic labyrinth are the utricle, three semicircular ducts which open into the utricle, the saccule, the cochlear duct, and the otic (endolymphatic) duct and sac. The otic labyrinth is filled with a clear endolymph (Scarpas fluid).

The periotic labyrinth is a filmy tissue that surrounds the otic labyrinth, filled with perilymph. It is divided into the vestibule, semicircular canals, scala vestibuli and scala tympani.

All end organs of the inner ear develop from terminal nerve fibers from the vestibular and cochlear ganglia cells (eighth nerve). The vestibular end organs are the maculae of the saccule and utricle, which serve to detect changes in head position, and the cristae of the semicircular ducts, which detect rotary head position changes. The cochlear end organ is the spiral organ of Corti. The many and varied theories of sound perception will not be considered here. It is agreed that the perilymph is put in motion by excursion of the stapes in the oval window, and that its movement eventually reaches the sensory hair cells in the organ of Corti, to be interpreted as sound.

The otic capsule is uniquely a single bone without suture lines and encloses the entire inner ear.

Chapter Sixty-Six

METHODS OF EXAMINATION

GAYLE G. ARNOLD, M.D.

Examination of the ear under direct vision may give much information as to anomalies, drainage from the external auditory canal, pre- and postauricular swellings, painful areas, skin involvement of the external canal, presence of furuncles, and so on.

With an infant or child in the supine position, an overhead or ceiling light should be directly over the ear that is to be examined. In this way, simple traction on the pinna can straighten the canal and the tympanic membrane can be visualized in many cases. If otoscopic speculum examination shows cerumen blockage or obstruction, this may be removed (Fig. 1) with a small, smooth cerumen spoon, using direct vision, as long as care is taken to have the child's hands and body restrained while the examiner is manipulating the head and ear. If the mother is given this responsibility, it

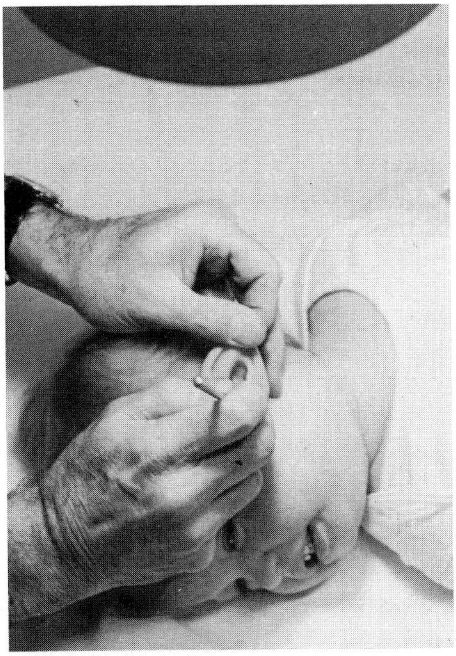

Figure 1.

must be made clear that the restraint is to be continued until the procedure is totally finished. Preferably, an assistant or office nurse can restrain the child.

If the child is to be examined in the upright position, it is frequently reassuring for the examination to be carried out while he is seated in his mother's lap (Fig. 2), his head resting against his mother, his hands again restrained. The head-mirror examination, manipulation, or treatment can be carried out this way.

If removal of cerumen by careful syringing is necessary, a metal syringe with a splatter collar on it is used with an emesis basin beneath the pinna. It has been recommended that a glass or plastic 20 ml. syringe be used, with a three-quarters of an inch #18 needle, which has a blunted tip, attached. By laying the needle gently along the external auditory canal floor, a small jet of fluid can be directed behind the occlusive cerumen more easily than is possible with the traditional flush technique with a larger metal syringe. The syringing fluid should be at body temperature.

After cleansing of the canal has been accomplished, the canal should be dried carefully, and the speculum examination, with head-mirror, can be continued.

Otoscopic examination of an infant or young child is best carried out with the child in the supine position, hands and body restrained by an assistant, and the head and ear area controlled by the examiner. Each examiner must evolve his own technique for this examination. I hold the otoscope handle near the child's head, so that if he moves unexpectedly the speculum is not driven deep, which would cause pain (Fig. 3). The balance of

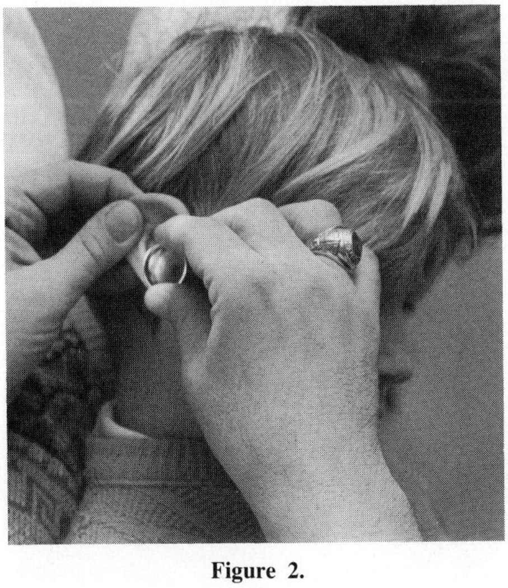

Figure 2.

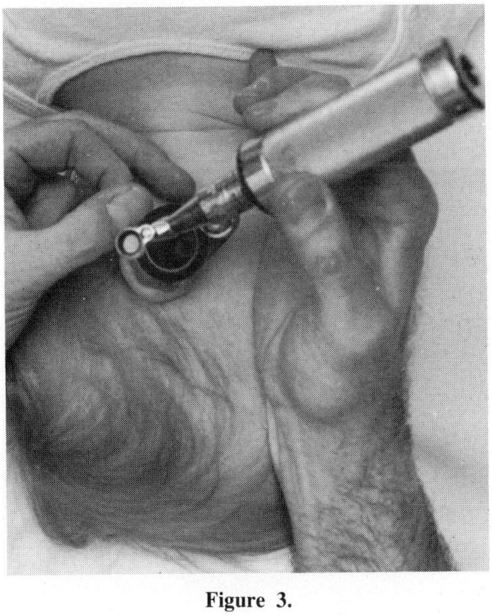

Figure 3.

the otoscope can be lightly held between the thumb and forefinger and the base of the hand can be used to steady the child's head. The other hand is then available for straightening the canal by retracting the pinna, or for instrumentation, cleaning or treatment.

This technique may also be used for an older child, but it is preferable to carry out the examination in an examining chair, with the child on his mother's lap.

The Siegle pneumatic otoscope (Fig. 4) is very helpful in evaluating the condition of the tympanic membrane and the middle ear. A small pin-point perforation of the drum, associated with persistent otitis media, can occasionally be observed by the use of alternating positive and negative pressure, made possible by the pneumatic scope. The flaccidity of the tympanic membrane is best observed with this scope. Differentiation between a thin, atrophic, but completely healed area in the drum and a perforation can be more readily made. Bubbles of fluid can often be noted with the use of positive and negative pressure. Lack of mobility of the tympanic membrane, using a properly fitted pneumatic scope, is suggestive of a continuing disease state in the middle ear.

The Weber test is easily carried out, using a 256 or a 512 c.p.s. tuning fork, placing it on the child's forehead (Fig. 5), and asking in which ear he hears the hum better.

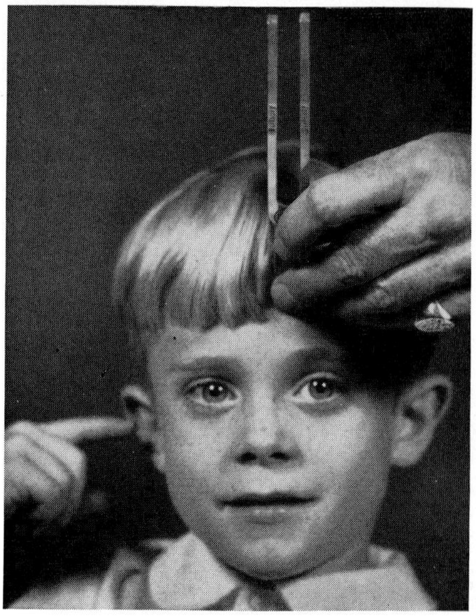

Figure 5.

Audiological testing is another important adjunctive method of examination of the ear and is thoroughly described in Chapter 73. Evidence obtained from this examination should be correlated with the results of all the other clinical evaluations of the ear mentioned previously, and a proper diagnosis may then be made.

After all these techniques of evalua-

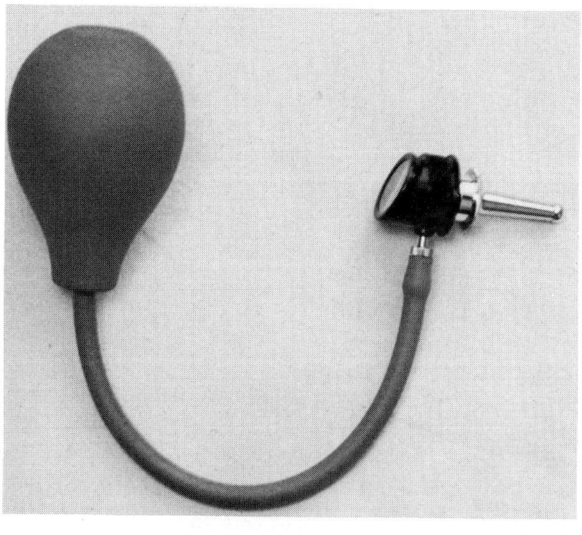

Figure 4.

tion have been used, there may still be a few cases in which the exact nature of the disease process is questionable. For completeness of examination, tympanotomy with microscopic examination of the middle ear structures may reveal pathology otherwise not diagnosable. Tumor, cholesteatoma, and congenital anomalies that were only suspected may thus be found and diagnosed. Corrective surgical treatment would then be possible.

Roentgen examination of the mastoid may be valuable. Where there is a suspicion of a mastoid reservoir as a source of chronic or recurrent middle ear disease, with or without cholesteatoma formation, x-rays should be obtained.

Examination by bacteriologic culture with sensitivity studies may be valuable in good management of a resistant or chronic otorrhea. Then, institution of the appropriate antibiotic, along with proper local treatment, may be effective.

Caloric or other vestibular tests should be carried out if there is a suspicion of vestibular disease (see Chapter 73).

Chapter Sixty-Seven

CONGENITAL MALFORMATIONS OF THE EAR

EDGAR M. HOLMES, M.D.

EMBRYOLOGY OF THE EAR

The development of the human ear closely follows the evolution of man. First there is a primitive end organ of balance, then an auditory sensor develops, and lastly a sound conduction mechanism is derived after leaving its watery environment. By midterm, the inner ear has reached adult size and shape. The middle ear and external ear continue to grow through puberty.

Inner Ear (Membranous Labyrinth)

The otic labyrinth differentiates early. By the end of the third week, the auditory placodes appear. Within a week the placode invaginates to form an auditory pit, which in turn dilates to form a sac, seals off and then becomes the otic vesicle.[2]

It has been shown recently that the acoustic ganglion is derived embryologically from the epithelium of the auditory vesicle and not from the neurocrest of the central nervous system. The future cells are innervated soon after the ganglion cells are formed from the vesicular wall and while the ganglion is intermittently associated with the auditory vesicle.[19]

By the tenth week, the endolymphatic sac and duct, the utricle, the semicircular ducts, the saccule and the cochlear duct have formed. Maturity in the labyrinth is reached at about the twenty-fourth week, by which time ossification of the surrounding cartilage has occurred.

The Middle Ear

The middle ear and its structures arise from the first endodermal pharyngeal pouch. The space within this pouch will form the middle ear and the eustachian tube. The malleus and incus are derived

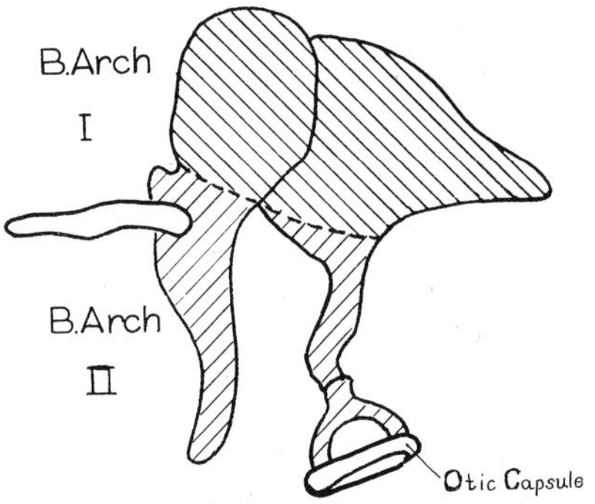

Figure 1. Embryologic development of the ossicles. This drawing schematically illustrates how the malleus and incus are derived from the first and second branchial arch, thus explaining why the ossicles are so deformed in faulty development.

from the upper end of the first visceral bar (Meckel's cartilage); the stapes is formed from the cranial end of the second visceral bar (the hyoid or Reichert's cartilage). By the fifth month, the ossicles are adult in shape and the rest of the cartilage regresses, except for the fibrous ligaments that hold the malleus and incus in place (Fig. 1).

The External Ear

The external ear grows out of the first mandibular and second hyoid branchial arches, and the branchial groove forms the primitive external auditory meatus. By the seventh month, the ectoderm has deepened to meet the expanding tympanic cavity. While the two approximate, the meatal plate is formed and becomes the bony part of the external auditory meatus. The membrana tympani is created by a thinning out of this mesodermal diaphragm. The auricle arises from the first brachial cleft. There are three mounds in the anterior border and three in the posterior border of the cleft that enlarge, migrate, fuse and develop into a mature auricle. The three anterior mounds apparently develop into the tragus. The posterior mounds expand and rotate to form the auricle as a whole.[24]

Considering how complicated the embryological development is, it is amazing that one does not see more abnormal birth defects. The abnormalities that are encountered include variation in shape and size of the auricle, from a rudimentary nubbin without any canal to an auricle larger than average and lacking the normal configurations and folds, permitting it to stand out prominently from the head (Figs. 2 and 3). Associated with lack of development of the auricle (called *microtia*), one may find an absent auditory meatus. Because Meckel's cartilage plays an important part in the development of the malleus and incus, the ossicles may be deformed, fused and nonfunctioning. The stapes, being formed separately from Reichert's cartilage, may be malformed and give rise to deafness without evidence of gross external abnormality (Fig. 4).

INNER EAR DEFORMITIES

Congenital hereditary deafness can be caused by a variety of defects. Some involve the auditory meatus, others are caused by abnormalities in the middle ear, and a lesser number are the result of faulty development in the cochlea. Some cases of deafness attributable to interference with sound conduction to the cochlea may be improved materially through microscopic surgery. Deafness due to neurosensory losses secondary to maldevelopment of the organ of Corti may be diagnosed, but treatment to date is limited to rehabilitation. Certain hereditary deafness develops insidiously and may not be noted until later in life. It has been estimated that hereditary deafness due to cochlear changes occurs in between 1 in 2000 and 1 in 6000 births.[19]

By audiometry and functional vestibular tests, one may determine the presence or absence of cochlear or labyrinthine function, but one has no specific knowledge as to its cause until the ear is sectioned and placed under the microscope. There have been sufficient cases so examined that one may report what has been found, and some of these histories from different authors show

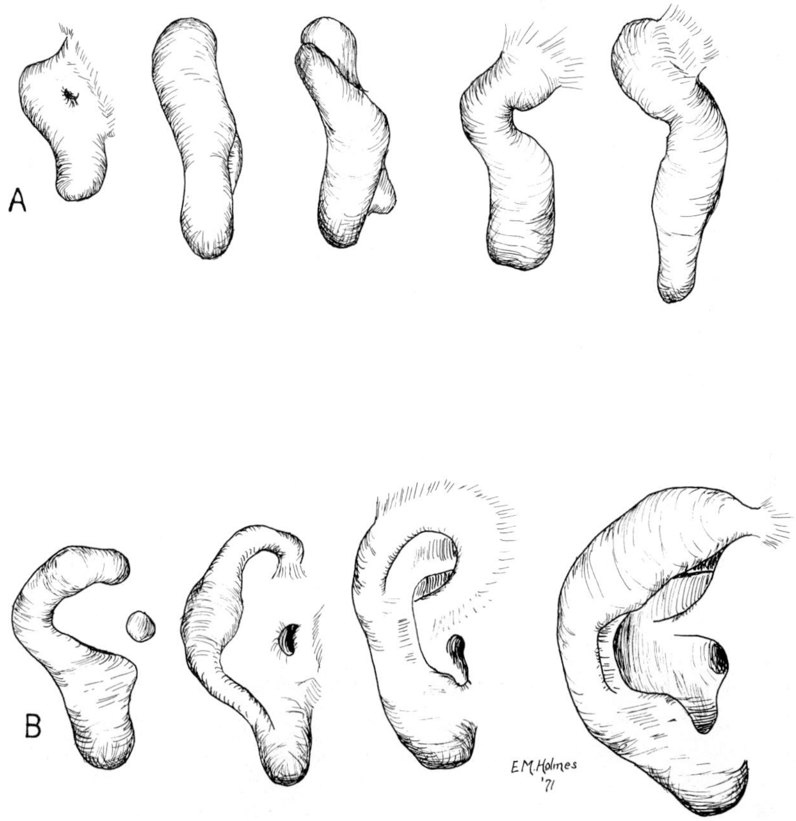

Figure 2. Various degrees of microtia. All those in Group A and the first one in B had no auditory meatus. The last three in Group B had a meatus.

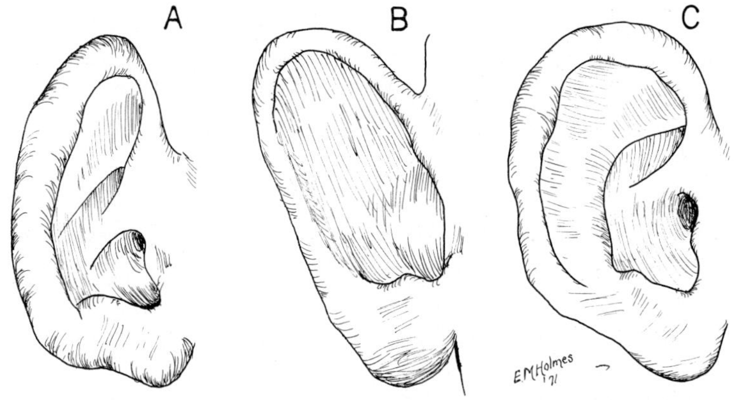

Figure 3. A prominent ear without an anthelix or a superior crus. *A,* The lateral view. *B,* The anterior view. *C,* Lateral view postoperatively after correction via the Holmes technique.

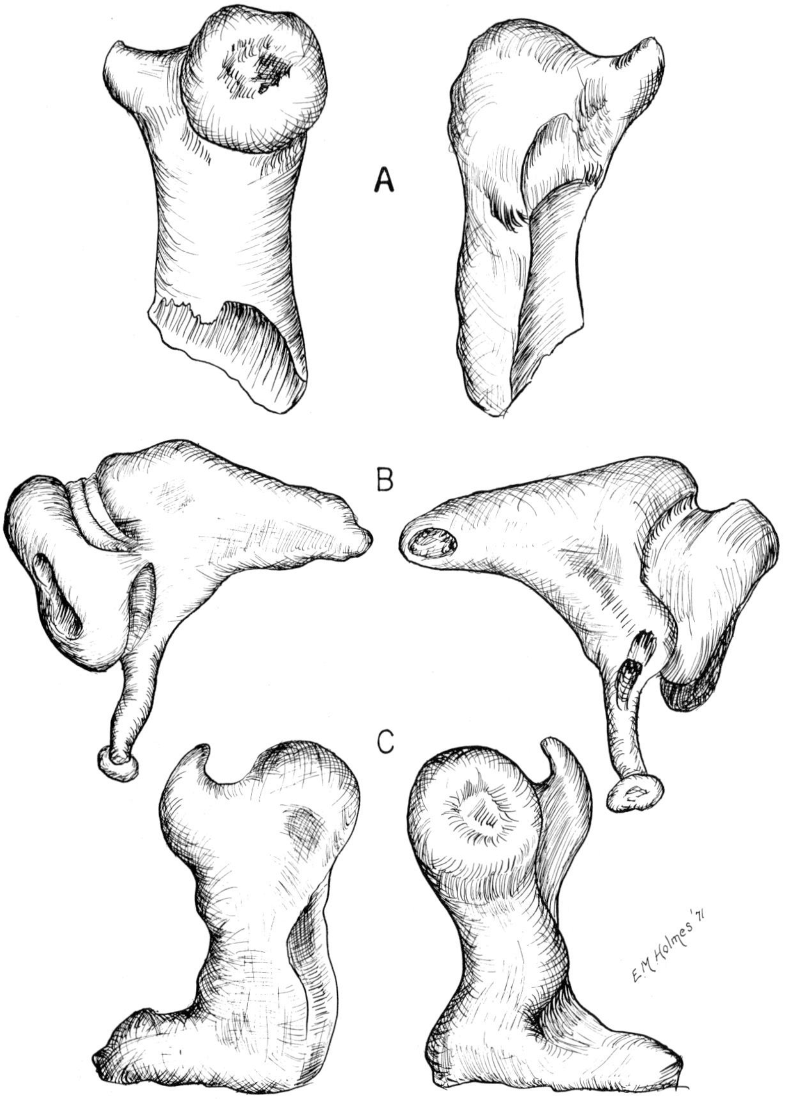

Figure 4. Three sets of congenitally deformed ossicles removed at operation in Type III microtia. It would be impossible to imagine just what the specimen in *A* and C was without having seen the ossicles in situ. Specimen *B* is quite readily identified from the incus, which is fairly normal in appearance. It is very apparent why the ossicular chain must be examined after exposure to determine the method which will be employed in an attempt to improve hearing.

that there has been an absence or flattening of crista in the semicircular canals and degeneration of hair and spiral ganglion cells. The macula and saccule have been seen to be abnormally developed and hydrops of the cochlear duct has been present. The organ of Corti and the tectorial membrane have been absent. The saccule has been collapsed and there has been a disarrangement of the epithelium of the macula.[3]

It has been observed that cases secondary to maternal rubella, measles and mumps showed a degeneration in the cochleo-saccula. Absence of the round and oval windows has been observed, as has absence of parts of the superior and horizontal semicircular canals.

Cochlear defects are frequently associated with a trisomy syndrome,[20] the genetic syndrome of retramelic deficiencies,[9] spiny hyperkeratosis and universal alopecia,[17] partial albinism and deaf-mutism, deafness associated with measles, mumps, syphilis, and other disorders.[11]

The new techniques of study in evaluating amniotic fluid are bringing to light much information concerning the fetus relative to congenital defects. It is barely possible that when the interrelationship of abnormal genes, enzymes and biochemical processes is better understood, some of our known probable defects that are familial may be treated in utero and thereby prevented. If untreatable, the disorder may be diagnosed and the parents may be given a chance to terminate the pregnancy.

CONGENITAL MALFORMATIONS OF THE MIDDLE EAR AND THEIR CORRECTION

Abnormalities of the middle ear may range all the way from a very small middle ear with an abnormality of one or all of the ossicles to a relatively normal-appearing middle ear with only some variation in the conductive mechanism from the drum to the oval window. Cases in this group that have a normal external auditory meatus and drum, if first seen when an adult, may be confused with

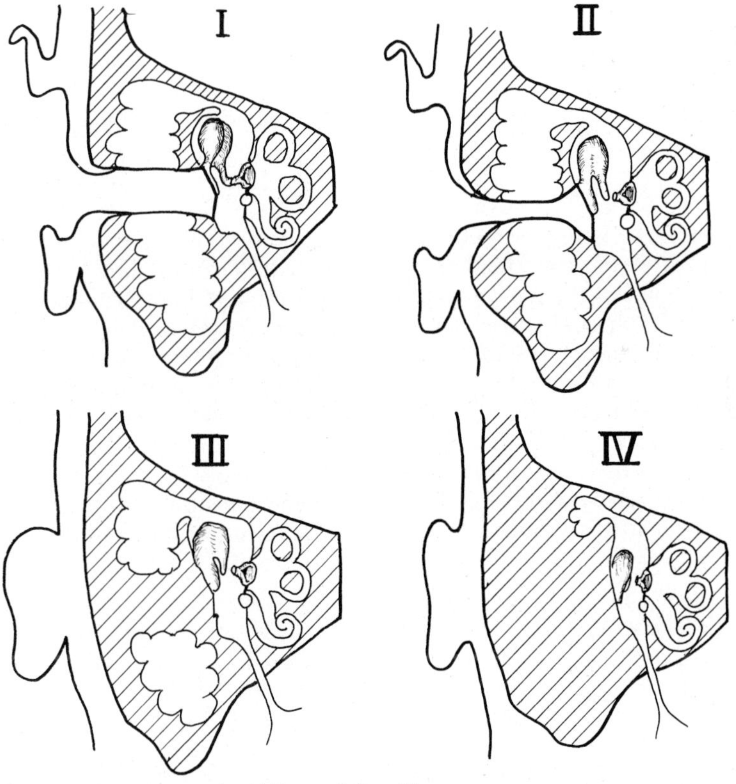

Figure 5. Classification of ear and middle ear deformities.

Class I. Schematic drawing of normal ear. Note the normal auricle, auditory meatus, ossicles and mastoid in a vertical plane.

Class II. The auditory meatus is narrowed. The mastoid is fully pneumatized. The drum is essentially normal, though it may be discolored. After entering the middle ear surgically, one would find a deformity of the malleus and the incus undoubtedly misshapen and probably fused with or without a connection to the stapes.

Class III. A microtic external auditory meatus associated with an absent auditory meatus and essentially normally developed mastoid. After one enters the antrum and removes the solid bone over the area of the tympanic membrane, no drum is found, merely the lining mucosa. The malleus and incus are fused and deformed, probably without connection to the stapes, and the eustachian tube may be narrowed.

Class IV. The same as Class III except for the fact that there is no mastoid development. The middle ear is usually smaller than normal and there is a very small eustachian tube. It is most difficult to reach the middle ear in this class and the facial nerve may be misplaced, exposing it to trauma.

otosclerosis. Most patients who have a normal-sized middle ear and a well-pneumatized mastoid can have their hearing restored to near normal using the techniques employed for stapes surgery.

These cases have been grouped into three classes by Hanner.[13] Class I may have a fairly normal-looking external ear, although the canal may be partially stenosed and markedly narrowed. The drum may be quite normal, although on occasion it is discolored. The mastoid, by x-ray, is usually well developed, and there may be anomalies in the ossicular chain that create an audiogram that is consistent with otosclerosis. The bone conduction is normal but the air conduction is down 50 to 60 decibels.

In Class II abnormalities, the mild effects mentioned in Class I may be more pronounced and associated with varying degrees of microtia. The auditory canal is usually absent, there is no bony canal and the drum is represented by a thick bony plate. The ossicles are usually deformed, sometimes being unrecognizable. The handle of the malleus is frequently attached to the lateral wall of the middle ear. The cochlea is usually normal in these cases. Audiometry is generally the same as in Class I. The stapes may be fixed or deformed, they may lack a tendon, or the footplate may be absent, so that there is no oval window. In about 70 per cent of the cases, it is possible to construct a canal down to the middle ear and reconstruct a tympanic membrane and ossicular chain.

Class III consists of cases that have all the problems of Class II plus undevelopment of the middle ear space, no mastoid development and occasionally facial paralysis and lack of a eustachian tube.

Before attempting to correct middle ear defects, it is imperative to evaluate all possible information that may be obtained. Examination should include a complete history and physical examination, audiometry and good x-rays, which preferably include laminograms.

Pneumatization of the mastoid must be present, because without it, not only is access to the middle ear difficult, but the facial nerve is probably in an abnormal position and difficult to avoid. I have seen a case in which the facial nerve took the course of the annulus tympanicus and went out in a supero-anterior portion of the field, apparently through the petrotympanic fissure (Fig. 6). The facial nerve may be found without bony covering, split and going around primitive crura in an abnormal stapes.[5] It is therefore imperative that there be x-ray evidence of pneumatization, so that the antrum may be found and the middle ear entered safely. Once the antrum is entered, exposure of the middle ear is safe and simple.

One does not know what one will encounter until the middle ear is explored.

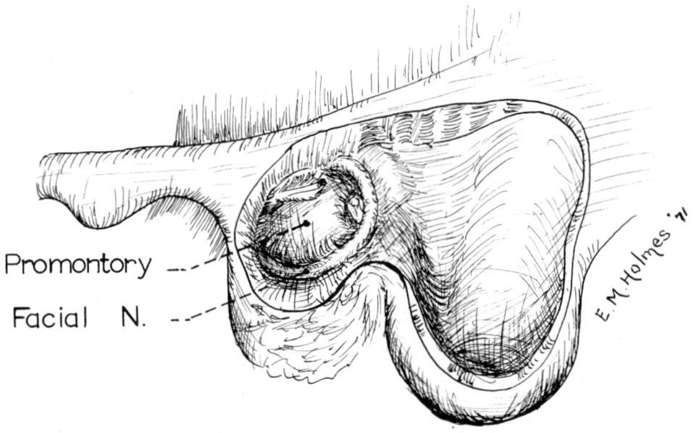

Figure 6. Abnormal position of the facial nerve. Abnormal position of the facial nerve observed at surgery on a microtic ear. Note that the facial nerve is in normal position from the geniculate ganglion in its course between the horizontal semicircular canal and the oval window. It then assumes the position of the annulus tympanicus and disappears anteriorly through the petrotympanic fissure.

Each case must be handled according to the anatomy found.

If a child has normal hearing in one ear and surgery can improve hearing in the other ear only to within 15 to 20 decibels of the normal ear, surgery does not seem justified. There are some otologists who will not agree with this. If one has an individual with bilateral microtia and severe deafness, it is imperative to help him to hear as early as possible. The first step is to have him wear a bone conduction hearing aid so that speech may be developed. This is important, because the development of speech occurs during the first year, and if one waits until surgery is performed, the child will have developed a handicap in speech formation that will be extremely difficult to overcome. In some clinics, surgical intervention is begun between two and three years of age; in others they prefer to wait until the child is three or more because the postoperative management is much more readily controlled.

Cases in which most of the pathology is in the middle ear are approached surgically through the auditory meatus, as one would for stapes surgery. If the bony canal is narrow but present, it may be enlarged, and the new canal is then lined with a graft. When there is complete atresia, our problem is more complex. In all these cases, to reach the middle ear one must go through the mastoid process.

When there is a microtic ear associated with middle ear pathology and deafness, there is another dimension to the problem. Should an attempt be made to construct an auricle as well as to improve the hearing? If the decision is yes, the otological surgeon should consult with the plastic surgeon prior to making his incisions to operate on the mastoid, as injudicious incisions will jeopardize the blood supply in plastic construction of an auricle.[1, 7, 12, 15, 21, 22]

In Class I abnormalities, one must assume that there is some abnormality in the ossicular chain, and so exposure of the middle ear contents is justified. The auditory meatus, being narrow, must be enlarged to enable visualization and work in the middle ear. The drum is then reflected as for stapedectomy and the middle ear examined. It will probably be found that the malleus and incus are fused, fixed and possibly not in communication with the stapes. The malleus and incus usually require removal, and then either a part of the bony ossicles or some prosthetic material is employed to create a columella effect between the drum and the stapes. The enlarged canal is then grafted. Following this corrective surgery, hearing should be materially restored.

In Class II deformities, an approach must be made through the pneumatized mastoid to the antrum. The solid bone over the tympanic plate must be removed and its lining mucosa left. The middle ear and its contents are then exposed and measures taken to re-establish a drum with its connection to the stapes. An exterior auditory meatus is established.

In Class III abnormalities, where there is no bony canal or pneumatization of the mastoid, no attempt should be made to improve the hearing in a unilaterally involved case. If both ears are involved, it is possible to drill through the solid mass, keeping high near the tegmen and forward near the glenoid fossa. One usually finds a small but malformed middle ear. The risk of encountering an abnormally placed facial nerve is ever present, and only those most skilled in microscopic surgery should consider attempting it. The likelihood of improving hearing sufficiently to offset the potential risk of complications rarely justifies surgical intervention. It is best to fit this type of case with a good bone conduction hearing aid.

RECONSTRUCTION OF THE ABNORMALLY FORMED AURICLE

If an ear is too large or too prominent, it is a comparatively simple matter to reduce its size or to create contours that will make the auricle fit into a normal pattern. When the ear is too small, our

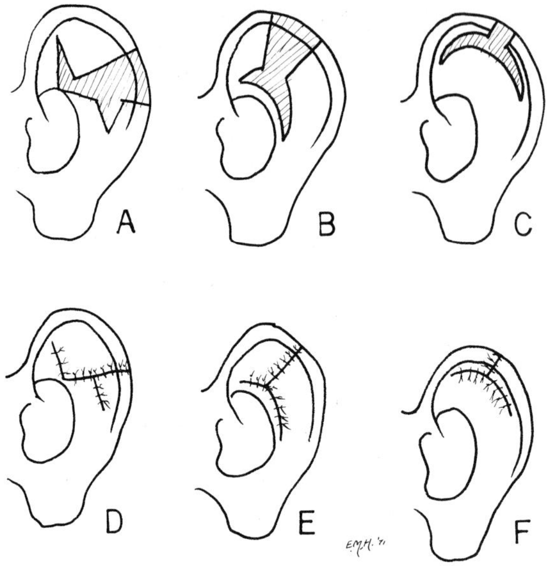

Figure 7. Correction of macrotia. Through-and-through sections are removed to decrease the circumference of the auricle. Any method creating the shortest radial scar is best; that in *C* is especially good.

problems are multiplied, and even the best of reconstructed ears are readily noticed as being abnormal.

Let us first consider the unusually large ear, which may be in normal relationship to the head. There are many procedures offered, each man usually developing a procedure that he hopes will overcome some defect left by other methods tried. Figure 7 shows the various procedures. It is always wisest to use a method that avoids a cut through the helix and the scapha, which is continuous, because when this is done, there is likely to be notching from contracture of the incisions. The last two diagrams show the methods of choice.

The prominent ear has many names, such as lop ear and mouse ear. The condition is basically the result of a lack of bending of the cartilage that creates an anthelix. Occasionally there is a failure of the helix itself to develop, so that the ear has very little contour from the concha to its rim. There are well developed ears that have a good anthelix but a very deep posterior wall of the concha. For details of the reconstructive problems

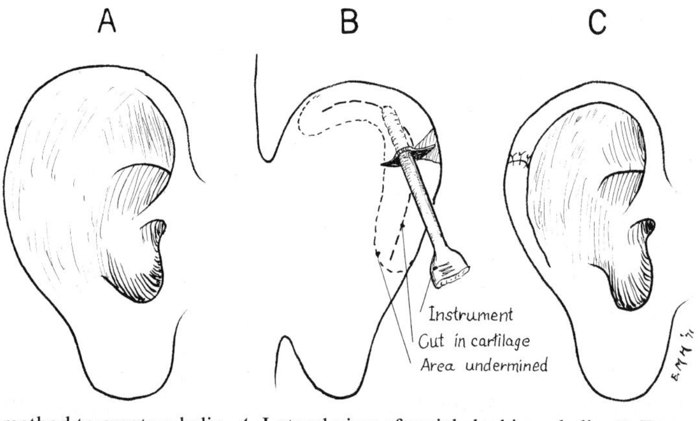

Figure 8. A method to create a helix. *A*, Lateral view of auricle lacking a helix. *B*, Exposure of posterior surface showing area undermined and instrument with short right-angle blade scoring cartilage along its line of desired forward bending. Shaded area indicates skin and cartilage to be removed. *C*, Closure and created helix.

and procedures pertaining to the ear, see Converse.[6]

When there is an underdeveloped helix, it is necessary to roll the cartilage along a predetermined line. This will create an excess of helical cartilage and skin that must be removed. A small incision is made on the posterior surface down to the cartilage adjacent to the periphery of the auricle. With the periosteum elevated along the line of the desired folding, the cartilage is then scored with a small right-angle instrument that permits the cartilage to bend forward of its own accord. It is then possible to determine the amount of excess skin and cartilage that must be excised to hold it in this position. The incision is then closed with interrupted sutures (Fig. 8).

When the prominence is due to lack of anthelix and superior crus bending, there are many possible procedures. All the successful ones have in common the fact that the cartilage must have its spring broken so that it will create the desired fold and yet avoid undesirable ridges and irregularities on the front surface. The earliest procedures broke the spring by cutting through and through the cartilage along the desired fold, making one, two, three or more cuts. The cartilage was then sewed back into position. Invariably a conspicuous and undesirable ridge would be left along this sharp cut line. To avoid this, a procedure was developed to free the cartilage to be folded by separating it from the surrounding cartilage and sewing it into a tube, thus creating more of a normal general contour (Fig. 9) (Becker, Converse). In 1959, Holmes described a technique of breaking the spring by using multiple gouge cuts through the posterior aspect of the cartilage. Using a gouge, rows of cuts were made into the cartilage attached to the anterior surface. These pieces of cartilage, resembling the scales of a fish, would permit the anterior surface to bend without sharp angulation; after healing, the multiple pieces of cartilage would hold the auricle in its new shape (Fig. 10).

Stenstrom used the principle that cartilage will bend away from a cut that breaks its surface. Therefore, he undermined the skin of the front of the auricle along the desired bend and, using a small instrument that could be inserted into this tunnel, he scratched or scored the area to be bent. This automatically folded the cartilage back into its new position (see Fig. 9 *D*). Ju et al. exposed the entire front face of the cartilage and then altered the size or shape of the auricle directly. Then the skin was resutured (see Fig. 9 *H* and *I*).

The simple technique of creating the fold by stay sutures placed through the cartilage postauricularly was tried years ago, but was given up because the sutures pulled out. In 1963, Mustarde reintroduced the technique, obtaining excellent results. He placed the sutures through the cartilage encompassing the perichondrium on the front surface but avoided perforating the anterior skin. When white, nonabsorbable sutures are employed in sufficient number, this procedure works well on selected cases.

Occasionally one will encounter a lobule that turns upward or outward. This deformity is caused by the cordate process of the auricular cartilage protruding forward. To correct this, the cordate process must be cut free. In some cases, this alone is not sufficient, and it is necessary to cut the lobule between the anterior and posterior surfaces (parallel to the anterior surface) and to permit the surfaces to slide on one another. The lobule is then sutured into the new desirable position by through-and-through stay sutures, which are later removed (Fig. 11).

When the ear stands out because of a deep concha, but the auricle is otherwise well formed, the conchal bed is exposed and the cartilage removed from the anterior conchal skin up to a point where it will permit the auricle to resume a normal attitude. One may also remove the postauricular tissue between the cartilage and the mastoid bone, thus permitting several more degrees of posterior positioning. The periosteum is not touched and the cartilage must be beveled so that it will not produce a sharp edge anteriorly. The cartilage is

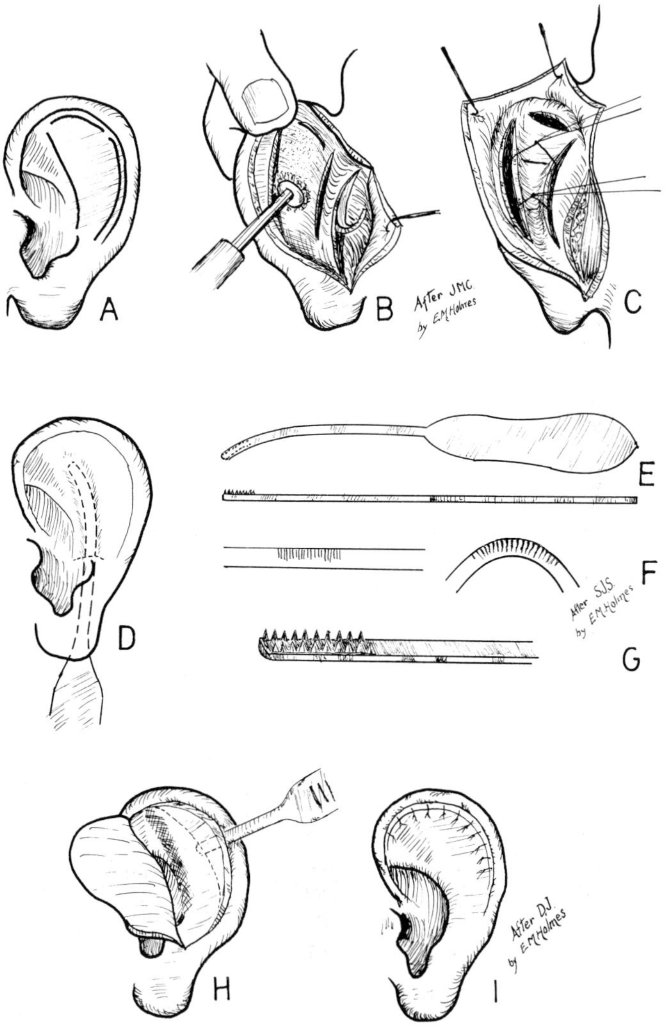

Figure 9. Accepted procedures of correcting prominent or "lop" ear. Converse and Becker's principle is shown in *A, B,* and *C. A,* Black line indicates incisions through the auricular cartilage from the posterior exposed surface. *B,* Thinning of the cartilage, if it is extremely thick, using a high-speed brush or a dermabrasion wheel. Note the strip of cartilage being removed just anterior to the retracting hook, which will permit the lowering of the anthelix into the concha. *C,* Permanent stay sutures that will hold the scapha and the anthelix in its desired contour. *D,* Stenstrom's technique shows the scarifying instrument having been inserted into a posterior insertion into a tunnel between the front surface of the cartilage and the perichondrium, where the cartilage is scarified, permitting it automatically to bend backward to a desired position. *E,* The instrument employed, AP and lateral views. *F,* A cross section of cartilage with parallel cuts through one surface, permitting that surface to open up, thus bending the cartilage away from the cuts. *G,* Magnification of the scarifying teeth of the instrument. *H,* Ju's method. The anterior surface of the cartilage is exposed by elevating subperichondrially. Scarification is performed where indicated (cross-hatching) to permit bending. The elevator is lifting out the scaphoid cartilage, which may be partially removed, thus decreasing the auricle as a whole. *I,* The skin flap resutured.

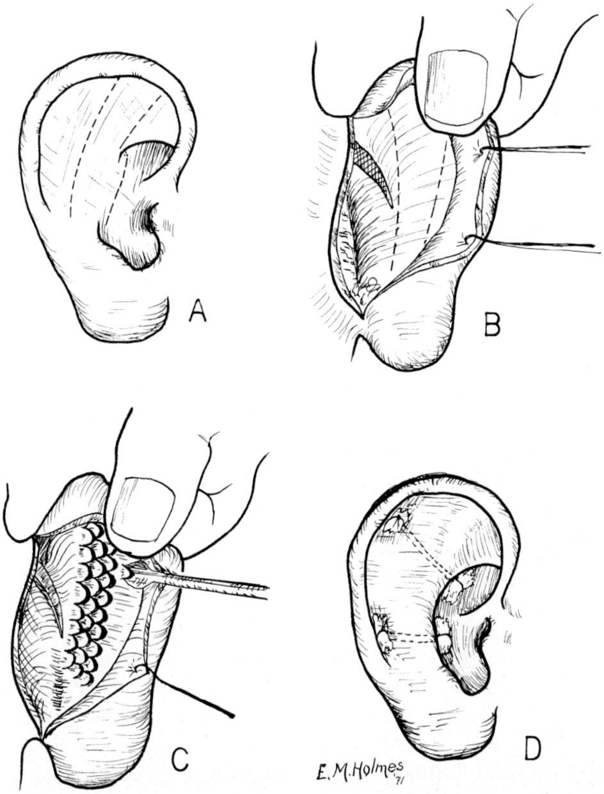

Figure 10. Holmes technique of otoplasty. *A*, Dotted line indicates the area that should have the spring of the cartilage broken to permit it to fold to a desired contour. *B*, Exposure of the posterior surface of the cartilage. Broken lines are the same as in *A*. *C*, Illustrates the creation of many pieces of cartilage, similar to the scales of a fish, which are attached to the anterior surface of the cartilage, permitting it to bend. After it has been held in the desired position, it will heal in this new position. *D*, Through-and-through stay sutures of fine absorbable gut. The postauricular incision is closed with a continuous subcutaneous suture of nylon, which is easy to remove.

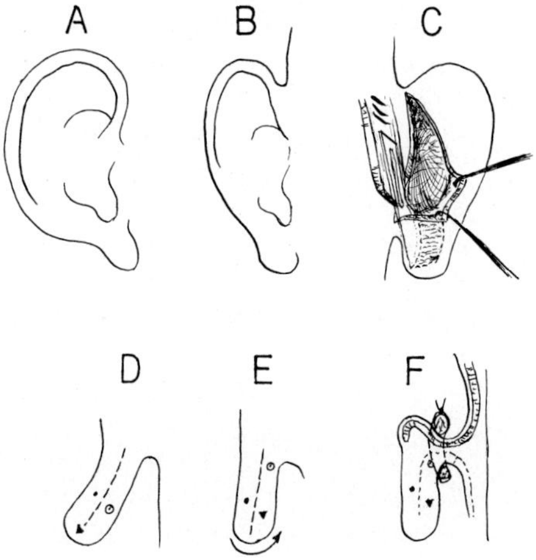

Figure 11. A method of correcting a forward protruding lobule. *A*, Lateral view of a prominent, partially cupped ear with forward protruding lobule. *B*, AP view of same ear. *C*, Posterior exposure illustrating how the anterior and posterior surfaces of the lobule are separated with a knife. This permits the surgeon to roll the skin backward, as in the cross sections *D*, *E*, and *F*. Once in position, it is maintained by a through-and-through stay suture, as indicated in *F*. Excess skin is excised.

then sutured back to the periosteum to hold it in place.

It is occasionally necessary to remove a strip of cartilage beneath the anterior crus of the anthelix. This may be done with impunity because any sharp ridge in this area is obscured from view by the anterior crus itself (see Fig. 9 *B* and Fig. 10 *B*).

The Underdeveloped Auricle

The underdeveloped auricle varies from a lack of development of the helix, with cupping of the auricle, to complete microtia, with so little ear presenting that it looks like a blob of cartilage and skin, with complete absence of the external auditory meatus, both bony and soft tissues. The problem of hearing has already been discussed; now the matter of appearance will be considered. If the child is a girl, all one really needs to do is to create a lobule, assuming that the remainder of the defect may be covered with her hair. In dealing with a male child, the appearance always used to be a problem, but with changing hair styles this no longer holds true.

In constructing an entire auricle, there are such a variety of abnormalities presenting that one cannot prescribe a particular procedure, but must understand the many possibilities and adapt them to the problem at hand. It is basic that skin of the proper thickness, color and texture be available to cover the reconstructed auricle. The utilization of local skin is always best, but occasionally it is necessary to borrow skin from the neck as a rotating or rope graft, or occasionally from behind the opposite normal ear as a free graft. The ear lobe is one of the easiest portions to reconstruct, as one may usually utilize a part of the hypoplastic ear that is present. If this is not adequate, local skin may be rolled up to augment any deficiency.

Auricular Framework

The auricular framework presents a problem, as it is impossible to get a material that will replace normal auricular cartilage. During the developmental period of reconstruction of the auricle, rib cartilage was employed in several ways. It was sculptured to imitate the absent auricular form. It was inserted in strips to lend support. It was diced and placed in a preconstructed vitalium mold, which was in turn placed subcutaneously in the abdomen for some weeks until fibroblasts had grown in through its sieve-like surface and formed a homogeneous mass of cartilage and connective tissue. When removed from the mold, it would hold its shape very well until it was used as a skeleton, at which time contraction of the skin over it and stresses on it would ultimately change its shape. Maternal auricular cartilage was first used by Gillies in 1937, but on the whole this was not sufficiently rigid, and it was frequently absorbed. Metals, plastics and silicone rubber have all been tried, but these are semirigid and nonviable and erode through many skin coverages, so eventually it has to be removed.

The method accepted today is to use rib cartilage, which may be carved. Using two or three blocks wired together, a satisfactory skeleton may be obtained. These have the least likelihood of absorption or extrusion.

The total reconstruction of an auricle has gradually developed into a pattern of steps developed by Tanzer (1967). He has produced some of the most acceptable reconstructed ears, and the follow-up of his cases has revealed that there has been the least amount of absorption of cartilaginous framework or loss of skin grafts. His results are so satisfactory that his technique will be offered as an acceptable technique (Fig. 12).

STAGE I. A tracing of the normal ear is made on x-ray film and a contour pattern of proposed cartilage grafts is made. At operation, a dye is used to indicate the outline on the affected side. The lobule is then rotated, employing a Z-plasty (Fig. 12 *A* and *B*).

STAGE II. After the scars have softened, blocks of cartilage are obtained from the sixth, seventh and eighth costal

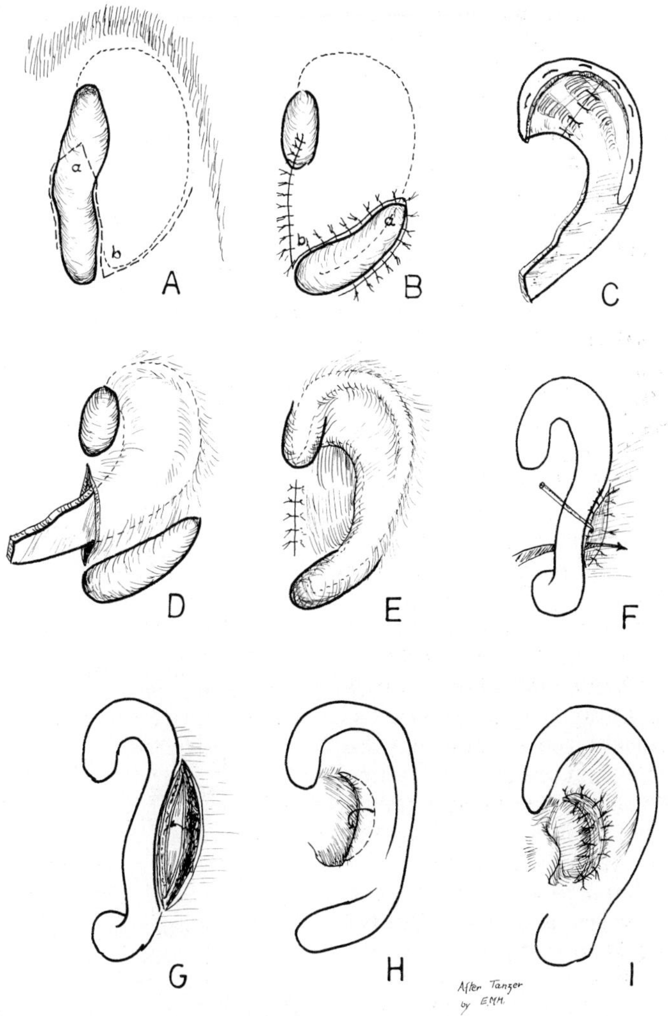

Figure 12. Steps in the otoplasty for reconstruction of an auricle developed by Tanzer. *A*, Fine dotted line indicates the desired shape of the auricle as determined by the normal ear on the opposite side. The long dotted lines show the incisions permitting a Z-plasty with transpositions of flaps a and b, which uses the rudiment of an auricle to create a lobule, as seen in *B*. *C*, A composite graft constructed from pieces of cartilage removed from the ribs and wired together with fine stainless steel wire, which is left in place. *D*, The scar of the first operation is removed and the skin undermined superficially, permitting the graft to be inserted into position, as shown in *E*. The skin was molded around the graft using multiple stay sutures placed over small rolls of cotton. *F*, The lower half of the auricle is elevated to create a tunnel. The reconstructed portion is covered with skin flaps that are created for the purpose and the defect against the head is covered with the skin graft. Some weeks later the same procedure is carried out on the upper half of the auricle. *G*, After several weeks of healing, when there is a good blood supply, the previously created tunnel is closed in one of two ways: In the first, the anterior surface of the concha is created by using local skin hinged above and below, and then the posterior surface is covered with a skin graft, lateral support being contributed by buried cartilage. *H*, In the second method, a skin covering is created for the posterior conchal wall from the skin of the anterior surface of the existing auricle. Support and creation of the rest of the conchal wall are obtained from a composite graft of the anterior skin and cartilage from the normal auricle on the other side. Sutures are in place as in *I*.

cartilages. The blocks are then shaped, wired together and sculptured to conform to the pattern first formed. The vertical scar from the first operation is then removed, the skin undermined and a pocket created to receive the sculptured auricular skeleton (Fig. 12 *C, D,* and *E*).

STAGE III. After at least four months of healing, the auricle is partially elevated from the head, avoiding exposure of the cartilage, and the bare areas are covered with skin grafts (Fig. 12 *F*).

STAGE IV. Two months later, the elevation started in Stage III is extended superiorly so that the entire auricle may be elevated, being attached at its upper and lower portions, and again the raw area is covered with a skin graft. This procedure is done in two stages to avoid any inadequacy of blood supply to the construction of the auricle (Fig. 12 *G*).

STAGE V. After three or four months have elapsed, one may proceed with the closure of the tunnel and construction of the posterior conchal wall (Fig. 12 *H*).

STAGE VI. The conchal floor may be deepened and a tragus formed. The tissue in the area of the concha may be used to create a tragus, and skin grafting used to create the deepened conchal floor, which will go down to the periosteum of the mastoid (Fig. 12 *I*).

The shortest time in which all this can be done is a year, and six operative procedures are necessary.

REFERENCES

1. Altman, F.: Malformations of the eustachian tube, the middle ear and its appendages. Arch. Otol., *54*:241, 1951.
2. Arey, L. B.: *Developmental Anatomy. A Textbook and Laboratory Manual of Embryology*, 6th ed., Philadelphia, W. B. Saunders Co., 1954.
3. Beal, D. O., Davey, P. R., and Lindsay, J. R.: Inner ear pathology of congenital deafness. Arch. Otol., *85*:134, 1967.
4. Bicker, O. B.: Surgical correction of the abnormally protruding ear. Arch. Otol., *50*:541, 1949.
5. Caparosa, R. J., and Klassur, D.: Congenital anomalies of stapes and facial nerve. Arch. Otol., *83*:420, 1966.
6. Converse, J. M.: *Reconstructive Plastic Surgery*, Vol. III. Philadelphia, W. B. Saunders, 1964, pp. 1073–1123.
7. Crabtree, J. A.: Tympanoplastic technique in ear atresia. *Arch. Otol.,* 88:63, 1968.
8. Erick, J. B.: Congenital cup-shaped deformity of the ear transmitted through four generations. *Mayo Clin. Proc.,* 40:597 (Aug.), 1965.
9. Freire-Maia, N.: A newly recognized genetic syndrome of tetramedic deficiencies, ectodermal dysplasia, deformed ears and other abnormalities. *Amer. J. Hum. Genet.,* 22:371, 1970.
10. Gillies, H.: Reconstruction of the external ear with special reference to the use of maternal ear cartilage as the supporting structure. *Rev. de Chir. Structive,* 7:169, 1937.
11. Gussen, R.: Delayed hereditary deafness with cochlear aqueduct obstruction. *Arch. Otol.,* 90:429, 1969.
12. Henner, R.: Congenital middle ear malformations. *Arch. Otol.,* 71:454, 1960.
13. Henner, R., and Buckingham, R. H.: Classification of middle ear defects. Recognition and surgical treatment of congenital ossicular defects. *Laryngoscope,* 66:522, 1956.
14. Holmes, E. M.: A new procedure for correcting outstanding ears. *Arch. Otol.,* 69:409, 1959.
15. House, H. P.: Management of congenital ear canal atresia. *Laryngoscope,* 63:916, 1953.
16. Ju, D. M. et al.: The surgical correction of protruding ears. *Plast. Reconstr. Surg.,* 32:283, 1963.
17. Mustarde, J. C.: The correction of prominent ears using simple mattress sutures. *J. Plas. Surg.,* 16:170, 1963.
18. Myers, E. N., Stool, S. E., and Koblausen, P. J.: Congenital deafness in spiny hyperkeratosis and universal alopecia. *Arch. Otol.,* 93:68, 1971.
19. Proctor, C. A., and Proctor, B.: Understanding hereditary nerve deafness. *Arch. Otol.,* 85:23, 1967.
20. Sando, I., Bergstrom, L., Wood, R. P., and Hemenway, W. G.: Temporal bone findings in trisomy 18 syndrome. *Arch. Otol.,* 91:552, 1970.
21. Scheer, A. A.: Correction of congenital middle ear deformities. *Arch. Otol.,* 85:269, 1967.
22. Shambaugh, G. E.: Developmental anomalies of the sound conducting apparatus and their surgical correction. *Ann. Otol.,* 61:873, 1957.
23. Tanzer, R. C.: Total reconstruction of the auricle—the evaluation of a plan of treatment. *Plast. Reconstr. Surg.,* 47:523, 1971.
24. Wood-Jones, F. W., and Wen, I. C.: The development of the external ear. *J. Anat.,* 68:525, 1934.

INTRODUCTION TO DISEASES OF THE EAR

"I am just as deaf as I am blind. The problems of deafness are deeper and more complex, if not more important, than those of blindness. Deafness is a much worse misfortune. For it means the loss of the most vital stimulus—the sound of the voice that brings language, sets thoughts astir and keeps us in the intellectual company of men."

These sentences were written by Helen Keller. They serve to put the seriousness of hearing loss in a more meaningful perspective. In order for the child to acquire understanding and use of language, hearing is necessary. The importance of hearing is paramount for the normal development of the child. Diseases which affect the organ of hearing, the ear, must be promptly recognized and correctly treated.

The process of hearing is dependent upon the ear and the central nervous system. The role of the ear in hearing can be thought of as threefold. The external and middle parts of the ear serve as the transformer mechanism; the inner ear, the cochlea, serves as the transducer; and the eighth cranial nerve is the connector.

Chapter Sixty-Eight

THE EXTERNAL EAR

ROBERT J. RUBEN, M.D.

The pinna and the external ear canal serve as a conduit for sound. Although absence of the pinna does not significantly affect the ability to hear, complete occlusion of the external auditory canal will result in a severe hearing loss. The congenital malformations of the pinna and external auditory canal have already been discussed in Chapter 67. Many of these malformations are associated with renal malformations. All patients who exhibit any malformation of the pinna should have an intravenous pyelogram (IVP) to rule out renal disease (Fig. 1).

GENETIC DISORDERS

There are several genetic disorders which affect the external ear. The most common of these is the *Treacher-Collins syndrome,* which is thought to be inherited as an autosomal dominant. The Treacher-Collins syndrome consists of one or any combination of the following signs: malformation of the pinna, external auditory canal or middle ear; hypoplasia of the mandible and the maxilla; an antimongoloid slant of the eyes; and coloboma. Another commonly seen ge-

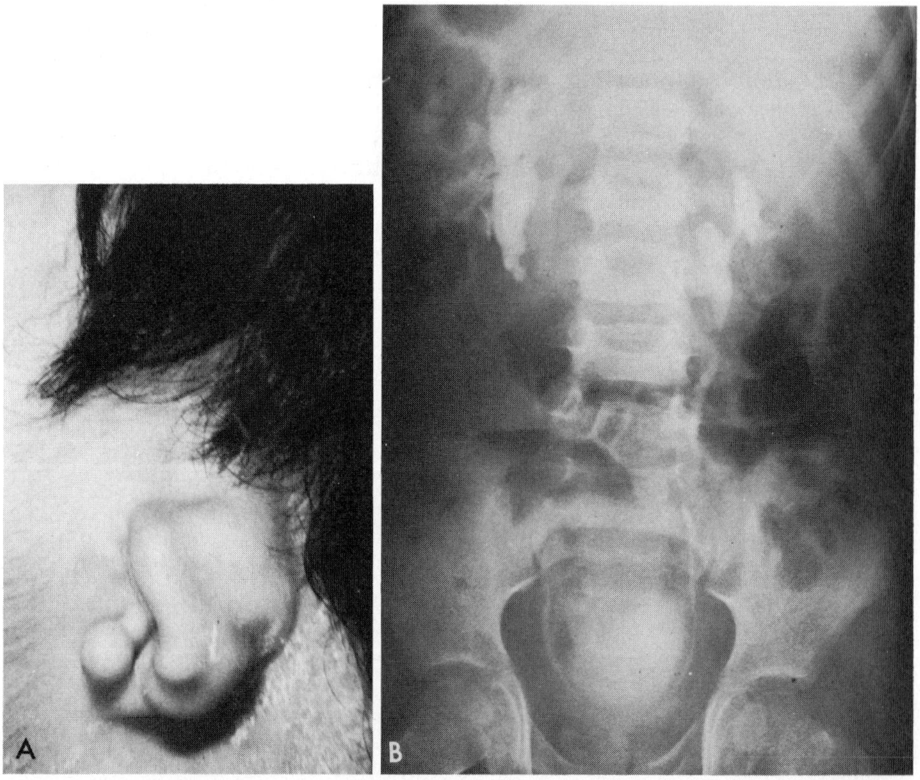

Figure 1. *A*, Abnormality of pinna. *B*, Abnormal intravenous pyelogram in same patient.

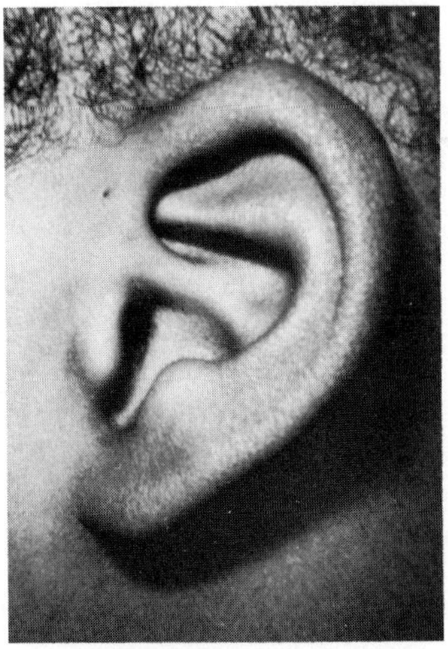

Figure 2. Preauricular branchial cleft cyst.

netic anomaly of the external ear is the presence of *branchial cleft cysts* anterior to the tragus (Fig. 2). These cysts can become infected and may then cause cellulitis of the pinna and the face. The cysts should be removed when they are free of infection. Occasionally, the tract of the cyst will lead into the middle ear.

ACQUIRED DISEASES

FOREIGN BODIES

In children, acquired diseases of the *external ear and canal* are quite common. Perhaps one of the diseases seen most frequently results from a *foreign body* which has been placed in the ear. This usually occurs in toddlers. The young child may place a piece of crayon, a bead or a dried vegetable, such as a pea, in his ear canal. The vegetable type of foreign body presents a special problem because the moisture of the external canal will cause it to expand. The removal of a foreign body from the ear canal is a simple procedure when done properly. Unfortunately, too many foreign bodies are removed improperly. Often the child is brought to a physician who attempts without proper instruments or anesthesia to remove the foreign body. The manipulation of the external auditory canal is extremely painful. The young child reacts to the pain and as the child struggles, the physician causes bleeding in the canal. The physician may persist and remove the contents of the external auditory canal; unfortunately on occasion, this will include the tympanic membrane and some of the ossicles of the middle ear. The child then is left with a hearing loss at the least, and possibly an infection as well.

Foreign bodies in the external auditory canal usually do not cause harm if they are allowed to remain for a short period of time. The proper and safe method for removing the foreign body requires, first, an evaluation of the child. If the foreign body looks as if it would be difficult to remove while the child is awake, and this will occur in the majority of cases, then arrangements should be made for general anesthesia. The child is put to sleep, and with the use of the operating microscope and proper instruments, the foreign body can be removed without damage to the external auditory canal, the middle ear, or the child's attitude toward physicians.

HEMATOMAS

Hematomas of the pinna should be drained before they become infected. Patients with cellulitis of the pinna should be given both systemic and local therapy. One of the most common pathogens is pseudomonas. The use of compresses of Burow's solution for cellulitis of the pinna in conjunction with systemic antibiotics will prevent or lessen the amount of perichondritis. Surgical drainage is needed, in addition to local and systemic therapy, when the infection has progressed to the stage at which there is pus underneath the skin of the pinna. Children with cellulitis of the pinna usually appear systemically ill. It is preferable to hospitalize these patients until the infection has been controlled.

Children who develop hematomas of the pinna secondary to trauma must also be examined for head injury. A significant number of children are found to have skull fractures, including fractures of the temporal bone, associated with trauma to the pinna.

ACCUMULATION OF CERUMEN

A common medical problem associated with the external ear canal is the accumulation of *cerumen.* Cerumen is, in itself, normal and harmless. However, some patients will accumulate enough cerumen to block their external auditory canal, and this must be removed. The removal of cerumen should be a simple and painless procedure. If there is no perforation of the tympanic membrane, a solution of ten parts water to one part hydrogen peroxide at body temperature can be gently flushed into the ear canal. This will remove almost all the cerumen. The same solution can also be used at home. Four to five drops should be placed in the child's ear each day. When the child then returns to the doctor's office the remaining softened cerumen is gently washed out. The technique of using a curette to remove cerumen from the ear canal of the child is usually unsatisfactory.

INFECTION

Infections of the pinna in children usually will occur when there is some predisposing factor. One of the most common factors is otitis externa. Another common cause of infection is the presence of the already discussed antitragus branchial cleft cysts. A third factor is trauma. When the pinna is traumatized a hematoma will form between the skin and the cartilage and can then become secondarily infected. If children's pinnae are bitten by animals, they can become infected. Infection of the pinna can be serious and can result in the deformity of the pinna which is called cauliflower ear (Fig. 3). The mechanism causing the ear deformity is the infectious process which destroys the delicate cartilage which maintains the pinna. The loss of cartilage results in the deformity.

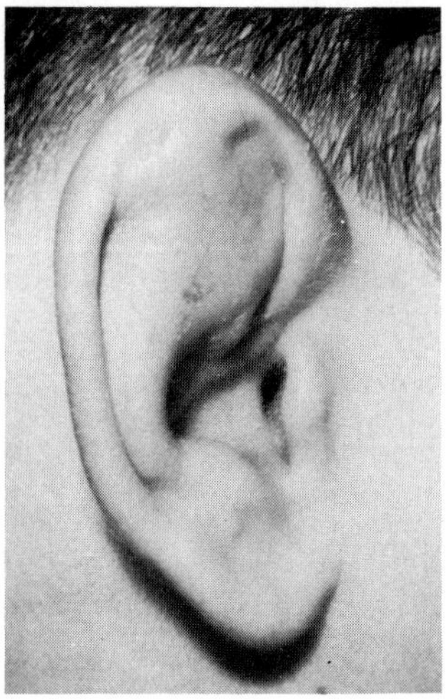

Figure 3. Cauliflower ear following trauma.

Otitis Externa

Otitis externa is a disease usually found in children over the age of 4 or 5. Most frequently it is secondary to a pseudomonas infection of the ear canal. The canal presents with swelling and is very tender. Any movement of the external auditory canal, such as pressure on the tragus, will cause significant pain. The canal may contain a foul-smelling, whitish debris and may also appear to be very inflamed. Occasionally an abscess of the external auditory canal will be seen and usually presents on the floor of the canal at its entrance. These abscesses should be incised and drained.

CAUSES. Otitis externa can be found after the ear canal has been traumatized with a curette, a sharp stick or a wire and also occurs when the ears have been wet. It is seen quite frequently in the summer months when children are swimming and is sometimes called *swimmer's ear.* Severe otitis externa is also seen when children have otitis media. Occasionally a young infant is seen with a long-term, low-grade otitis externa, which may also be associated with an otitis media. If the otitis media is adequately treated, then the otitis externa will also resolve.

TREATMENT. The treatment for otitis externa usually consists of two stages. The initial therapy, when the canal is swollen and tender, is to reduce the swelling. During the first twenty-four hours, a small cotton wick, soaked in Burow's solution, is placed in the ear canal. This wick is kept wet with the Burow's solution. After one day it is removed, and ear drops containing antibiotics and steroids are used for approximately one week. The ear canal should be gently cleaned of debris four to seven days after the swelling has subsided. Most cases of otitis externa will resolve within two weeks' time with this type of therapeutic regime. If the otitis externa does not resolve, then other predisposing factors, such as middle ear infection, allergy or repeated trauma, should be sought. Occasionally, an otitis externa will cause a widespread cellulitis, involving either the pinna or the face. These patients require systemic antibiotics and are usually hospitalized.

Ramsey-Hunt Syndrome

An uncommon infection of the external ear canal or the pinna and lateral surface of the tympanic membrane is called the *Ramsey-Hunt syndrome*. This is thought to be a viral infection similar to herpes. It results in otitis externa and paralysis of the facial nerve of the ipsilateral side. Both the external otitis and the facial nerve paralysis will resolve with conservative therapy.

The lateral aspect of the tympanic membrane must be included in discussion of diseases of the external canal, for its epithelium is contiguous with that of the ear canal. *Bullous myringitis* is another probable viral disease which affects this area of the tympanic membrane, which will present with a number of large blebs on its lateral wall. These blebs are filled with blood or serous fluid, sometimes both. This disease will usually present with ear pain and some hearing loss. It can be treated with local antibiotic steroid ear drops. If it is very painful, the blebs can be opened with a small myringotomy knife.

TUMORS

There are few *tumors of the external ear and ear canal,* and they occur rarely. The most common tumor of the external ear canal is the *canal cholesteatoma* (Fig. 4), a benign epithelial growth. This presents as a whitish mass, usually in the superior aspect of the external auditory canal. This will continue to grow, and therefore must be removed, since it can result in permanent hearing loss, facial paralysis and possible central nervous system infection.

Bony tumors of the external auditory canal are also sometimes seen in children. Osteoma of the external auditory canal can present as round, hard, skin-covered masses growing in the superior wall of the canal. *Fibrous dysplasia* (Fig. 5), either monostotic or polystotic, may often involve the external auditory canal. This will result in a hearing loss and will also isolate the middle ear, which will become infected. The bony growth must be removed. Cases of *ossifying fibroma* have also been seen. These also must be surgically removed from the external canal, and the middle ear must be exteriorized.

Polyps

The most common mass presenting in the external auditory canal, a *polyp* is usually located in the middle ear or tympanic membrane. The appearance of a polyp in the external auditory canal usually means that there is serious disease in the middle ear.

Malignant Tumors

Malignant tumors of the external auditory canal rarely occur in children. The most common of these is rhabdomyosarcoma; occasionally, *reticular cell sarcomas* are found. Any mass in the external auditory meatus must be examined. Complete examination of the ear includes the medical history, noting the patient's physical appearance, a hearing test and x-rays. The hearing test and x-rays can greatly increase the

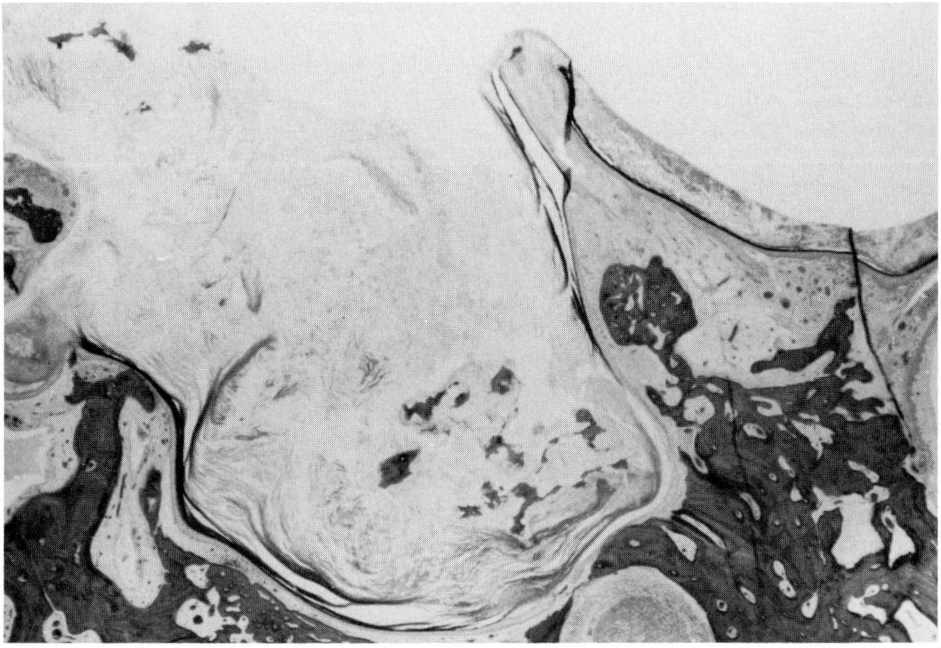

Figure 4. Cholesteatoma growing in external auditory canal.

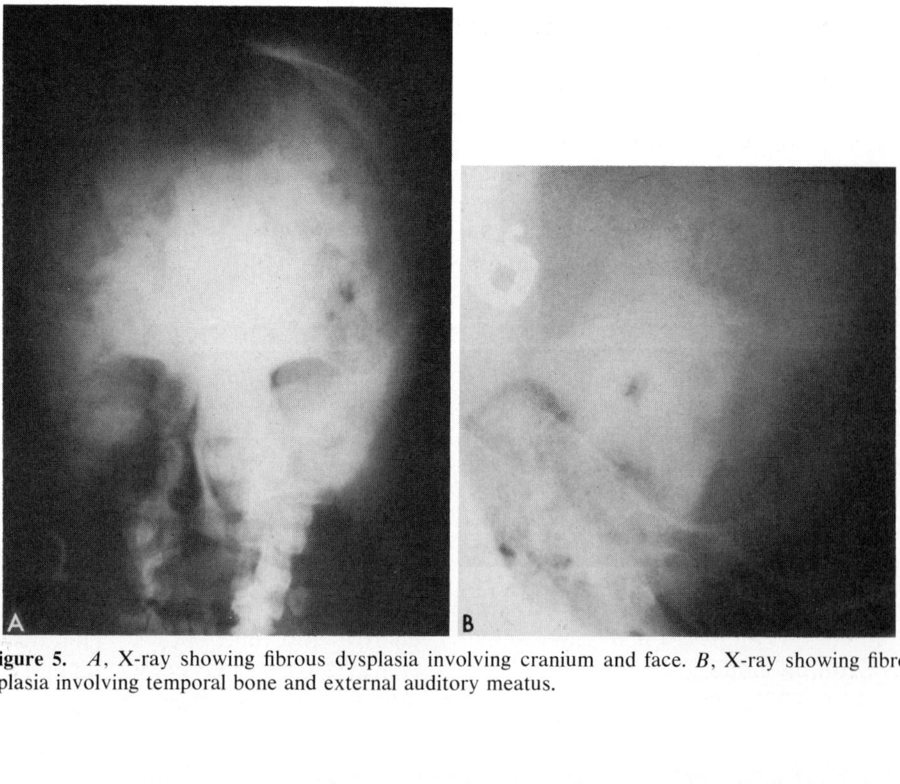

Figure 5. *A*, X-ray showing fibrous dysplasia involving cranium and face. *B*, X-ray showing fibrous dysplasia involving temporal bone and external auditory meatus.

knowledge of the extent of a lesion. This becomes extremely important in devising proper therapy for the individual child.

REFERENCES

The references for Chapter 68 appear at the end of Chapter 72.

Chapter Sixty-Nine

THE MIDDLE EAR AND MASTOID

ROBERT J. RUBEN, M.D.

The three anatomic regions of the middle ear are the mastoid cell system; the middle ear cleft, which contains the three ossicles; and the eustachian tube. During the period of growth from infancy to maturity, the relative sizes and anatomic relationships of these three parts of the middle ear change. The tympanic membrane is more horizontal in infants and gradually attains a more vertical position by the age of 6.

Mastoid Cell System

At birth there is usually a single mastoid cell, called the antrum, which is connected to the middle ear cleft by a small channel, known as the aditus ad antrum. The mastoid cells increase in number until adolescence. There is a significant variation in the number, size and location of these mastoid cells in different people. Their clinical importance lies in the areas in which they are contiguous. This usually includes the anterior border of the sigmoid sinus, the anterior aspect of the posterior cranial fossa, the floor of the middle cranial fossa, the posterior aspect of the zygomatic process and the petrous tip of the temporal bone. The tip lies deep within the cranium and touches the fifth, sixth, seventh and eighth cranial nerves. As will be discussed later in this chapter, diseases of the mastoid can present with symptoms and signs involving those structures which are next to the mastoid cells.

The mastoid cells are lined with a modified type of respiratory mucosa and are all interconnected with the antrum. The antrum is connected to the middle ear by means of the aditus ad antrum. The middle ear is in turn connected to the pharynx through the eustachian tube. The mastoid cells are part of the respiratory system. Infections of the upper respiratory system can and often do spread into the middle ear.

Middle Ear Cleft

The middle ear cleft contains the tympanic membrane (ear drum); three ossicles (the malleus, incus and stapes) with their associated ligaments and muscles; and the facial nerve and its branch for taste, the chorda tympani. The eustachian tube and the aditus ad antrum are located posterosuperiorly and anterosuperiorly, respectively, in the middle ear. The medial wall of the middle ear cleft is composed of the cochlea and its two windows—the oval window, in which the foot plate of the stapes is found, and the round window.

PHYSIOLOGIC FUNCTIONS

TRANSMISSION

The middle ear has two major *physiologic functions*. The first of these is to transmit airborne sound to the inner ear, which is contained in fluid. The transfer of sound energy from air to fluid could result in a loss of sound energy. The tympanic membrane and the three middle ear ossicles prevent this loss by acting as a type of transformer. The tympanic membrane and the ossicles work like a hydraulic transformer (Fig. 1) at an approximate ratio of 18:1. The sound that is received at the tympanic membrane is concentrated and transmitted to the stapes foot plate. The difference in the surface areas of the tympanic membrane and the foot plate and other lever factors of the ossicles cause the sound to be concentrated approximately 18 times by the time it reaches the cochlea at the oval window. Since the middle ear is similar to a mechanical transformer, it is characterized by an optimal impedance which can be clinically measured.

Any disturbance of the ability of the tympanic membrane or the ossicles to function properly will result in a conductive hearing loss. There are two general types of pathology which can affect the hearing function of the middle ear. The most common of the two are those disorders which cause an increase in the impedance of the middle ear. If the middle ear is filled with fluid, or if the ossicular chain is fixed by adhesions or bony growth, then the sound cannot be properly transmitted; this results in a conductive hearing loss. If the tym-

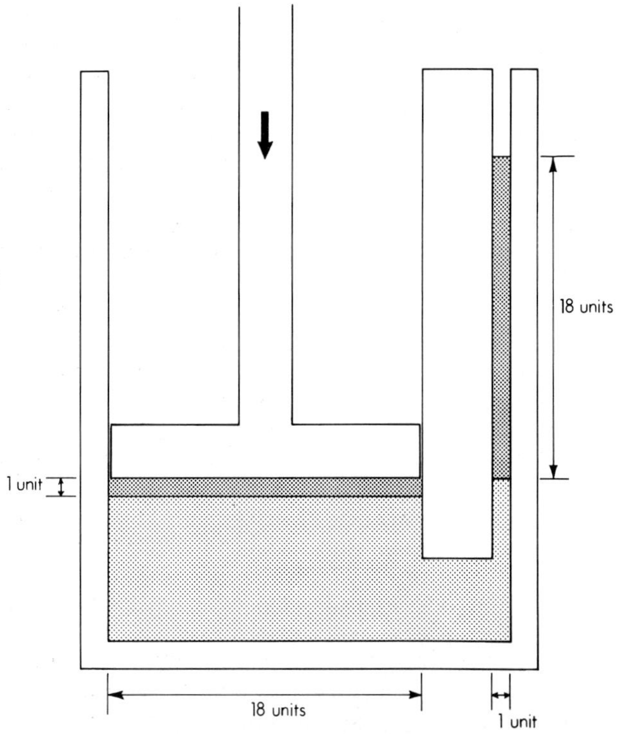

Figure 1. Schematic diagram to show the transformer principle of the middle ear. The large area, 18 units, represents the tympanic membrane; the small area, 1 unit, represents the footplate of the oval window.

panic membrane or an ossicle is missing or broken, the impedance will also be decreased, and this will again result in a conductive hearing loss.

EQUALIZATION OF AIR PRESSURE

The Eustachian Tube

The second major physiologic property of the middle ear concerns its relationship to the upper respiratory tract. The connection of the middle ear to the nasopharynx via the eustachian tube allows for equalization of air pressure between the middle ear and the external environment. If the pressure within the middle ear differs significantly from the atmospheric pressure, the eustachian tube opens and equalizes the pressure. If the eustachian tube cannot open because of either mechanical or physiological blockage, then the pressure cannot be equalized. If air is trapped in the middle ear, the oxygen will be absorbed. This will cause a decrease in the air pressure within the middle ear. The mucosa lining the middle ear will react by forming a sterile transudate, which will accumulate and result in an increase in the impedance of the middle ear. This will cause a marked conductive hearing loss. Some situations, such as scuba diving, will create a large increase in the external pressure. If the middle ear cannot accommodate rapidly for this increase, the ear drum can be ruptured. If the pressure in the middle ear is greatly increased, or if the external pressure is decreased and the middle ear cannot accommodate for it, then again, the ear drum can be ruptured.

The modified respiratory mucosa which lines the mastoid, the middle ear cleft and the eustachian tube contains cilia and mucus secretory cells, both of which become more numerous in the region of the eustachian tube. The mucus serves as a vehicle for the cilia to remove debris from the middle ear. When infection occurs, the respiratory mucosa must work properly so that the pus can be cleared. If the respiratory mucosa is not functioning properly or the eustachian tube is blocked, then pus will remain in the middle ear. The superficial infection of the mucosa will then become more serious. Pressure will build up in the middle ear, and this will result in venous thrombosis, followed by infection of the bony portion of the ear, which is called mastoiditis.

PHYSICAL EXAMINATION

The middle ear is examined by means of direct viewing of the tympanic membrane, a hearing test and x-rays. The *normal tympanic membrane* (Fig. 2) should be a transparent-to-translucent membrane through which most of the following structures can be seen: The long process of the malleus is observed in the middle of the pars tensa of the ear drum. The most superior portion is slightly posterior, and the inferior portion is slightly anterior. Directly anterior and a little inferior to this is the light reflex, which is a triangular area of high light reflex. The apex of the light reflex triangle points superiorly and posteriorly.

Posterior to the superior portion of the malleus, another bony structure can be seen. This is the long process of the incus. Occasionally the incudostapedial joint may also be seen. Running horizontally over the incus behind the malleus, the chorda tympani can be noted. The most superior portion of the tympanic membrane is called the pars flaccida. It is somewhat less translucent than the pars tensa.

The posteroinferior quadrant will on many occasions exhibit a dark circular shadow. This is the round window niche. Anteriorly and superiorly another dark circular shadow can be seen, and this is the middle ear orifice of the eustachian tube.

Most tympanic membranes will not reveal all of these structures. This is because disease causes the tympanic membrane to lose its transparency. Often there will be small white spots in

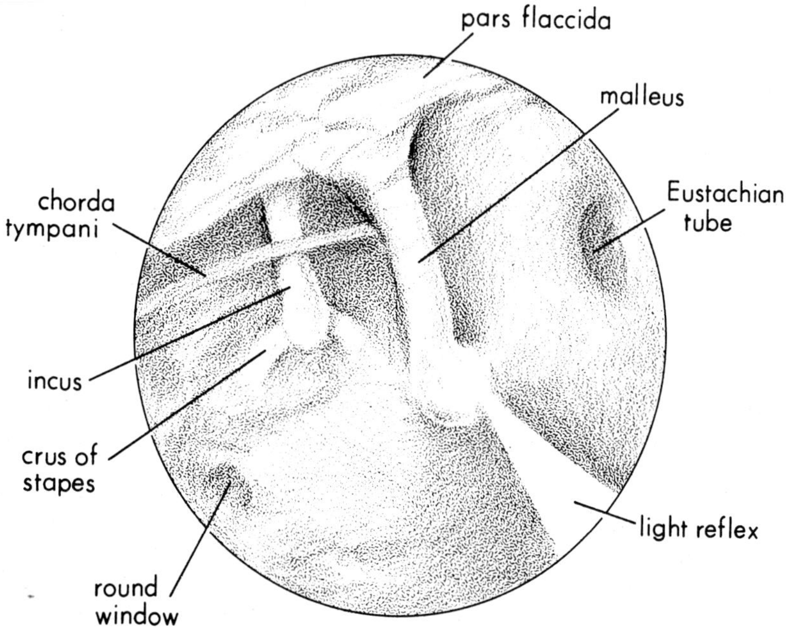

Figure 2. Diagram of tympanic membrane illustrating the landmarks which should be seen through the normal translucent tympanic membrane.

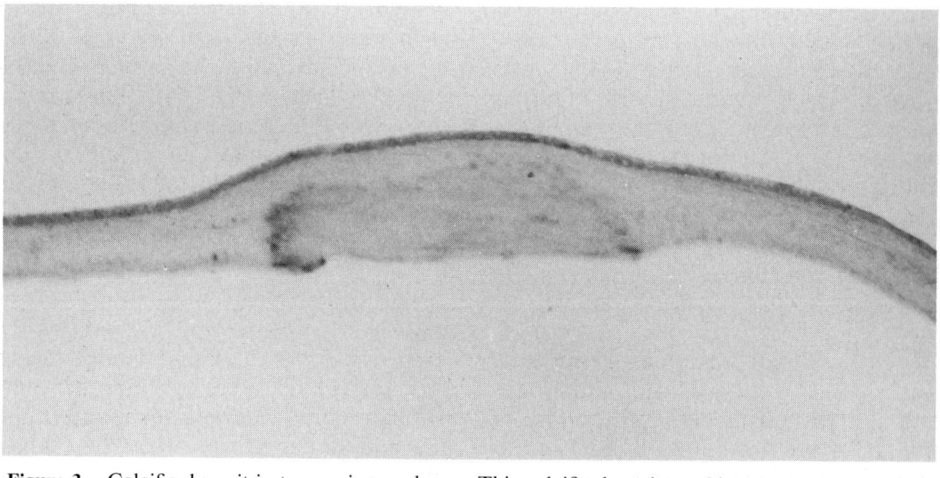

Figure 3. Calcific deposit in tympanic membrane. This calcific deposit would appear as a white plaque in the tympanic membrane on otoscopic examination.

the tympanic membrane (Fig. 3); these are calcium deposits secondary to infection and usually are of no significance.

Each tympanic membrane should be carefully examined. The examination of the tympanic membrane is difficult, and it takes time to note all the normal structures. A tympanic membrane in which only the malleus and the light reflex can be seen is not normal. Thickening of the drum can represent significant middle ear disease and hearing loss.

ACUTE OTITIS MEDIA

Acute otitis media is one of the most common infections in children. It will occur most frequently in children from 2 to 6 years old. Various studies have indicated that more than 20 per cent of all children are affected each year. The incidence is seasonal; greatest occurrence is in the winter months and in early spring. Otitis media does occur in the newborn and infant. If otitis media is found in the newborn, a check of the aseptic techniques of the newborn nursery should be undertaken.

Etiology

The *etiology* of acute otitis media has been repeatedly studied. The most common organism is pneumococcus, and the second most common organisms are *Haemophilus influenzae*, occurring especially in infants, and pneumococcus. One or both of these pathogens can usually be cultured from more than 70 per cent of the middle ears examined in which there is growth of a pathogen. Other common pathogens which are found are the β-hemolytic streptococci, Nisseria and occasionally *Pseudomonas klebsiella,* Proteus, *Escherichia coli* or *Escherichia freundii.*

The relationship of viral infection to acute otitis media has been studied. Some of these studies have occasionally revealed the growth of virus in the middle ear. About 10 per cent of the patients studied will have a rise in antibody titer, but it will not be possible to isolate the virus from the middle ear fluid. Most often the bacterial pathogen can be cultured from the middle ear in association with the patient's rise in antibody titer. It is felt that many times viral infection will precede the bacterial infection and serve as an underlying cause for the bacterial otitis media.

Predisposing Factors

There are several predisposing factors in children which result in an increase in the incidence and severity of otitis media. The most common of these is either anatomic or physiologic dysfunction of the eustachian tube. Children with midfacial or base of skull malformations appear to have eustachian tube dysfunction. They have a much greater incidence of acute otitis media. This group includes children with cleft palate, Crouzon's disease, Apert's disease, Klippel-Feil disease and Turner's syndrome.

Occlusion of the pharyngeal orifice of the eustachian tube also results in an increase in the incidence of otitis media. This occurs in children with large nasopharyngeal masses occluding the eustachian tube orifice. Most commonly the mass is the adenoid. Adenoids should be removed if they occlude the eustachian

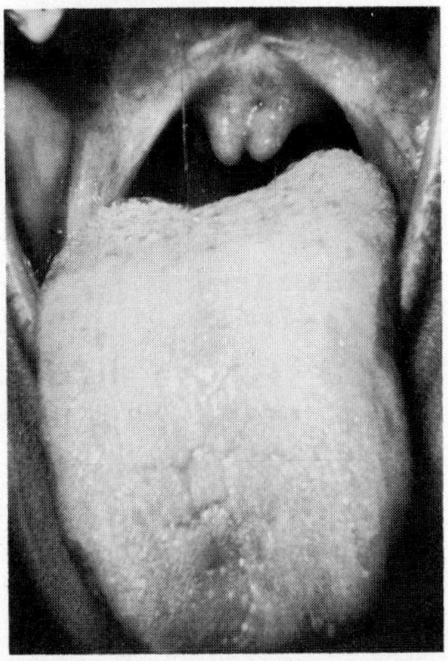

Figure 4. Patient with a bifid uvula. Patients with bifid uvulae may develop velopharyngeal incompetence after adenoidectomy.

tube orifice and if the child has a significant increase in the number or severity of attacks of acute otitis media. Before they are removed, the function of the velopharyngeal sphincter must be ascertained. Velopharyngeal insufficiency is characterized by hypernasal speech or the escape of liquid from the nose. Children in whom there is a cleft palate, submucosal palatal cleft, bifid uvula (Fig. 4) or other signs of velopharyngeal insufficiency should not have their adenoids removed. If they are removed, the velopharyngeal insufficiency is made much worse because the adenoid tissue helps to close the velopharyngeal sphincter. A lateral soft tissue x-ray of the nasopharynx often can show the relative size of the nasopharyngeal mass (Fig. 5). Cineradiography can be useful in demonstrating velopharyngeal function. Velopharyngeal insufficiency can be tested clinically by having the patient blow up a balloon or just puff out his cheeks. If he cannot do this and has air escaping from his nose, he may have velopharyngeal insufficiency.

There are other growths in the nasopharynx which can cause occlusion of the eustachian tube and subsequent acute otitis media. The most common of these is a choanal polyp which has grown from either the nasal turbinate or a paranasal sinus. A patient with a polyp may have a systemic allergy or cystic fibrosis. The physician must then treat three problems: the acute otitis media, the choanal polyp and the underlying disease.

Angiofibroma is a benign but destructive tumor which is found in the nose and nasopharynx of young boys. Occasionally, an encephalocele or craniopharyngioma will present in the nasopharynx and occlude the eustachian tube orifice.

All patients with recent infectious or noninfectious otitis media must have the function of the eustachian tube evaluated. This can be done in part by the use of impedance audiology. However, when eustachian tube dysfunction is found, the nasopharynx orifice must be examined. Direct examination can be done by

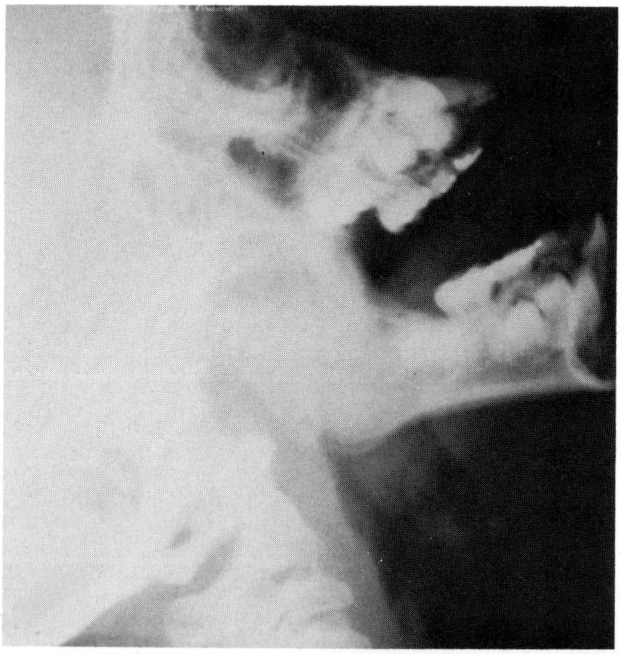

Figure 5. Lateral neck x-ray showing a large adenoid filling the nasopharyngeal space.

means of a nasopharyngoscope or a small laryngeal mirror. Most patients under 4 years of age are difficult to examine this way. The use of lateral x-ray (Fig. 5) is recommended for determining whether or not there is a significant tubal obstruction secondary to a nasopharyngeal mass.

Another group of factors predisposing to acute otitis media are the blood dyscrasias. Acute otitis media is seen in children with sickle-cell disease, leukemia, agranulocytosis and generalized anemias. There is also an increased frequency of the disease in children who have defects in their ability to produce antibodies. Children with various conditions which result in mucus discharge tend to have an increased incidence of otitis media. This group includes children with severe allergy and cystic fibrosis.

Some ethnic groups, such as Eskimos or American Indians, appear to have a greater incidence of acute otitis media. It is sometimes felt that in the United States poverty may be another predisposing factor. It is not known whether this is due to poor nutrition, borderline anemia, inadequate housing and sanitation, or poor medical services.

Symptoms and Signs

The *symptoms of acute otitis media* vary somewhat with age. The acute infection causes pain. The presenting signs of an acute otitis media in an infant may be either lethargy or irritability, and the infant may pull on his ear. The physician must examine the infant to locate the souce of this infection. Older children will complain of ear pain and also may state that their hearing has decreased in one ear. They may also have a feeling of fullness or hear a gurgling sound in the ear. Nevertheless, the predominant symptom in all age groups is pain.

The *signs of an acute otitis media* are found upon examination of the tympanic membrane. The tympanic membrane will no longer be transparent to translucent, as previously described. The drum will be thick, and all or most of the landmarks will be obscured. The color of the drum varies from a dull white to a very red, blood-engorged membrane. The normal tympanic membrane is dry. The tympanic membrane of acute otitis media is wet and will be covered with pus and mucus. Fluid levels, either single or multiple, may be seen behind the drum. Free pus can sometimes also be seen behind the drum.

Many times the tympanic membrane will bulge laterally. If treatment is delayed or the infection is particularly severe, the tympanic membrane will spontaneously rupture. This will cause the pus which has accumulated behind the tympanic membrane to drain into the external auditory canal. The patient will have relief from the pain, and the external auditory canal will be filled with pus and cellular debris. The drum will still appear thick but will not be bulging. The area of perforation may be seen, and on many occasions pus and mucus will also be seen coming from this area; the discharge will be pulsatile.

The clinical appearances of acute otitis externa and an otitis media with perforation can be quite similar. However, the acute otitis media patient will have little or no pain associated with movement of the external auditory canal, whereas the patient with acute external otitis will have considerable pain with such movement. The patient with acute otitis media will also have more general septic manifestations of the infection.

Children with acute otitis media may have systemic signs of fever and malaise. Many times an acute otitis media will be associated with upper respiratory infection or pneumonia. The infection in the middle ear can cause vestibular disturbance, and the patient may have severe vertigo, vomiting and nystagmus.

Treatment

The aim in treatment of acute otitis media is to stop the infection and restore the normal function of the ear as soon as possible. Most cases of acute otitis media respond well to antibiotics and some form of decongestant. The antibiotic used in most cases is ampicillin and is initially given intramuscularly. The pain associated with an acute otitis media will be reduced within four to six hours after initial therapy. A *myringotomy* is seldom performed unless an associated complication of acute otitis media is present. Occasionally, in cases of severe pain which has been unresponsive to antibiotics, a myringotomy will be performed. Myringotomy is indicated in those patients in whom the ear drum does not return to normal after several weeks and can also be done as a diagnostic procedure in an infant with fever and in whom an acute otitis media is suspected. Cultures of the infection should be taken. Since myringotomies are not routinely done, the culture will not be taken from the middle ear. The culture should be taken from the nasopharynx in the vicinity of the eustachian tube. If the tympanic membrane has ruptured, the culture can be taken from the external auditory canal.

Local or systemic decongestants should be used for the first three to five days after onset of the disease but should be discontinued after this time, since they probably lose their effectiveness. Indeed, in the case of nose drops, prolonged use can result in a chronic change of the nasal mucosa and can produce a condition called rhinitis medicamentosus.

Acute otitis media will usually respond well when adequate therapy is used. The fever and pain should be relieved within twenty-four hours, and the ear drum should return to normal within two to four weeks or sooner.

COMPLICATIONS OF ACUTE OTITIS MEDIA

There are many *complications of acute otitis media.* One of these is chronic otitis media and mastoid disease which is discussed in the next section of this chapter. Children can develop meningitis from acute otitis media. Any child with meningitis and an abnormal ear drum should have a myringotomy. The myringotomy will serve three purposes: (1) the presence of acute otitis media can be established; (2) if acute otitis media is present, the pus can be drained and the pressure will be relieved; and (3) a culture of the organism can be obtained through the myringotomy. Mastoid films should also be obtained. If the x-rays show clouding or an absence of the bony trabeculae of the mastoid, the patient may have a subacute or coalescent mastoiditis and will require further surgery.

Facial nerve paralysis can sometimes be seen with acute otitis media and usually occurs because of a defect in the bony covering, the fallopian canal or of the middle ear portion of the facial nerve. This defect occurs in more than 10 per cent of the population, but fortunately, the occurrence of facial nerve paralysis with acute otitis media is rare. Acute otitis media is treated in the usual manner, but a myringotomy is performed to relieve the pressure in the middle ear. The facial nerve paralysis should be followed by means of electromyography. Most of these paralyses will resolve in three to four weeks and will not require further surgical treatment. Another complication of acute otitis media is labyrinthitis, which occurs when the infection spreads into the cochlear and the vestibular apparatus. The patient will become profoundly deaf in the infected ear. He also will have marked vertigo, usually accompanied by nystagmus. Labyrinthitis is also treated with antibiotics and a myringotomy. There is usually no recovery of the hearing and a slow adaptation to the loss of the vestibular function.

There are significant *long-term sequelae* associated with acute otitis media. It has been found that approximately 17 per cent of children who have had acute otitis media will have significant hearing loss in one to ten years after the infection. It is advisable that all children with acute otitis media have a hearing test several months after the infection. If the hearing loss persists, appropriate treatment must be instituted. This usually consists of a myringotomy and the placement of a middle ear ventilating tube, as discussed in the paragraphs dealing with serous otitis media later in this chapter.

Mastoid Disease

Mastoid disease is an infection of the bony portion of the middle ear and is a complication of an acute otitis media. The pathophysiology has already been discussed. There is one anatomic factor which contributes to mastoid disease. As previously mentioned, the mastoid cell system is connected to the middle ear by a narrow passage called the aditus ad antrum. If this passage is occluded by mucosal edema, a tumor mass or cellular debris, then pus cannot drain into the middle ear from the mastoid cells. The blockage of pus in the mastoid cells will cause osteitis and death of the bone. The pus can then drain into any of the areas which are contiguous with the mastoid cell system. This will result in abscesses in these various areas.

Acute Mastoiditis

Acute mastoiditis is still seen. If a child develops an acute otitis media, then, usually one to two weeks later, he will develop swelling behind the pinna, displacing it inferiorly and anteriorly (Fig. 6). The cause of this swelling is pus which has broken through the mastoid and formed an abscess beneath the temporalis muscle (Fig. 7). These patients will usually have systemic signs of infection. The tympanic membrane may be dull, and its landmarks are usually missing. There is seldom drainage from the middle ear. The pus may drain into the zygomatic cells or tunnel under the skin of the superior portion of the external auditory canal. Either of these conditions will result in an abscess presenting anterosuperiorly to the pinna. The abscess will be over the posterior root of the zygomatic process. X-rays of the mastoid will show clouding of the cells, but the bony septa may still be present.

TREATMENT. The treatment of acute mastoiditis is systemic antibiotic therapy and surgical drainage of the mastoid, which is done by performing a simple mastoidectomy. This operation consists

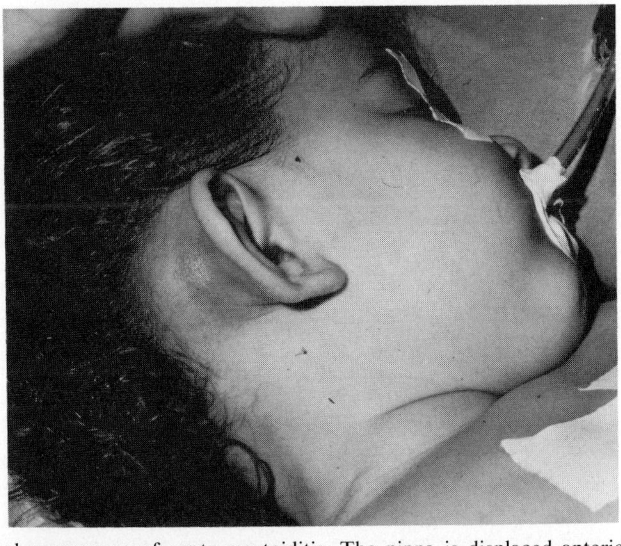

Figure 6. Clinical appearance of acute mastoiditis. The pinna is displaced anteriorly and inferiorly. There is a fluctuant mass behind the pinna.

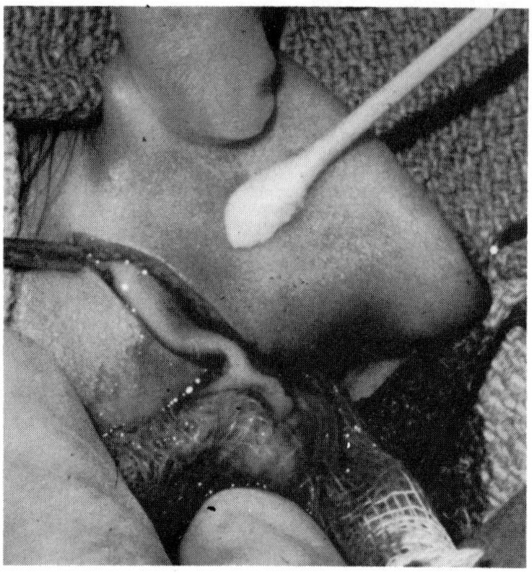

Figure 7. Postauricular incision in patient illustrated in Figure 6. Free pus is seen coming from the postauricular abscess, in this case because of acute mastoiditis.

of a postauricular incision which is followed by removal of all of the mastoid cells lateral to the labyrinth. If the perilabyrinthine cells are infected, they, too, must be removed. The posterior canal wall and the middle ear are left intact. It is important to make sure that the aditus ad antrum is patent. This is done by performing a large posteroinferior myringotomy. A saline solution is put in the external auditory canal and must be able to flow into the mastoid cavity through the aditus. Usually the mastoid cavity is allowed to close by granulation and is not primarily closed.

Subacute Mastoiditis

Subacute or coalescent mastoiditis is another form of mastoid disease which is encountered in children. The diagnosis of this condition is difficult. Cases will usually present with long-standing, low-grade fever or temperature spikes. The patient will have had a history of acute otitis media some weeks before. The tympanic membrane will be dull, and the landmarks are obscured. The patient may also present with signs of meningitis. He will have a stiff neck, and a lumbar puncture will reveal an increase in protein with several lymphocytic and polymorphic nucleated cells. The cerebrospinal fluid may be sterile. X-rays of the mastoid will show a diffuse clouding, and the delicate bony trabeculae of the mastoid cells will not be seen. Treatment of these patients is the same as that for those with acute mastoiditis. The surgical findings usually are a mastoid cavity in which the bone is soft with pus and granulation tissue in the remaining mastoid cells. As the cells are removed, the area of the tegmen—i.e., the floor of the middle cranial fossa—will be covered with granulation tissue and pus. This will extend to the dura of the middle cranial fossa and is the probable cause of the meningitis. This process has been noted to extend to the mastoid cells bordering the sigmoid sinus. Epidural and subdural abscesses and sigmoid sinus thrombosis must be ruled out in these cases.

Chronic Mastoiditis

The most common symptom of *chronic mastoiditis* is long-standing ear drainage, and the most common pathogen involved is pseudomonas. X-rays will usually reveal a small sclerotic mastoid in the affected ear (Fig. 8). There are seldom any systemic signs of infection, such as fever or malaise. A hearing test will usually reveal a large air conduction type of hearing loss. Physical examination will show an ear canal which has filled with pus and cellular debris. After

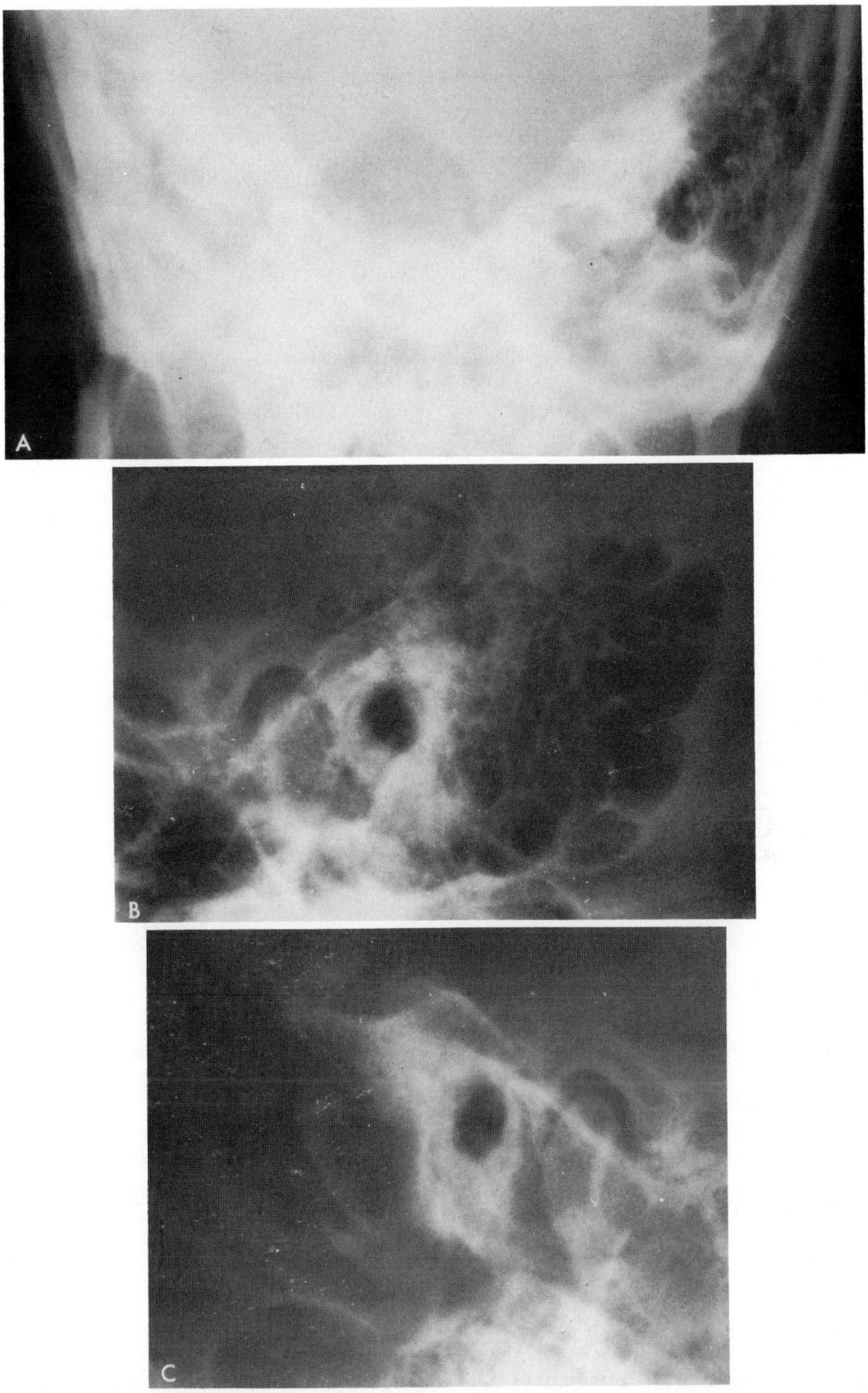

Figure 8. *A*, X-ray showing the cloudy sclerotic mastoid on the left and normal mastoid on the right. *B*, Lateral view of normal mastoid showing the large number of well-aerated mastoid cells. *C*, Lateral view of chronic mastoiditis showing lack of mastoid air cells.

this is cleaned, the tympanic membrane will be visible and will have a perforation. It may be a small superoposterior perforation, indicating a possible cholesteatoma, or there may be a large, subtotal perforation in which most of the drum is missing. Chronic mastoiditis can result in the destruction of a portion of the ossicular chain.

Chronic mastoiditis can be thought of as osteitis of the temporal bone. This chronic infection can spread to the structures contiguous to the mastoid. Either the bone can erode posteriorly and laterally or a postauricular abscess similar to that of acute mastoiditis will be found. Likewise, a zygomatic abscess can be formed. The infection may erode the external tip of the temporal bone, and an abscess will be formed in the mastoid head of the sternomastoid muscle. This is called *Bezold's abscess* and can be mistaken for a deep neck abscess. Infection may be present in the structure of the mastoid cells at the petrous tip of the temporal bone. This would cause inflammation of the fifth, sixth and seventh cranial nerves. The syndrome consisting of facial pain and paralysis of the internal rectus muscle of the eye, with or without facial paralysis and deafness, is called *Gradenigo's syndrome*. This infection of the tip of the mastoid can also lead to thrombosis of the cavernous sinus, which may present as exophthalmos on the affected side.

The mastoid infection can erode the tegmen and result in an epidural, subdural or temporal lobe abscess. It may also erode posteriorly and cause a sigmoid sinus thrombosis or a cerebellar abscess. Anteriorly, it can enter the fallopian canal and cause facial paralysis. Chronic mastoiditis can also cause labyrinthitis and subsequent deafness.

PREDISPOSING FACTORS. The predisposing factors to chronic mastoid disease are the same as those for acute otitis media. Added to this is the occurrence of any tumor of the middle ear which may result in blocking of the eustachian tube or the aditus ad antrum.

TREATMENT. Treatment of chronic mastoid disease is by surgery. All of the infected portions of the mastoid must be removed. This is done by means of various operative procedures. The objective in children is to create a safe, uninfected ear. There has recently been great emphasis on trying to restore hearing function in chronically infected ears through operations called tympanoplasties, but the role of tympanoplasty in children is limited.

If the mastoid disease is due to cholesteatoma, the primary aim of the surgeon must be to remove the disease. This will usually include removal of the posterior canal wall, the malleus and the incus. The cavity should remain open so that it can be epithelialized. If there is no cholesteatoma, or if the cholesteatoma is very small, tympanoplasty may then be considered. Results of tympanoplasty are only fair; most cases will result in a closure of the tympanic membrane perforation. However, in less than half of the cases in children will there be significant restoration of the hearing function. Usually tympanoplasty is performed as a second procedure after the ear has been free of infection for at least a year. If only one ear is affected and the other ear has normal hearing, there is little urgency to attempt to restore hearing in the affected ear. It is, however, possible to close most perforations after the ear is dry. This will protect the ear from infection and will allow the child to go swimming.

It is most important to remember the very serious sequelae which can develop from mastoid infection in children. An inadequate operation for infection to improve hearing should not be performed. In unilateral disease, the restoration of hearing is of little practical significance. If the disease is bilateral, a hearing aid can be used with excellent results.

TUMORS

Tumors of the middle ear in children represent an important aspect of pediatric otolaryngology in that they all represent a probable permanent hearing loss and a potential threat to life. The most common tumor of the middle ear is the cholesteatoma. These are epithelial growths. They are benign but cause disease by their anatomic position. As they grow they secrete collagenase, which causes bony erosion.

CONGENITAL CHOLESTEATOMA

Clinically, cholesteatomas can be classified into three groups. The first of these is the *congenital cholesteatoma*, which is thought to be a congenital rest of epithelial tissue. These usually occur deep within the temporal bone and may only secondarily enter the middle ear cleft. They are rare and many times present primarily as intracranial tumors. They should be removed surgically. Many times a combined mastoid and intracranial procedure will be needed to completely remove them.

PRIMARY ACQUIRED CHOLESTEATOMA

There are two types of acquired cholesteatoma. Both are quite common in children. The first is primary acquired cholesteatoma, which is believed to form as a result of metaplasia or the retraction of the pars flaccida into the middle ear. A piece of epithelium is detached from the tympanic membrane and grows in the middle ear (Fig. 9). The cholesteatoma becomes large and causes destruction of the ossicles. The tympanic membrane will usually be intact, and a white mass can be seen through a relatively translucent tympanic membrane. Hearing loss may or may not be present, depending on the involvement of the ossicles.

The primary acquired cholesteatoma occurs in children with retracted ear drums and negative middle ear pressure. After the small primary cholesteatoma is removed, provision must be made for the proper aeration of the middle ear cleft. This is usually done by inserting a middle ear ventilating tube, with or without an adenoidectomy.

SECONDARY ACQUIRED CHOLESTEATOMA

The most common type of cholesteatoma is the secondary acquired cholesteatoma. This is always associated with a perforated tympanic membrane. The perforation is commonly a small, innocent-appearing superoposterior perforation in the pars flaccida. The squamous epithelium may come from the drum, or

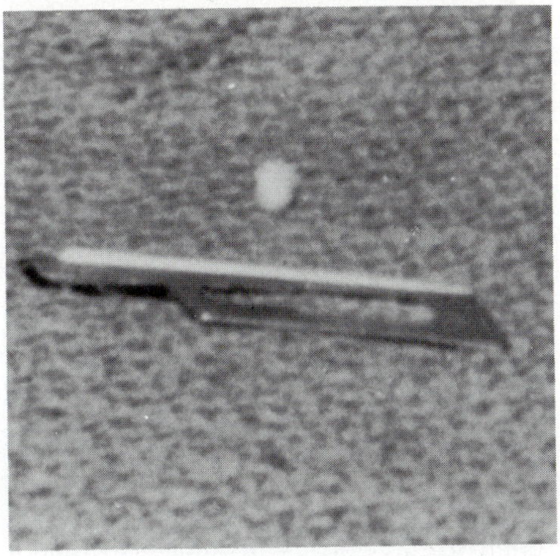

Figure 9. A small primary acquired cholesteatoma removed from behind the ear drum in a 2-year-old.

the epithelium of the middle ear may undergo metaplasia and become squamous. These cholesteatomas usually grow into the attic of the middle ear and involve the incus and malleus. They then grow into the aditus and eventually involve the mastoid. Sometimes the cholesteatoma will be contained in a small sac. This type of small cholesteatoma may only involve part of the ossicular chain and can be dissected free; then a more conservative operative procedure, such as a modified radical mastoidectomy, can be performed.

Most secondary acquired cholesteatomas will invade the cells of the mastoid. This type of cholesteatoma must be completely removed. There is a strong tendency for cholesteatomas to recur, and the ear should be so prepared that any recurrence can be easily observed. Most cholesteatomas in children should be removed by means of a radical mastoidectomy.

Tympanoplasty should not be attempted for moderate and large-sized secondary acquired cholesteatomas in children because of the possibility of recurrence. The ear should be observed for approximately one year. If the ear is dry and there are no signs of recurrence when the ear is examined under the operating microscope, a secondary procedure in some instances could be considered.

Polyps are commonly associated with secondary acquired cholesteatomas of the middle ear and are produced by the mucosa of the middle ear in response to chronic infection. Polyps usually present as red, friable masses in the external auditory canal. They should be removed under general anesthesia with provision being made for possible mastoid surgery, since a cholesteatoma will almost always be found behind the polyp.

BENIGN BONY TUMORS

There are several benign bony tumors which can be found in the temporal bone in children; they include monostotic and polyostotic fibrous dysplasias and fibrous osteomas. Such tumors can present as hard masses in the external auditory canal. They will invade the middle ear and destroy the eustachian tube orifice or block the aditus ad antrum. These tumors must be removed in such a fashion that their possible recurrence will not cause isolation of the middle ear cleft.

Eosinophilic granulomas of the middle ear are also seen in children and will present as a chronic mastoid disease with ear pain, ear discharge and a loss of hearing. The x-ray findings are quite typical of those showing an area of radiolucency. If there is a solitary lesion, it should be surgically removed. If there are multiple lesions, they are treated with low dosage x-ray. Rhabdomyosarcoma and reticular cell sarcoma also occur in the middle ear. Leukemia may present as a middle ear problem with hearing loss and aural discharge.

SEROUS OTITIS MEDIA

The middle ear cleft is affected by the noninfectious process called *serous otitis media*. The name serous otitis media is somewhat misleading, since the fluid within may vary greatly in its viscosity. This fluid can be either a very thin, waterlike transudate or a very thick, gelatinous material. When the thick fluid is formed it is called *glue ear*, since it is gluelike in consistency. The most common sign of serous otitis media is a marked conductive hearing loss. Behavioral problems or learning difficulties often signal such a hearing loss in children. The etiology of the disease is probably abnormal eustachian tube function. Patients with cleft palates are particularly prone to this disease.

Physical Examination

Physical examination will reveal an abnormal tympanic membrane which may be bulging or retracted. The drum will be thick, and the usual landmarks will not be seen. Occasionally, air-fluid levels can be seen behind the drum. The incidence of this disease is quite high. Studies have shown that about 25 per cent of young children in urban ghetto areas have moderate hearing loss secondary to serous otitis media.

The hearing loss may result in retardation of language and verbal ability. For disadvantaged children who attend poor schools and who are often bilingual a hearing loss must reduce the possibility of normal development of verbal language and learning skills.

Pathology

The pathophysiology underlying serous otitis media is thought to be abnormal function of the eustachian tube. Air becomes trapped in the ear, the oxygen is absorbed and the pressure in the middle ear is decreased; the ear is then filled with a transudate from the mucosal lining of the middle ear. Studies show mainly a negative middle ear pressure. The fluid in serous otitis media is sterile but can become a good culture medium. These ears usually have retracted ear drums. This culture medium, together with the retracted ear drum, can lead to acute infection and possibly the formation of cholesteatoma.

Treatment

Treatment of chronic serous otitis media is directed toward equalizing the air pressure. When the condition is first noticed, an attempt is made to open the eustachian tube by using systemic or local decongestants. If this does not succeed and the condition remains for four to six weeks, surgical therapy must be used.

The surgical therapy consists of performing a myringotomy in the postero-inferior quadrant of the tympanic membrane. The fluid or gel is removed with suction, and a ventilating tube is put in place (Fig. 10) to equalize the pressure. Most of the plastic tubes used will remain in place for three months. The patient may require reinsertion of the tube on several occasions. These patients must be followed periodically to make sure that the tube is still in place and does not fall into the middle ear. Infections following operations occur in about 10 per cent of the patients and can usually be treated as an ordinary otitis media or an otitis externa. Systemic topical antibiotics should be used. The tube should be left in place to promote ventilation and possible drainage from the middle ear.

Adenoidectomy for the treatment of serous otitis media must be carefully considered. Many children with serous otitis media already have some predisposing nasopharyngeal factor, such as cleft palate or submucosal cleft palate. The velopharyngeal sphincter must be assessed before an adenoidectomy is done. If there is any possibility of creating velopharyngeal insufficiency, then the adenoidectomy should not be performed. Cleft palate children can be handled very satisfactorily by means of a ventilating tube without an adenoidectomy.

There are several other groups of patients in whom serous otitis media plays a significant role. Children with mucopolysaccharidosis or children who are mongoloid will have increased secretions, and the middle ear will be filled with fluid. These children also are mentally retarded. There can be little question that a child with mental retardation should have access to his maximum environmental input so that he may optimalize his already limited intellectual capacity. It is imperative, therefore, that these children have optimal hearing. They are best treated with the more permanent types of middle ear ventilating tubes. Another group of children significantly affected are those with neurosensory hearing losses. These losses can be aggravated by serous otitis media. A moderate loss can be turned into a severe loss, and a severe loss may become a profound loss. All children with neurosensory hearing loss must have their ears examined and a hearing test several

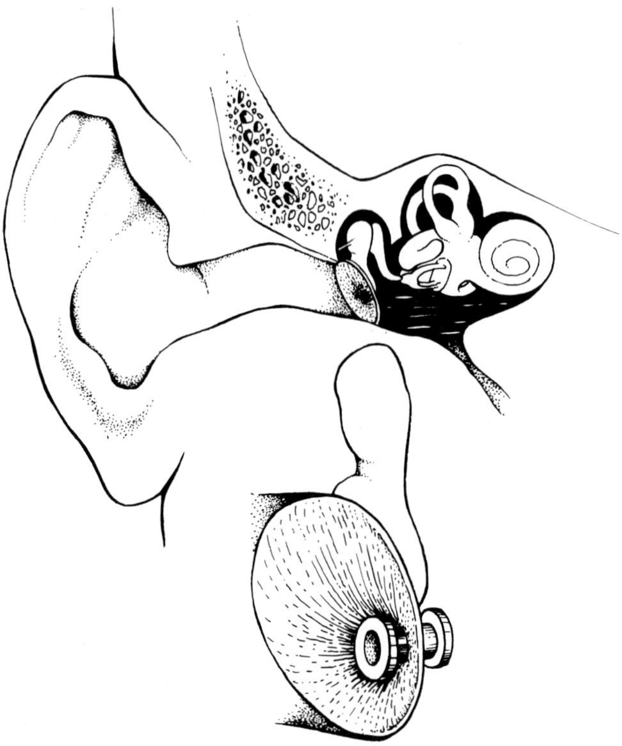

Figure 10. *Above,* Diagram illustrating fluid behind the tympanic membrane. *Below,* A ventilating tube is placed through the tympanic membrane to treat this condition.

times a year. If a serous otitis media is found, it is treated with a ventilating tube. A hearing aid can be worn while the tube is in place.

GENETIC BONE DISEASE

Genetic bony diseases can affect the middle ear in childhood. *Otosclerosis,* an autosomal dominant disease, will occasionally manifest itself in children who are 10 to 15 years old. These children will present with progressive, conductive hearing loss and a normal tympanic membrane. There will usually be a family history of deafness. If the hearing loss is severe enough, operative correction can be considered. However, if the child still has episodes of otitis media, a hearing aid should be used until the child has grown to an age at which his ear infections and upper respiratory infections are less frequent.

Most operations for otosclerosis involve stapes surgery and opening of the labyrinth. The oval window is usually healed over by a thin layer of fibrous tissue. This fibrous tissue is not considered to be the best protection against infection for the inner ear. An infection of the inner ear would result in total deafness and even meningitis. It is felt that for several years a hearing aid will do quite adequately, and when the chances for serious complication are lessened, an operation could be considered.

Children with *osteogenesis imperfecta,* an autosomal dominant disease, can also have hearing loss. A hearing aid is preferable in the treatment of these children because the disease will progress. Both the middle and inner parts of the ear are affected.

Osteoporosis, an autosomal dominant

disease, can also cause considerable hearing loss and may be associated with blindness and central nervous system difficulties. These children can have a very limited life expectancy. The lesion not only involves abnormalities of the middle ear but also abnormalities of the bone in the middle ear. It is most advisable to use a hearing aid for the habilitative therapy of these children.

REFERENCES

The references for Chapter 69 appear at the end of Chapter 72.

Chapter Seventy

THE INNER EAR

ROBERT J. RUBEN, M.D.

The physical function of the inner ear, the cochlea, is to transduce sound into biological signals. The cells which do this are called the hair cells. A loss of hair cells results in a hearing loss. If the cells are missing from the apex of the cochlea, there is a low tone loss; if the cells are missing from the basal end of the cochlea, there is a high tone loss. If there is only a moderate loss of hair cells, there is most probably only a decrease in the sensitivity of the cochlea. However, as more hair cells are lost, there is a decrease in the ability to discriminate sounds as well as a loss of sensitivity.

The hair cells are end-state cells and are formed during the first three months of gestation. Once the hair cell dies, it is not replaced. A hair cell in the cochlea must last a lifetime. If the hair cell dies prematurely, then that person is left with impaired hearing.

CONGENITAL MALFORMATIONS

Congenital malformations of the inner ear are rare, and they usually result in severe to profound hearing losses. They involve malformations of the bony labyrinth. Embryological observations indicate that in order for the bony labyrinth to develop normally, there must be a normal neural tube. Clinically, the bony malformations of the inner ear are frequently associated with central nervous system malformations (Fig. 1). Bony malformations of the labyrinth are usually associated with hair cell loss. A bony malformation of the cochlea can be clinically diagnosed by the use of x-ray. Stenver's and Towne's views of the young infant will usually reveal enough of the bony labyrinth to determine whether or not it is normal (Fig. 2). Polytomography should be used for precise definition of any abnormality. It is important to establish the presence of a normal bony labyrinth in a child who has a neurosensory deafness, as there is a good possibility, if the bony labyrinth is abnormal, that the child may have a central nervous system malformation as well.

GENETIC DISORDERS

There are numerous *genetic disorders* which affect the inner ear in children. The genetic diseases are dominant, re-

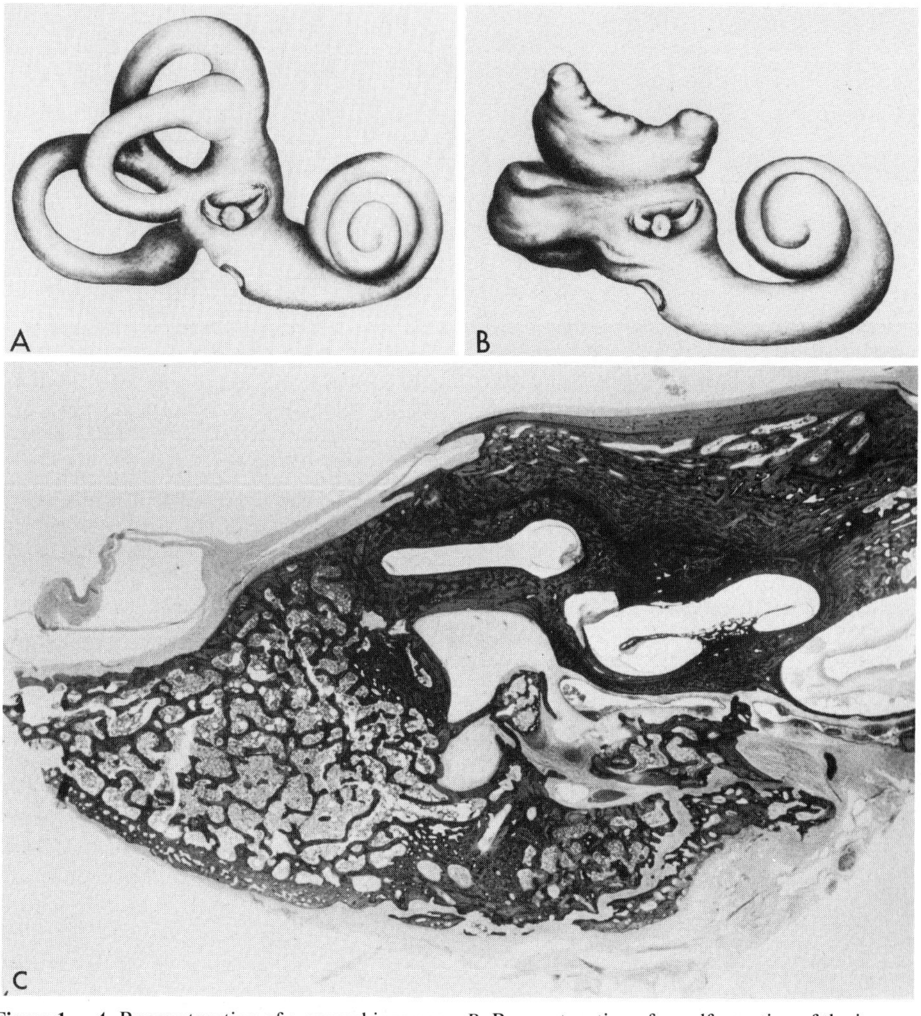

Figure 1. *A*, Reconstruction of a normal inner ear. *B*, Reconstruction of a malformation of the inner ear. *C*, Horizontal histological section through the inner ear represented in *B*.

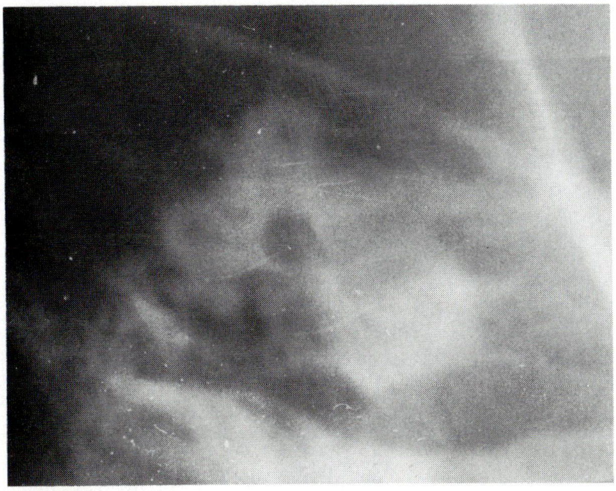

Figure 2. X-ray showing normal bony labyrinth. The superior and horizontal semicircular canals, the cochlea and internal auditory meatus can be seen in this x-ray.

cessive and sex-linked. The deafness syndromes which are transmitted by means of a dominant mode of inheritance can be quite variable. Each syndrome of dominantly inherited diseases will be presented in the following paragraphs as a complete syndrome. Many patients may be affected with only one or two of the multiple stigmata associated with each of these syndromes.

The Waardenburg Syndrome

The *Waardenburg syndrome* (Fig. 3) is autosomal dominant and is one of the most common inherited diseases of the

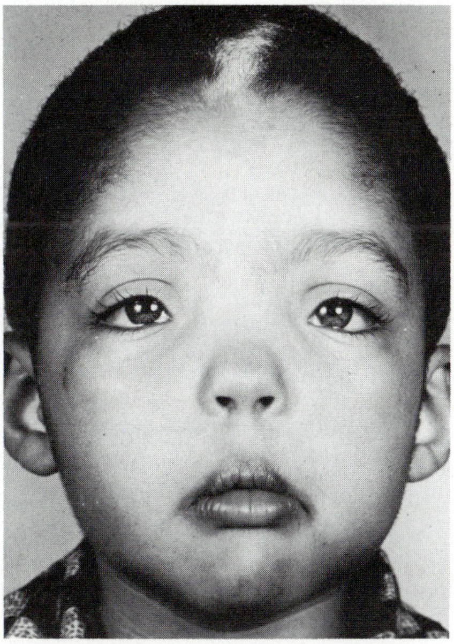

Figure 3. A boy with Waardenburg's syndrome. The white forelock, antimongoloid slant of the ears and increased distance of the bridge of the nose are seen. The patient has a bilateral, severe sensory neural hearing loss. He does not have heterochromia of the irides.

ear. The syndrome consists of either unilateral or bilateral neurosensory deafness, a white forelock, broad nasal root, confluent eyebrows, heterochromia of the iris and displaced medial canthi of the eye. In addition to the deafness the patient may also have hypoactive vestibular labyrinths. One pair of temporal bones studied in a patient with Waardenburg's syndrome showed a lack of hair cells.

Albinism With Deafness

Albinism with deafness is transmitted by an autosomal dominant gene. This syndrome consists of albinism of the entire body except the iris and the optic fundi.

The Leopard Syndrome

The *Leopard syndrome* is another autosomal dominant type of deafness. It acquires its name from the multiple lentigines (freckles) which are associated with this syndrome. The patients have a spotted appearance. The syndrome consists of a variable amount of neurosensory deafness; multiple lentigines (freckles) covering the entire body; cardiac defects, which can include an abnormal QRS complex; bundle branch block; pulmonary stenosis; hypogonadism; ocular hypotelorism; and retardation of growth.

Alport's Disease

Alport's disease may be an autosomal dominant with variable penetrance. It appears to affect males more often than females. This is a progressive neurosensory deafness with onset after the age of 10. The disease is associated with a severe and progressive glomerulitis. The patients will have hematuria and proteinuria. Urinalysis and measure of the blood creatinine should be performed in all cases of neurosensory deafness so that glomerulitis and other forms of renal disease can be diagnosed and treated.

Profound congenital deafnesses, unilateral deafnesses and progressive deafnesses, which are inherited in a manner consistent with autosomal dominant transmission, also have been observed. These diseases have not yet been associated with any other system abnormality. Likewise, severe and progressive deafnesses have been observed which are inherited in a manner consistent with autosomal recessive transmission.

Pendred's Syndrome

Pendred's syndrome is an autosomal recessive deafness associated with a thyroid defect. The patients will be deaf and euthyroid. A goiter will develop usually after the age of 4 or 5 because of the inability of the thyroid to absorb inorganic iodine. The perchlorate test will be positive in patients with this syndrome.

The Jervell and Lange-Nielsen Syndrome

The *Jervell and Lange-Nielsen syndrome* consists of severe neurosensory deafness and cardiac malfunction. The syndrome is inherited as an autosomal recessive. The cardiac syndrome includes periods of syncope and then sudden death. The disease is characterized by a prolonged Q-T interval on the electrocardiogram. The sudden death is suspected to be secondary to cardiac arrhythmia.

Usher's Syndrome

Usher's syndrome consists of retinitis pigmentosa and congenital deafness and is inherited as an autosomal recessive. The child is born with a severe to profound hearing loss. The child appears well otherwise until the onset of the second or third decade. At this time the visual field begins to constrict, and the visual acuity is decreased. The disease progresses more rapidly in some patients than in others. The progressive loss of vision in patients with Usher's syndrome must be kept in mind when doing follow-up studies in deaf children. The visual acuity and a funduscopic examination should be evaluated at least once a year in any child with deafness of unknown etiology or in whom genetic disease is suspected.

There are also sex-linked forms of inherited hearing loss. Some of these are associated with other systemic defects, such as albinism. Others are not associated with any other systemic disease. These inherited disorders of the inner ear are only the more clinically significant ones of a larger number of syndromes. It is felt that a great number of patients with idiopathic disease may actually have autosomal recessive disease.

Chromosomal Abnormalities

Chromosomal abnormalities will cause malformation and loss of hair cells in the inner ear. This has been reported in Trisomy 18 and Trisomy 13–15.

ACQUIRED DISEASE

VIRAL INFECTION

Viral infection is one of the most significant causes of acquired diseases of the inner ear. *Congenital rubella infection* causes significant hearing loss in more than 25 per cent of exposed fetuses. The pathology involved in hearing loss secondary to rubella infection can involve the entire hearing chain. It can affect the middle ear and the central nervous system as well as the inner ear. The inner ear pathology consists of a loss of hair cells and other variable findings.

Two pairs of temporal bones from infants with *cytomegalovirus* have both shown changes which would be compatible with severe to profound neurosensory deafness. However, a direct clinical correlation in a deaf patient with a history of cytomegalovirus infection and abnormal temporal bone has not been made. It is strongly suspected that cytomegalovirus may be another cause of congenital deafness.

Mumps virus is a well-known cause of neurosensory deafness in childhood. The mumps infection usually results in a unilateral profound neurosensory deafness, but it can also result in a profound bilateral neurosensory deafness.

BACTERIAL INFECTION

Bacterial infections of the inner ear, labyrinthitis, are relatively uncommon. They can be secondary to acute otitis media, chronic mastoiditis or meningitis. In patients with deafness following meningitis, the infection is thought to enter the inner ear through one of four pathways: the endolymphatic duct, the perilymphatic duct, the internal auditory meatus or the vascular system.

Bacterial labyrinthitis can also follow a fracture of the temporal bone which involves the cochlea (Fig. 4). The infection destroys the entire inner ear, resulting in a profound deafness. The inner ear is then replaced by granulation tissue and new bone formation.

FRACTURES

Fractures of the temporal bone which involve the inner ear can result in profound deafness without labyrinthitis. Fractures which run from posterior to anterior are called transverse fractures and may not involve the middle ear. Longitudinal fractures, running from lateral to medial, almost invariably involve the middle ear. When a fracture involves the middle ear, blood will be seen either in the external auditory canal or behind the drum. There also may be a cerebrospinal fluid leak. The blood or the cerebrospinal fluid can drain through the eustachian tube and can be seen on the posterior pharyngeal wall.

Temporal bone fractures are treated conservatively unless there is facial nerve paralysis. If there is no infection, antibiotics are not given. Because of the possibility of meningitis, the patient

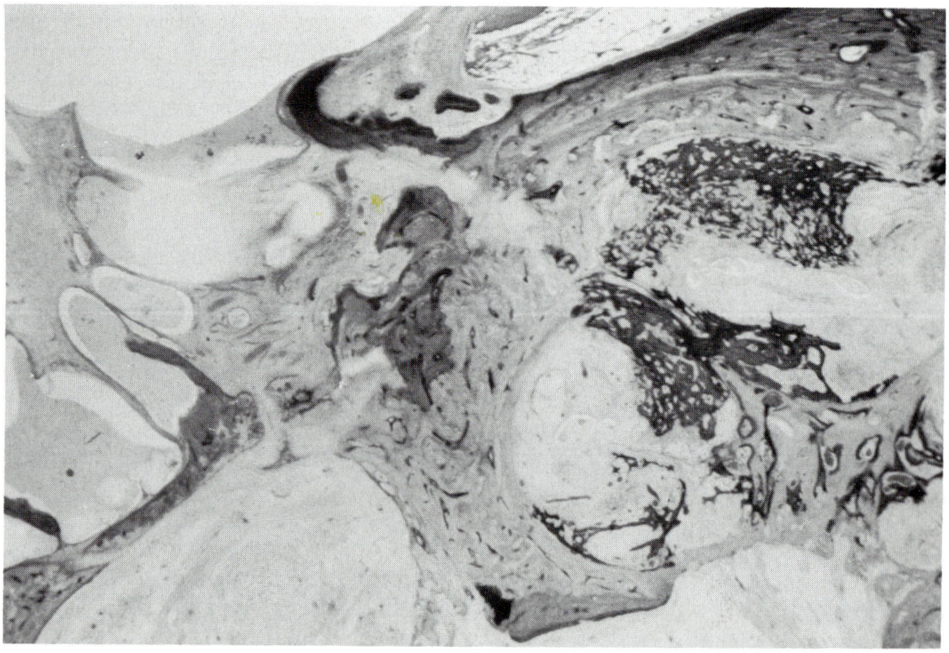

Figure 4. Histological section showing a fracture through the temporal bone with subsequent labyrinthitis. The inner ear has been replaced by granulation tissue and new bone formation.

should be carefully observed for about three weeks. The patient should also be studied for possible intracranial injury. After the blood has been absorbed from the middle ear, the patient should be assessed for both conductive and neurosensory hearing loss. Fractures of the labyrinth heal only by a fibrous union. This fibrous union does not afford good protection against bacterial infection of the middle ear to the central nervous system. The child with a temporal bone fracture must be carefully followed, and all episodes of acute otitis media must be thoroughly treated.

DRUGS

Ototoxic drugs, such as kanamycin, streptomycin, dihydrostreptomycin, bacitracin, neomycin, gentamicin, quinine and etherinic acid, can cause death of the hair cells and subsequent deafness. Quinine and streptomycin have been thought to cross the placental barrier and cause a congenital hearing loss. Whenever an ototoxic drug is used, the hearing of the child must be periodically tested while on the drug. If there are signs of hearing loss, the drug should be stopped. Some drugs, such as neomycin, are also nephrotoxic. If there are signs of reduced renal function, the possibility of hearing loss from the drug is greatly increased.

BLOCKING OF THE LABYRINTHINE ARTERY

Another form of deafness which can occur in children is secondary to emboli blocking off the labyrinthine artery. The blood supply of the inner ear is dependent on this artery, which is part of the vertebral system. Emboli are noted in children who have been on cardiac bypass for correction of a cardiac defect. Occasionally an embolus will lodge in the labyrinthine artery, causing a unilateral deafness.

LOUD SOUND

Extremely loud sound can also cause a hearing loss. This occurs when a gun or a firecracker explodes next to a child's ear. Hearing loss has also been reported in teen-agers who are exposed to loud music. Fortunately, before there is a permanent hearing loss there may be a temporary hearing loss. The patient will have symptoms consisting of reduced hearing and tinnitus immediately following the noise exposure and lasting from minutes to hours. The patient should be advised to avoid loud sounds or, if this is not possible, to use some type of ear protection to reduce the amount of sound reaching his ear.

DISEASE OF VESTIBULAR APPARATUS

The *vestibular apparatus* is also contained in the inner ear and consists of the three semicircular canals, the saccule and the utricle. Their function is to maintain orientation in space. Disease of the vestibular apparatus will cause the child to have difficulty orienting in space while his eyes are closed. The major symptom of vestibular abnormality is the sensation that either he or his environment is moving. This is called vertigo and may be associated with spontaneous or induced nystagmus.

It is sometimes difficult to differentiate between vertigo caused by disease of the vestibular apparatus and its nerve and that which originates in the central nervous system. Clinically, a vertiginous attack lasting from several minutes to hours is usually an indication of disease of the vestibular apparatus. Vestibular testing will usually reveal a hypoactive labyrinth. Lesions of the vestibular nerve will cause momentary episodes of unsteadiness but seldom cause true vertigo. True vertigo is seldom experienced in central nervous system disease. Vestibular testing usually will not show labyrinthine hypofunction but will be characterized by directional preponderance. Also, the induced nystagmus in central nervous system disease can be paradoxical, whereas in peripheral disease of either the nerve or the labyrinth itself the nystagmus is in the expected direction.

Ménière's Disease

Diseases which affect the vestibular apparatus are similar to those which affect the cochlea. *Ménière's disease* is a disease of unknown etiology occasionally found in children. The syndrome consists of periodic episodes of long-lasting vertigo associated with a peripheral neurosensory hearing loss. The hearing loss is characterized predominantly by a low-frequency loss, good speech discrimination, recruitment and a lack of tone decay. There is no effective treatment for Ménière's disease. Various operative procedures have been proposed, most of which destroy the affected ear. These should not be used in children, since the disease has a propensity for occurring in the other ear.

Vestibular Dysfunction

Congenital absence of vestibular function, associated with and without deafness, has been observed. It is felt that a lack of vestibular function may result in motor retardation.* Therefore, children with motor retardation should be tested for vestibular function. If such function is absent, a prognosis of more general retardation should be postponed.

REFERENCES

The references for Chapter 70 appear at the end of Chapter 72.

*Rapin, I.: Personal communication.

Chapter Seventy-One

THE EIGHTH CRANIAL NERVE

ROBERT J. RUBEN, M.D.

The eighth cranial nerve consists of four parts. Three of these are afferent and include the cochlear nerve, the superior vestibular nerve and the inferior vestibular nerve. The fourth segment is the efferent nerve running to the cochlea. The function of the afferent portion of the eighth cranial nerve is to connect the cochlear and vestibular apparatus to the central nervous system.

Patients with severe malformations of the inner ear will also have agenesis or aplasia of the eighth cranial nerve. Many of the diseases which cause destruction of the hair cells in the cochlea also result in destruction of the cochlear division of this nerve.

TUMORS

Tumors of the eighth cranial nerve are found in children. They are usually neurofibromatous and may occur either sporadically or as part of a genetic disease. They are frequently found in Recklinghausen's neurofibromatosis. There is also a well-described autosomal, dominantly transmitted, genetic disease con-

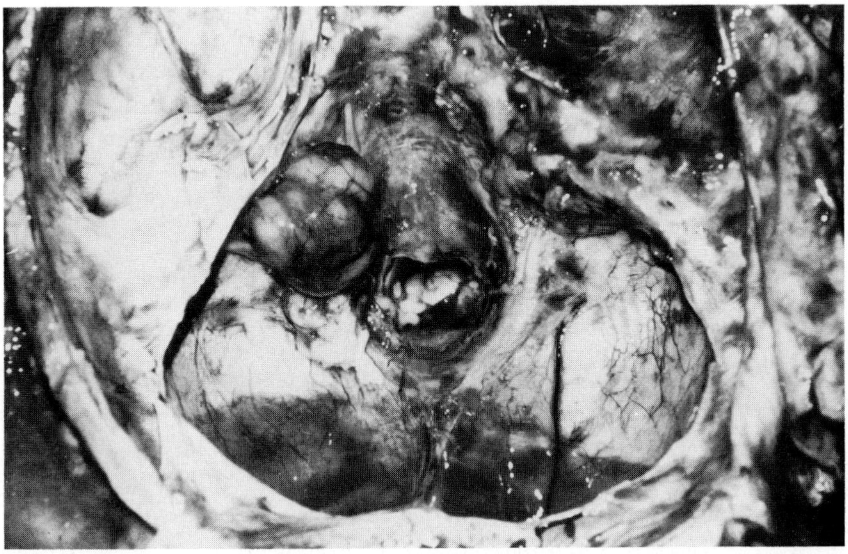

Figure 1. A large acoustic neuroma extruding from the left internal auditory meatus in a 14-year-old child. A similar tube was removed several years earlier from the right side. The child also had a tumor in the frontal lobe and another tumor in the brain stem.

sisting of bilateral acoustic neuromas. These tumors can grow to such a size as to cause increased intracranial pressure and eventual death (Fig. 1).

Symptoms

The presenting symptom of an eighth cranial nerve tumor is usually a progressive unilateral hearing loss. When a child is seen at age 5 or 6 with a total unilateral hearing loss, it is very difficult to determine whether or not it is progressive. All children with unilateral hearing loss should have an audiogram; a set of mastoid films, which include views of the internal auditory meatus; and a vestibular test.

Diagnostic Findings

The audiological findings in eighth cranial nerve tumors are a sensorineural hearing loss with tone decay and usually poor speech discrimination. Hypofunction of the vestibular apparatus on the ipsilateral side is also characteristic of this type of tumor. X-rays of the internal auditory meatus should be symmetrical. If there is more than a 2- or 3-mm. difference in the inferosuperior dimension of the internal auditory meatus, there is a high probability that a tumor is present. If the clinical picture indicates the possible presence of a tumor, further studies involving a lumbar puncture and contrast radiography should be performed. Before any procedure is performed, the fundi are examined to determine if there is any papilledema. Early diagnosis of acoustic tumors in a child is important. The removal of small tumors involves considerably less morbidity and mortality than the removal of the larger tumors.

REFERENCES

The references for Chapter 71 appear at the end of Chapter 72.

Chapter Seventy-Two

CLINICAL MANAGEMENT OF HEARING LOSS

ROBERT J. RUBEN, M.D.

INCIDENCE

The incidence of severe to profound hearing loss is approximately 1 per 1000 live births. The incidence of moderate hearing loss in the pediatric population is much higher. Findings are varied, depending on the criteria used. The incidence range is from 15 to 250 per 1000, depending on the age and, to some extent, the socioeconomic group.

The problem of hearing loss in a child is very common, and the results are extremely serious. As noted in the Introduction to Diseases of the Ear, a severe hearing loss results in the child's inability to acquire speech and use language. These defects have a twofold effect on the child. The first is a retardation of the child's ability to learn and to use his intelligence optimally. The second is a profound effect on the child's personality. Many times deaf children are mistakenly thought to be autistic, and many deaf children have severe personality problems which further decrease their ability to reach their full potential. It is felt that early habilitative therapy, consisting of hearing aids and special education, will improve the prognosis for the normal development of the deaf child. Proper habilitative therapy can be instituted in the first few months of life.

DIAGNOSIS

Early diagnosis of hearing loss is the most important aspect of the management of the deaf child. There are two approaches to early diagnosis of deafness in children. The first of these is the use of infant screening programs, and the second is the establishment of a high-risk registry.

INFANT SCREENING PROGRAMS

Infant screening programs are based upon the ability of the infant to react to sound. The normal reactions of an infant to sound are listed in Table 1. Screening testing can be done in the newborn nursery, using calibrated speakers and objectively measuring the startle responses of the infant. An informal type of screening can be performed in the clinic or office. A quiet area should be found. The infant is seated on the mother's lap. One examiner stands behind the infant and presents the appropriate stimuli, using both loud and soft sounds. Loud sounds are characterized by squeak toys, hand clapping and tambourines. Soft sounds can be the tapping of a cup, a whispered voice, a bell or the crumpling of a piece of paper. A second examiner stands in front of the infant and observes the reactions to the stimuli. This type of testing should be done at birth and every six months during the first two to three years of life. There are a number of children with progressive hearing loss, and these can be found only if screening is performed throughout the first years of life. If the child does not pass the screening test, then he must be extensively tested at a properly equipped hearing

TABLE 1. RESPONSE TO SOUND IN INFANTS WITH NORMAL HEARING

Age	Loud Sounds*	Soft Sounds*
0–3 mos.	Eye blink and muscle jerk	Very little reaction to sound
3–8 mos.	Small eye blink and minimal muscle jerk which is inhibited after repetition of sound	Familiar sounds will cause the infant to turn his eyes or head to the sound; unfamiliar sounds will cause the same reaction but response will quickly be extinguished
>8 mos.	Turn and localize the sound	Quickly localize the sound; understand simple commands

*See text for examples of both loud and soft sounds.

TABLE 2. HIGH-RISK REGISTRY

I. Prenatal
- A. Family history of deafness
- B. Consanguinity
- C. Rubella infection or exposure during pregnancy
- D. Rising Rh titer
- E. Other viral infection during pregnancy
- F. History of maternal use of ototoxic drugs
- G. Maternal syphilis

II. Perinatal
- A. Prolonged or precipitous labor
- B. Traumatic delivery
- C. Maternal infection
- D. Meningitis
- E. Use of ototoxic drugs
- F. Kernicterus
- G. Prematurity
- H. Anoxia

III. Neonatal Examination
- A. Head and Neck
  1. Abnormal skull
  2. Short neck
  3. Microcephaly
  4. Macrocephaly
- B. Musculoskeletal
  1. Polydactyly
  2. Fusion of fingers and/or toes
  3. Absence of clavicle
  4. Osteogenesis imperfecta or osteoporosis
- C. Ear, Nose and Throat
  1. Abnormal or absent pinna (unilateral or bilateral)
  2. Fails hearing screening test
  3. Low-set ears
  4. Cleft lip or cleft palate
  5. Choanal atresia
  6. Facial abnormality
- D. Eyes
  1. Chorioretinitis
  2. Blindness
  3. Cataract
  4. Subluxation of lens
  5. Heterochromia iridis
  6. Micro-ophthalmia
  7. Coloboma
  8. Widening of intercanthal distance
  9. Antimongoloid slant
- E. Cardiac
  1. Abnormal EKG
  2. Pulmonary stenosis
  3. Mitral insufficiency
  4. Atrial septum or ventricular septum defect
- F. Pigmentation
  1. Albinism
  2. Piebaldness
  3. Lentigines
  4. White forelock
- G. Renal
  1. Genitourinary malformation
  2. Abnormal renal function
- H. Neurologic
  1. Cranial nerve paresis or paralysis, especially facial
  2. Motor abnormality
  3. Muscle abnormality
  4. Generalized convulsions
- I. Metabolic
  1. Hypothyroidism
  2. Mucopolysaccharidosis
- J. Chromosomal abnormality

center. If the child responds to the stimuli, he still may have a hearing defect, as the screening test can rule out only the more severely and profoundly deaf children. The clinician must evaluate the patient by obtaining a history from the parents. If a parent feels that the child is not responding to sound as he should, the child should be considered as having a probable hearing impairment. This child must have definitive audiological assessment at a hearing center even if he passes the hearing screening test. All children who have not developed speech at 2 years of age should also be considered to have a possible hearing defect and are in need of definitive testing. It must be noted that profoundly deaf children will continue to make a babbling type of noise until about the seventh or eighth month of life. After that age they make fewer and fewer vocalizations. A normal child will increase vocalizations after the seventh to eighth month.

HIGH-RISK REGISTRY

The use of infant auditory screening has proved to be only moderately successful in finding cases of severe and profound deafness. The second approach to finding a large portion of deaf infants is the use of a high-risk registry. This method has been very successful in some countries. The registry is based upon the known causes of deafness in children. Studies have shown that the etiology of congenital deafness is approximately 40 per cent acquired, 20 per cent genetic and 40 per cent unknown. The unknown group probably contains many cases of autosomal recessive deafness which cannot be definitely assigned to the genetic category. These cases either do not have a sufficient pedigree or are not associated with a known syndrome. Using our knowledge of genetic and acquired etiologies, a check list can be established. If any items on the check list are associated with the newborn infant, then the infant should have a definitive audiological evaluation. Table 2 presents an outline for a high-risk registry. The use of both infant auditory screening and a high-risk registry should result in the detection of serious and profound hearing losses, in 90 per cent of cases before the age of two.

ASSESSMENT

After a child is diagnosed as having a hearing loss, there is a need for a complete assessment of the physical, mental and social conditions of the affected child. As has been pointed out, many types of deafness are associated with other significant diseases. The physician must have a complete assessment of the child's physical state. It is also important to ascertain the etiology of the child's deafness. This is needed in

TABLE 3. OUTLINE FOR WORK-UP OF A HEARING IMPAIRED CHILD

I. History
- A. Complete history
- B. Genetic pedigree
- C. If there is a history of neonatal difficulty, hospital records should be reviewed

II. Physical Examination
- A. Ear, nose and throat
- B. Ophthalmological, including funduscopic
- C. Head measurement
- D. Neurologic examination

III. Laboratory Studies
- A. Hearing test—including impedance audiometry
- B. Electronystagmographic vestibular examination
- C. Mastoid x-rays—including, if indicated, tomography
- D. Rubella antibody titer of mother and child
- E. Fluoroscopic studies for Treponema antibody
- F. Blood urea nitrogen and/or serum creatinine
- G. Urinalysis, including albumin and microscopic
- H. Leukocyte count
- I. Hemoglobin
- J. Hematocrit
- K. Differential
- L. Serum protein and albumin globulin ratio
- M. Electrocardiogram
- N. Psychometrics
- O. Speech and language evaluation
- P. Hearing test of relatives in cases of unknown etiology or suspected genetic etiology

order to establish a prognosis and to offer proper genetic counseling. As noted above, there are a number of children in whom the etiology of the deafness is unknown. It is assumed from population studies that many of these children have recessive genetic disease. Clinically, the genetic counseling of the child with deafness of unknown etiology should stress the possibilities that the parents may have another affected child and also that the child can have deaf children if he marries another person who is heterozygous or homozygous for the same gene.

Table 3 outlines the studies and tests which should be done in all cases of significant hearing loss in children. The only types of hearing loss which are excluded from this are those secondary to middle ear infections.

HABILITATION

After the medical work-up has been completed, the child must be started on an habilitative program. This will require the use of a social worker and special educational facilities. State programs usually exist which will accept children for this special education. The ability to carry out a complete work-up and to provide the child with a hearing aid and proper education varies greatly throughout the United States. Ideally, the child should be diagnosed before the first year of life, have a hearing aid provided, and be exposed to infant auditory training. The child should then progress to a nursery school which includes both hearing and deaf children. The child should receive special education while in the nursery school which would prepare him, with the use of his hearing aid, to enter a normal elementary school which has facilities for special instruction. The segregation of deaf children in schools for the deaf is to be avoided. Unfortunately, in the United States there are few such comprehensive programs to serve children with hearing impairment.

The deaf child needs to be closely followed by the otologist. The child should be seen by the otologist at least twice a year, and the child's hearing should be reassessed at each visit. The educational, social and psychological progress of the child should also be evaluated at each visit. Often a further decrease in hearing will develop. Sometimes this is due to a serous otitis media which can be easily corrected. If the hearing loss has further sensorineural degeneration, then the hearing aid may have to be adjusted. Children with idiopathic deafness or with a history of autosomal recessive disease should also have yearly eye tests and urinalyses. The otologist is in the best position to become the *ombudsman* for these children.

Fortunately, the greatest number of children with hearing losses have only moderate hearing losses. These children, however, can have serious sequelae in retardation of language and verbal ability. It would be advisable for all children at age 3 to have audiograms done by routine bone and air conduction, and impedance audiometry also should be done at this time. A check should be made every three years until age 12. This type of testing calls for participation by the otolaryngologist in the area of public health. All nursery and elementary school children should have accurate tests performed every three years. Once the hearing losses are found, there is need to provide the proper medical care for these patients.

REFERENCES FOR CHAPTERS 68 TO 72

Altmann, F.: Malformations of the auricle and external auditory meatus: A critical review. *Arch. Otolaryng.*, 54:115, 1951.

Altmann, F.: Malformations of the eustachian tube, middle ear and its appendages: A critical review. *Arch. Otolaryng.*, 54:241, 1951.

Asbed, R. A., Masland, M. W., Sever, J. L., and Weinberg, M. M.: Early case findings of children with communication problems. Part I: Report of a community screening program. *Volta Rev.*, 72, No. 1, 1970.

Begley, J. W., Jr.: Acute and subacute mastoiditis necessitating mastoidectomy in the antibiotic era: Report of 10 cases. *J. Indiana Med. Ass.*, 48:496, 1955.

Birrell, J. F.: *Ear, Nose and Throat Diseases of Children.* Philadelphia, F. A. Davis Co., 1960.

Black, F. O., Bergstrom, L. V., Downs, M., and Hemenway, W.: *Congenital Deafness: A New Approach to Early Detection of Deafness Through a High Risk Register.* Boulder, Colorado Associated University Press, 1971.

Davison, F. W. (Guest Editor): Symposium on Pediatric Otolaryngology. *Otolaryng. Clin. North Amer.,* Vol. 3, No. 3, 1970.

Eagles, E. L., et al.: Hearing sensitivity and related factors in children. Monograph. Univ. Pittsburgh Graduate School of Public Health. *Laryngoscope,* 1963.

Ewing, A. W. G.: The ascertainment of deafness in infancy and early childhood. *J. Laryng.,* 59:309, 1944.

Ewing, A., and Ewing, F. C.: *Teaching Deaf Children to Talk.* Washington, D.C., The Volta Bureau, 1967.

Frazier, G. R.: Profound childhood deafness. *J. Med. Genet.,* 1:118, 1964.

Gronroos, J. A., Vihma, L., Salmivalli, A., and Berglund, B.: Coexisting viral (respiratory syncytial) and bacterial (pneumococcus) otitis media in children. *Acta Otolaryng.,* 65:505, 1968.

Harrison, K.: Exudative otitis media in children (the glue ear). *Practitioner,* 159:744, 1967.

Hemenway, W. G. (Guest Editor): Congenital Deafness. *Otolaryng. Clin. North Amer.* Vol. 4, No. 2, 1971.

Holm, V. A., and Kunze, L. V. H.: Effect of chronic otitis media on language and speech development. *Pediatrics,* 43:833, 1969.

Howie, V. M., Ploussard, K. A., and Lefter, R. L.: Otitis media: A clinical and bacterial correlation. *Pediatrics,* 45:29, 1970.

Konigsmark, B. W.: Hereditary deafness in man.
(Part 1) *New Engl. J. Med.,* 281:713 (Sept. 25), 1969.
(Part 2) *New Engl. J. Med.,* 281:774 (Oct. 2), 1969.
(Part 3) *New Engl. J. Med.,* 281:827 (Oct. 9), 1969.

Marcus, E. B.: Ototoxic medication in premature children. *Arch. Otolaryng.,* 77:198, 1963.

McConnell, F., and Ward, P. H.: *Deafness in Childhood.* Nashville, Vanderbilt University Press, 1967.

McLellan, M. S., and Struck, A.: Ear studies in the premature infant: A statistical description of otoscopic landmarks. *J. Pediat.,* 67:122, 1965.

Myklebust, H. R.: *Auditory Disorders in Children.* New York, Grune and Stratton, 1954.

Olmstead, R. W.: A study of the pattern of hearing in children following acute otitis media. *Amer. J. Dis. Child.,* 100:772, 1960.

Olmstead, R. W., et al.: Pattern of hearing following acute otitis media. *J. Pediat.,* 65:252, 1964.

Omerod, F. C.: Pathology of congenital deafness. *J. Laryng.,* 74:19, 1960.

Paradise, J. L., Bluestone, C. D., and Felder, H.: The universality of otitis media in 50 infants with cleft palate. *Clin. Pediat.,* 44:35, 1969.

Rapin, I.: Evoked responses in normal, brain damaged and deaf infants. *Neurology,* 117:881, 1967.

Rapin, I., Ruben, R. J., and Lyttle, M.: Diagnosis of hearing loss in infants using auditory evoked responses. *Laryngoscope,* 80:712, 1970.

Robinson, J. C., and Cambon, K. G.: Hearing loss in infants with tuberculosis mothers treated with streptomycin during pregnancy. *New Engl. J. Med.,* 271:949, 1964.

Ruben, R. J.: Development of the inner ear of the mouse. *Acta Otolaryng.,* Supplement 220, 1967.

Ruben, R. J., et al.: External and middle ear malformations associated with mandibulo-facial dysostosis and renal abnormalities: A case report. *Ann. Otol.,* 73:605, 1969.

Ruben, R. J., and Rozycki, D.: Diagnostic screening for the deaf child. *Arch. Otolaryng.,* 91:429, 1970.

Ruben, R. J., and Rozycki, D.: Clinical aspects of genetic deafness. *Ann. Otol.,* 80:255-263, 1971.

Saunders, W., and Paparella, M.: *Atlas of Ear Surgery.* St. Louis, C. V. Mosby Co., 1968.

de Schweinitz, I., Miller, A. C., and Miller, J. B.: Delays in the diagnosis of deafness among preschool children. *Pediatrics,* 24:462, 1959.

Shambaugh, G. E., Jr.: *Surgery of the Ear,* 2nd ed. Philadelphia, W. B. Saunders Company, 1967.

Stevens, S. S., and Davis, H.: *Hearing—Its Psychology and Physiology.* New York, John Wiley & Sons, 1938.

Tilles, J. G., et al.: Acute otitis media. Serologic studies and attempts to isolate viruses and mycoplasmas from aspirated middle ear fluids. *New Engl. J. Med.,* 277:613, 1967.

Wedenberg, E.: Auditory training of deaf and hard of hearing children. *Acta Otolaryng.,* Supplement 94, 1951.

Wever, E. G., and Lawrence, M.: *Physiological Acoustics,* Princeton, N. J., Princeton University Press, 1954.

Whetnall, E., and Fry, D. B.: *The Deaf Child.* Springfield, Ill., Charles C Thomas, Publishers, 1964.

Chapter Seventy-Three

PEDIATRIC AUDIOLOGY

ALLAN C. GOODMAN, Ph.D.

This chapter will discuss the principles and procedures for the study and evaluation of hearing in a pediatric population. Most of the considerations apply to the general study of hearing, without respect to age. Audiometric methods will be presented as a description of current clinical practice, set in a frame of reference that implies and suggests directions for new development and improvement. Discussion of nonmedical remedial efforts will also be presented.

SIGNIFICANCE OF HEARING LOSS

Impairment of hearing has developmental, social, educational, emotional and economic significance. When impairment is severe and occurs in the first few years of life, the effects on development of language and speech are profound. Hearing is the primary sensory input relevant to this development. Even mild hearing loss early in life may have adverse effects on development of language (Holm and Kunze, 1969). When hearing loss occurs after about age 3, the consequences, although frequently severe, are less dramatic. Nevertheless, even mild and moderate degrees of hearing loss in preschool and school-age children often result in significant behavioral and educational impairment (Goetzinger et al., 1964). In many instances, the chief complaint is poor school performance or behavioral disturbance. Effects on behavior of the hearing loss concomitant with recurrent otitis media are frequently underestimated.

Failure to compensate for reduced hearing early in life, perhaps even in the first year of life, reduces the probability of adequate speech and language development. Insufficient or inappropriate management promotes the development of maladaptive social and listening behavior. Furthermore, the effects of delay may be irreversible. These are important considerations, based in part on clinical observations and in part on hypotheses concerned with sensitive periods for language development and the possible effects of sensory deprivation (Davis, 1965; Davis and Silverman, 1970; Wiesel, 1971).

Adequate methods now exist for evaluation early in life. The audiologist usually can classify an infant as having grossly normal hearing, severely impaired hearing, or some intermediate degree of impairment as early as age 4 to 8 months.

FRAME OF REFERENCE FOR EVALUATION

Lack of response to sound does not necessarily imply abnormal hearing, nor do normal thresholds for detection of sound necessarily imply normal auditory function. Clinical studies should operate within a conceptual frame of reference that considers the plurality of purposes served by auditory function, the plurality of auditory functions that permit meeting these purposes and the effects on auditory function of systems other than the auditory. Hearing is not a unitary phenomenon, and if the clinical endeavor is to be effective and relevant, it must recognize this explicitly.

The primary purposes served by hearing are alerting, orientation, and communication. These functions require detection of signals and discrimination of signals in terms of background-foreground and in terms of identification or association of the signal with the object or action responsible for it. They appear to require a decision process related to the significance of the auditory signal and a change of state or set from "passive" hearing to "active" attending or listening. For communication, more precise discriminations appear to be necessary more often, and more complex perceptual and motor processes are invoked that involve association, memory and learning.

It is reasonable to expect, and clinical experience confirms the expectation, that defects may occur in any one of these aspects of function independently of or concomitant with defects in one or more other aspects. For example, ability to detect sound and make certain discriminations may appear normal, but over-all function may be impaired by a disability of higher processes having to do with memory or with attending; ability to detect sound may be normal, but discrimination and identification may be impaired; ability to detect sound may be impaired, but provided the signal is loud enough, there are no impairments of discrimination. All such combinations are logically possible and many have been observed clinically.

If we operate within such a conceptual scheme, depending upon how insightful, imaginative and fortunate we are in our sampling of auditory and other than auditory functions for measurement and appraisal, we can provide a clinical assessment that will be specifically appropriate to the needs of our patients. Ideally, the assessment would be descriptive, predictive and prescriptive. It would describe with some precision the residual normal functions and the malfunctions as the basis for prediction and prescription and would do this in a context that would elucidate the natural history of the disease processes for potential prevention or reduction of their effects. It would be predictive of the capacity of the patient to cope with his world on the basis of the relations between specific impairments of function, residual normal function and the patient's present and future needs. It would be prescriptive of the specific treatment (medical, prosthetic and educational) necessary for habilitation or rehabilitation.

This presentation is obviously simplified, but simplification is necessary for perspective. The rationale presented suggests a model and strategy for evaluation of disorders of communication for therapeutic procedures and for evaluation of the effectiveness of therapy. Not all of these considerations are invoked in present clinical practice, and when they are employed there is, theoretically, room for improvement. Measurement of the phenomena of interest is difficult at best, and some functions are more amenable to measurement than others. The rationale presented can thus also suggest an agenda for research concerned with those aspects of evaluation not presently done or not done well enough.

PURPOSES OF AUDIOMETRY

Before discussion of assessment, it will be helpful to comment further on purposes of audiometry in the more traditional vocabulary of diagnosis, prognosis, monitoring and screening.

Diagnosis

In the context of medical diagnosis, the purposes are to identify or corroborate the presence or absence of a disease and to provide information that will help to specify the probable locus of the pathology and thus provide guides for the specifics of medical or surgical treatment. One must try to determine whether the characteristics of the auditory function suggest a disturbance of middle ear function, a cochlear malfunction, a disease process affecting middle ear and cochlea, or a disease process that interferes with eighth nerve function, the brainstem, or high neural processes. The nature of the anatomy, the physiology and the pathologies and the uncertainties of measurement of hearing frequently preclude precise definition, and such interpretations are not always made with certainty. In pediatric audiology, the younger the child, the greater the uncertainty.

Prognosis

Purposes of prognosis are interwoven with the diagnostic purposes, but they go a step further. The concern is with the effects of the impairment on the patient's ability to communicate and its probable effects on interpersonal relationships and on social, emotional and intellectual development. One tries to answer the general questions, How much of a handicap is there? In what ways is there handicap? and What is to be done? Primary variables are the severity of the hearing loss, the age at onset, and the nature and degree of concomitant impairments. The more specific set of questions to be answered from this point of view are: How successful is an otological surgical procedure likely to be in alleviating the impairment of communication ability? How much and what kinds of help can be expected from use of a hearing aid? Does the patient need one or more forms of special teaching and educational treatment? and What are the specifics of the skills that need to be taught or redeveloped for optimal language and speech development and for success in processing auditory input?

Monitoring

Monitoring audiometry is a term usually applied in industrial or military audiology when the concern is observation of the effects of potentially hazardous noise exposure. The term seems appropriate in clinical audiology to describe the purpose of determination of changes in hearing that may occur over a period of time. The most frequent conditions are a progressive disease affecting hearing, as in some hereditary syndromes and in some forms of nephritis; fluctuations in hearing, frequently found in otitis media; spontaneous recovery of hearing following presumed viral or vascular insults; effects of ototoxic drugs administered for overriding concerns of health; and effects of mastoidectomy, tympanoplasty, adenoidectomy, myringotomy and decongestants.

Screening or Identification

The population of concern, whether infant, preschool or school-age, will influence the method of evaluation in terms of type and precision of audiometry or choice of audiometry versus some form of questionnaire about history and behavior as well as the architectural space employed (physician's office, school room, well-baby clinic). The purpose is to study some large population to detect those who have a significant impairment of hearing that requires further evaluation and care. Additional objectives are to accomplish this quickly and inexpensively, with a minimum of false positives and false negatives, and to identify the appropriate individuals before the impairment of hearing has interfered seriously with development or performance.

MEASUREMENT OF HEARING

We talk about measurement of hearing, and it is convenient to do so. We do not, however, measure hearing. Whatever the methods employed, measurements are restricted to stimuli and to responses. Stimuli are specified in terms of measurable physical attributes; responses are specified in terms of observable verbal, motor or electrophysiological events. Only inferences are made about hearing, and these inferences are drawn only after consideration of the stimulus-response relations and of variables that may alter these relations.

Stimulus Characteristics

Ideally, stimuli should be powerful elicitors of response that are pertinent to purposes of description, prediction and prescription and that are amenable to precise specification of their physical properties. Of these objectives, specification of stimulus properties is the easiest to attain, although in most clinical practices it is incomplete. The need for stimuli to be "meaningful" or familiar to the infant or young child when yes-no descisions about response are the data sought is at best a moot point.

The relevant dimensions for pure tones are frequency, intensity, duration and rise-fall time. These properties may be specified without difficulty when laboratory quality electroacoustic systems are used and when the sound source at the patient's ear is an earphone or insert receiver. When the transducer is a loudspeaker in a reflective sound field or when a tuning fork is the source, specification of the stimulus properties at the patient's ear is less precise. Specification of intensity and spectrum of frequency-modulated tones ("warble tones") in a sound field is usually difficult and imprecise. Bone-conduction vibrators present a special set of problems in terms of spectral purity and intensity calibration and also in terms of biophysical variables. Careful and frequent calibration of audiometric systems is essential. Performance characteristics of commercial pure-tone audiometers may be particularly labile (Thomas et al., 1969).

White noise and recorded environmental sounds can be specified with respect to over-all intensity, duration, rise-fall time, and frequency band width. Band width can be varied and controlled with filters. Narrow bands can provide more specific audiometric information than wide bands.

When speech is used as a stimulus to elicit an alerting response or to determine, with some conditioning procedure, the lowest intensity level at which the child detects the signal, specification of the over-all intensity appears sufficient for present practice and can be reasonably precise. However, when the response desired is not merely detection of the stimulus, but rather some form of identification or other action that implies use and understanding, there are additional problems that require careful consideration. These difficulties occur because the talker is an important variable, as is the vocabulary selected and the linguistic sophistication of the patient (Egan, 1948; Silverman and Hirsh, 1955; Davis and Silverman, 1970). These considerations are particularly pertinent in measurements of identification or discrimination of speech at levels above threshold. When the variable of talker is not controlled, as in live-voice presentation, the physical characteristics of the speech differ from talker to talker. Results obtained by different examiners and in different clinics are not comparable and cannot be duplicated. Reports in the literature that describe discrimination abilities in relation to auditory malfunctions or disease entities are reduced in value when standardized recorded tests are not used. This also limits interpretation of results in terms of diagnosis and prediction of communicative adequacy. Specification or control of the message set or response choices also alters the stimulus properties and influences the predictive value of identification and discrimination tests (House et al., 1965; Speaks, 1967).

Response Indicators

It is convenient to view response indicators in three categories: the reflex and orienting responses, the behavioral responses and the electrophysiological responses. In simple outline with respect to age, reflex and orienting responses are observed with infants up to about age 12 months, and perhaps to 24 months. These include startle reactions, changes in motor activity and turning to localize the source of sound. With children 30 to 36 months of age and older, one or more behavioral responses are selected, for example, placing a block in a box, moving a bead on a counting frame or raising a hand. Reflex and behavioral motor responses may be conditioned, at least theoretically, with an infant or child of any age. Electrophysiological responses represent a different class of events and a different approach for eliciting responses. Measurement of acoustic impedance reflects the physical properties of the middle ear and provides an entirely different methodology for assessment of auditory function.

Stimulus-Response Relations

It is easy to be misled and to accept the child's raised hand or his moving a bead as a response to a tone when in fact he responded to the expectation of a tone because the presentation occurred in a predictable rhythmic sequence. Alternatively, he may have responded to the movement of the examiner's hand on the tone-presentation control or to a visual clue provided by the examiner, such as looking at the child after each presentation of tone.

It is equally easy to be misled and to accept responses at some abnormal values of hearing threshold level because the child's understanding of what constitutes a "very faint tone" differs from the examiner's. In addition, because of his desire to please or to avoid "failure," the child may employ criteria for response such that he will respond only when he is entirely certain that he has heard the tone and thus will respond at some value of hearing level clearly above threshold. If the examiner accepts a false response, that is, a response when no tone was presented, he is uncertain of the truth of most of the child's responses. If he reinstructs or admonishes the child after a "false" response, he is likely to increase the child's need to be certain and thereby may obtain responses only at relatively high hearing threshold levels, resulting in an audiogram that represents greater deviation from normal than actually exists.

In measuring a threshold of intelligibility for speech by having the child repeat words or identify pictures, fear of "failure" or the need to be certain may influence the child's responses in much the same way as with the task of identification of presence or absence of a tone.

When the response indicator is reflex or electrophysiological, state of alertness and psychological set of the patient influence the responses. Responses may fail to occur to signals that previously were effective. In audiometry in which the EEG is observed, myogenic electrical activity or electrophysiological correlates of epilepsy may distort or obscure the responses.

The foregoing comments may be stated in general terms. Whether the response indicator is reflex, behavioral or electrophysiological, specification of the stimulus properties must be precise and complete, and the audiologist must identify, control and evaluate events and processes which are other than auditory and which influence the stimulus-response relations. Failure to do so may lead to erroneous inferences about hearing and to inappropriate clinical interpretations and recommendations. The nonauditory events and processes derive from several sources. Among these are insufficient procedural control, in which nonauditory stimuli occur more or less concomitant with the auditory stimulus; response artifacts, which include coincidental response to some other stimulus or in which failure to respond reflects state or set; and unknown or unmeasured variables that affect the patient's criteria and motivation for response.

The examination in audiology is essentially a series of psychophysical experiments done under less than ideal experimental conditions. Subjects (patients) are not usually selected to meet criteria of intelligence or motivation. The clinician simply takes them as they come. For several reasons, time is frequently a greater constraint in the clinic than in the laboratory. Patients have fears and concerns about the test results that are unlikely among subjects in an experiment. The difficulties are usually greater with pediatric than with adult patients; the fears are greater because "doctor" frequently has unpleasant connotations and because "tests" are associated with unpleasant events in schools. Motivation may be weak because the purposes and the significance of the examination are not clearly understood. The listening tasks may call for more sustained attention than the child is able or willing to provide. The effect of the instructions and of the manner of the examiner on the patient's criteria for response becomes particularly obvious with children. Intuitively, criterial variables appear to be more significant more often in pediatric than in adult audiology. It often appears that most of the special effort, ingenuity and technique in audiology for children of about age 3 to 7 is concerned with optimizing motivation and performance.

A metric that takes the effect of motivational and criterial variables into account is highly desirable. Procedures based on the theory of signal detectability can account for these variables separately from the measurements of auditory sensitivity and also provide for precise specification of stimuli (Clarke and Bilger, 1963; Bilger, 1964). Application of the theory has been restricted so far to experimental laboratory procedures. A vastly greater amount of time is needed with these procedures than with conventional methods, and this appears as the principal bar to applications in pediatric audiology. This is not to say that methods derived from the theory of signal detectability should not be the source of experiments pertinent to pediatric audiology, whether concerned with determinations of some threshold of detectability or with some measurement of differential sensitivity.

In the absence of these potentially excellent controls, we have to make the analog of political compromise in the clinic. The burden falls upon the audiologist to apply as effectively as possible the controls and safeguards of traditional experimental methods of psychophysics, including calibration of equipment before and during evaluation. We can only guess about criteria for response, but we can evaluate latency of response and repeatability of response within and between sessions. With many infants and young children we must recognize the need for successive evaluations. Other important checks and means for estimating the probable magnitude of error of measurement lie in observation and evaluation of the consistency of results within a test battery—correlation between the results of tests, the reports of clinical history and behavior, the less formal observations of behavior during the interview, the characteristics of the patient's speech and voice, and the quality of his school performance. We can then evaluate the degree of imprecision and the significance of the imprecisions in relation to the nature and importance of the clinical decisions that have to be made.

ASSESSMENT OF FUNCTION

Tests of hearing alone do not provide sufficient information. We need to know not merely how much additional intensity the child needs in order to hear, but how he hears, how he responds, how consistently he responds, how he communicates and how he relates to others. With present methods, much of this information for the infant and the child with severely impaired hearing who has little ability in communication is available only from the history, the reports of behavior and informal observations of behavior. When such information is available from examination of hearing, corroborative information from the clinical and developmental history remains highly desirable.

Many of the children referred for audiological evaluation also have impairments of function other than hearing. Since lack of response to sound and failure to develop speech and language do not necessarily imply abnormal hearing or abnormal hearing alone, the evaluation procedure must also address itself to questions about mental retardation, developmental aphasia and severe emotional disturbance as contributing or primary factors. More extended discussion of these considerations is available elsewhere (Davis, 1965). Evaluation in the areas of otology, audiology, speech pathology and psychology are desirable in order to detect and understand these and other probable impairments in relation to the child's potential for developing communication skills and to provide a reasonable basis for treatment.

Recent reports on genetic etiologies of hearing loss indicate a high prevalence of concomitant eye, renal, cardiac and thyroid malfunctions (Ruben and Rozycki, 1971; Konigsmark, 1971). These observations provide additional cogent reasons for comprehensive evaluation. Ruben suggests that an in-patient setting may be good for such evaluation, and I agree. There are additional advantages in the ease with which psychiatric and neurologic consultations may be obtained when needed, in the availability of the child for multiple sessions of audiological evaluation, and in the reduction of parental anxiety by providing well-informed interpretations and counseling within a few days of admission. The practicalities of so comprehensive an inpatient evaluation for all or most children who appear to have a severe communication disorder present obvious economic and logistic problems that are yet to be solved.

Indications for Referral

When parents observe that the infant or young child is frequently not responsive to environmental sounds or is responsive only to very loud sounds, suspicion of impairment of hearing is justified and referral for audiological evaluation is reasonable. At about age 3 months the normal child will usually be awakened by his mother's voice and at about 8 months will try to imitate speech. At 1 year he will begin to understand simple phrases and by 18 months more complex requests. Although the norms are widely variable, failure of this development is cause for suspicion. A frequent indication is the observation by the parents or other relatives that the child pays remarkably close attention to the talker's face.

Some children have normal or near-normal hearing in low frequencies but markedly abnormal hearing at 500 Hz or at 1000 Hz and above. These children will appear to respond normally to most environmental sounds, and the indications for referral will be inappropriate response to speech and impaired or delayed development of speech. Again, the norms are widely variable, but a reasonable criterion to provide early detection, although not as early as is desirable, is to view as suspect those children who at age 2 show little or no spontaneous speech. This is a more certain reason for referral if the child's speech and language development differs from that of his siblings.

Most children with mild or moderate hearing loss, that is, hearing levels better than about 45 dB (ISO), will not be suspected of hearing loss on the basis of marked aberrations in speech or gross unresponsiveness to sound. Difficulties will be observed when the talker is at a distance; they may require repetition of verbal requests or comments, responses to comments may be inappropriate, and they may appear unusually reluctant to participate in discussion. In school-age children, the hearing impairment may be manifest in inattention, daydreaming, poor school work and behavior disturbances.

Early detection and assessment are highly desirable. To this end, there has been substantial effort in neonatal screening for hearing impairment. The value of these efforts, however, has been viewed by many professionals as open to question (Goldstein and Tait, 1971; Downs, 1970; Rosenblith, 1970; Hardy et al., 1970; Davis, 1970a). A joint committee of the American Academy of Ophthalmology and Otolaryngology, the American Academy of Pediatrics, and the American Speech and Hearing Association, after review of data from neonatal auditory screening programs, issued a statement that advises that "...results of mass screening programs are inconsistent and misleading" and concludes that "...despite our recognition of the urgent need for early detection of hearing impairment, we urge increased research efforts, but cannot recommend routine screening of newborn infants for hearing impairment" ("Neonatal screening," 1970).

On the basis of experience, a number of prenatal, perinatal and postnatal circumstances have been identified that may impair hearing in a newborn. Infants who have been exposed to these situations should be observed carefully during the first months of life, and perhaps most should be referred for audiological evaluation at about age 6 months. The most prominent high risk conditions are as follows.

Prenatal hazards include a family history of deafness; parental blood incompatibility (Rh, ABO); a virus infection during early pregnancy, especially rubella; maternal bleeding, especially during the first trimester, and treatment of the mother with drugs, notably any of the mycin group. Premature delivery and either prolonged or precipitate labor can cause problems. Fetal distress due to maternal shock or other conditions may impair hearing, as can a difficult delivery requiring traction on the neck, or any birth injury. Neonatal problems include apnea or cyanosis; cerebral birth injury; jaundice with hyperbilirubinemia (15 mg. per 100 ml. and above); multiple anomalies; possible acoustic trauma, as noise from a defective incubator; and ototoxic drugs given for infections.

All of these conditions do not necessarily result in hearing loss. They may, however, result in other severely handicapping conditions, with or without concomitant hearing loss, that interfere with development of adequate communication skills. Conversely, application of these risk criteria will not identify all children with severe hearing impairment. More extended discussion of the problems associated with neonatal screening and of alternatives, including the use of a high risk register, is available (Davis and Silverman, 1970).

TESTS OF HEARING

For purposes of discussion, we may classify tests in accordance with either the age of the child or the response indicators and auditory signals employed. In this presentation, classification is by age of the child. Neither classification scheme is entirely satisfactory because hard and fast categories cannot be drawn with validity in view of variation in maturation and other factors that affect ability or desire to cooperate. Evoked or electric response audiometry and acoustic impedance tests have roles as special procedures for any age group and will be discussed separately.

Birth to Age Twenty-four Months

Reasonably definitive estimates of hearing loss can be obtained for a full-term infant by age 3 or 4 months, and more certainly by age 6 months. The most desirable response is an orienting response in which the child turns his head toward the source of sound. The optimal age for a clear orientation response is 6 to 9 months. Response may be to the onset as well as to the cessation of the sound. Response to the same sound in a given sequence of presentation may not occur more than once or twice even at a higher intensity because it is no longer an alerting signal to him; he has habituated to that sound. Later presentation, after other signals have been presented, is likely to elicit a response again.

A variety of signals is necessary. In addition to speech, these usually include white noise and environmental sounds such as doorbells, running water, sirens, bells, whistles and toy noisemakers. Specification of frequency range and intensity permit more useful interpretation of auditory function. This can be achieved when the signals are recorded on disc or tape, when filters are used to restrict the frequency band width and when presentation is via loudspeaker in a controlled acoustic environment. Control of duration and rise-fall time may also be desirable.

If the child is about age 6 months, he is usually seated in a highchair or on his mother's lap. One examiner holds the child's attention forward with a suitable toy while the other examiner presents the acoustic signals from the control room, and usually both evaluate the events of the pre- and post-stimulus intervals to decide whether or not a response occurred.

When the child is younger than 6 months, he may be placed in a crib. The procedure is essentially the same. Children who are about 4 months old or younger are less likely to respond with a full head turn. In the first week or two of life the response may be a Moro reflex or startle response; later it may be an increase or cessation of ongoing movement, blinking, or eye movement that may be directed toward the source of sound.

When one observes for alerting and orienting responses, what appears as a response may be subtle, and it must be evaluated in the context of the infant's activity and state prior to presentation of the stimulus. An apparent response may be a coincidental movement. The infant may be so absorbed in the play task or the object used to hold his attention forward that he may not be alerted at that moment by a low intensity signal that otherwise would result in a response. He may fail to respond because he is generally unresponsive at the time of examination as a result of some mild illness or fever or discomfort. At an extreme, he may be slow to respond or generally unresponsive to most stimuli in the environment most of the time because he is intellectually retarded or emotionally disturbed.

Prior to presentation of the acoustic signals by loudspeaker, many audiologists observe for responses, using toy noisemakers, bells, gongs, wooden blocks, squeeze toys and speech (calling the child's name, or saying "Hi," or babbling) while standing directly behind the child in the examining room. Again, the child's attention is held forward. These observations provide additional information and, with knowledge of the approximate intensity of the signals, can give the audiologist a gross estimate of hearing levels and may suggest the levels at which to start the more formal tests. It is usually better to start with faint rather than loud signals; this is one means of avoiding habituation. Essentially the same procedure may be used in the physician's office or in the well-baby clinic as a screening test for hearing impairment. Care must be taken to avoid being in the child's field of peripheral vision and to avoid puffs of air from movement of the noisemakers.

Clear and repeatable responses within a fairly narrow range of intensities to a variety of auditory signals permit a reasonably secure interpretation of the over-all degree of hearing impairment. The infant may be classified as having grossly normal hearing, a severe to profound hearing loss, or impaired hearing at one or perhaps two intermediate levels of severity. If the auditory signals are wide-band, as is most often the case in present practice, no reasonable prediction can be made about the severity of hearing loss in relation to frequency region. That is, the shape of the audiogram cannot be predicted, and one may be misled in assessment of significance of impairment when the hearing is very much better at frequencies below about 500 or 1000 Hz compared to frequencies above this range. Hearing loss in the central speech frequencies of 500 to 2000 Hz results in greater handicap than impairment above 2000 Hz.

It is also important to remember that in these procedures we have not determined a threshold of detectability or a hearing threshold level in the sense of signal versus silence, as we would in plotting an audiogram for an adult or older child. Rather, we have observed the intensity levels at which we can reliably distract the child from some task or toy. This "distraction level" is probably at a higher intensity than the hearing threshold level would be. Furthermore, when we test with signals presented in a sound field by loudspeaker, we have information only about the better ear.

Observation should also be made of the infant's reaction to light and to touch. His affect and his social responsiveness to his parents and to the examiners should also be observed. Interpretations will obviously be different for the child who fails to respond to auditory signals alone than for the child who is unresponsive in general.

Despite its limitations, enough information is usually obtained from this examination procedure to decide on the need for therapy procedures. It is not unusual, however, to require more than one session.

Age Eighteen Months to Thirty-six Months

At the earlier ages in this period, the procedures for evaluation may be essentially the same as those just described. At age 36 months (and sometimes as young as age 30 months), one or another variation of play audiometry is usually successful. If the hearing loss is not very severe or if onset is later in this period, significant information may be obtained from the child's ability to respond to speech. Generally, however, children in the age range of 12 or 18 months to 30 months present very difficult problems in testing. On one hand, they are too young for conditioning in play audiometry, and on the other hand, the orientation reflex becomes obscured after about age 12 months.

For many of these children, audiologists have reported success in determining an audiogram by one or another variation of conditioning a visual orienting response (Suzuki and Ogiba, 1961; Reddell and Calvert, 1967; Miller and Rabinowitz, 1969; Lidén and Kankkunen, 1969). An illuminated toy or a projected picture or a simple light bulb is used as the visual stimulus. An auditory signal is presented, followed immediately by the visual signal. The illuminated toy is placed so that the child must turn his head or clearly move his eyes to look at it. In some clinics two light signals are used, each placed at about a 45-degree angle from the child's position. After several pairings of tone and light, the child looks toward the light after presentation of the tone. Usually the child is "rewarded" by presentation of the light after each response to a tone. The auditory signal may be a pure tone, speech, noise or a frequency-modulated pure tone ("warble tone"). Presentation of signal may be by loudspeaker, earphones or bone-conduction vibrator.

Age Thirty Months to Six Years

For this age group, most audiologists use play audiometry, selecting from a wide variety of objects to devise games that will interest and motivate the child in performance of the required task. The child is taught to place a ring on a peg, to move a block from one box to another or to move a bead on a counting frame when he hears a tone. There are many variations. The examiner may start by testing himself or testing the child's mother to encourage the child to play the game. He presents the first tone to the child at a level loud enough to be heard easily and then gradually reduces the intensity. He always rewards the child with praise for a correct response, and moving of the block becomes a reward. The procedure requires a cheerful and friendly atmosphere, an examiner who can relate well and easily to the child, and considerable patience, imagination and insight to keep the child interested and to keep his attention focused appropriately and long enough. At this age, most children will accept earphones and most will play the game.

It may take more than one session to plot an audiogram, and the number of frequencies tested may be restricted. Speech or noise may also be used and are desirable as additional information to corroborate the audiogram. If the child is emotionally disturbed or mentally retarded, or if he has little residual hearing and little or no language, it may not be possible to obtain reliable and interpretable results. Some children cannot or will not cooperate or play the game according to the examiner's rules for reasons that are not clear. When the child appears unable to learn the game when sounds are used, it may be helpful to try to teach him with a tactile stimulus, using the bone-conduction vibrator at a high output at 250 or 500 Hz., and then return to tones. Obviously memory, attention and ability to learn are involved. The child's ability to perform the task with reliability and how he relates to the examiner are important behaviors for interpretation.

There are many variations of these play and conditioning procedures, including "peep-show" techniques and the use of pop-up toys. The simpler games are usually more appropriate at the younger end of this age range. Hardy (1965) provides a detailed description and discussion of these procedures. Frisina (1963) discusses pertinent clinical research.

With many children in this age group it is possible to obtain bone-conduction hearing levels as well as air-conduction levels. Sometimes masking can be used, but frequently it confuses the child. Useful information can often be obtained by holding the bone-conduction vibrator on the child's forehead and asking him to point to the ear in which he hears the tone—in other words, by using a Weber test, but with intensity controlled, and thus also providing an estimate of the bone-conduction hearing levels.

Age Seven and Older

Although there are exceptions, it is usually possible with older children to obtain reliable air and bone-conduction audiograms, and with masking when needed. For the 7- or 8-year-old child, it is desirable to offer a choice of responding with a hand signal or moving a bead on a counting frame. Praise for good performance is always helpful and a pleasant atmosphere and manner remain essential. Standardized recorded tests can be used for determination of hearing levels for speech and for suprathreshold identification of speech. Loudness balance and tone decay tests can be done. If the mental age is about 7, Bekesy audiometry can be done. Obviously, when there are behavioral disturbances or the child is mentally retarded, an approach to the examination more or less as with an adult will be less than entirely successful. With the older child, it is usually helpful to take the history and the description of the difficulties of communication from the child as well as from the parents. This becomes particularly desirable with adolescents.

SPECIAL PROCEDURES

The two testing procedures discussed—acoustic impedance tests and evoked or electric response audiometry (ERA)—require no overt or learned response on the part of the patient. For that reason, the age of the patient and his willingness or ability to cooperate present fewer problems than with other methods. They are particularly valuable with infants and young children, the mentally retarded and those with psychiatric problems and nonorganic hearing impairments. Prior experience with electrodermal audiometry (EDA) and recent experience with ERA indicate the need to emphasize that these methods are not foolproof, that neither is a panacea and that failure is to be expected with some proportion of patients. They are not simply techniques, nor are they simple techniques; considerable expertise is required. Each provides different kinds of information, and both must be viewed as examination procedures that are complementary to, not substitutes for, other tests of function.

Electrodermal audiometry (EDA) and electroencephalic audiometry (EEA) are not discussed in this presentation. There are many difficulties and limitations with EDA, and it is not now in frequent clinical use with infants and young children. EEA has fewer disadvantages, but its limitations and the development of ERA, which may be viewed as a refinement of EEA, have reduced its clinical application. Davis and Goldstein provide more extended commentary on these considerations (Davis and Silverman, 1970). Earlier literature is discussed by Goldstein (1963) and by Hardy (1965).

Acoustic Impedance Tests

Acoustic impedance tests provide information indicative of the transmission characteristics of the middle ear structures. Their most certain and special contributions at present are that they assess the integrity and function of the middle ear in ways not provided by audiometry or by otoscopic examination and yield information predictive of causes of conductive hearing loss.

LIMITATIONS OF OTOSCOPY AND AUDIOMETRY. Otoscopic examination may be falsely negative or inconclusive, particularly with young children. It is usually informative of middle ear fluid, of retractions and perforations of the tympanic membrane and of marked limitations of mobility. Stapes fixation, adhesions, and ossicular discontinuity are usually not detected. With audiometry, we usually can classify hearing loss as conductive, sensorineural or mixed. At times we can differentiate between sensory and neural malfunctions. However, we cannot differentiate between kinds of middle ear malfunction. Acoustic impedance tests provide information that significantly reduces these limitations of audiometry and otoscopy. In addition, the amplitudes and frequencies employed as stimuli to elicit the mechanical response of the middle ear system are within the range of those normally experienced in hearing. This is in contrast to the large amplitudes of motion induced for tests of mobility in otoscopic examination, which may not provide information that is valid with respect to hearing (Zwislocki, 1961; Zwislocki, 1963; Zwislocki and Feldman, 1970).

DIFFERENTIATION OF MIDDLE EAR PATHOLOGIES. Normative values are reported for the compliance and resistance components of the acoustic impedance. Comparison of the measurements of normal ears with those obtained on patients with middle ear pathologies indicates that separate measurement of compliance and resistance permits differentiation of ossicular separation, stapedial fixation and fixation of the larger ossicles. Adhesions, retraction of the tympanic membrane and fluid are not separable. When fixation of the stapes and ossicular separation or massive adhesions are concomitant, fixation of the stapes is not detected (Zwislocki and Feldman, 1970).

Bilateral contraction of the middle ear muscles in response to a tone of 70 to 90 dB hearing level delivered to one ear is detectable and measurable as a change in acoustic impedance. When considered together with the measurements of absolute impedance, evaluation of the acoustic reflex provides additional information. Given abnormally low or high compliance, the absence or marked reduction of the reflex is corroborative of middle ear pathology. If the compliance is abnormally low but overlaps with a portion of normal compliance values, the presence of the reflex essentially rules out fixation of the stapes. Presence of the reflex implies a normal middle ear except when the ossicular chain is separated at the stapedial crura (Zwislocki and Feldman, 1970).

The observations reported by Jerger differ in detail from those of Zwislocki and Feldman. He employs different measurements and different instrumentation. The general clinical applicability, however, is essentially the same. Jerger finds that measurement of the absolute acoustic impedance is too variable for accurate prediction and, therefore, is not sufficient alone. His test battery consists of measurement of the threshold for the acoustic reflex, measurement of the acoustic impedance at the tympanic membrane and measurement of changes in acoustic compliance at the tympanic membrane as a function of alteration of the air pressure in the external auditory canal. In the latter measurement (tympanometry), characteristically different pressure-compliance functions are observed in cases of negative middle ear pressure, serous or adhesive otitis and otosclerosis; otosclerotic and normal ears are not differentiated. When the results of these impedance tests are related to the results of audiometry, a reasonable estimate of degree and type of hearing loss may be made in all but a small percentage of children (Jerger, 1970).

RESOLUTION OF AMBIGUITIES IN AUDIOMETRY. In addition to providing information predictive of the pathology in middle ear impairment, measurements of absolute acoustic impedance and observation or measurement of the acoustic reflex permit resolution of ambiguous clinical observations. There are many times, particularly with children, when audiometry is unreliable, making it difficult to interpret air-bone differences. When air-conduction hearing levels are within or close to normal limits, it may not be possible to differentiate between conductive and sensorineural hearing loss on the basis of air-bone differences. Detection of a possible conductive component in a severe sensorineural hearing loss may also be difficult because of output limitations of the bone-conduction vibrator and confusion of tactile with auditory sensation. In such circumstances, on the basis of the data described in the preceding sections, measurements of acoustic impedance can permit a decision about the presence or absence of middle ear disturbance and in this way will provide a basis for deciding whether the hearing loss is sensorineural, conductive or mixed.

Applications of the Acoustic Reflex. The acoustic reflex is usually readily observed in normal ears and usually is not observable in the presence of middle ear pathology or pathology of the facial nerve. It reflects sensorineural function as well as middle ear function. The average threshold for the reflex in normal ears is at 70 to 90 dB hearing level. There is an extensive literature on these observations and their clinical applications. Only a partial review is presented in this discussion. Zwislocki and Feldman (1970) and Jerger (1970) provide additional review and comments. More extensive summaries and discussion are presented by Jepsen (1963), by Lamb and Norris (1969) and by Lilly (1972). The principal clinical applications have been observation of the reflex to detect the presence of middle ear pathology, to estimate hearing threshold levels and as an indicator of loudness recruitment. There are many uncertainties in such interpretations. Absence of the reflex does not necessarily indicate middle ear dysfunction (Zwislocki and Feldman, 1970; Jerger, 1970), and its presence does not necessarily exclude abnormality of the middle ear (Zwislocki and Feldman, 1970). Although the mean or modal values of levels above the threshold of normal hearing necessary to elicit the reflex fall within a narrow range in most studies, variability in the same subject and among subjects is high (Lamb and Norris, 1969; Jerger, 1970). Prediction of hearing threshold levels on the basis of the reflex threshold is therefore uncertain. The reflex may not be observed in presumably normal ears for unknown reasons (Robertson et al., 1968; Jerger, 1970), and clinical application as an indicator of loudness recruitment has not yet been clearly established (Davis and Silverman, 1970).

Other than use as part of a battery of acoustic impedance measurements, as described by Zwislocki and Feldman (1970) and by Jerger (1970), it appears at present that the most reasonable application of tests for the acoustic reflex employs patients who are essentially untestable with audiometry because of age, retardation or emotional disturbance. When an acoustic stimulus is used to elicit the reflex in such patients, observation of the reflex will permit an interpretation of the presence of hearing and a reasonable assumption of a normal middle ear. Absence of the reflex would be inconclusive.

THE BASIS FOR MEASUREMENTS OF ACOUSTIC IMPEDANCE. The physical basis for the clinical application of measurements of acoustic impedance at the tympanic membrane are derived from the following. When a tone is introduced into the external auditory canal it impinges on the tympanic membrane, and most of its energy is transmitted by the ossicular chain to the cochlea. Very little energy is dissipated by the normal middle ear. Some energy is reflected by the tympanic membrane. The frequency of the reflected wave is the same as the original wave, but its amplitude and phase are determined by the mechanical characteristics of the middle ear structures, including the round and oval windows, and to a small degree by the mechanical properties of the cochlea. Thus, the reflected wave is indicative of the integrity and state of the middle ear. The mobility of the system is expressed in terms of its opposition or resistivity to movement—its acoustic impedance. The acoustic impedance is dependent upon the compliance or stiffness, mass, and resistance of the middle ear system. When, for example, the system is abnormally stiff or heavy, its mobility is reduced and it is less compliant; less of the energy in the incident wave is transmitted through it, and more energy is reflected. Fixation of the stapes and adhesions are conditions which increase the compliance and the resistance. Conversely, when there is ossicular discontinuity the system is more compliant than normal, and the stiffness and resistance are reduced. The measurements of acoustic impedance at the tympanic membrane express the acoustic properties of the middle ear system and are sensitive to pathological conditions. These principles are discussed in greater detail by Zwislocki (1961) and by Tonndorf (1965).

INSTRUMENTATION. The mechanical acoustic bridge as modified and developed by Zwislocki (Metz, 1946; Zwislocki, 1963) is the basic instrument for measurement of acoustic impedance at the tympanic membrane. It permits precise measurement of the compliance and resistance components of the impedance without undue difficulty in the clinic. Details of procedure have been reported (Zwislocki and Feldman, 1970). The instrument is available commercially (Grason-Stadler Company). Electroacoustic counterparts to mechanical acoustic bridges have also been developed (Klockhoff, 1961; Møller, 1958; Terkildsen and Nielsen, 1960). The electroacoustic instruments are more suitable for use with children because the essential tight seal between the probe and the ear canal is obtained with greater comfort and is less easily disturbed by movement of the head than the mechanical bridge. Electroacoustic bridges are available commercially (Grason-Stadler Company Otoadmittance Meter Model 1720, Madsen Electro-Acoustic Impedance Meter Model ZO 70).

Electric Response Audiometry (ERA)

Many designations for this testing procedure are used, such as evoked response audiometry, auditory evoked potentials, cortical evoked response audiometry, cortical audiometry, auditory evoked response, averaged electroencephalic audiometry, and averaged electroencephalic response. In conference and discussion at the 1970 International Symposium of the ERA Club there was consent to "electric response audiometry" ("Round-table-conference," 1971).

ERA provides a reliable and broadly applicable electrophysiological means of determining hearing threshold levels. It is reasonable to infer that the observed responses reflect neural activity in or near the cerebral cortex resulting from an acoustic signal (Davis and Silverman, 1970; Vaughan and Ritter, 1970). No inferences are justifiable with respect to discriminations or cognition. Future applications may permit such interpretations, and some of the literature is provocative in this respect. These are research questions at this time, however, and clinical application does not appear practical. Some of the pertinent references are Ritter et al. (1968), Vaughan and Ritter (1970), Sutton et al. (1967), Haider et al. (1968), Davis (1964), Vaughan (1969), Cohen (1969), and Sutton (1969). Thresholds obtained with ERA are not necessarily the equivalent of psychophysical thresholds determined with behavioral audiometry. The relations between the electrophysiological response and sensation or perception are not known, and the subject is not necessarily aware of a given auditory signal that yields a clear response. For practical purposes of audiometry, there is very good correspondence between ERA thresholds and behavioral thresholds with both normal and hearing-impaired listeners. Price (1968) summarizes these data.

The special clinical contribution of ERA is that it permits determination of hearing threshold levels, although not always with ease, for most of those patients who cannot be evaluated adequately with behavioral procedures. These are infants and young children, emotionally disturbed infants and children, the severely retarded, hyperactive and distractible children, and those with probable nonorganic hearing loss. For those infants who can be evaluated with more or less precision by behavioral methods, ERA permits an additional set of observations and potentially more precise determination of hearing levels for each ear individually.

For hyperactive and distractible children and most infants, ERA appears as the most suitable procedure, provided they are in deep sleep. Drug-induced sleep is the most convenient. Chlorpromazine, secobarbital sodium, and pentobarbital sodium are reported to be effective (Davis, 1970b). Suzuki and Origuchi (1969) report good agreement between behavioral thresholds and ERA thresholds obtained during sedated sleep for 42 of 47 children with normal hearing and for 92 of 133 children with impaired hearing. Of the latter group, no responses were obtained with either behavioral audiometry or ERA at maximum output levels for 30 children with severe impairment. In general, the correspondence between ERA and behavioral thresholds was closer for the children with greater hearing loss.

Whether the child is awake or asleep, there are limitations imposed by time. When tested awake, the young child cannot be kept reasonably quiet, nor can drowsiness be avoided for longer than an hour. When asleep, the necessary high-voltage slow wave stage is not constant and may not be present for more than 30 or 45 minutes (Davis, 1971).

This method of testing is also limited by the responsiveness of infants. Although responses have been observed in infants at hearing levels within 10 or 20 dB of normal adult psychophysical thresho.ds, there are insufficient data to generalize this. In addition, experience to date indicates that with infants younger than 6 months whose hearing is presumably normal, it is difficult to observe clear responses below about 40 dB hearing level (McCandless, 1971). Barnet makes a similar observation. Her data indicate, however, that several repetitions may elicit an observable response close to normal adult threshold (Barnet, 1971).

Other limitations are imposed by cost. Instrumentation costs range from about ten or twelve thousand dollars to more than fifty thousand. Usually two highly skilled and experienced people are needed for an examination.

Complexity and versatility of equipment vary considerably from one laboratory or clinic to another. Decisions need to be made in choice of instrumentation because ERA is still very young and not all the pertinent parameters of testing are fully understood. The practical decision involves a choice between flexibility for research and making use of reported research observations on the one hand, and ease, convenience and speed of operation for clinical purposes on the other. Some trade between flexibility and convenience is necessary.

The essential instrumentation includes an audio signal source, a physiological amplifier, write-out for the raw EEG, an averaging computer, and a write-out or other visual display for viewing the averaged response. The procedure, in brief, involves taking the EEG from an electrode on the vertex to the averaging computer. This is done in response to each of 50 or 60 brief tonal stimuli (usually 200 or 300 milliseconds with a 10 to 20 millisecond rise-fall time) presented with an interstimulus interval of one or two seconds (usually one second for the awake child and two seconds for the sleeping child). The EEG voltage is sampled at each of 50 or 100 (or more) points in time, usually for a period of 500 milliseconds. The voltage at each point in time is summed for each of the 50 or 60 responses. The ongoing electrical activity unrelated in time to the stimuli is more or less random and is canceled out in the algebraic averaging process. The write-out represents a waveform time-locked to the stimulus series.

Price provides an excellent summary and discussion of instrumentation, details of procedure, and interpretation of responses (Price, 1969). Davis (1971) and Davis and Silverman (1970) should also be consulted, particularly for their comments on interpretation of responses, interpolation or extrapolation to threshold and strategy for testing.

Most of the clinical literature is concerned with responses which occur between 50 and 300 or 400 milliseconds after onset of the stimulus. The reports of Mendel and Goldstein suggest that the components with latency less than 50 milliseconds may be reliable indicators of threshold and less influenced by state of the subject than the later components (Mendel and Goldstein, 1969a; 1969b; 1971).

LIMITATION OF PRESENT TESTS

The primary concern is not with how effective present tests for infants and young children are for estimation of thresholds of hearing, although certainly there is room for improvement in several dimensions. Within the limits already indicated they usually provide acceptable descriptions of how great an increase in intensity, compared to an established normal reference, the child needs before an observable response occurs and whether this represents a hearing level for a pure tone, for speech, or a level sufficient to distract the child and cause him to orient to the sound. The most significant limitation is that present methods provide little more than one or another threshold of detectability. This is useful but limited information. We know little or nothing about the ability of the infant to make discriminations that are pertinent to development of language and speech or his ability to make meaningful or purposeful use of auditory information. On the basis of experience with adults, and at least on the basis of informed speculation with young children, we know that suprathreshold discriminations may be impaired in varying degrees from no impairment to severe and in the presence or absence of elevation of thresholds of detectability.

With present evaluation procedures, after determining that the infant or young child has a severe hearing loss, we begin to learn something about his abilities to make useful discriminations only after there has been considerable effort in preschool teaching or therapy. In addition, we fail to define adequately the problems, auditory and other, for the child whose language and speech are severely delayed and who appears to have normal hearing threshold levels in the absence of evidence of mental retardation or psychotic behavior. In the context of the conceptual scheme for evaluation presented at the beginning of this chapter, present methods in pediatric audiology appear insufficiently descriptive and far less predictive and prescriptive than is desirable. This appears so with restriction of the comments to auditory function, saying nothing and implying little about memory and attending, let alone visual function or combined auditory and visual function. Present methods, although very helpful, fall far short of the ideal.

It is beyond the scope of this presentation and beyond the limits of present knowledge to write the prescription that will make all well. Stating the case, even briefly, however, may have a salutary effect. In addition, there are indications in the literature of what may be productive approaches. Some of these are now discussed.

There are published data pertinent to an understanding of normal infant capacities and development which are suggestive of means for closing some of these gaps in the clinic. One study (Eimas et al., 1971) indicates that infants at age 1 month not only respond to speech sounds but are also capable of making fine discriminations of acoustic cues in the speech sounds along the same dimensions as employed by adults. Furthermore, since the infants have had only limited exposure to speech and no experience in producing the speech sounds, the data are interpreted as implying that the means by which perception of speech is accomplished may be part of the biological makeup of the child and are functional very early in life.

In a series of experiments with infants in which stimulus parameters, response characteristics and prestimulus state have each been carefully specified, Eisenberg has observed differences in responsiveness, in magnitude of response and in the response characteristics in consistent relations to the stimulus properties. In very brief summary, frequencies below 4000 Hz result in different responses than those above 4000 Hz. Each stimulus class evokes different response behaviors. Signals which change in frequency during presentation, as opposed to constant signals, result in differences in latency of response and magnitude of response. The responses also appear to reflect differences in the direction of the tonal sequence. These response characteristics appear related to other than simple arousal behavior (Eisenberg, 1970).

What is most provocative in these studies is that high level functions of attending and of discrimination appear to be present very early in life. These functions seem relevant to development of language and speech, and with appropriate experimental procedure they are observable and appear amenable to study in the clinic. Eisenberg's experiments and those of other observers are discussed in the context of the capacity of the infant for development of language by Menyuk (Menyuk, 1971).

AURAL REHABILITATION

When corrective treatment is not feasible, as with sensorineural hearing loss, or when there is residual hearing loss after otologic treatment, aural rehabilitation is necessary. Comprehensive rehabilitation includes use of hearing aids, auditory training, instruction in visual communication, speech and language therapy, and educational counseling. Whether all or only some of these remedial efforts are indicated depends primarily on the severity of the hearing loss, the age at onset, and the duration of the hearing loss before initiation of treatment.

Hearing aids are necessary with the more severe hearing losses and are helpful with infants and children whether the hearing loss is mild or apparently severe. Our experience with many school-age children indicates that there is obvious handicap imposed by mild hearing loss of the order of 30 to 35 dB (ISO). Use of a hearing aid, at least in the classroom, has resulted in less shyness, more active participation in group discussion, and more desirable behavior and habits of attention.

With sensorineural hearing loss, particularly when it is severe, hearing aids do not restore normal hearing. For many patients, the severity of the hearing loss and the disabilities in discrimination are such that only limited help is to be expected. Nevertheless, use of an appropriate hearing aid, even with very little residual hearing, can make audible a signal of danger or a signal that someone is talking and should be looked at. In addition, the amplification provides useful information about the temporal, stress and intonation patterns of speech. When this information is added to the information from the visual channel, the total information appears to be greater than the sum of its parts; the ambiguous auditory signal becomes clearer when additional information is provided by visual input. As previously discussed, experience with deaf and hard-of-hearing infants attests to the desirability of use of amplification as soon as a reasonable assessment is made and by age 12 months, if possible.

Discussion of the acoustic characteristics of speech and perception of speech in relation to hearing aid design and design of visual aids for the hearing handicapped are beyond the scope of this section. Informative discussion and review of pertinent research and development are provided by Pickett (1971), Risberg (1971), Erber (1971) and Sanders (1971).

Auditory training, training in visual communication and efforts designed to foster language and speech development are essential for the deaf and hard-of-hearing child. Parent counseling, parent education, and educational guidance are also of great importance. When hearing loss occurs later in childhood or adolescence, depending primarily on severity and age of onset, similar training and counsel are necessary. These subjects are merely identified in this chapter. They are far too important to be treated in a cursory manner and are too complex to be summarized briefly. Thorough discussion of principles and practice and a review of pertinent literature are provided by Sanders (1971), and by Davis and Silverman (1970).

REFERENCES

Barnet, A. B.: Evoked response audiometry in 241 normal and hearing impaired children under three years. *Arch. Klin. Exp. Ohr. Nas. Kehlkopfheilk.,* 198:154, 1971.

Bilger, R. C.: Viewpoint, evolution in psychophysics? *J. Speech Hearing Res.,* 7:105, 1964.

Clarke, F. R., and Bilger, R. C.: The theory of signal detectability and the measurement of hearing. *In* Jerger, J. (Ed.): *Modern Developments in Audiology.* Academic Press, New York, 1963.

Cohen, J.: Very slow brain potentials relating to expectancy: the CNV. *In* Donchin, E., and Lindsley, D. B. (Eds.): *Average Evoked Potentials.* National Aeronautics and Space Administration, Washington, D.C., 1969.

Davis, H.: Enhancement of evoked cortical potentials in humans related to a task requiring a decision. *Science,* 145:182, 1964.

Davis, H. (Ed.): The young deaf child: Identification and management. *Acta Otolaryng.,* Suppl. 206, 1965.

Davis, H.: Summary. Symposium: conservation of hearing through neonatal testing. *Trans. Amer. Acad. Ophthal. Otolaryng.,* 74:1238, 1970a.

Davis, H.: Evoked response audiometry. *Trans. Amer. Acad. Ophthal. Otolaryng.,* 74:1236, 1970b.

Davis, H.: Is ERA ready for routine clinical use? *Arch. Klin. Exp. Ohr. Nas. Kehlkopfheilk.,* 198:2, 1971.

Davis, H., and Silverman, S. R. (Eds): *Hearing and Deafness,* third edition. Holt, Rinehart and Winston, New York, 1970.

Downs, M. P.: The identification of congenital deafness. *Trans. Amer. Acad. Ophthal. Otolaryng.,* 74:1208, 1970.

Egan, J. R.: Articulation testing methods. *Laryngoscope,* 58:955, 1948.

Eimas, P. D., Siqueland, E. R., Jusczyk, P., and Vigorito, J.: Speech perception in infants. *Science,* 171:303, 1971.

Eisenberg, R. B.: The organization of auditory behavior. *J. Speech Hearing Res.,* 13:453, 1970.

Erber, N. P.: Evaluation of special hearing aids for deaf children. *J. Speech Hearing Dis.,* 36:527, 1971.

Frisina, D. R.: Measurement of hearing in children. *In* Jerger, J. (Ed.): *Modern Developments in Audiology.* Academic Press, New York, 1963.

Goetzinger, C. P., Harrison, C., and Baer, C. J.: Small perceptive hearing loss: its effect on school age children. *Volta Rev.,* 66:124, 1964.

Goldstein, R.: Electrophysiologic audiometry. *In* Jerger, J. (Ed.): *Modern Developments in Audiology.* Academic Press, New York, 1963.

Goldstein, R., and Tait, C.: Critique of neonatal hearing evaluation. *J. Speech Hearing Dis.,* 36:3, 1971.

Haider, M., Groll, E., and Studynka, G.: Orienterungs und Bereitschaftspotentiale bei unerwarteten Reizen. *Exp. Brain Res.,* 5:45, 1968.

Hardy, J. B., Hardy, W. G., and Hardy, M. P.: Some problems in neonatal screening. *Trans. Amer. Acad. Ophthal. Otolaryng.,* 74:1229, 1970.

Hardy, W. G.: Evaluation of hearing in infants and young children. *In* Glorig, A. (Ed.): *Audiometry: Principles and Practices.* Williams and Wilkins, Baltimore, 1965.

Holm, V. A., and Kunze, L. H.: Effect of chronic otitis media on language and speech development. *Pediatrics,* 43:833, 1969.

House, A. S., Williams, C. E., Hecker, M. H. L., and Kryter, K. D.: Articulation-testing methods: consonantal differentiation with a closed-response set. *J. Acoust. Soc. Amer.,* 37:158, 1965.

Jepsen, O.: Middle ear muscle reflexes in man. *In* Jerger, J. (Ed.): *Modern Developments in Audiology.* Academic Press, New York, 1963.

Jerger, J.: Clinical experience with impedance audiometry. *Arch. Otolaryng.,* 92:311, 1970.

Klockhoff, I.: Middle ear muscle reflexes in man. *Acta Otolaryng.,* Suppl. 164, 1961.

Konigsmark, B. W.: Hereditary congenital severe deafness syndromes. *Ann. Otol.,* 80:269, 1971.

Lamb, L. E., and Norris, T. W.: Acoustic impedance measurement. *In* Fulton, R. T., and Lloyd, L. L. (Eds.): *Audiometry for the Retarded.* Williams and Wilkins, Baltimore, 1969.

Lidén, G., and Kankkunen, A.: Visual reinforcement audiometry in the management of young deaf children. *Internat. Audiol.,* 8:99, 1969.

Lilly, D. J.: Acoustic impedance at the tympanic membrane. *In* Jerger, J. (Ed.): *Modern Developments in Audiology,* revised edition. Academic Press, New York, 1972.

McCandless, G. A.: Electroencephalic audiometry. *In* Rose, D. E. (Ed.): *Audiological Assessment.* Prentice-Hall, Englewood Cliffs, New Jersey, 1971.

Mendel, M. I., and Goldstein, R.: The effect of test conditions on the early components of the averaged electroencephalic response. *J. Speech Hearing Res.,* 12:344, 1969a.

Mendel, M. I., and Goldstein, R.: Stability of the

early components of the averaged electroencephalic response. *J. Speech Hearing Res.*, 12:351, 1969b.

Mendel, M. I., and Goldstein, R.: Effect of sleep on the early components of the averaged electroencephalic response. *Arch. Klin. Exp. Ohr. Nas. Kehlkopfheilk.*, 198:110, 1971.

Menyuk, P.: *The Acquisition and Development of Language.* Prentice-Hall, Englewood Cliffs, New Jersey, 1971.

Metz, O.: The acoustic impedance measured on normal and pathological ears. *Acta Otolaryng.*, Suppl. 63, 1946.

Miller, M. H., and Rabinowitz, M.: Audiological problems associated with pre-natal rubella. *Internat. Audiol.*, 8:90, 1969.

Møller, A.: Intraaural muscle contraction in man examined by measuring acoustic impedance of the ear. *Laryngoscope,* 68:48, 1958.

"Neonatal screening." *Trans. Amer. Acad. Ophthal. and Otolaryng.*, 74:1352, 1970.

Pickett, J. M.: Some applications of speech analysis to communication aids for the deaf. *Volta Rev.*, 73:147, 1971.

Price, L. L.: Cortical-evoked response audiometry. *In* Fulton, R. T., and Lloyd, L. L. (Eds.): *Audiometry for the Retarded.* Williams and Wilkins, Baltimore, 1969.

Reddell, R. C., and Calvert, D. R.: Conditioned audio-visual response audiometry. International Conference on Oral Education of the Deaf. Proceedings I. A. G. Bell Association for the Deaf, Washington, D.C., 1967.

Risberg, A.: A critical review of work on speech analyzing hearing aids. *Volta Rev.*, 73:23, 1971.

Ritter, W., Vaughan, H. G., Jr., and Costa, L. D.: Orienting and habituation to auditory stimuli: a study of short term changes in average evoked responses. *Electroenceph. Clin. Neurophysiol.*, 25:550, 1968.

Robertson, E., Peterson, J., and Lamb, L.: Relative impedance measurements in young children. *Arch. Otolaryng.*, 88:162, 1968.

Rosenblith, J. F.: Are newborn auditory responses prognostic of deafness? *Trans. Amer. Acad. Ophthal. Otolaryng.*, 74:1215, 1970.

"Round-table-conference," *Arch. Klin. Exp. Ohr. Nas. Kehlkopfheilk.*, 198:167, 1971.

Ruben, R. J., and Rozycki, D. L.: Clinical aspects of genetic deafness. *Ann. Otol.*, 80:255, 1971.

Sanders, D. A.: *Aural Rehabilitation.* Prentice-Hall, Englewood Cliffs, New Jersey, 1971.

Silverman, S. R., and Hirsh, I. J.: Problems related to the use of speech in clinical audiometry. *Ann. Otol.*, 64:1234, 1955.

Speaks, C.: Performance-intensity characteristics of selected verbal materials. *J. Speech Hearing Res.*, 10:344, 1967.

Sutton, S.: The specification of psychological variables in an average evoked potential experiment. *In* Donchin, E., and Lindsley, D. B. (Eds.): *Average Evoked Potentials.* National Aeronautics and Space Administration, Washington, D.C., 1969.

Sutton, S., Tueting, P., Zubin, J., and John, E. R.: Information delivery and the sensory evoked potential. *Science,* 155:1436, 1967.

Suzuki, T., and Ogiba, Y.: Conditioned orientation reflex audiometry. *Arch. Otolaryng.*, 74:84, 1961.

Suzuki, T., and Origuchi, K.: Averaged evoked response audiometry (ERA) in young children during sleep. *Acta Otolaryng.*, Suppl. 252:19, 1969.

Terkildsen, K., and Nielsen, S. S.: An electroacoustic impedance measuring bridge for clinical use. *Arch. Otolaryng.*, 72:339, 1960.

Thomas, W. G., Preslar, M. J., Summers, R. R., and Stewart, J. L.: Calibration and working condition of 100 audiometers. *Public Health Rep.*, 84:311, 1969.

Tonndorf, J.: Introduction to acoustics. *In* Glorig, A. (Ed.): *Audiometry: Principles and Practices.* Williams and Wilkins, Baltimore, 1965.

Vaughan, H. G., Jr.: The relationship of brain activity to scalp recordings of event-related potentials. *In* Donchin, E., and Lindsley, D. B. (Eds.): *Average Evoked Potentials.* National Aeronautics and Space Administration, Washington, D.C., 1969.

Vaughan, H. G., Jr., and Ritter, W.: The sources of auditory evoked responses recorded from the human scalp. *Electroenceph. Clin. Neurophysiol.*, 28:360, 1970.

Wiesel, T. N.: Effects of monocular deprivation on the cat's visual cortex. *Trans. Amer. Acad. Ophthal. Otolaryng.*, 75:1186, 1971.

Zwislocki, J.: Acoustic measurement of the middle ear function. *Ann. Otol.*, 70:599, 1961.

Zwislocki, J.: An acoustic method for clinical examination of the ear. *J. Speech Hearing Res.*, 6:303, 1963.

Zwislocki, J., and Feldman, A. S.: *Acoustic Impedance of Pathological Ears.* ASHA Monographs No. 15. American Speech and Hearing Association, Washington, D.C., 1970.

SECTION III

NOSE AND ACCESSORY SINUSES

Chapter Seventy-Four

EMBRYOLOGY, APPLIED ANATOMY AND PHYSIOLOGY

WILLIAM E. LAUPUS, M.D.

EMBRYOLOGY

The skin and mucous membranes of the nose are of ectodermal origin and derive from the nasal placodes which appear very early in embryonic development. Through growth and differential proliferation of surrounding mesoderm the nasal placodes form the nasal, or olfactory, pits which are present as early as the fourth week when the embryo is approximately 5 mm. in length. The nasal pits deepen, now being termed the nasal sacs, or fossae, which establish continuity with the pharynx by rupturing through the bucconasal membrane, thus forming the nasal passages.

Meanwhile, the frontonasal, nasal and maxillary processes, of mesodermal origin, are developing and fusing to produce the palate, nasal septum and probably the central portion of the upper lip. By the end of the seventh week, the basic anatomy of the nose has been established. The lateral nasal wall is, at first, smooth but soon develops folds and furrows which become, in turn, the turbinates and meatuses. The sinuses arise as diverticula in the mucosa of the lateral nasal wall at the appropriate meatuses.

The maxillary sinus precursor can be seen as early as the tenth week; the sphenoid appears at about the sixteenth week, and the ethmoids become evident somewhat later. Some ethmoid and other sinus cells are represented only by dimples or pits in the lateral nasal wall at the time of birth. The maxillary and sphenoid sinuses are present at birth; however, the maxillary sinus at this time is merely a slitlike indentation on the lateral nasal wall, and the sphenoid sinuses are similarly small and are not yet positioned within the sphenoid bone. As the mass of the maxilla between the orbital plate and the alveolar process increases with growth, the maxillary sinus enlarges, reaching its full size in early adult life. The sphenoid sinuses throughout childhood increasingly occupy the central portion of the sphenoid bone; they are well defined by 6 years of age and continue to grow until adulthood.

The ethmoid sinuses are present as evaginations without penetration into the ethmoid bone as early as the thirtieth week of gestation, but the ethmoid bone retains its solid structure until sometime after birth when the bony ethmoidal labyrinth forms to accommodate the developing ethmoidal sacs. Pneumatization of the ethmoidal cells continues throughout childhood, producing labyrinths varying considerably in size and number of cells.

Although the rudimentary frontal sinuses may be identifiable at birth or even in late fetal development, they do not begin to ascend into the frontal bone until the eighteenth to twentieth month of age and remain so small throughout the first six years of life that they are difficult to identify radiographically; thereafter, pneumatization proceeds and increases until early adulthood. In some persons the frontal sinuses may never develop (agenesis).

APPLIED ANATOMY

The external structure of the nose is given shape and support by the paired nasal bones, the maxillae and the nasal portions of the frontal bones. The paired lateral, greater and accessory alar, vomeronasal and the sesamoid cartilages contribute further to the form of the external nose and to the size of the fossae.

The internal nose consists of the nasal cavity, which is divided by the septum into the generally symmetrical nasal fossae. Each fossa is further subdivided by the turbinates into nasal meatuses and is considered to extend into the surrounding bones via the paranasal accessory sinuses.

The inferior turbinate (or concha) defines the upper limit of the inferior meatus which consists of the portion of the lateral nasal mucosa between the nasal floor and this turbinate. The nasolacrimal duct ostium is usually found in the inferior meatus. The mucosal space between the inferior and middle turbinates is termed the middle meatus and contains the ostia of the anterior ethmoidal cells and the frontal and maxillary sinuses. A third turbinate, the superior nasal concha, forms the upper limit of the superior meatus in which the openings of the posterior ethmoidal cells are located. The sphenoethmoidal recess into which the sphenoidal sinus opens is the most superiorly situated of the meatal divisions of the lateral nasal wall.

PHYSIOLOGY

The olfactory function of the nose is not highly developed in man, being primarily utilized in distinguishing odors which are pleasing from those which are not. The senses of taste and smell are so interrelated that foods may have an unpalatable flavor when nasal disease interferes with olfaction. Temporary distaste for food and anorexia may follow temporary reduction in olfactory acuity, thus accounting in part for the diminished appetite commonly present in nasal disorders.

In conditions of health the nose is admirably adapted for its other functions of controlling the temperature and humidity and for removing the minute foreign substances and bacteria in inspired air. The nose may contribute as much as 1000 ml. of water daily to inspired air in the adult. After passage through the nose in the short time of 0.25 second or less, the air reaching the nasopharynx will have been conditioned to a relative humidity of 75 to 80 per cent and to approximately normal body temperature. The specialized ciliated pseudocolumnar epithelium is covered by a continuous layer of mucus (the "mucus blanket") which collects dust particles, pollens, bacteria and other tiny air contaminants on its surface. The cilia move the mucus blanket toward the pharynx at a rate of 10 mm. or more per minute, providing for replacement of the mucus coating about six times in each hour. Ciliary movement is continuous unless impeded by infection or other noxious influences such as tobacco and other smoke pollutants which slow ciliary activity; interruption of the moist mucous surface covering rapidly leads to injury of the underlying ciliated cells.

The pH of the nasal secretions is maintained at a nearly constant level of 7; infection or local medication may alter the pH and reduce the effectiveness of natural barriers to infection. Although Sir Alexander Fleming described a bactericidal enzyme, a lysozyme, capable of destroying bacteria on contact, present opinion differs as to the importance of the protection afforded by this substance. Other secretory enzymes may provide significant, though nonspecific, antimicrobial effects upon pathogenic organisms. Secretory IgA antibodies, 11S immunoglobulins synthesized in plasma cells in the mucous membranes and in secretory glands, have been shown to be of importance in specific immunity to many respiratory viruses; they are not known to be active against mycoplasma and bacterial organisms. Cellular immunity, phagocytosis, other secretory substances and nonspecific humoral factors are considered to contribute substantially to immunity but have not been studied to the extent of the more accessible antibodies.

The principal contributions of the nose to defense against infection appear to be physical in nature: mucus, which separates infectious agents from the underlying mucosal cells, and ciliary action, which rapidly propels the mucus and its entrapped organisms to the pharynx, where it is swallowed and thence eliminated through the gastrointestinal tract.

The paranasal sinuses communicate with the nasal fossae via the sinal ostia. The nasal and sinal mucosae are continuous, and the secretions of the sinal mucosa contribute to the total secretory output of the nose. From the earliest days of medical knowledge the following list of "functions" ascribed to the sinuses has been accumulating. They have been said to

1. Impart resonance to the voice;
2. Humidify and warm inspired air;
3. Increase the surface area of the olfactory membranes, thus contributing to olfactory sensitivity;
4. Absorb shock applied to the head and protect the sensory organs;
5. Secrete mucus to assist in keeping the nasal chambers moist;
6. Provide thermal insulation for the nervous centers;
7. Aid facial growth and architecture;
8. Lighten the weight of the bones of the head for maintenance of proper balance; and
9. Exist as evolutionary remains or unneeded air spaces.

Despite 2000 or more years of speculation, no satisfactory functional explanation for the sinuses has been produced, and the role, if any, played by the sinuses in nasal function remains obscure.

REFERENCES

Blanton, P. L., and Biggs, N. L.: Eighteen Hundred Years of Controversy: The Paranasal Sinuses. *Amer. J. Anat.*, 124:135, 1969.

Proctor, D. F.: Physiology of the Upper Airway; in W. O. Fenn and H. Rahn (Eds.): *Handbook of Physiology*, Section 3, Respiration. Washington, D.C., American Physiological Society, 1964.

Schaeffer, J. P.: *The Nose, Paranasal Sinuses, Nasolacrimal Passageways, and Olfactory Organ in Man*. P. Blakiston & Co., Philadelphia, 1920.

Turner, A. L.: *The Accessory Sinuses of the Nose*. Longmans, Green & Co., New York, 1902.

Chapter Seventy-Five

EXAMINATION OF THE NOSE AND PARANASAL SINUSES

NORMAL M. WOLDORF, M.D., and PETER N. PASTORE, M.D.

The nose and paranasal sinuses should be examined in an orderly, routine manner to avoid missing pertinent physical findings. This examination, although systematic, is by no means inflexible. The order and extent of the examination is in part predicated upon the patient's complaints and the physician's findings. A few descriptive statements and suitable diagrams about these findings are of aid for future reference.

Instruments

For routine examination, the examiner needs a 100-watt lamp light source, a head mirror, a polished metal tongue blade, a nasal speculum, nasopharyngeal mirrors, bayonet forceps, nasal probes, a nasal suction tip, an Atomizer, 4 by 4 squares of gauze, cotton, pHisoHex, 0.25 per cent Neo-Synephrine solution, 1 per cent Xylocaine solution, 5 per cent cocaine solution and 2 per cent Pontocaine solution,* and a transilluminator (sinus). For special examination, one needs a nasopharyngoscope, biopsy forceps, French catheters, a sinus irrigation tray, small glass slides for smear or stain specimens, special stains and culture tubes.

*The use of any topical anesthetic agent requires extreme care, especially in children.

Order and Methods of Examination

In a routine systematic examination, one begins with inspection and palpation of the external nose. The use of a metal breathing plate (polished tongue blades) may be helpful. Then one proceeds to anterior rhinoscopy, posterior rhinoscopy and transillumination of the sinuses. For special examination, one may perform nasal probes, take smears and cultures of nasal secretions, perform direct nasopharyngoscopy, perform a digital examination of nasopharynx, or order a biopsy. X-ray studies may be indicated, as may sinus irrigation and endoscopic evaluation.

EXAMINATION OF THE EXTERNAL NOSE

Examination of the nose actually begins by noting the patient's facial expression, taking his or her state of mind and health into consideration. Naturally, the appearance of the eyes, lips, and facial skin as well as the nasal form and symmetry are included in the initial evaluation.

Inspection is performed with good illumination provided by indirect overhead lighting, a lamp placed posteriorly and laterally, and a head mirror. Usually the patient is seated in an examining chair with the physician either standing or sitting. General nasal contour and symmetry are evaluated from directly in front of the patient as well as from both sides and from above and below the level of the head. The nasal skin is scrutinized for color, texture, turgor, inflammation, tumors and other abnormalities. Starting superiorly and proceeding inferiorly, one notes the contours of the forehead, orbits, glabella, dorsal nasal bones and cartilages, nasal tip, alar cartilages, nares and columella. The appearance of any exudate is noted. The exudate may be collected by having the patient blow his nose onto wax paper. The exudate is then smeared onto microscopic glass slides and later stained for differential cell count.

Nasal patency is evaluated visually by inspecting for flaring of the cartilages and nares. In addition, placement of a polished metal tongue blade or breathing plate under the nostrils should result in the appearance of two areas of condensed water vapor. These areas are indicative of the volume of air flow and serve as an index of patency when compared to one another. By gently occluding first one and then the other nostril, one can further compare relative air flow visually by this method and also by listening for any change of pitch between the two sides. Should it become necessary, the passage of rubber or plastic catheters through the nostrils to the level of the oropharynx and the use of visual or radiopaque dyes with x-ray studies can help to establish the presence or absence of patency (choanal atresia or stenosis). These special studies are performed only after thorough examination of the nasal interior.

Palpation of the nose is undertaken with the physician standing beside the seated patient, both facing the same direction. Typically, a right-handed examiner stands to the right of the patient and uses his left hand to palpate. The base of the nose is examined from below, looking up at the nares and columella. The thumb of the right hand is placed on the columella and may gently move it from side to side when evaluating the caudal end of the septum.

By palpation of the external nose, one can further diagnose the causes of dorsal, lateral, tip and caudal deformities, be they bony or cartilaginous. Also, one can evaluate the length of the nasal bones and cartilages, the support and resiliency of the cartilages and the quality of the skin. This is important for the evaluation of obstruction, especially if cosmetic or functional surgery is contemplated in the older patient.

EXAMINATION OF THE INTERNAL NOSE AND SINUSES

ANTERIOR RHINOSCOPY. Examination of the nasal fossae (spaces) from the anterior aspect is known as anterior rhinoscopy. Basic instruments include the 100-watt lamp as a light source, a head mirror and a nasal speculum. Generally, the examiner stands to one side of the patient with the light source posterior and lateral to the patient's head. Looking through the mirror hole with one eye but using binocular vision, the examiner then focuses the reflected light onto the patient's nose. The nasal speculum blades are inserted into one nostril with the blades closed. These blades are then opened in the superior inferior axis to avoid trauma to the sensitive nasal spine and caudal septum. The reflected light is directed through the open speculum into the nasal interior. The examination starts inferiorly and proceeds superiorly and posteriorly, always looking both medially and laterally. After completing the examination of one nasal chamber, one examines the other chamber in a similar manner (Fig. 1).

The first area visualized inferiorly is the vestibular skin, which is typically hair-bearing. Attention is directed to this skin and its vasculature; one looks for follicular infections, abscesses, papillomas and other abnormal changes.

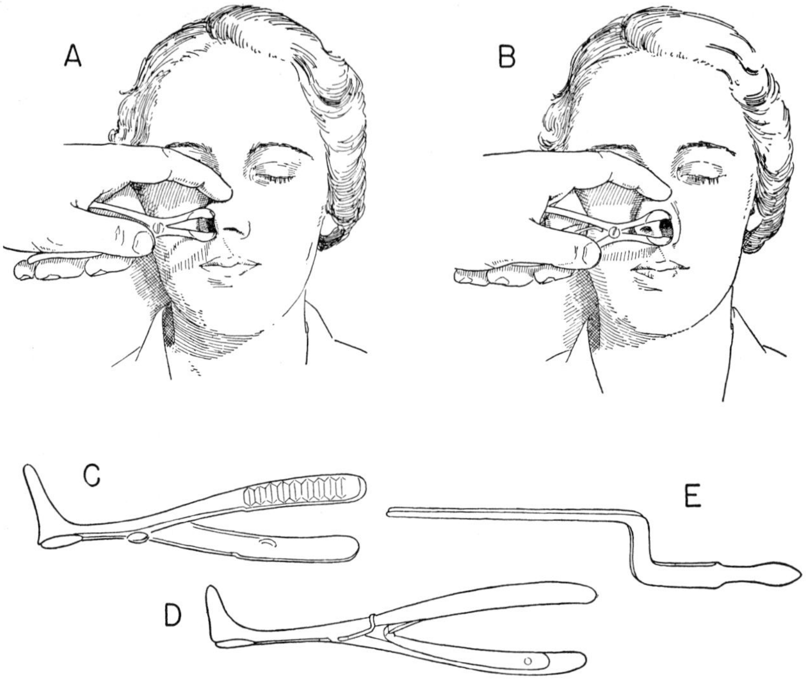

Figure 1. Examination of the nose with a speculum. *A* and *B*, Method of holding speculum. *C*, Adolescent's nasal speculum. *D*, Child's nasal speculum. *E*, Bayonet forceps (From Richards, L. G.: *Otolaryngology in General Practice,* Macmillan Co., 1939.)

Also, the examiner reconfirms the location of the cartilaginous septum where it joins the columellar skin and nasal spine. Next, one looks further into the nose, carefully noting the valve areas where the distal ends of the upper lateral cartilages are overlapped by the superior border of the alar cartilages. The angle between the medial and lateral crura of the alar cartilages is inspected.

The patent nasal fossae are generally equal in size but narrower than one would expect. Looking upward, one notes the anterior cartilaginous septum medially and the larger inferior turbinate and smaller middle turbinate laterally. The anterior inferior cartilaginous septum (Kiesselbach's area) is the most common site of nosebleeds in children and adults. The nasal mucosa is normally smooth, nonredundant and deep pink in color. Markedly edematous mucosa may be pale and bluish grey in color. When infected, the swollen mucosa may be red and injected. Pitting of the mucosa upon gentle pressure with a cotton-tipped nasal probe is indicative of edema.

Little, if any, mucus is seen in the normal nose, and when present, it is clear and slightly tenacious. Copious, clear, watery or tenacious mucus is generally indicative of allergic or viral rhinitis, whereas purulent secretions are more likely to denote acute bacterial rhinitis or rhinosinusitis. These secretions may be collected with a sterile cotton-tipped swab and sent for culture and sensitivity tests.

As one continues to examine the nasal septum superiorly and posteriorly, it is noted to be variable in thickness. It is frequently deviated to one or both sides in the manner of a C or S curve, but should not impinge on the turbinates. Inferiorly, near the floor of the nose, the cartilaginous septum joins the bony maxillary crest. At this junction, there is often a horizontal shelf or ridge, commonly called a spur. These spurs should not impinge on the inferior turbinate.

By looking laterally, one again notes the wing-shaped inferior turbinate projecting into the nasal fossa. The turbinates are generally wider anteriorly than posteriorly. They join the side walls of the nose by lateral extensions running the length of their superior borders. The inferior meatus, middle meatus and superior meatus are clefts found respectively under the inferior, middle and superior turbinates. To see the turbinates and their meati, one must look progressively upward. In so doing, one looks for exudates on the superior surface of the inferior turbinate, in the middle meatus, and on the superior border of the middle turbinates. These secretions are suggestive of sinus infection or stagnant mucus collections, such as noted in various stages of dryness or atrophy of the mucous membrane.

Only the anterior one-third of the nose can be visualized easily. In order to obtain further visualization, secretions must be suctioned away and shrinking solutions applied. This allows visualization of the remainder of the inferior and middle turbinates and their meati, the superior turbinate and meatus, the superior and posterior portions of the septum, the posterior choanae, the nasopharynx and portions of the nasal surface of the soft palate. Any polyps should be noted, especially if the history is suggestive of cystic fibrosis.

Mucosal shrinkage by vasoconstriction can be accomplished by spraying the nasal interior with 0.25 per cent Neo-Synephrine solution, using an atomizer and nasal speculum. Further vasoconstriction may be obtained by carefully placing cotton pledgets slightly moistened with a 5 per cent cocaine solution in the desired areas. One may prefer to use cotton-tipped nasal probes in a similar manner. Cocaine also provides topical anesthesia for any manipulation deemed necessary. Because cocaine and Pontocaine are extremely potent drugs, one may prefer to use 1 per cent xylocaine solution for topical anesthesia in children. By the judicious use of these anesthetic agents, painless biopsy of suspicious masses can be performed with a nasal biopsy forceps. This should be deferred until after posterior rhinoscopy and nasopharyngoscopy so as not to obscure the field with abnormal mucus flow or blood.

Posterior Rhinoscopy. Posterior rhinoscopy is by definition an examination of the nose from its posterior aspect, i.e., the nasopharynx. The light source, positioning, and use of the head mirror are as in anterior rhinoscopy. In some individuals this examination requires the use of a topical anesthetic, such as 2 per cent Pontocaine solution, applied with an atomizer to the oropharynx, tonsillar pillars and soft palate. One begins by warming a small postnasal (nasopharyngeal) mirror with an alcohol lamp (see Chapter 93). A safer method to prevent condensation of water vapor from expired air is to place a few drops of PhisoHex on the mirror and wipe it dry with a tissue or compress. This eliminates an open flame and thereby prevents accidental burns.

Next, one instructs the patient to open the mouth without protruding the tongue and to breathe through the mouth. Then a tongue blade is placed two-thirds of the way back on the tongue and depressed with gentle but firm pressure. Some examiners prefer a wooden tongue blade to a steel blade, for if it slips it will not chip the enamel of a tooth. One must not go too far posterior on the tongue, or he will gag the patient. The nasopharyngeal mirror with its reflecting surface upward is inserted into the mouth far posteriorly, avoiding contact with all structures. The patient is instructed to try to breathe through the nose and is reassured that he is doing a good job, even though it is nearly impossible to breathe through the nose with the mouth wide open. By attempting to breathe in this manner, the soft palate drops, and the examiner is afforded a view of the posterior nasal fossa and nasopharynx.

It is impossible to see all the structures at once in the mirror, so one must proceed systematically. One should first look for the posterior choanae and the vomer. The posterior ends of the inferior and middle turbinates can be seen first on one side and then the other. By relocating the vomer, one can follow it superiorly to look at the roof of the nasopharynx. Now the posterior pharyngeal wall is visualized. Finally one inspects the eustachian tube orifices and the fossae of Rosenmüller behind the tubal openings. It may be necessary to pass French catheters through the nares, pulling them out through the mouth. The catheters act as palate retractors, allowing excellent visualization of the posterior nose and nasopharynx. This procedure is quite uncomfortable for the patient, as is digital examination of the nasopharynx. Consequently, such procedures are not routinely performed, and at times they require general anesthesia for their accomplishment.

NASOPHARYNGOSCOPY. Nasopharyngoscopy is not routinely performed by most examiners. It does provide however a magnified but limited view of the fossae of Rosenmüller, the eustachian tube orifices and posterior portions of the inferior meatus and septum. In order to perform this examination, the floor of the nose is treated with cotton pledgets moistened with a topical anesthetic. The scope is then advanced along the floor of the nose to the posterior nasopharyngeal wall. One thus examines the structures by rotating and slowly withdrawing the scope.

EXAMINATION OF THE PARANASAL SINUSES

After inspecting the external nose and nasal fossae, further study of the paranasal sinuses is often necessary. As previously stated, visualization of the forehead, glabella and orbits is part of the initial evaluation. Tenderness, fullness and tumefaction of these areas as well as of the canine fossae are at times detected by palpation and percussion. Infraorbital paresthesia may result from trauma or tumor.

Transillumination of the paranasal sinuses is of limited value. It is performed in a dark room, using the least current necessary to transilluminate the frontal and maxillary sinuses (Fig. 2). The frontal sinuses are examined by placing the bulbs of the instrument against the floor of the frontal sinuses bilaterally. The area of contact is deep to the superior orbital margins along their medial aspects. Both sides can be illuminated simultaneously and compared to each other. The preferred method of transilluminating the maxillary sinuses is as follows. A clear plastic or glass hood that can be sterilized is placed over the bulbs and barrels of the transilluminator. This in turn is placed inside the mouth with the lips and jaws gently closed. Both infraorbital areas are normally illuminated and can be compared simultaneously. If there is a difference in the two sides, the less translucent side is suspected of harboring disease. Proper evaluation requires knowledge of the degree of development of each sinus at different ages.

Sinus x-rays are important when sinusitis or tumor is suspected. A standard sinus survey consists of four views. The Caldwell view is good to demonstrate the frontal and anterior ethmoid sinuses. The Waters view best demonstrates the maxillary sinuses. A lateral view shows the frontal and maxillary sinuses but is ordered primarily to demonstrate the sphenoid and posterior ethmoid sinuses, and a base view likewise is primarily for these sinuses. An upright view may show the fluid level. Radiologic findings such as mucosal thickening, soft tissue densities, air-fluid levels, and bony erosion are at times diagnostic, but more frequently they must be interpreted in the light of the history and physical examination.

The methods of sinus irrigation are more properly discussed under such topics as the diagnosis and treatment of acute and chronic sinusitis. Suffice it to say that after sinus x-rays are obtained, sinus irrigation may be utilized as a diagnostic and therapeutic modality.

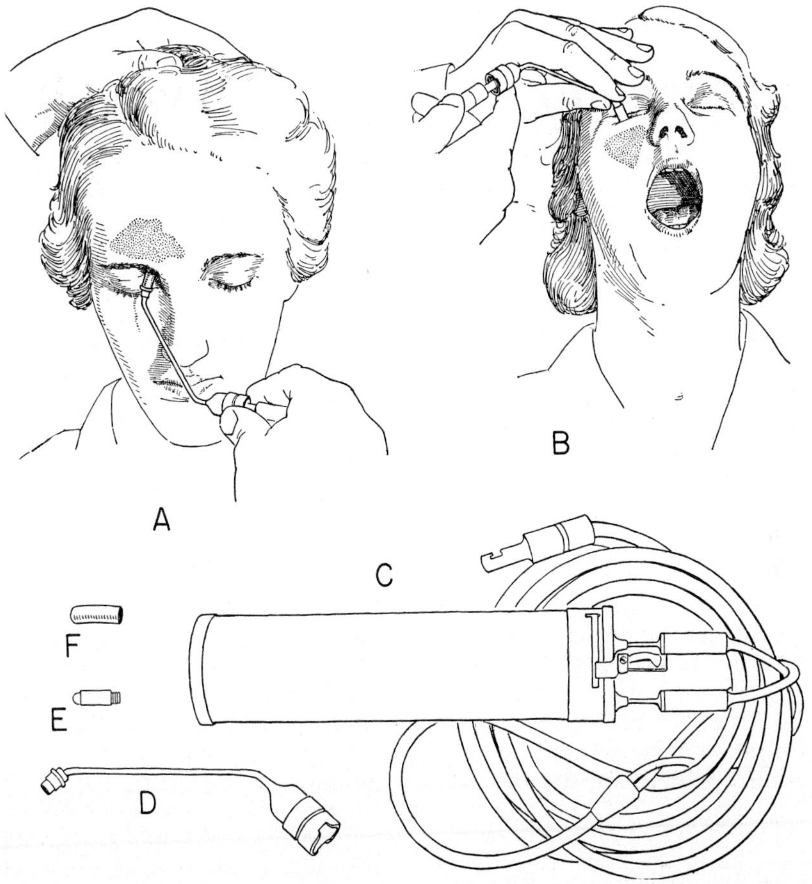

Figure 2. Transillumination of the nasal sinuses. *A*, Frontal sinus. *B*, Maxillary sinus (antrum). Note that the palate is illuminated on the examined side. *C*, Battery and cord. *D*, Briggs' transilluminator. *E*, Lamp (2.5 volt). *F*, Rubber sleeve for bulb to prevent dispersion of rays. (From Richards, L. G.: *Otolaryngology in General Practice*, MacMillan Co., 1939.)

Endoscopy through a previously made nasoantral window may be performed as an office procedure. If one is in doubt about the diagnosis, an operative procedure such as a nasoantral window or a Caldwell-Luc approach should be performed. At times this is the only way to diagnose early carcinoma of the sinus interior before bony erosion of the sinus wall occurs.

REFERENCE

Boies, L.: *Fundamentals of Otolaryngology.*, Philadelphia, W. B. Saunders Co., 1964.

Chapter Seventy-Six

CONGENITAL MALFORMATIONS

GEORGE H. GIFFORD, JR., M.D., and DONALD W. MacCOLLUM, M.D.

ANATOMY

The nose occupies the central and most conspicuous portion of the face. It is made up of bony and cartilaginous framework represented by the paired nasal bones above and the upper lateral cartilages below, meeting in the midline and supported by the bony and cartilaginous septum. Inferior to the upper lateral cartilages, the alar cartilages (lower lateral) are paired with a medial and lateral crus surrounding each nostril and giving it support and shape. The two medial crura are adjacent and contained in the columella between the two nostrils.

EMBRYOLOGY

The nose develops rostral to the oral fossa, and the first (mandibular) branchial arch. The major contribution of the dorsum is from the frontal prominence. At the beginning of the second month the medial and lateral nasal processes separate to circle the paired olfactory pits, which in turn become deepened, breaking through into the upper part of the oral cavity by the middle of the second month (Patten, 1968). At about the ninth week, the septal process, growing inferiorly, meets the two palatine processes, growing medially, in the midline. Fusion of these three processes progresses posteriorly from the primary palate at the incisive foramen, separating the nasal cavity from the oral cavity and dividing the anterior nasopharynx into halves. Comprehension of the embryology of the nose helps explain some of the rather bizarre congenital anomalies discussed in this chapter.

MALFORMATIONS

Complete Nasal Absence

Complete absence of the nose and nasal airway is extremely rare (Wahby, 1903-4; Davis, 1919; Walker, 1961). The authors have treated two such cases, both of whom had high-arched anterior palates in place of the completely absent anterior nasopharynx. Both of these children learned to mouth-breathe, but feeding was a problem. A nasal airway was established in each case (Fig. 1). A prosthetic nose will be replaced by complete nasal reconstruction after full growth has been attained.

Partial Absence

Partial absence of the nose (unilateral alar notching or alar coloboma) is rare, but it is relatively more common than complete nasal absence. In a report of rare facial clefts in 1965, Fogh-Andersen noted an experience of four nasal coloboma deformities out of 3988 consecutive cases of facial clefts seen over 30 years. Repair is by either composite auricular graft or flap reconstruction, depending on the amount of tissue required. This deformity is often associated with hypertelorism (increased distance between the eyes) (Fig. 2).

Unilateral hypoplasia with stenosis of one nostril is occasionally seen (Fig. 3). After revision, the use of an indwelling

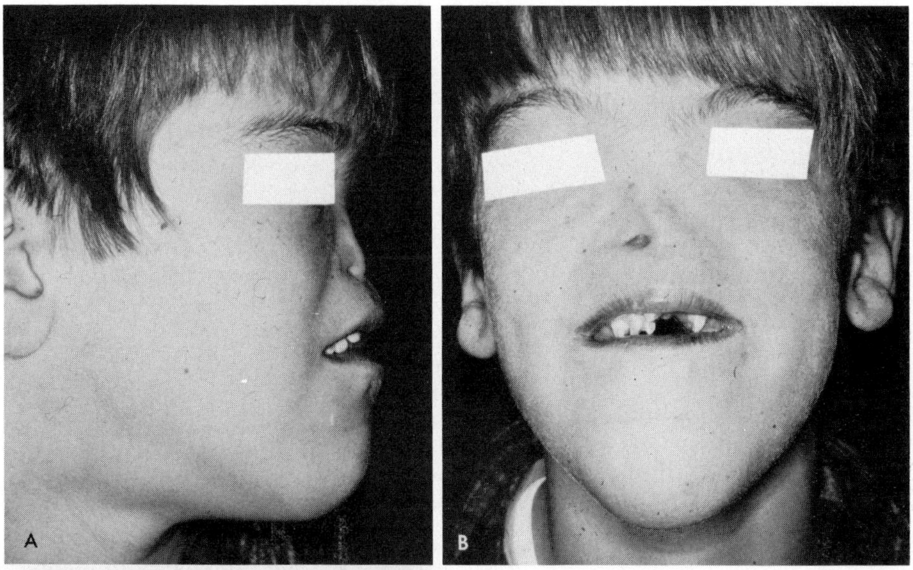

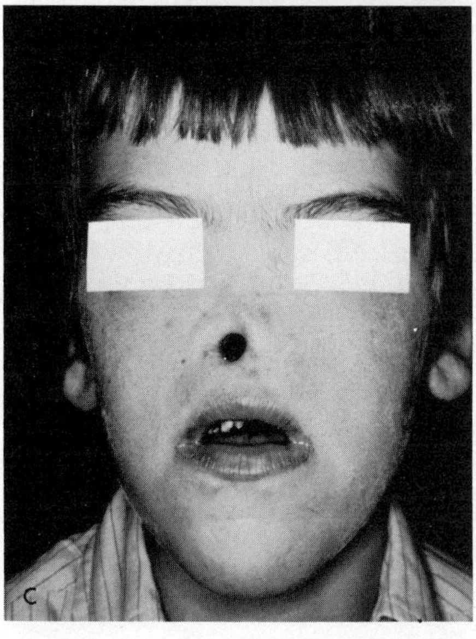

Figure 1. *A* and *B*, Complete absence of nose and nasal airway (congenital). *C*, Postsurgical reconstruction of airway.

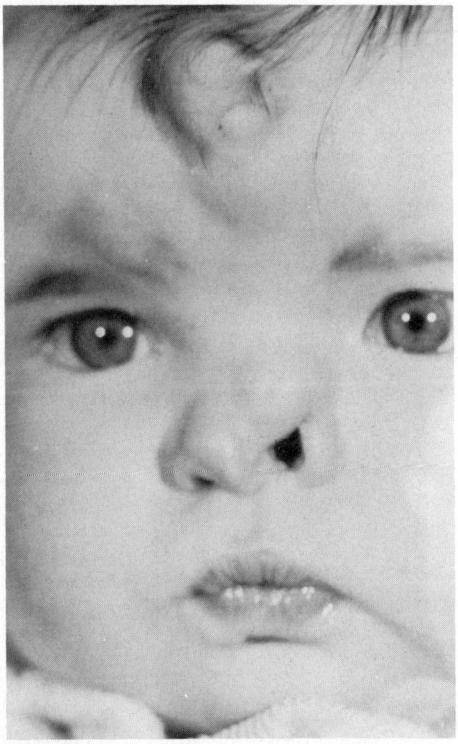

Figure 2. Unilateral alar notching (alar coloboma).

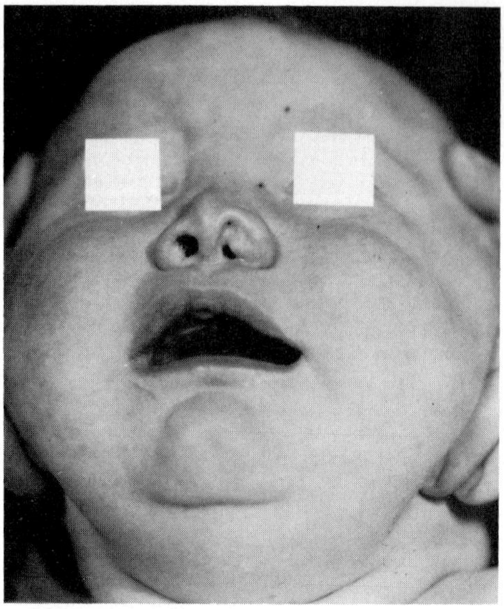

Figure 3. Congenital stenosis of left nostril.

molded prosthesis protects against restenosis (Bajaj, 1946).

Cleft (or Paired) Nose

Median clefts of the nose are as rare as lateral clefts (Fogh-Andersen, 1965). They range in severity from a simple cleft of the tip of the nose, with bifid alar cartilages (Fig. 4) (Burian, 1960), to a more severe separation frequently associated with hypertelorism (Webster, 1950), to association with a midline cleft of the lip (Fig. 5) (Weaver, 1946), to complete absence of the premaxilla with hypertelorism and separation of the paired nasal halves by a wide midline cleft of both lip and nose (Kazajian, 1959).

According to DeMyer (1967), if orbital hypertelorism is associated with cleft deformity, the likelihood of normal or near normal mentality is high. If extreme hypertelorism is present unassociated with a facial cleft, or associated with extracephalic anomalies such as brevicollis, then the probability of mental retardation is high. Soft tissue repair with closure of associated midline cleft lip sometimes requires wedge-shaped excision of midline tissue in order to approximate the paired alar and upper lateral cartilages. This may be done in infancy, although in more severe cases further plastic surgery may be required. Direct operative attack on the underly-

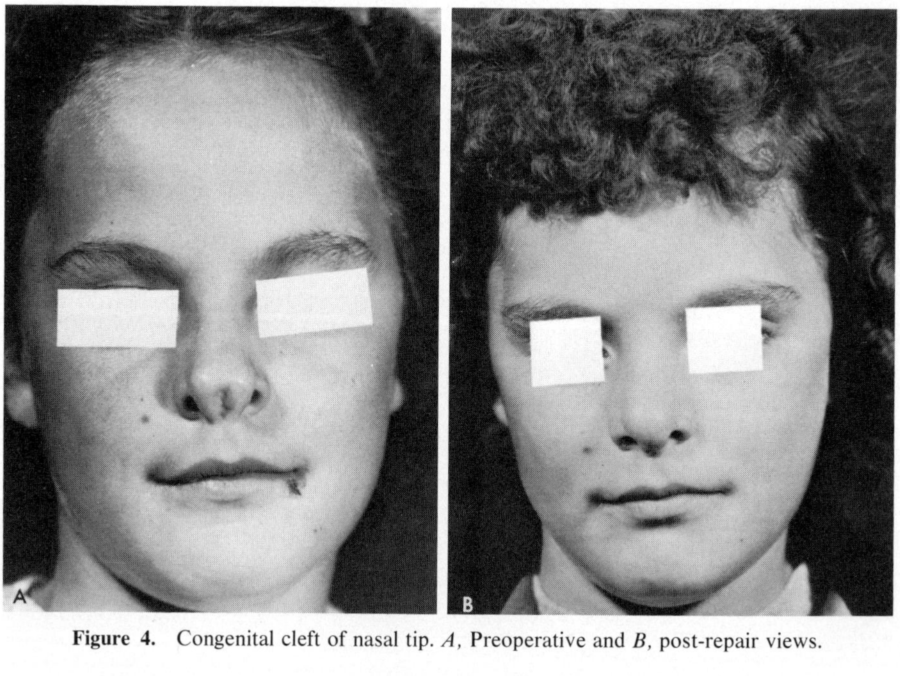

Figure 4. Congenital cleft of nasal tip. *A*, Preoperative and *B*, post-repair views.

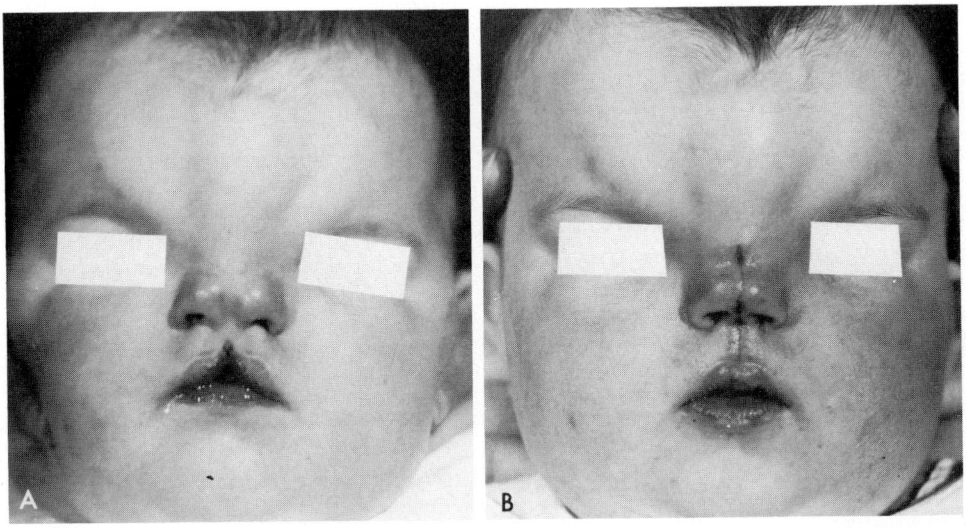

Figure 5. *A*, Congenital midline cleft of both lip and nose. *B*, Same patient shortly after surgical repair.

ing bone malformation with hypertelorism usually is not carried out until the patient has gained full growth.

Proboscis Lateralis

Proboscis lateralis, a congenital tubular prominence arising from the inner canthus of the eye and associated with hypoplasia of the ipsilateral side of the nose, is very rare (Biber, 1949; Rao, 1963; Coetzee, 1964; Binns, 1969). It is difficult to determine the exact embryologic explanation of this bizarre anomaly; however, it is probably related to imperfect mesodermal proliferation in the frontonasal and maxillary processes after the olfactory pits have formed, so that the nasolacrimal apparatus never connects with the nose. A strange skin-lined tube is the result (Fig. 6). Most authors advise using the tissue of the

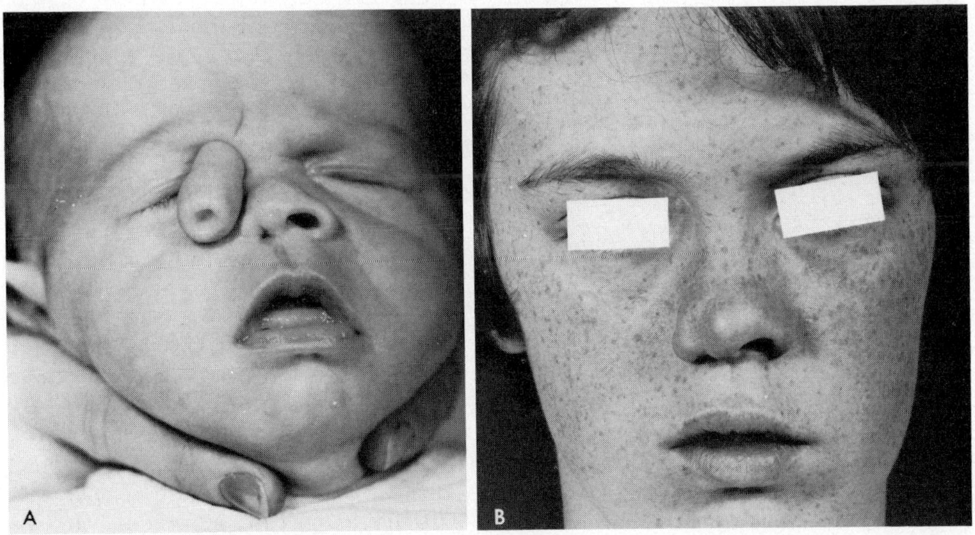

Figure 6. *A*, Congenital tubular prominence (proboscis lateralis), age 3 weeks. *B*, Postoperative staged reconstruction, age 15 years.

tubular prominence to reconstruct the ipsilateral hypoplastic nose that usually accompanies the deformity.

Central Hypoplasia

Complete absence of prolabium and premaxilla (primary palate) may give the appearance of a wide midline cleft of the lip with absent columella and lack of nasal support (Fig. 7). Fogh-Andersen (1965) reports such a case. With any such severe cleft, particularly if associated with polydactyly and microphthalmus, one should suspect a chromosomal abnormality such as Bartholin-Patau syndrome (13–15 trisomy). (Patau, 1960; Warburg, 1963). If a 13–15 trisomy does exist, prognosis for the child is poor, and surgery is not indicated. However, this severe type of deformity can exist in an otherwise normal child. Reconstruction is difficult because of a lack of nasal framework and a paucity of tissue. Silicone tubes in the reconstructed nostrils during the postoperative period may be life-saving in order to maintain a satisfactory airway.

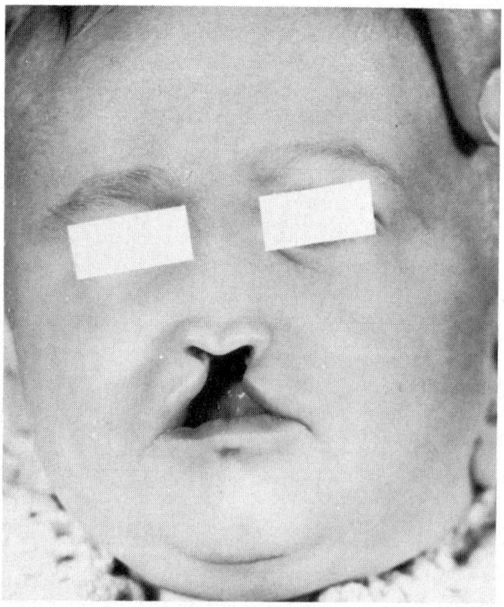

Figure 7. Congenital absence of prolabium and premaxilla (age 7 months).

Generalized Facial Dysostoses

Generalized congenital facial deformities, such as Treacher-Collins syndrome, show the characteristic nasal deformity of a deficient frontonasal angle and a depressed nasal tip, giving the characteristic fishlike profile, Crouzon's disease (hereditary craniofacial dysostosis) has a characteristic parrot's-beak nose. These two hereditary dysostoses will be discussed in greater detail elsewhere. Apert's syndrome (acrocephalosyndactylism) produces a nose deformity not unlike that in Crouzon's disease. Cosmetic rhinoplasty after full growth can be of significant benefit in improving facial appearance in these three syndromes.

Cleft Lip and Nose Deformity

Unilateral congenital cleft lip is seen in approximately 1 of 10,000 live births. Depending on the severity of the cleft, there is a greater or a lesser degree of associated nasal deformity. As the nose and lip are formed by fusion of five components (the median frontonasal process, and paired maxillary and lateral nasal processes converging from each side), it is understandable that the nose shares in the deformity caused by this anomaly of embryogenesis with the subadjacent lip.

The original simple cleft lip repairs described by Rose (1912) and Thompson (1921) were later largely replaced by flap repairs such as those performed by Blair-Brown-Mireault (1950) and Hagedorn-LeMesurier (1955). Later innovations and modifications of cleft repair were made by Skoog (1958), Millard (1958) and Randall (1958). The earlier cleft repairs, although frequently giving a very satisfactory lip repair, left something to be desired with regard to the nose in the more severe cases. More recent repairs have devoted much more attention to the nose, and the initial results have been much more satisfactory (MacCollum, 1957). Skoog (1970) advocates reposition of the deformed alar cartilage as part of the original cleft lip

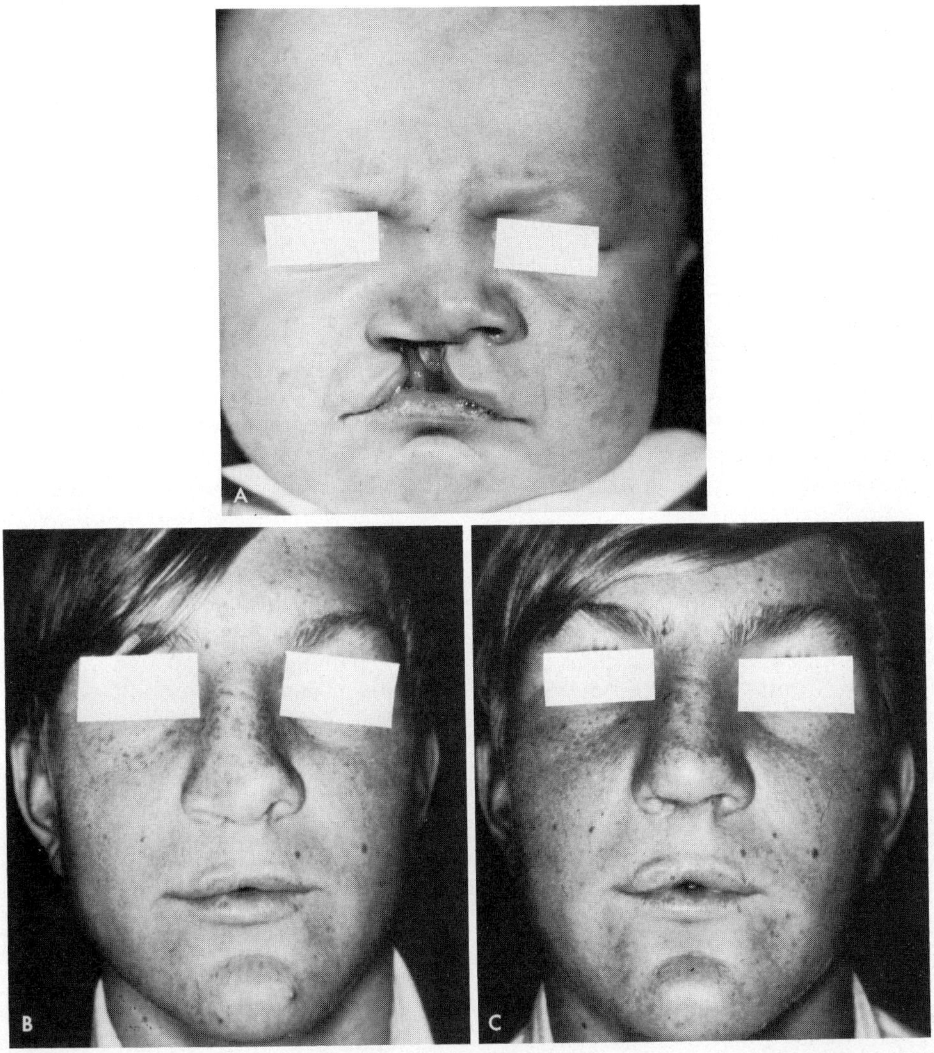

Figure 8. *A*, Right complete cleft lip deformity, age 5 weeks, preoperative lip repair. *B*, Residual cleft lip–nose deformity, age 16 years. *C*, Postoperative alar cartilage suspension with cartilage graft.

repair. It is unlikely, however, that a completely satisfactory primary repair of the cleft lip nose will ever be achieved in the more severe cases. McIndoe (1959) pointed out that even if perfect positioning of the alar cartilages were possible, the surgeon would still be confronted by the uncertainties of changes with growth. It is indeed a very real possibility that too aggressive primary surgery with extensive cartilage dissection to attain satisfactory anatomic positioning would cause scarring, and there is the possibility of decreased blood supply, which might in itself be an adverse factor affecting future growth.

The pathologic anatomy of the unilateral cleft lip nose described by Huffman in 1949 is represented by prolapse of the involved alar cartilage so that it occupies a position inferior and lateral in comparison to its normal neighbor. The junction of the alar portion of the nose with the face is frequently lateral and inferior in the degree dependent on the skill with which the original cleft lip repair was performed. The septum may be significantly deviated, causing posterior obstruction, usually on the side of the deformity, although the foot of the septum may present in the normal nostril anteriorly, causing asymmetry of the columella. The floor of the involved nostril is frequently wide and depressed.

The double cleft lip nose has a characteristic porcine deformity with a blunted nasal tip, relative absence of the columella, obliteration of the normal nasolabial angle, and wide, flaring nostrils.

The time for secondary repair of these deformities depends on the degree of the deformity and the psychological effect on the growing child. In general, a severe deformity justifies corrective surgery at an earlier age, even though with growth a secondary revision may be necessary. Correction of a less severe deformity can wait until growth of the nose is complete.

A variety of procedures to correct unilateral cleft lip–nose deformities have been described, with excellent contributions by Straith (1946), Erich (1953), Musgrave (1960) and Rees (1966). The double cleft lip–nose deformity can be ingeniously corrected by a columella lengthening procedure, using a forked flap as described by Millard (1958) (Fig. 9). Brauer (1966) advocates a bipedicle flap procedure to lengthen the columella and narrow the nasal tip. McIndoe (1959) describes an extensive revision combined with osteoplastic rhinoplasty and should therefore be reserved until the patient has attained full growth. Converse (1964) advocates combining columella lengthening with a lip switch flap as originally described by Abbe (1898). If necessary, he augments the nasal dorsal ridge with a split rib bone graft. A great deal can and should be done for these children with cleft lip–nose deformities. Each case varies considerably, and the plastic surgeon must have a wide choice of procedures, and be willing to individualize his approach to suit the circumstances.

Dermoid Cysts of the Nose

Congenital dermoid cysts or sinuses involving the nose are relatively rare (12.9 per cent of head and neck dermoids in a series reported by New in 1937). They usually present at birth or in the first few months of life (Taylor, 1967; McLean, 1964; Littlewood, 1961; Crawford, 1952; Johnson, 1964).

Luongo explained formation of the cysts as a defect occurring in the third month of embryonic development when bony transformation of the cartilaginous portion of the frontonasal process was taking place. He felt that small portions of epithelium became sequestrated, developing into a cyst or a sinus, depending on whether or not an external communication existed. Brunner (1942) reported a case of dermoid associated with midline dermoid of the forehead and glabella as well as a bifid nasal tip. New (1937) had one case associated with a midline cleft lip. These associated deformities would seem to indicate an embryologic pathogenesis for dermoid cysts. Although cases are usually isolated, a familial incidence has been reported (New, 1937; Khan, 1970).

One should suspect the possibility of a dermoid cyst in any discrete swelling of the nose in the newborn infant. The usual location is midline, overlying the nasal bones, often causing depression and distortion of the nasal framework (Fig. 10). Occasionally, however, the lesion can be asymmetrical, and even present in a nostril, causing airway obstruction (Fig. 11). The lesion is usually relatively mobile, and not fixed to the skin. When a sinus tract exists, the diagnosis may be easily made if sebaceous material can be expressed, or if hairs present in the opening of the tract.

Complete excision may be difficult because of deep extension of the lesion, which often extends into the region of the nasal septum (Crawford, 1952). McLean (1964) found extension to the cribriform plate in six of ten nasal dermoids. Intracranial extension has also been reported (Tiwari, 1967), although this complication is much less common than in occipital dermoids (Matson, 1969). New (1937), McLean (1964), Crawford (1952) and Taylor (1967) all

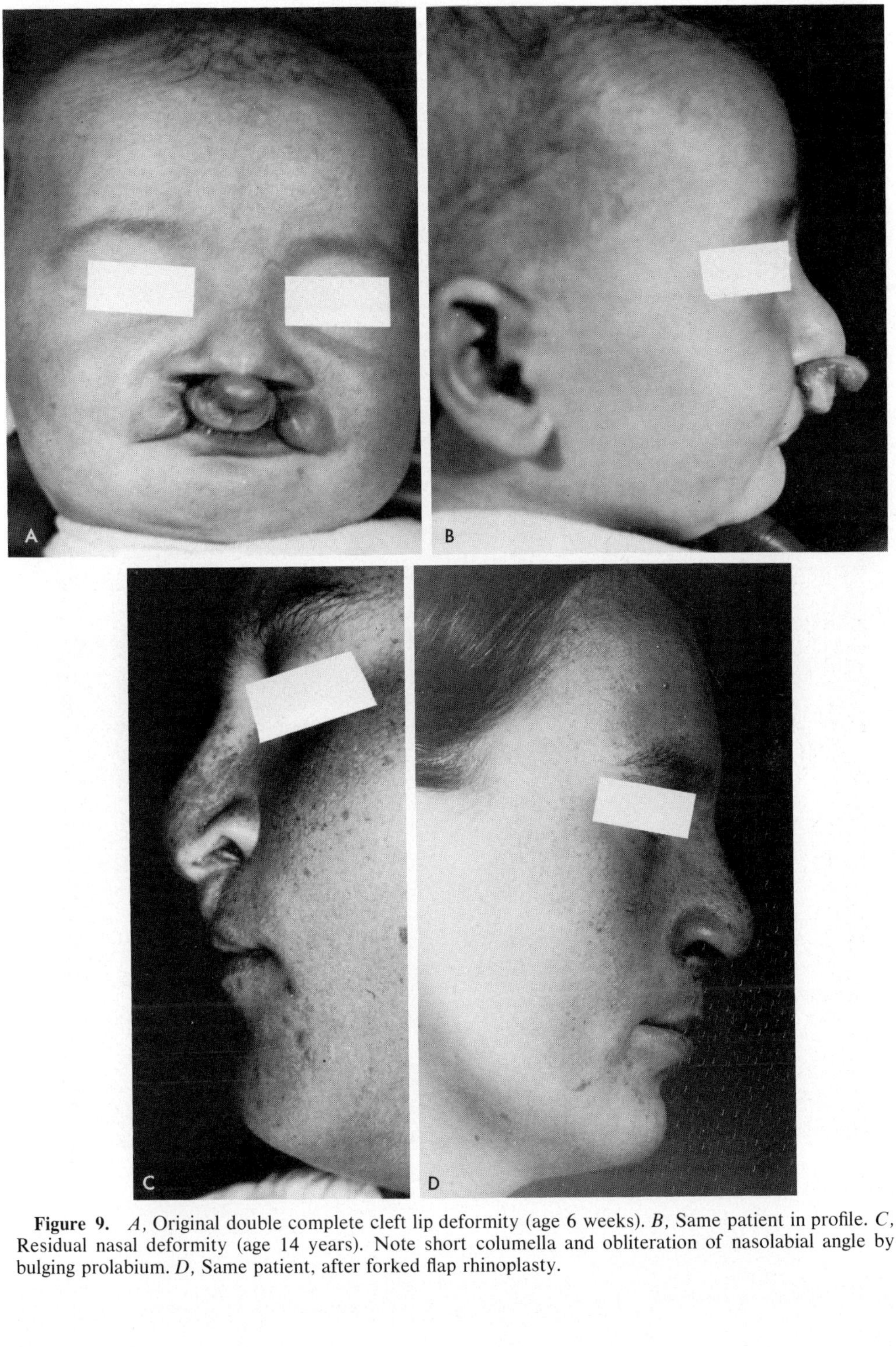

Figure 9. *A*, Original double complete cleft lip deformity (age 6 weeks). *B*, Same patient in profile. *C*, Residual nasal deformity (age 14 years). Note short columella and obliteration of nasolabial angle by bulging prolabium. *D*, Same patient, after forked flap rhinoplasty.

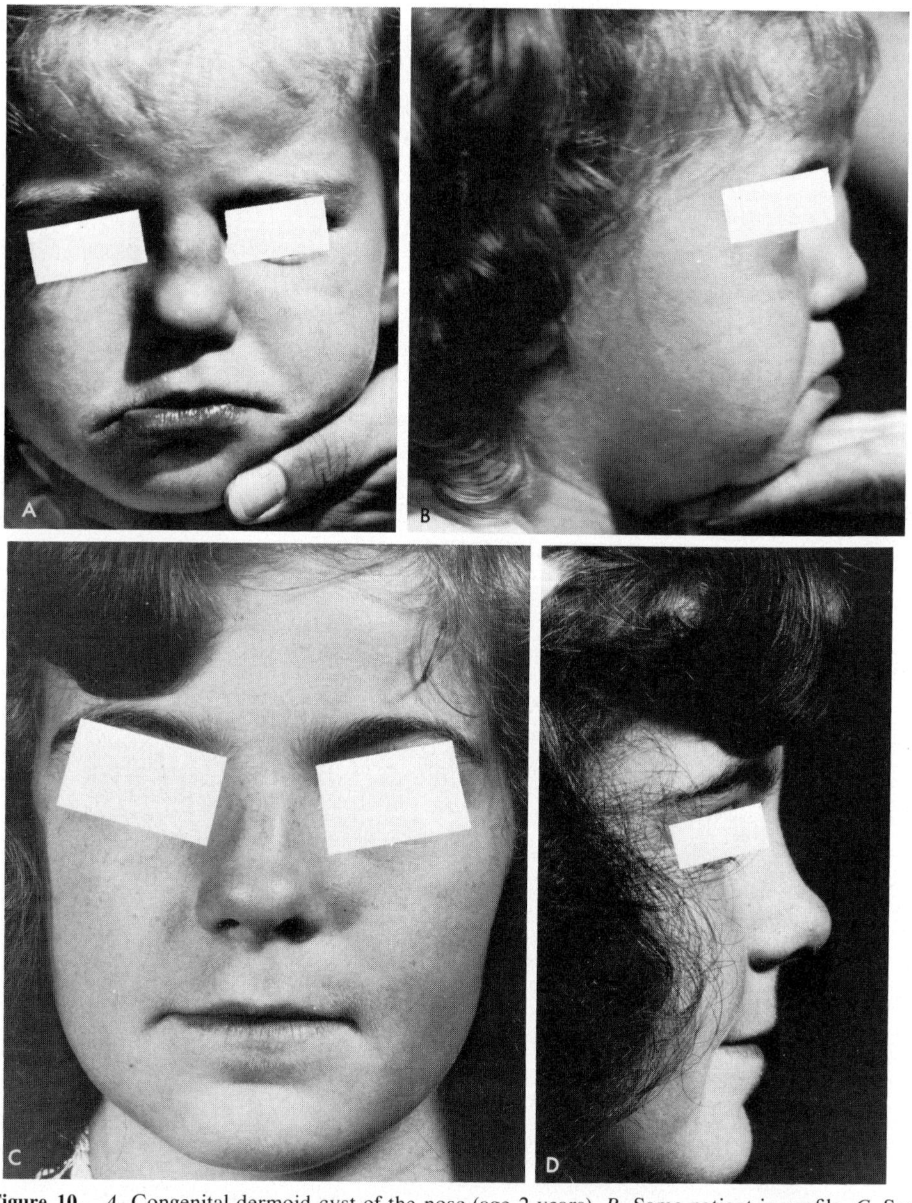

Figure 10. *A,* Congenital dermoid cyst of the nose (age 2 years). *B,* Same patient in profile. *C,* Same patient after operative excision (age 10 years). *D,* Same patient in profile.

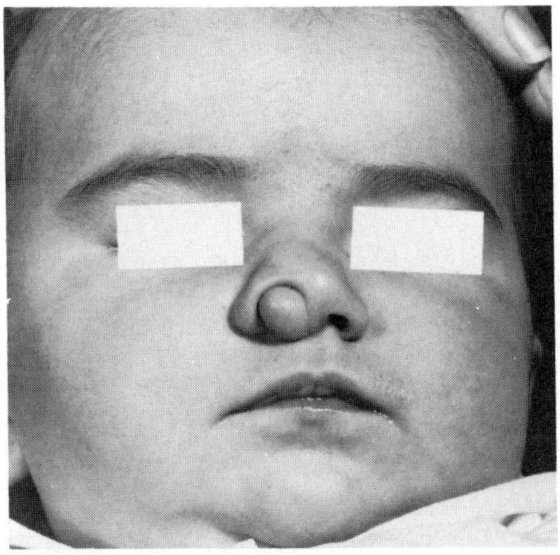

Figure 11. Dermoid cyst, obstructing the right nostril.

found a high incidence of previous surgery in their series, which seemed to underline the importance of complete surgical resection.

As Khan (1970) pointed out, x-rays should be ordered, as they may show separation of the nasal bones, bone destruction or broadened or bifid septum. Matson (1969) noted that a cyst with an intracranial extension shows a characteristic smooth, rounded area of decreased density. Radiopaque injection of the sinus tract may be helpful, but it is often difficult to delineate the full extension of involvement. Excision should be complete even if it requires multiple step-ladder incisions to give adequate exposure to follow a sinus tract to its termination.

Encephaloceles

Nasal encephaloceles are extra protrusions of meningeal-lined brain substance that communicate freely with intracranial ventricular substances or subarachnoid area (Bloomfield, 1965). The incidence is rare. Matson notes that of 1157 spinal lesions viewed at the Children's Hospital Medical Center there were only 187 encephaloceles, and of these, only 21 were nasofrontal. Bloomfield quoted the incidence of encephaloceles in general as 1 in 4000 births, with only 10 per cent being of a nasal variety. Of nasal encephaloceles, 60 per cent present on the bridge of the nose (Fig. 12), 30 per cent are internal high in the nasal vault, and 10 per cent are a combination of both (Ziter, 1969). The anomaly seems to be somewhat more common in Southeast Asia (Suwanwela, 1966), and it is postulated that perhaps the flat, widened intercanthal area of the

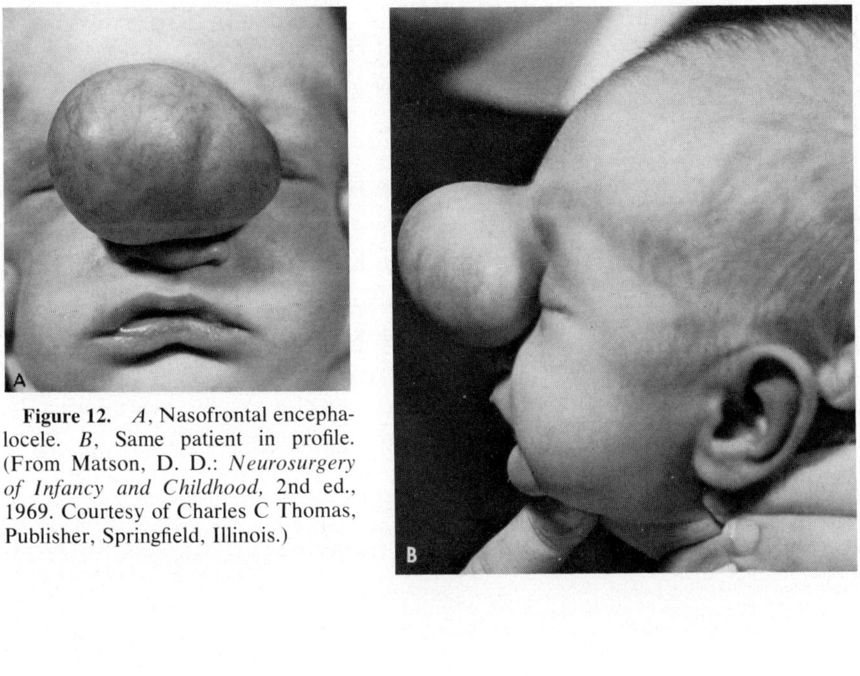

Figure 12. *A*, Nasofrontal encephalocele. *B*, Same patient in profile. (From Matson, D. D.: *Neurosurgery of Infancy and Childhood,* 2nd ed., 1969. Courtesy of Charles C Thomas, Publisher, Springfield, Illinois.)

Oriental skull is somewhat predisposed to the anomaly. Odeku (1967) feels that encephaloceles are more common in the Nigerian population.

The lesion seems to be the result of defective closure of the anterior neuropore occurring at the beginning of the fourth week after fertilization (Millen, 1963). Applying pressure to the extranasal lesion may cause somnolence or even seizure. Hypertelorism is usually present, but this does not necessarily rule out nasal dermoid, which also can show this finding.

Appropriate x-rays may be helpful. A basal (submental vertical) projection may show a transsphenoidal type of bony defect at the base of the skull, often associated with intranasal encephaloceles (Pollock, 1969). Transethmoidal communications may be more difficult to demonstrate, requiring tomography and pneumoencephalography (Pollock, 1968; Bierbaum, 1968).

McGillicuddy (1942), Jones (1962), and Luyendijk (1969) have all mentioned the possibility of rhinorrhea after intranasal "polypectomy." If a rare intranasal encephalocele has been amputated unwittingly, with a resultant cerebral spinal fluid leak, meningitis will certainly occur unless antibiotic treatment and closure of the dural leak is performed.

Treatment involves complete excision of the lesion with plastic surgical closure for the external deformity. Neurosurgical closure of the dural defect, if large, may require a fascial graft. The best exposure for dural closure seems to be through an intracranial approach via a bifrontal craniotomy (Davis, 1959).

REFERENCES

1. Abbe, R.: A new plastic operation for the relief of deformity due to harelip. *Med. Rec.*, 53:477, 1898.
2. Bajaj, P. S., and Bailey, B. N.: Stenosis of the nostrils: A report of three cases. *Brit. J. Plast. Surg.*, 22:269, 1969.
3. Bierbaum, L. M., and Owsley, J. Q., Jr.: Frontonasal tumors of neurogenic origin. *Plast. Reconstr. Surg.*, 41:462, 1968.
4. Binns, J. H.: Congenital tubular nostril (proboscis lateralis). *Brit. J. Plast. Surg.*, 22:265, 1969.
5. Blumenfeld, R., and Skolnik, E. M.: Intranasal encephaloceles. *Arch. Otolaryng.*, 82:527, 1965.
6. Brauer, R. O., and Foerster, D. W.: Another method to lengthen the columella in the double cleft patient. *Plast. Reconstr. Surg.*, 38:27, 1966.
7. Brunner, H., and Harned, J. W.: Dermoid cysts of the dorsum of the nose. *Arch. Otolaryng.*, 36:86, 1942.
8. Burian, F.: Median clefts of the nose. *Acta Chir. Plast.*, 2:180, 1960.
9. Coetzee, T.: Proboscis lateralis: A rare facial anomaly. *South African J. Lab. Clin. Med.*, 10:81, 1964.
10. Converse, J. M., Horowtiz, S. L., Guy, C. L., and Woodsmith, D.: Surgical-orthodontic correction in the bilateral cleft palate. *Cleft Palate J.*, 1:153, 1964.
11. Crawford, J. K., and Webster, J. P.: Congenital dermoid cysts of the nose. *Plast. Reconstr. Surg.*, 9:235, 1952.
12. Davis, C. H., Jr., and Alexander, E., Jr.: Congenital nasofrontal encephalomeningoceles and teratomas. Review of seven cases. *J. Neurosurg.*, 16:365, 1959.
13. Davis, J. S.: *Plastic Surgery: Its Principals and Practice*. Philadelphia, Blakiston Co., 1919, pp. 490–491.
14. DeMyer, W.: The median cleft lip syndrome: Differential diagnosis of cranium bifidum occultum, hypertelorism and median cleft nose, lip and palate. *Neurology*, 17:961, 1967.
15. Erich, J. B.: A technique for correcting a flat nostril in cases of repaired harelip. *Plast. Reconstr. Surg.*, 12:320, 1953.
16. Fogh-Andersen, P.: Rare clefts of the face. *Acta Chir. Scandinav.*, 129:275, 1965.
17. Huffman, W. C., and Lierle, D. M.: Studies on the pathologic anatomy of the unilateral harelip-nose. *Plast. Reconstr. Surg.*, 4:225, 1949.
18. Johnson, C. F., and Weisman, P. A.: Radiological features of dermoid cysts of the nose. *Radiology*, 82:1016, 1964.
19. Jones, R. E., Bennington, J. L., and Warner, N. E.: Encephalocele masquerading as nasal polyp. *J.A.M.A.*, 181:640, 1962.
20. Kazanjian, V. H.: Treatment of dermoid cysts of the nose. *Plast. Reconstr. Surg.*, 21:169, 1958.
21. Kazanjian, V. H., and Holmes, E. M.: Treatment of median cleft associated with bifid nose and hypertelorism. *Plast. Reconstr. Surg.*, 24:582, 1959.
22. Khan, M. A., and Gibb, A. G.: Median dermoid cysts of the nose, familial occurrence. *J. Laryngol.*, 84:709, 1970.

23. Littlewood, A. H. N.: Congenital nasal dermoid cysts and fistulas. *Plast. Reconstr. Surg.,* 27:471, 1961.
24. Luongo, R. A.: Dermoid cyst of the nasal dorsum. *Arch. Otolaryng.,* 17:755, 1933.
25. Luyendijk, W.: Intranasal encephaloceles. A survey of eight neurosurgically treated cases. *Psychiat. Neurol. Neurochir.,* 72:77, 1969.
26. MacCollum, D. W., and Richardson, S. O.: Management of the patient with cleft lip and cleft palate. *Pediatrics,* 20:573, 1957.
27. Macomber, W. F., and Wang, M. K.: Congenital neoplasms of the nose. *Plast. Reconstr. Surg.,* 11:215, 1953.
28. Matson, D. D.: *Neurosurgery of Infancy and Childhood.* Springfield, Ill., Charles C Thomas, 1969.
29. McGillicuddy, O. B.: Encephalomeningoceles in the nasal cavity. *Ann. Otol. Rhinol. Laryngol.,* 51:516, 1942.
30. McIndoe, A., and Rees, T. O.: Synchronous repair of secondary deformities in cleft lip and cleft nose. *Plast. Reconstr. Surg.,* 24:150, 1959.
31. McLean, G. E., Broadbent, T. R., and Woolf, R. M.: Dermoid cysts of the nose. *Amer. Surg.,* 30:203, 1964.
32. Millard, D. R., Jr.: Columella lengthening by a forked flap. *Plast. Reconstr. Surg.,* 22:454, 1958.
33. Millen, J. W.: Timing of human congenital malformations. *Develop. Med. Child Neurol.,* 5:343, 1963.
34. Musgrave, R. H., and Dupertuis, S. M.: Revision of the unilateral cleft lip and nostril. *Plast. Reconstr. Surg.,* 25:223, 1960.
35. New, G. B., and Erich, J. B.: Dermoid cysts of the head and neck. *Surg. Gynec. Obstet.,* 65:48, 1937.
36. Odeku, E. L.: Congenital malformations of the cerebrospinal axis seen in Western Nigeria. The African child with "encephaloce." *Int. Surg.,* 48:52, 1967.
37. Patau, K., Therman, E., Smith, D. W., Inhorn, S. L., and Wagner, H. P.: Multiple congenital anomaly caused by an extra autosome. *Lancet,* 1:790, 1960.
38. Patten, B. M.: *Human Embryology,* 3rd Ed. New York, McGraw-Hill, 1968.
39. Pollock, J. A., Newton, T. H., and Hoyt, W. F.: Transsphenoidal and transethmoidal encephaloceles. *Radiology,* 90:442, 1968.
40. Pratt, L. W.: Midline cysts of the nasal dorsum: Embryologic origin and treatment. *Laryngoscope,* 75:968, 1965.
41. Rees, T. D., Guy, C. L., and Converse, J. M.: Repair of the cleft lip–nose. *Plast. Reconstr. Surg.,* 37:47, 1966.
42. Skoog, T.: Repair of unilateral cleft lip deformity: Maxilla, nose and lip. *Scand. J. Plast. Reconstr. Surg.,* 2:109, 1969.
43. Straith, C.: Elongation of the nasal columella. *Plast. Reconstr. Surg.,* 1:79, 1946.
44. Suwanwela, C., and Hongsatrabhas, C.: Frontoethmoidal encephalomeningocele. *J. Neurosurg.,* 25:172, 1966.
45. Taylor, B. W., and Erich, J. B.: Dermoid cysts of the nose. *Proc. Mayo Clin.,* 42:488, 1967.
46. Tiwari, R. M.: Dermoid cyst with tubular bifurcation and dermal sinus. *Post-Grad. Med. J.,* 43:550, 1967.
47. Wahby, B.: Congenital absence of the nose and premaxilla. *J. Anat.,* 38:49, 1903–04.
48. Walker, D. G.: Malformations of the Face. Edinborough, E. & S. Livingstone, Ltd., 1961.
49. Warburg, M., and Mikhelaen, M.: A case of 12–15 trisomy or Bartholin-Patau's syndrome. *Acta Ophthal.,* 41:321, 1963.
50. Weaver, D. F., and Bellinger, D. H.: Bifid nose associated with midline cleft of the upper lip. *Arch. Otol.,* 44:48, 1946.
51. Webster, J. P., and Deming, E. G.: Surgical treatment of the bifid nose. *Plast. Reconstr. Surg.,* 6:1, 1950.
52. Ziter, F. M. H., and Bramwit, D. N.: Nasal encephaloceles and gliomas. *Brit. J. Radiol.,* 43:136, 1970.

Chapter Seventy-Seven

TUMORS OF THE NOSE AND PARANASAL SINUS

GEORGE H. GIFFORD, JR., M.D., and DONALD W. MacCOLLUM, M.D.

BENIGN TUMORS

Nasal Gliomata

Nasal glioma in the newborn may present with a picture like that of nasal encephalocele or congenital dermoid cyst (Fig. 1). It is rare; in 1950 Black found only 34 documented cases, and in 1963 Smith found 55.[4, 50] O'Brien[39] estimated the number at 100, with five cases added by Lowe.[27] As with encephalocele, the majority of gliomas present extranasally (55 per cent), 35 per cent are seen intranasally, and 10 per cent are a combination of the above.[27]

Willis felt that the embryology of this congenital tumor is closely allied to that of an encephalocele (see Chapter 76) and that it is a primary anomaly of growth and separation of the neural tube.[57] Gliomas are different from congenital encephaloceles in that they do not freely communicate with either the ventricular system or the subarachnoid space. During development, the neural tissue presumably becomes completely sequestrated, and separates from the rest of the central nervous system. In a certain percentage of patients, however, there is a stalk of cells that passes through a hole in the cribriform area and is connected to the brain.

Smith felt that 14 of the 48 cases he studied had intracranial connections.[50] He submitted tissue from both intracranial and extracranial portions of one such lesion to both light and electron microscopy, which showed the tissue to be remarkably similar, strongly suggesting a common origin.

There is no evidence of malignancy or malignant transformation in any of these cases. There is some difference of opinion as to whether the lesion should be considered a congenital anomaly or a benign neoplasm. Many authors have observed the phenomenon of recurrence.[4, 27, 50] Presumably this was due to inadequate primary excision, but it does seem to indicate that this benign tumor has some capacity for neoplasia.

The extranasal glioma is a firm, slightly movable subcutaneous mass that may be attached to the skin of the nose but does not transilluminate, pulsate or change in size with pressure. There is a variable degree of distortion of cartilage and bone. The intranasal glioma (as with the intranasal encephalocele) may cause total or relative obstruction and can be confused with a nasal polyp, although polyps are so rare in early childhood (except in cystic fibrosis) that this confusion probably should not arise.

As with encephaloceles and dermoids, if there is a question of intracranial communication, careful x-ray examination of the cribriform plate area should be done, including laminograms if necessary. If communication exists, treatment should involve intracranial exposure through a bifrontal lobotomy, so that the stalk may be divided without cerebrospinal fluid leak. The lesion itself may then be removed entirely at a second operative procedure.[50] If there is no evidence of intracranial communication,

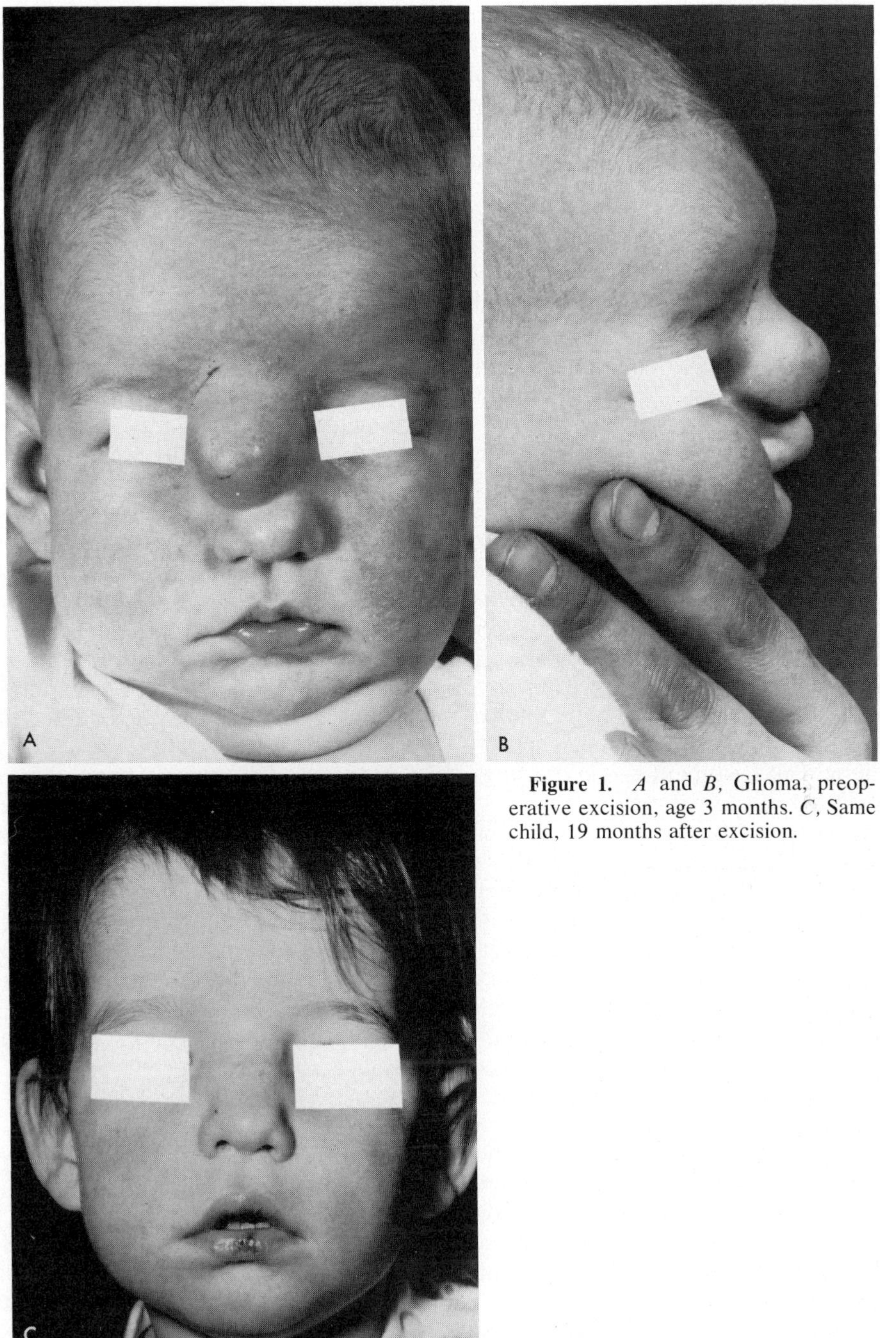

Figure 1. *A* and *B*, Glioma, preoperative excision, age 3 months. *C*, Same child, 19 months after excision.

the lesion can be excised through the direct external approach. Care should be taken to remove all the tissue, which may extend well into the cartilage of the septum.[27] For intranasal lesions or where more extensive exposure is necessary, other approaches have been reported.[15, 39] The tumor does not appear to be radiosensitive,[15] and it would seem to be unwise to use x-ray treatment in a growing child.

Pigmented Nevi

According to Spitz, pigmented nevi are the most common tumors of childhood.[52] Any of these commonly found cutaneous tumors can be present on the nose.

BLUE NEVUS. A blue nevus is histologically made up of spindle-shaped melanoblasts in the lower two-thirds of the dermis. The lesion is not considered premalignant, and according to Anderson[2] malignant change has not been reported in children. The lesion is sharply circumscribed, round or oval, and is smooth. The color may vary from slate grey to blue-black to pure blue. Indication for treatment in children is purely cosmetic, and treatment should be surgical excision.

JUNCTIONAL NEVUS. The junctional nevus is so called because of the microscopic finding of active proliferating nevus cells at the junction of epidermis and dermis. It appears to be level or very slight y raised, smooth, and nonhairy. The color varies from brown to black. This type of lesion is associated with the potential for malignant change.[40] However, there is no great threat of malignant change prior to puberty. According to Stegmaier, all nevi in children show junctional proliferation,[53] and Spitz noted that true malignant melanoma in children is a rarity.[51] However, this type of nevus should be removed prior to the hormonal stimulus of puberty.

COMPOUND NEVI. A compound nevus has the histological features of both dermal and junctional nevi. Spitz noted that 98 per cent of children's moles had this pattern, in contrast to only 12 per cent in adults.[52] The compound nevus is usually uniform brown and elevated, and may or may not have hair growth. The lesion is so common in childhood that the indication for removal is cosmetic, unless there is a reason for excision because of chronic irritation.

HALO NEVUS. A halo nevus is a small round spot with a central brown macule surrounded by a white halo of relative depigmentation. In time the pigmented portion disappears, leaving a spot of leukoderma. The lesion does not have malignant potential and no treatment is indicated, except for cosmetic reasons.

VON RECKLINGHAUSEN'S DISEASE. Von Recklinghausen's disease (neurofibromatosis) is a congenital anomaly which is represented by multiple neurofibromata and cutaneous pigmentation. Both of these can involve the nose. When the lesion is wide-spread, it is impossible to remove all of it, nor is it wise to do so. However, the lesions do have the potential for sarcomatous transformation, and for this reason patients with such lesions should be followed closely, so that a sudden change in one lesion may be treated.

NEVUS SEBACEOUS OF JADASSOHN. The sebaceous nevus of Jadassohn is a relatively common skin lesion in children. It is usually present at birth, and may become more evident after the first or second month of age. The lesion is not darkly pigmented, but has an irregular consistency and is yellow in color because of a rich supply of sebaceous glands (Fig. 2). Excision is indicated because of the reported incidence of malignant degeneration.[7] When this lesion is located in linear fashion in the midline, such as on the forehead and nose, it may be associated with convulsions and mental retardation.[17, 25, 30, 36]

GIANT HAIRY NEVUS. The giant hairy nevus has a well-known incidence of malignant degeneration. Conway,[8] Russell,[45] and Greeley[21] have shown a 10, 13, and 11 per cent incidence of malignancy in a series of 40, 53 and 56 cases, respectively. Malignant transformation is known to occur in childhood,[18]

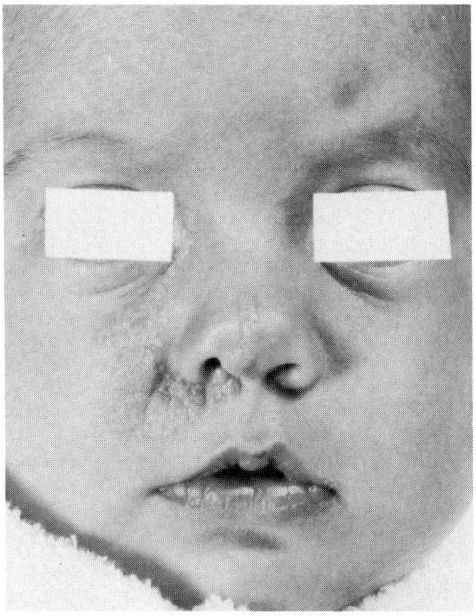

Figure 2. Sebaceous nevus (age 6 weeks).

but it is rare. Treatment of choice is complete excision with skin graft coverage (Fig. 3).[41] Dermabrasion has been tried with initially satisfactory results. Unfortunately, late results are very disappointing.[10] Mottled hyperpigmentation returns, which is in some respects more grotesque than the original lesion. Also, with a lesion known to be premalignant, irritative therapy is not appealing.

Hemangiomas

The hemangioma (a common benign tumor of infancy and childhood) may well be considered a hamartoma. It is composed of a collection of endothelial cells similar to those that line the vascular system. The nose is not an infrequent site for hemangioma, and in this obvious position, there may be considerable pressure placed on the surgeon by parents, grandparents, and pediatricians to embark upon various courses of therapy. In most cases, therapy is misguided and detrimental to the welfare of the child. The surgeon must be armed with complete knowledge of the natural history of the process to enable him to withstand this well-meaning, but misguided, pressure.

Neonatal Staining. Neonatal staining may not be a true hemangioma. It is noted at birth as a small area of capillary discoloration that is sharply demarcated. It often involves the occiput, but it also can involve the glabella and upper nose. It disappears within a few months and should not be treated.

Port Wine Stain (Nevus Flamius). This capillary hemangioma can vary from a dark purple port color (as the name implies) to a light rose. The consistency of the skin is usually entirely normal, but the lesion is clearly demarcated, and colored by blood flowing through an abnormally rich capillary dermal circulation (Fig. 4). It frequently involves the face and nose. When present, it is noted immediately at birth, and although the shade of color may change somewhat with time, it cannot be expected to regress. Various forms of treatment have been tried including dry ice and sclerosing agents. Unfortunately, both of these are relatively ineffective, and tend to cause scarring.[28]

Excision of a small lesion with primary closure may be the treatment of choice, but all too frequently the lesion may be too large to treat in this fashion. A tight closure must be avoided, particularly in the growing child, as it may contribute to growth deformities. Excision with grafting may be beneficial for the very deep-colored lesions, but all too frequently what is gained in color is lost in texture. Tattooing over the lesion may give some improvement,[6, 11] but multiple treatments are necessary, and often the results fall short of expectation, so that application of makeup is required. Skillful application of makeup without surgery often gives very satisfactory results, particularly in the female who would use makeup in any case. Advice from a cosmetologist can be very helpful.

Strawberry Hemangioma. Strawberry hemangioma is so named because of its color and raised lobular characteristics. It is usually a combination of capillary and deeper cavernous elements. Usually there is little or no sign of abnormality at birth, but at the age of about two weeks the lesion may appear as a

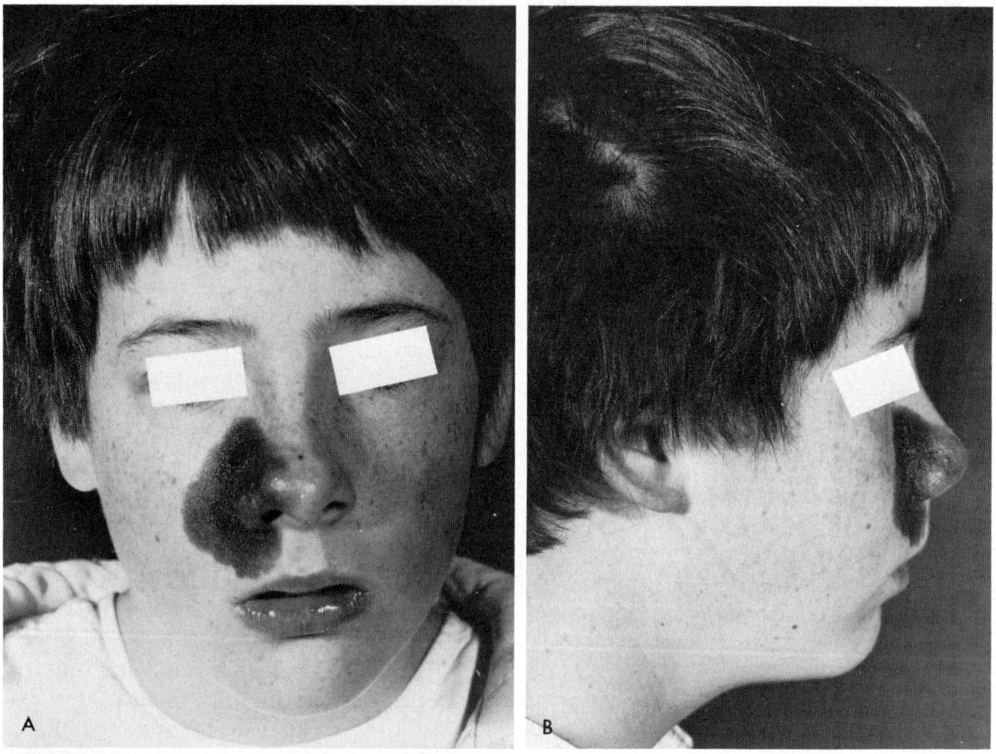

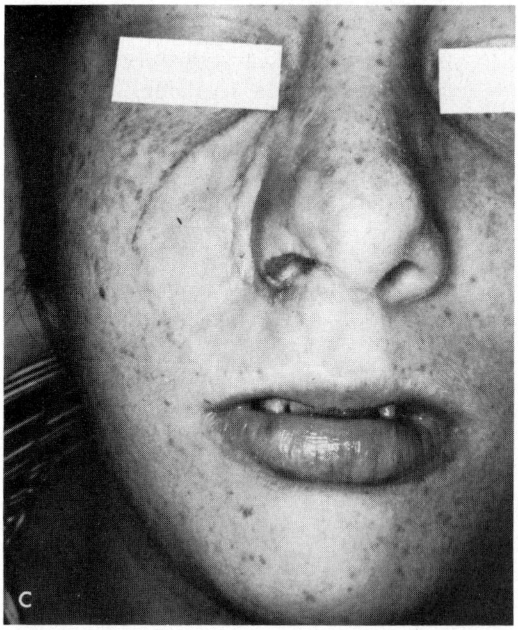

Figure 3. *A* and *B*, Giant nevus involving nose. *C*, Same patient shortly after stage excision and full thickness skin grafting.

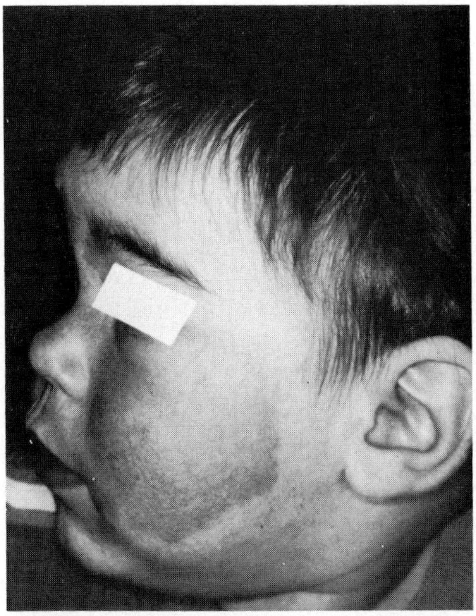

Figure 4. Port wine stain involving cheek and nose.

faint bluish mark and then shortly starts to grow. It may increase in size out of proportion to the child's own growth up to three, four or five months of age. From this time on, however, it will not grow out of proportion to the child's own growth, and it starts to show signs of regression (patches of grey color).

If a lesion regresses rapidly, it may ulcerate and require a protective dressing. During the period of ulceration it should be cleaned frequently with Zephiran chloride and covered lightly with ointment to keep the lesion from drying or crusting to the dressing. With this treatment, infection is rare, and even a large ulceration will re-epithelialize remarkably rapidly.

Eventually, regression and resolution will occur, with complete obliteration of all vascular components, but this may take several years (Fig. 5). The best result is obtained by a "hands-off" policy, as originally noted by Lister in 1938,[26] and confirmed by others later.[5, 24, 31, 32, 33, 46] The conservative approach cannot be emphasized too strongly. A distressing number of surgeons, presumably due to lack of patience, refuse to observe the natural course of the lesion and advocate surgery or other form of treatment.

After regression is complete, there may be some residual redundancy to the skin, or residual fibrofatty tissue, which will require a minor revision. However, frequently patience is rewarded, and no revision is necessary.

CAVERNOUS HEMANGIOMA. This lesion frequently involves the tip of the nose, giving the patient a Cyrano de Bergerac type of profile. As mentioned earlier, it may be associated with capillary component giving a typical strawberry appearance, but if the skin is not involved it has a typical blue hazy appearance, imparted by a network of veins showing through. It can be reduced by pressure and fills like a sponge. Large veins may at times be seen radiating from the lesion in the subcutaneous tissues. These may be dramatically demonstrated with infrared photography.

As with strawberry hemangiomata, regression is the rule, but the timetable is somewhat slower. Regression may not be complete until the child is 10 years old or more. Matthews advocates injection with hypertonic saline,[32, 33] but in most surgeons' hands sclerosing agents give disappointing results. Systemic corticosteroid treatment has also been advocated.[58] It is possible that this form of treatment may speed up the natural process of resolution. However, this is difficult to judge in a lesion that normally resolves anyway at a rate that varies from child to child. There are also significant hazards to prolonged systemic use of steroids in the growing child.

Local x-ray therapy (one to three treatments of 200 R. each) may be indicated in selected cases. X-ray seems to hasten the natural process of resolution, presumably by causing edema of the endothelium lining the sinusoids. X-ray treatment is probably justified only when there is a risk of tissue destruction or compromise to a vital structure. A nasal hemangioma involving the orbit or causing significant pressure on the nasal framework might be such an example.

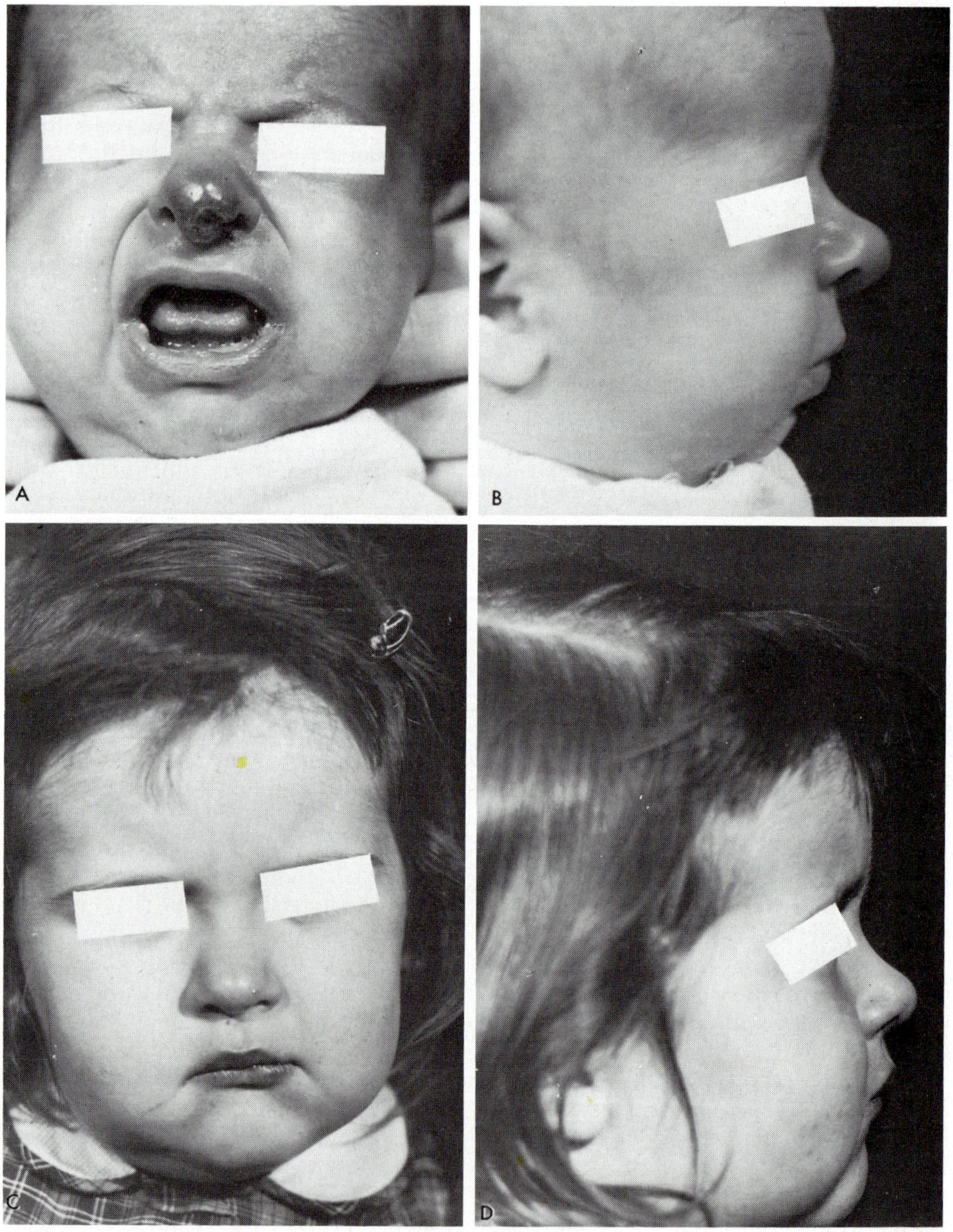

Figure 5. *A* and *B*, Capillary-cavernous (strawberry) hemangioma with ulceration (age 7 weeks). *C* and *D*, Same patient after resolution (age 2 years 4 months).

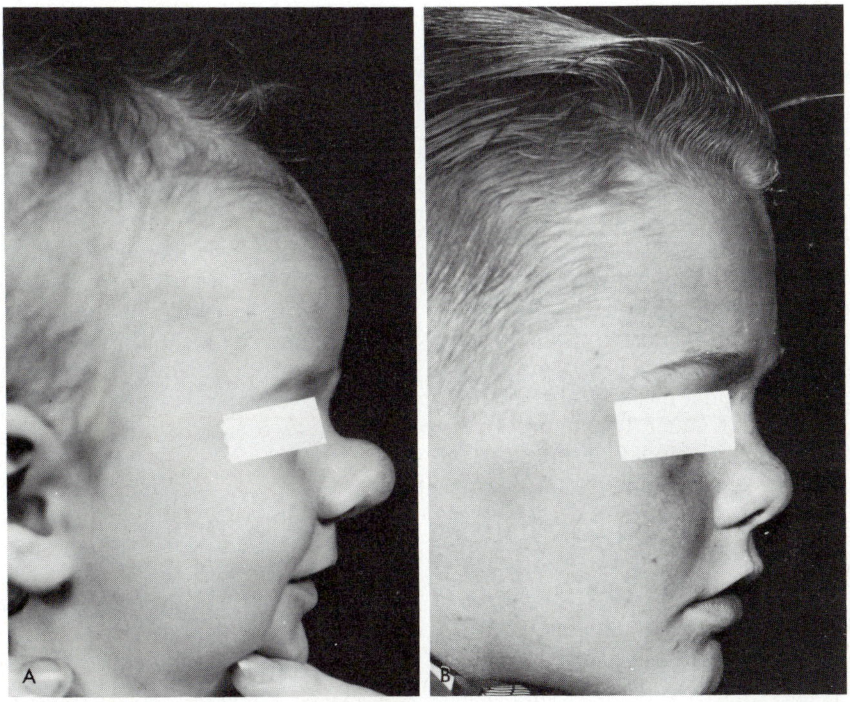

Figure 6. *A*, Cavernous hemangioma (age 3 months). *B*, After resolution (age 10 years).

Thrombocytopenia, although rare, can be caused by a hemangioma, and can be cured by its resection.[23] The coagulation defect probably is more complicated than can be explained on the basis of the low platelet count alone. It is probably a form of consumption coagulopathy.

Juvenile Nasopharyngeal Angiofibroma

Juvenile angiofibroma is a disease of pubertal males. The lesion is nonmalignant in that it does not metastasize or infiltrate, but it appears to be locally destructive from pressure.[20] It can cause obstruction to the nasal airway, and bleeding may be serious. Friedberg advocated treatment by a combination of x-ray and electrocoagulation. He felt that surgery was too dangerous because of attachment to and involvement with bones.[20] MacComb[29] and Apostol[3] advocated a surgical resection, pointing out that adequate exposure is necessary because of the size and the firm attachments of the tumor. Apostol advocated a transantral approach through a modified Weber-Ferguson incision.[3] MacComb found that pretreatment with stilbestrol reduced the size and vascularity of the tumor for surgery.[29] Prolonged use of stilbestrol is not wise because it has undesirable side effects.

Cysts and Polyps of the Sinus Cavities

The sinus cavities, particularly the maxillary sinus, can develop symptomatology in association with both cysts and polyps. The maxillary sinus may have an independent polyp or several polyps associated with nasal polyposis. These polyps develop as the result of irritation of the sinus mucosa from an allergic or long-standing toxic exudate from an infected sinus. If a polyp blocks the osteum of the sinus, it may be a significant factor in continued purulent sinusitis.

Cysts may be single or multiple, and may be very small or large enough to fill the entire sinus cavity. Nonsecreting cysts contain clear, straw-colored fluid and are presumably allergic in origin.

Mucus-secreting cysts are, in effect, dilated glands of sinus mucosa backed up behind an obstructed duct. Symptomatology from both of these cysts tends to be somewhat vague, such as fullness or numbness of the cheek or frontal headaches on the affected side. Diagnosis can often be made by x-ray (Waters and lateral views). At times, however, tomography and the use of a radiopaque medium may be helpful.[55]

Successful treatment with obliteration of cysts can sometimes be accomplished at the same time as nasoantral fenestration. However, frequently the direct exposure through a sublabial incision is best for intra-antral polyps and large cysts.

Miscellaneous Benign Tumors

Other benign neoplasms may affect the tissue of the nose, nasopharynx or sinus cavities, such as osteoma, fibroma, papilloma, chondroma, lymphoma and myxoma.[22] However, the incidence of these lesions in childhood is so small that a full discussion is not warranted. Involvement with neurofibromata in von Recklinghausen's disease (congenital neurofibromatosis) is somewhat more common.[13] This has been previously referred to in this chapter because of the associated pigmented lesions of the skin. The nose and face are particularly susceptible to the plexiform variety of neurofibromata, which has no discrete boundaries, and tends to be progressive and difficult to treat. However, if the deformity is extreme, surgery may well be justified. Results are often disappointing because of the difficulty of complete resection and the propensity for residual elements to progress.

MALIGNANT TUMORS OF THE NOSE AND SINUSES

Fortunately, cancer of the nose and sinuses is very rare in childhood. Out of 416 patients, Frazell found only three cases in the first decade of life.[19] The youngest child in his series was 22 months old, with adenocarcinoma of the nasal cavity (apparently associated with nasal polyps). Pointon had only two cases under 15 years of age out of 428 reported;[42] Pollack had one 3-year-old boy with a malignant teratoma.[43] As a general rule, treatment for true malignancy is similar to that in the adult. A primary malignancy of the maxillary sinus should be treated by complete resection through wide exposure via a Weber-Ferguson incision.[43]

Rhabdomyosarcoma

Rhabdomyosarcoma (a highly malignant tumor of childhood) can involve the nasopharynx[47] or the external nose.[12] Treatment of this lesion should be aggressive. It often involves chemotherapy and x-ray therapy as well as radical surgical resection.

Basal Cell Cancer

The nose is a common site for basal cell cancer, it does occur in childhood, but very rarely. Cholnoky had only two cases under 19 years of age in a series of 1062 cases of facial cancer. Murray, however, reported five cases.[37]

Malignant Melanoma

As mentioned previously in the discussion of pigmented nevi, Spitz[51] and Allen and Spitz[1] showed that true malignant melanoma in childhood is very rare. A few cases, however, have been reported.[49, 54]

Olfactory Neuroepithelioma

A rare group of nasal neoplasms of neurogenous origin (olfactory neuroepithelioma) has been reviewed by Skolnick.[48] The cases included every age group, including several in adolescent children. The tumor is a true malignancy and should be treated aggressively by surgery. McGavran reports only 50 per cent five-year survivors with surgical resection, with or without postoperative x-ray treatment.[34] Postoperative follow-up of catecholamine secretion should be done as an index of residual or metastatic tumor with secretory capacity.

Malignant tumors of the nose of salivary gland origin have been reported,[35] but must be exceedingly rare.

REFERENCES

1. Allen, A. C., and Spitz, S.: Malignant melanoma: A clinical pathological analysis of the criteria for diagnosis and prognosis. *Cancer,* 6:1, 1953.
2. Anderson, N. P.: Moles and melanomas and epitheliomas in children. *Calif. Med.,* 78:17, 1953.
3. Apostol, J. V., and Frazell, E. L.: Juvenile nasopharyngeal angiofibroma. A clinical study. *Cancer,* 18:869, 1965.
4. Black, B. K., and Smith, D. E.: Nasal glioma. *Arch. Neurol. Psychiat.,* 1964:614, 1950.
5. Blackfield, H. M., Torrey, F. A., Morris, W. J., and Low-Beer, B. V. A.: The management of visible hemangiomas. *Med. J. Surg.,* 94:313, 1957.
6. Brown, J. B., Cannon, B., and McDowell, F.: Permanent pigment injection of capillary hemangiomata. *Plast. Reconstr. Surg.,* 1:197, 1953.
7. Connor, A. E.: Nevus sebaceous of Jadassohn. *Amer. J. Dis. Child.,* 114:626, 1967.
8. Conway, H.: Bathing trunk nevi. *Surgery,* 6:585, 1939.
9. Conway, H.: Tattooing of nevus flammeus for permanent camouflage. *J.A.M.A.,* 152:666, 1953.
10. Conway, H., and Jerome, A. P.: Nevi and melanomata of the face. *Plast. Reconstr. Surg.,* 14:200, 1954.
11. Conway, H., McKinney, P., and Climo, M.: Permanent camouflage of vascular nevi of the face by intradermal injection of insoluble pigments (tattooing): Experience through 25 years with 1022 cases. *Plast. Reconstr. Surg.,* 40:457, 1967.
12. Crosby, J. F.: Unusual nasal tumors in children. *Plast. Reconstr. Surg.,* 19:143, 1957.
13. Davis, W. B., Edgerton, M. T., and Hoffmeister, S. F.: Neurofibromatosis of the head and neck. *Plast. Reconstr. Surg.,* 14:186, 1954.
14. DeCholnoky, T.: Cancer of the face: A clinical and statistical study of 1062 cases. *Ann. Surg.,* 122:88, 1945.
15. Deutsch, H. J.: Intranasal glioma. *Ann. Otol. Rhin. Laryng.,* 74:637, 1965.
16. DeVenecia, G., and Lobeck, C. C.: Successful treatment of eyelid hemangioma with Prednisone. *Arch. Ophthal.,* 84:98, 1970.
17. Feuerstein, R. C., and Mims, L. C.: Linear nevus sebaceous with convulsions and mental retardation. *Amer. J. Dis. Child.,* 104:675, 1962.
18. Fish, J., Smith, E. B., and Canby, J. P.: Malignant melanoma in children. *Surgery,* 59:309, 1966.
19. Frazell, E. L., and Lewis, J. S.: Cancer of the nasal cavity and excessory sinuses: A report of the management of 416 patients. *Cancer,* 16:1293, 1963.
20. Friedberg, S. A.: Vascular fibroma of the nasopharynx (nasopharyngeal fibroma). *Arch. Otol.,* 31:313, 1940.
21. Greeley, P. W., Middleton, A. G., and Curtin, J. W.: Incidence of malignancy in giant pigmented nevi. *Plast. Reconstr. Surg.,* 36:26, 1965.
22. Handousa, A. B.: Primary benign neoplasms of the nose. *J. Laryng. Otol.,* 66:421, 1952.
23. Hill, G. J., II, and Longino, L. A.: Giant hemangioma with thrombocytopenia. *Surg. Gynec. Obstet.,* 114:304, 1962.
24. Lampe, I., and Latourette, H. B.: Management of hemangiomas in infants. *Pediat. Clin. N. Amer.,* 6:511, 1959.
25. Lantis, S., Thew, M., and Heaton, C.: Nevus sebaceous of Jadassohn. *Arch. Derm.,* 98:117, 1968.
26. Lister, W. A.: Natural history of strawberry naevi. *Lancet,* 1:429, 1938.
27. Lowe, R. S., Robinson, D. W., Ketchum, L. D., and Masters, F. W.: Nasal gliomata. *Plast. Reconstr. Surg.,* 47:1, 1971.
28. MacCollum, D. W., and Martin, L. W.: Hemangiomas in infancy and childhood. A report based on 6479 cases. *Surg. Clin. N. Amer.,* 36:1647, 1956.
29. MacComb, W. S.: Juvenile nasopharyngeal fibroma. *Amer. J. Surg.,* 106:754, 1963.
30. Marden, P. M., and Venters, H. D., Jr.: A new neurocutaneous syndrome. *Amer. J. Dis. Child.,* 112:79, 1966.
31. Margileth, A. M., and Museles, M.: Cutaneous hemangiomas in children. *J.A.M.A.,* 194:523, 1965.
32. Matthews, D. N.: Treatment of hemangiomata. *Brit. J. Plast. Surg.,* 6:78, 1953.
33. Matthews, D. N.: Hemangiomata. *Plast. Reconstr. Surg.,* 41:528, 1968.
34. McGavran, M. H.: Neurogenous nasal neoplasms. *Ann. Otol.,* 79:547, 1970.
35. Mortada, A.: Malignant salivary gland tumors of the nose and exophthalmos in children. *Bull. Ophthal. Soc. Egypt,* 62:329, 1969.
36. Moynahan, E. J.: A new neurocutaneous syndrome (skin, eye, brain) consisting of linear nevus, bilateral lipo-dermoid of the conjunctiva, cranial thickening, cerebral

cortical atrophy, and mental retardation. *Brit. J. Derm.*, 79:651, 1967.
37. Murray, J. E., and Cannon, B.: Basal cell cancer in children and young adults. *New Eng. J. Med.*, 262:440, 1960.
38. Newman, B. A.: Cutaneous tumors of children. *Calif. Med.*, 86:1, 1957.
39. O'Brien, P.: The surgical approach to nasal glioma. *Brit. J. Plast. Surg.*, 23:30, 1970.
40. Pack, G. T., and Ariel, I. M.: *Tumors of the Soft Somatic Tissues.* New York, Paul B. Hoeber, 1958, p. 681.
41. Pilney, F. T., Braodbent, T. R., and Woolf, R. M.: Giant pigmented nevi of the face: Surgical management. *Plast. Reconstr. Surg.*, 40:469, 1967.
42. Pointon, R. C.: Neoplasia of the nose and sinuses. *J. Laryng.*, 83:407, 1969.
43. Pollack, R. S.: Carcinoma of the maxillary sinus. *Ann. Surg.*, 145:68, 1957.
44. Ross, D. E.: Skin manifestations of von Recklinghausen's disease and associated tumors (neurofibromatosis). *Amer. Surg.*, 31:729, 1965.
45. Russell, J. L., and Reyes, R. C.: Giant pigmented nevi. *J.A.M.A.* 171:2083, 1959.
46. Sachatello, C. R., and McSwaine, B.: Regression of cutaneous capillary hemangioma. *Amer. J. Surg.*, 116:113, 1968.
47. Shands, W. C.: Soft tissue sarcomas in children and adults. *Amer. Surg.*, 29:811, 1963.
48. Skolnik, E. M., Massari, F. S., and Tenta, L. T.: Olfactory neuroepithelioma: Review of the world literature, and presentation of two cases. *Arch. Otolaryngol.*, 84:644, 1966.
49. Skov-Jensen, T., Hastrup, J., and Lambrethsen, E.: Malignant melanoma in children. *Cancer,* 19:620, 1966.
50. Smith, K. R., Schwartz, H. G., Luse, S. A., and Ogura, J. H.: Nasal gliomas: A report of five cases with electron microscopy of one. *J. Neurosurg.*, 20:968, 1963.
51. Spitz, S.: Melanomas of children. *Amer. J. Path.*, 24:591, 1948.
52. Spitz, S.: Cutaneous tumors of childhood, disparity between clinical behaviour and histologic appearance. *J. Amer. Med. Women's Assn.*, 6:209, 1951.
53. Stegmaier, O. C., and Montgomery, H.: Histopathologic studies of pigmented nevi in children. *J. Invest. Dermat.*, 20:51, 1953.
54. Traux, K. F., and Page, H. G.: Prepubertal malignant melanoma. *Ann. Surg.*, 137:255, 1953.
55. Van Alyea, O. E.: Management of nonmalignant growths in the maxillary sinus. *Trans. Amer. Laryng. Assoc.*, 77:104, 1956.
56. Watson, W. L., and McCarthy, W. D.: Blood and lymph vessel tumors: Report of 1056 cases. *Gynec. Obstet.*, 71:569, 1940.
57. Willis, R. A.: *The Borderland of Embryology and Pathology.* London, Butterworth, 1958.
58. Zarem, H. A., and Edgerton, M. T.: Induced resolution of cavernous hemangiomas following Prednisolone therapy. *Plast. Reconstr. Surg.*, 39:76, 1967.

Chapter Seventy-Eight

FRACTURES OF THE NOSE, SINUSES AND FACE

RICHARD T. FARRIOR, M.D., DAVID R. BEAM, M.D., D.D.S., and JOHN M. HODGES, M.D.

INTRODUCTION

It is difficult to discuss fractures of the nose and paranasal sinuses without discussing fractures of the adjacent bones. However, to discuss all facial fractures would be too lengthy. Thus, fractures of the mandible and frontal sinuses will not be included. Fractures of the middle third of the face will be discussed primarily as they differ in children and in adults. Facial fractures in children are different from those in adults because the face is growing, and injury sometimes produces a disturbance in the normal growth and development of bones, which can result in developmental deformities in later life. This could be due to neglect or improper management on the part of the practitioner or surgeon, but deformities can occur in spite of proper treatment.

Fortunately, even with more frequent trauma to the face, facial fractures in children are less common than those in adults. The child has several things in his favor to produce relative immunity from middle third facial fractures. First, the facial bones of the child occupy a much smaller area, particularly when compared with the cranium. Secondly, the growth centers of cartilage and the high degree of elasticity of the bone of the child permit a considerable amount of bending before fracturing actually takes place. It is probable that a force sufficient to create a craniofacial dysjunction in the very young child would probably produce enough intracranial damage as to be incompatible with life.

Typical injuries to the middle third of the facial skeleton in the young child are usually fractures of the nasal bones. In the older child, the zygoma fractures have an increased incidence. Injuries to the anterior teeth are also very common in children.

The physical examination and principles of management of facial injuries in the child are not different from those utilized in the management of the adult patient with similar injuries, particularly as the child comes closer to having the full development of the face. They respond well to the simplest techniques that result in proper alignment of the bones and occlusion of the teeth. Although cervical spine injuries are relatively uncommon in children, the cervical spine must be carefully evaluated in facial trauma cases.

The difficulty encountered in the management of children's fractures is related to the condition, development and number of teeth available for application of wires or arch bars. The greatest period of difficulty is during the time of mixed dentition when there are unerupted teeth present within the bodies of the maxilla and mandible. Open reductions in children should be approached much more cautiously and much more conservatively to avoid damaging the unerupted teeth.

Fractures of the facial skeleton should be repaired as soon as possible because of the rapidity of healing with fixation and malposition, which can occur within five to seven days.[1] For the same reason, an intermaxillary immobilization does not need to be for more than two to four weeks, depending on the age of the child.

It is very important to have full cooperation of the child in managing his facial fracture. Sedation may be imperative, even while taking x-rays, and general anesthesia may be in order for the simplest problem requiring precise manipulation.

BIRTH INJURIES

Injuries to the middle third of the face during labor and delivery do occur and can cause developmental deformities. Dislocations, slight fractures and other trauma may influence the development of the premaxillary, maxillary and septal elements, producing facial asymmetries,

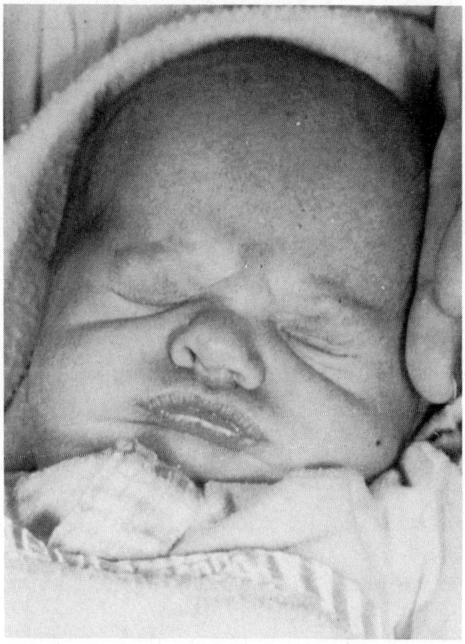

Figure 1. Birth injury. This newborn infant exemplifies a cartilaginous dislocation with associated external nasal deviation. A closed reduction using blunt instrument pressure was carried out.

sagittal and dental malalignments and malocclusion.[2] Prolonged labor with a marginal pelvis and forceps delivery may well contribute to injuries during this period (Fig. 1).[3] Injuries received during birth and in the early period of development are more likely to be cartilaginous than bony.

The frequency of prenatal injury in children is a somewhat theoretical consideration, although congenital malformation, intrauterine or pelvic pressure, and abnormal fetal positions are important considerations.[4, 5] The majority of the prenatal and perinatal injuries involve the nose, and they are usually due to septal dislocation or twisting. Some of them clear spontaneously; many can be corrected by simple closed reduction, or even finger manipulation. If these measures fail to correct the deformity, time should be given a chance. Many such deformities disappear, or at least have no functional or respiratory component, after three to six months.[3]

NASAL INJURIES

Seemingly minor injuries to the nose of a child may leave their mark in later life. Mild injuries that have a minimal amount of edema and ecchymosis and no hematoma or mucosal tears may produce a later deformity. This problem is perplexing and must be dealt with. It is believed that in some of these cases there may be a greenstick septal fracture with minimal extravasation of blood and serum along the fracture line, with healing by fibrous union, producing angulation and deformity.[6] If the injury is minor or questionable, early consultation may be the wisest approach.

Hematoma of the nasal dorsum is less common than hematoma of the nasal septum and is usually associated with a direct blow with tearing of the upper lateral cartilage from the nasal bones. It has been reported to cause pressure necrosis of the nasal bone and cartilage on the injured side of the nose.[7] Early diagnosis with drainage and packing is a key to preventing a post-traumatic nasal deformity.

A septal hematoma is usually due to a laceration, fracture or dislocation of the septal cartilage and can often occlude both nostrils. It must be diagnosed and drained early to prevent destruction of the septal cartilage by pressure and avascularity. Furthermore, a septal abscess may develop in the septal hematoma, producing more rapid destruction of the cartilaginous septum and upper lateral cartilages, leading to a saddle-nose deformity.

Bleeding from the nose of a child who has had a nasal injury should strongly suggest a nasal fracture or dislocation of the nasal bones or cartilages. If a fracture is present, it is best to place a young child under general anesthesia for closed reduction of the fracture and packing. A reliable x-ray examination is difficult because the nasal fracture is still in the cartilaginous or only partly ossified area of the nasal bone and maxilla. The nasal tissues heal rapidly, and unless they are repositioned within two or three days, reduction may be difficult and results are not very good.

Kazanjian and Converse point out that fractures of the nasal bones in children may frequently be unilateral because they do not have the bony midline attachment to each other as is found in the adult.[8]

The kind of fracture most frequently seen is the open-book type, with splaying out of the fractured segments over the frontal process of the maxilla. In cases of severe trauma, the bony nasal bridge is dislocated into the ethmoid sinuses, producing a naso-orbital injury. Frequently, the frontal sinuses are involved. With a severe naso-orbital injury, there is tearing of the medial palpebral ligament on one or both sides, which results in hypertelorism with narrowing of the palpebral fissures and widening of the distance between the medial canthi. These fractures are reduced by the usual methods and many will need open reduction and direct interosseous wiring. Fixation with through-and-through wires over soft

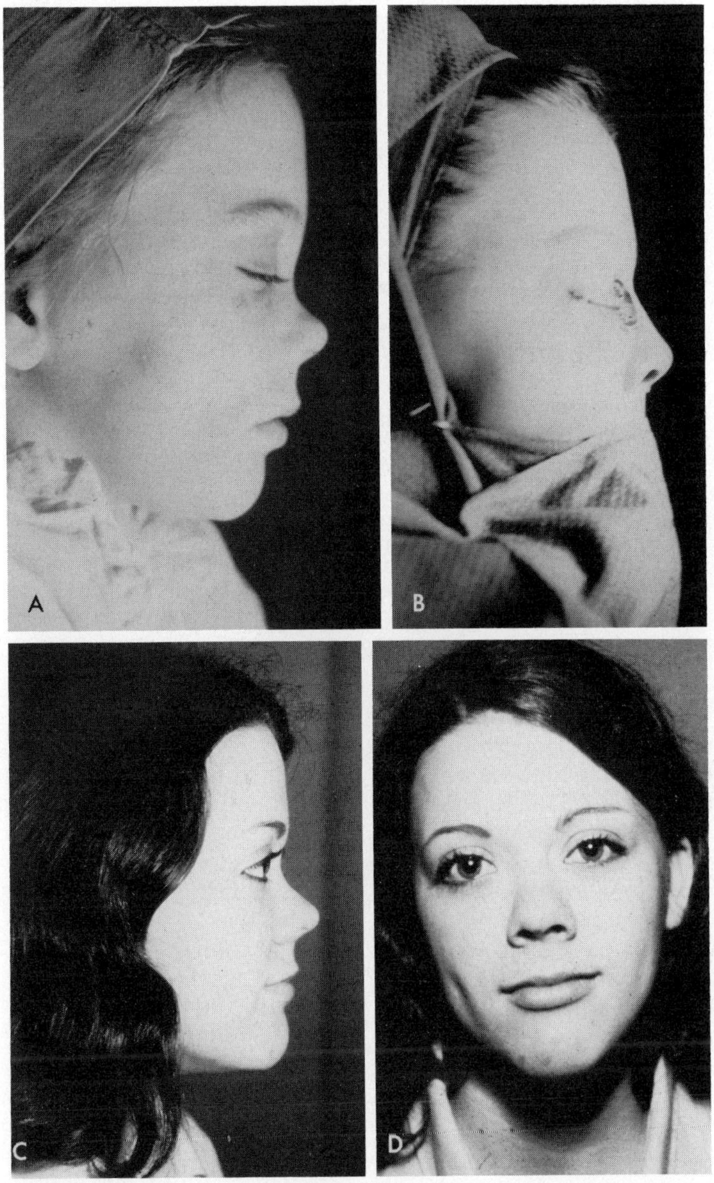

Figure 2. Soft metal plates. This 11-year-old girl was involved in an automobile accident and suffered multiple facial fractures including comminution and depression of the nasal bones. She underwent open reduction with direct interosseous wiring of the right maxillary, nasal, and frontal bones and transnasal wiring with soft metal plates. *A*, Lateral view at surgery demonstrating the telescoping of the nasal bones. *B*, Postoperative view demonstrating the soft metal plates and acceptable profile. *C*, Profile view five years later. A dorsal implant is planned. *D*, Frontal view demonstrating absent hypertelorism.

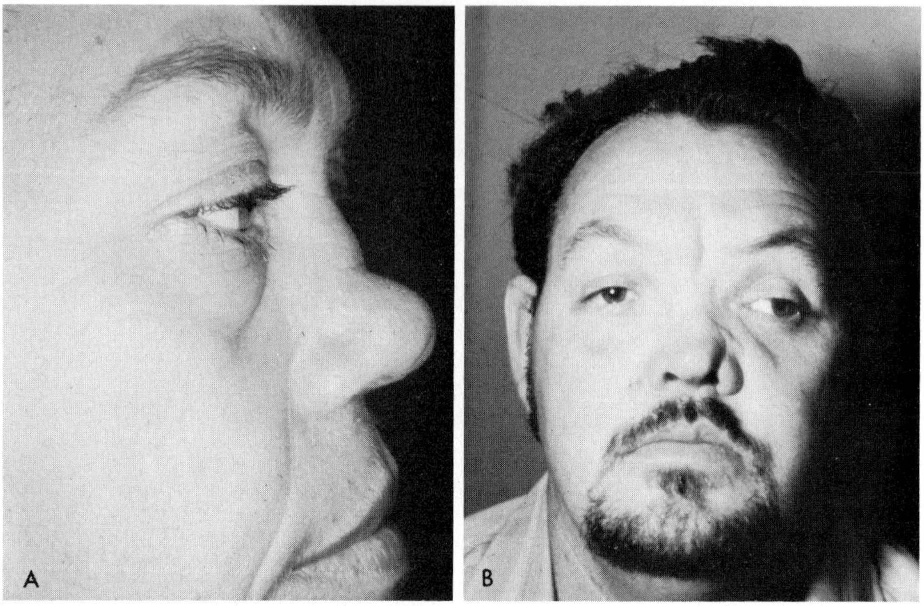

Figure 3. Long-term effects of childhood injuries. *A*, This 45-year-old female had a saddle nose "all her life," attributed to a severe "nasal" injury at the age of 3, for which no medical consultation was obtained. Notice the dish-face deformity. The nasal dorsum was corrected with a hip graft implant. The maxilla was built out with cancellous bone implants along the pyriform rim. *B*, This 32-year old male was involved in an automobile accident at the age of 16 and suffered severe intracranial and facial trauma. Notice the hypertelorism, narrowing of the palpebral fissures and external strabismus with the obvious frontal and nasal defects.

metal plates may be indicated (Fig. 2).

Failure to recognize and manage the nasal and interorbital fractures may lead to late developmental deformities that produce serious functional and cosmetic deformities (Fig. 3). When seen late, nasal deformities in children should not be corrected unless this can be done by a simple procedure. Extensive reconstruction procedures for a deformity of the nose in children are inadvisable. If, however, there is significant deformity of a septum producing airway obstruction, surgical intervention may be wise.[1]

There are many questions still left unanswered concerning the effect of surgery and injury on the growth and development of the facial bones. Disturbances in growth and development are seen sometimes in patients who have sustained severe injury and following surgery. It is interesting that in severe comminuted fractures, which are likely to extend across growth centers, correct reduction in many cases does not lead to external deformity. This would lead to arguments that corrective surgery when accurately done should produce minimal disturbances in growth. However, almost every author cites instances of underdevelopment of the nose following premature nasal surgery. Contrary to this, however, are the frequently quoted statements that nasal humps are overgrowths due to injury.[2, 9] It is perhaps more appropriate to describe the results of trauma or surgery as a disturbance of growth rather than a retardation of growth or a stimulation of growth.

In any event, conservatism and repositioning without removal of tissue or with minimal tissue disturbance seem to be the wisest approach (Fig. 4). Any disturbance from trauma or surgery can create scar tissue, and thus, loss of normal tissue elasticity or a disturbance of cartilage resilience. Correction of cosmetic deformities definitely should be delayed until age 16 or 17 in boys, or 15 to 17 in girls. Even these deformities in certain

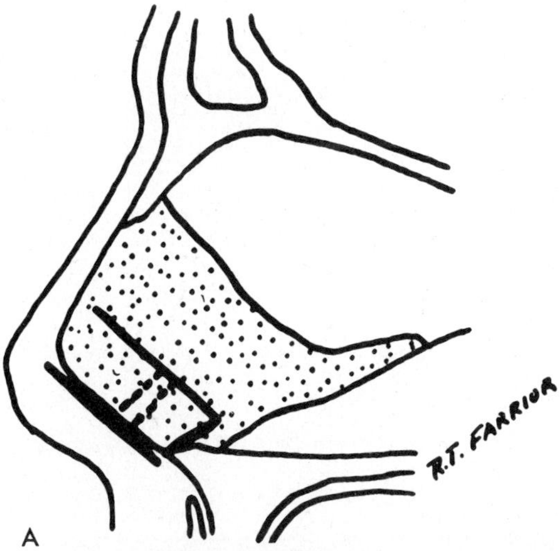

A

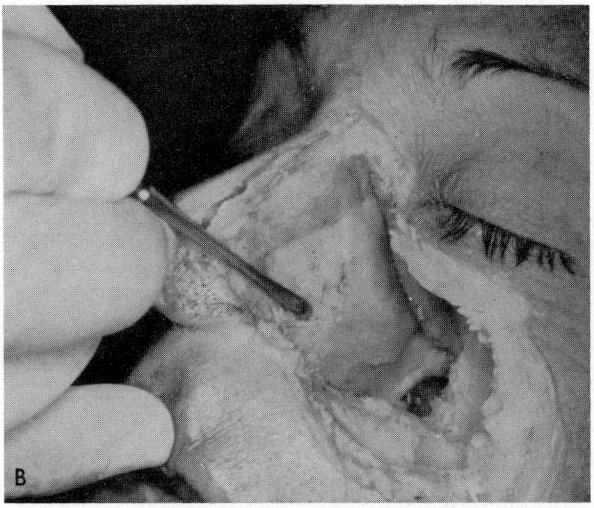

B

Figure 4. Septal reconstruction. *A*, Metzenbaum method (1929). Elevation of mucous membrane on one side and simple repositioning of the caudal septum without removal of tissue. *B*, Cadaver dissection showing teasing of the septal cartilage from the perpendicular plate of the ethmoid without removal of cartilage or bone. Mucous membrane remains attached on the opposite side.

instances may be operated on at a slightly earlier age, particularly in girls (Fig. 5). The rationale for this statement is, first, that development is completed earlier in girls and, second, that slight differences or cessation of further development of the nose in the female is often pleasing in our culture. Males develop later, and in later teen years, up to age 25, considerable growth occurs in the nose as well as the rest of the face.[4]

Many generalists and pediatricians have followed the dictum that no corrective surgery of the nasal framework should be performed until full growth has occurred. Early corrective surgery in specific instances may be indicated and desirable, and the importance of careful evaluation of each deformity and the application of physiologically sound surgical techniques cannot be overemphasized. Early examination by the qualified consultant should be provided for all nasal deformities, rather than delaying and allowing either abnormal facial development or the development of other complications. The surgeon must balance the need and timing of the correction with restoration of function against the degree of tissue disturbance and possible residual nasal and facial deformities.

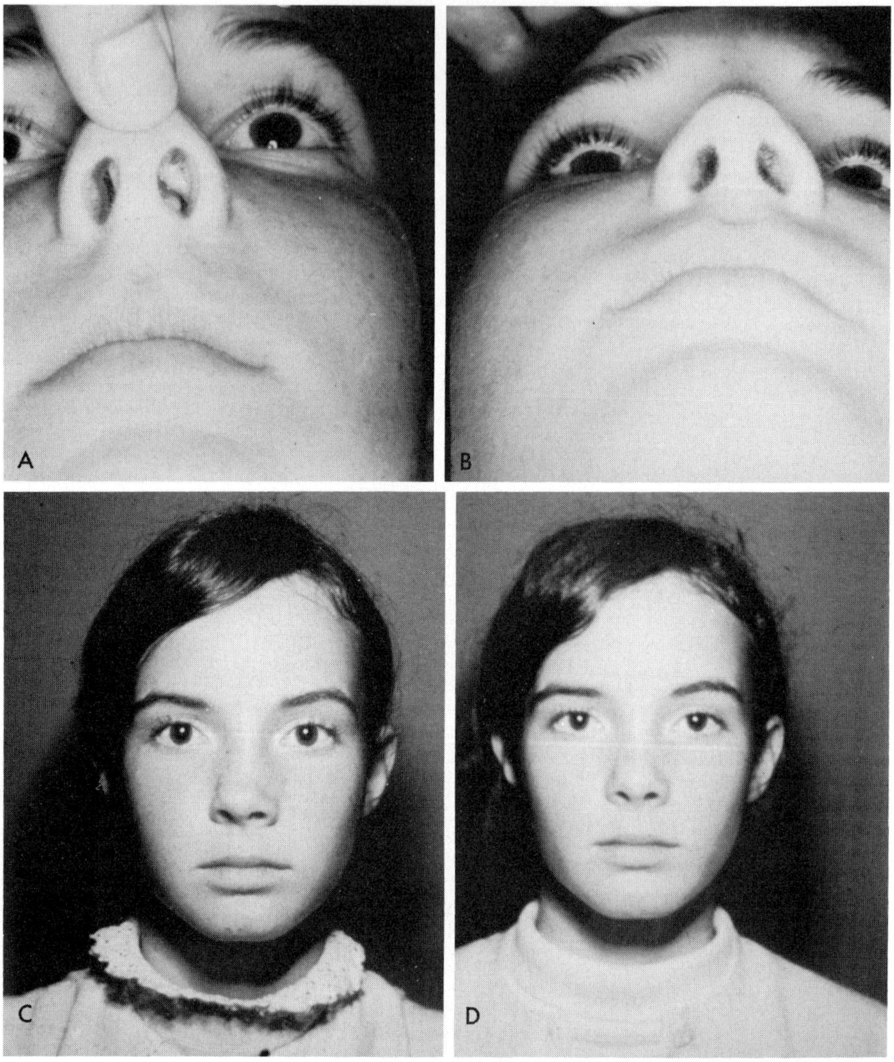

Figure 5. Cosmetic and functional deformity at an early age. In this 13-year-old patient, there is a severe septal deflection and caudal dislocation with twisting and deviation of the tip and cartilaginous dorsum. Advanced septal reconstruction without osteotomies was performed. Despite a radical takedown of the septum, dorsal support was maintained. *A,* Preoperative view, nasal base demonstrating caudal deflection of the septum. *B,* Postoperative view after septal reconstruction and modified rhinoplasty. *C,* Preoperative anterior view demonstrating twist with deviation of cartilaginous dorsum and tip. *D,* Postoperative. No osteotomies.

ZYGOMATIC AND MAXILLARY FRACTURES

Fractures of these bones are relatively rare in children, and their treatment is essentially the same as that for an adult patient. Many maxillary factures will respond to reduction and fixation with chin support or temporary headcap appliances.[1]

The paranasal sinuses are small in young children and need no practical consideration in the management of fractures of the maxilla, but as the child grows older, their importance increases.[10] At birth, the maxillary sinus is about 1 cm. high, 1 cm. wide, and 2 cm. long, and the floor of the sinus is above the level of the floor of the nose. By the age of 12, the floor of the sinus is level with the floor of the nose, and as the secondary teeth erupt, the sinus expands into the alveolus and reaches its final growth after the completion of dentition. The frontal sinus begins to develop after the age of 6 and is clinically significant about age 10 or 12. The growth of all sinuses ceases at about puberty or early adulthood.

Fractures of the zygoma in children are relatively rare and their treatment is essentially the same as that for the adult. They are associated frequently with fractures of the maxilla and of the orbital structures. Direct wiring is the treatment of choice. One must be extremely careful with the closed methods of reduction of the fractured zygoma in children because of the consequences of the inadequate reduction due to the "greensticking" of fractures (Fig. 6).

Unless gross displacement exists, unilateral fractures of the maxilla do not warrant open reduction, for this may inflict further damage on the growing bone and the unerupted dentition (Fig. 7). This does not apply when the orbit is fractured. With craniofacial dysjunction,

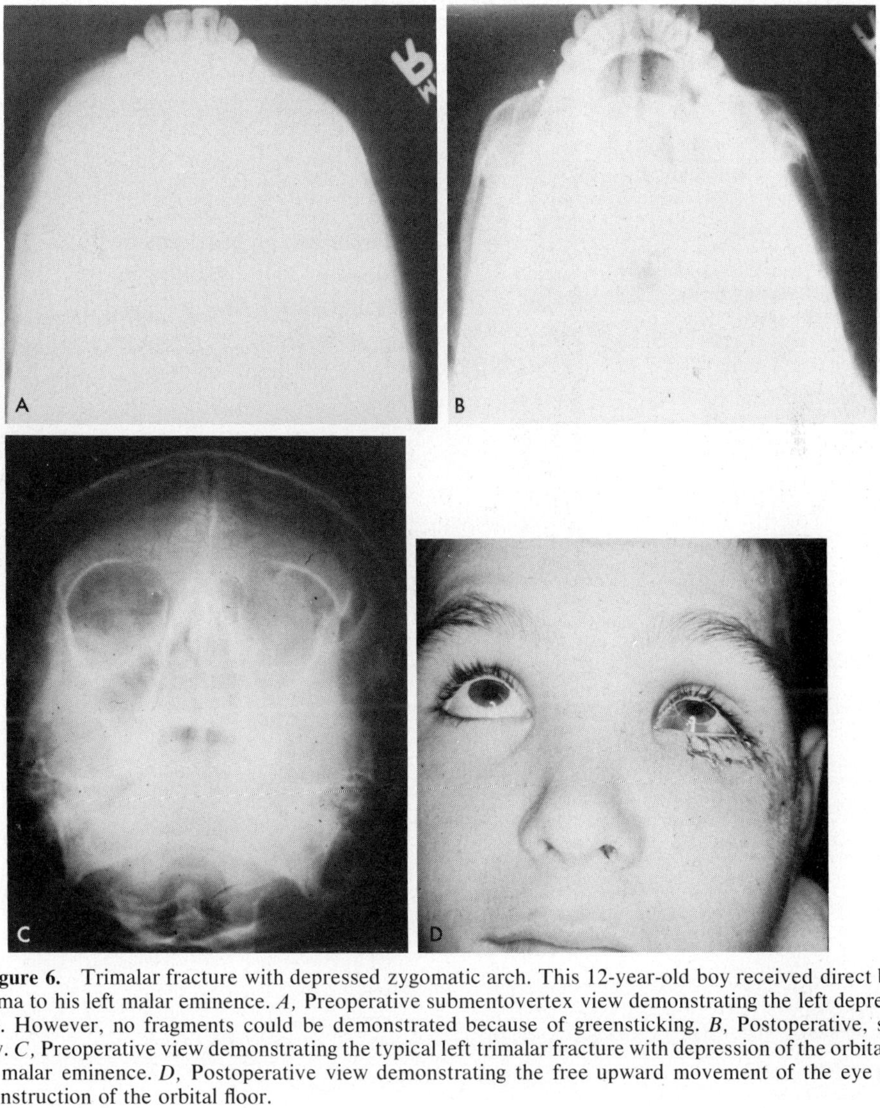

Figure 6. Trimalar fracture with depressed zygomatic arch. This 12-year-old boy received direct blunt trauma to his left malar eminence. *A*, Preoperative submentovertex view demonstrating the left depressed arch. However, no fragments could be demonstrated because of greensticking. *B*, Postoperative, same view. *C*, Preoperative view demonstrating the typical left trimalar fracture with depression of the orbital rim and malar eminence. *D*, Postoperative view demonstrating the free upward movement of the eye after reconstruction of the orbital floor.

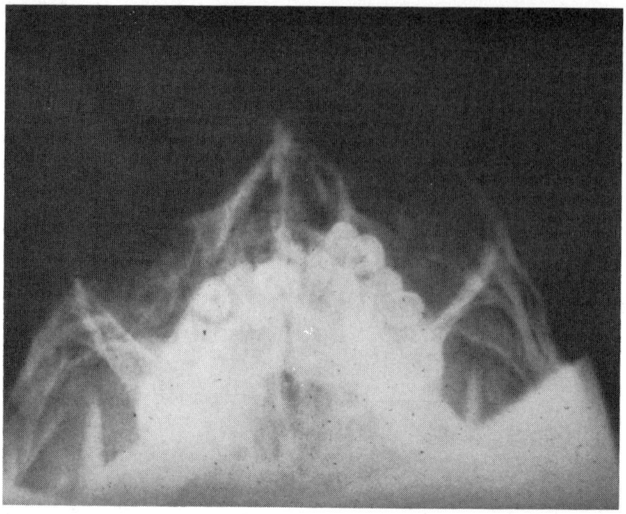

Figure 7. Vertical fracture of the maxilla. Submental x-rays showing fracture of the palate with marked posterior displacement of entire alveolar arch and left side of mid-face with orbital involvement. (This patient is shown in Figure 8 as well.)

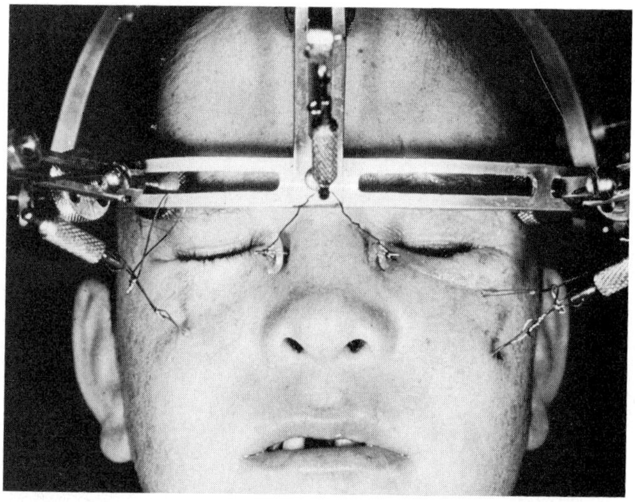

Figure 8. External appliance utilizing mechanical springs on nasal bones and maxilla. Kirschner wire is passed through nasal bones for pulling superiorly and outward. Wire on the right passes directly to the dental arch bar. On the left, wires combined from dental arch bar to infra-orbital rim. The headcap has been most satisfactory when used. (Farrior, R. T.: J. Mississippi State Med. Assoc., *2*:431, 1961.)

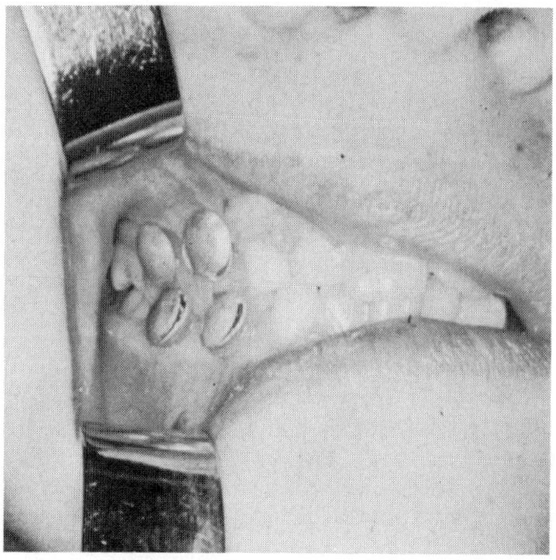

Figure 9. Intermaxillary fixation. Demonstrating the use of "clams" on a 9-year-old girl. The rubber bands are around the clams. The clams are neat, comfortable and unobtrusive, and they function well.

open reduction and interosseous wire fixation or suspension is indicated.

As in the adult, the mandible may be utilized as a guide for the proper positioning of the maxilla, and good occlusion must be obtained. Ophthalmologic and dental consultations should be used very readily, especially when the eye and teeth are involved.

In the past, middle third facial fractures in particular stimulated the inventiveness of the physician in developing elaborate headcaps and external appliances. Some of these appliances are still necessary and are useful to keep in reserve, but the trend in the management of these injuries is toward open reduction, direct interosseous wiring and fixation to the cranium. Figure 8 shows an external appliance used in past years.

The difficulty in utilizing the deciduous teeth for the purpose of immobilization of jaw fragments is that the height of contour is nearer the root on deciduous teeth, so that greater care is needed to get the ligature wire past this point. The Erich arch bar, because it is malleable, is preferred when the stability of an arch bar is required. With the use of "clams,"[12] #26 stainless steel wire and elastics, we have had minimal problems with intermaxillary wiring in children (Fig. 9).

INJURIES TO THE ANTERIOR TEETH

Children in the general age range of 6 to 12 years are in the stage of mixed dentition, which leads to some special problems in facial fractures and intermaxillary wiring. During these ages, the roots of the deciduous teeth are being resorbed, making some of them unsuitable for wiring. The permanent teeth erupting into the mouth during this period are undergoing development, and many of these teeth are unsuitable for wiring because of short roots or insufficient eruption of crown. During the stage of mixed dentition, some of the posterior teeth may not be in occlusion, and if these teeth are wired, they can be extruded. Knowing the approximate times of eruption of the various permanent teeth and the approximate ages at which the various deciduous teeth are usually shed, as well as having good x-rays, is a great aid in determining which teeth are most suitable for wiring with whichever method the surgeon chooses.

The deciduous teeth can withstand greater trauma than the usual permanent teeth and not lose their vitality, because they have a larger apical foramen, and therefore, the blood supply is less apt to be compromised. The primary incisors also seem to be displaced more frequently than fractured. A primary tooth that has been pushed out of its normal alignment by a blow frequently can be readjusted in position with little difficulty if the child is seen soon after the accident. These repositioned primary teeth, in many instances become firm again without subsequent discomfort and devitalization. The erupting permanent dentition also has a greater recuperative power of the pulp than the permanent tooth that has its apex and root fully formed; because they, too, have a large opening at the apical end and the blood supply is less easily compromised, with less subsequent pulpitis progressing to devitalization of the tooth.

Most teeth that are pushed out of normal alignment, but are still relatively firmly attached in the alveolar socket, can be saved even if the tooth later becomes devitalized and requires endodontic treatment. This is especially true of permanent dentition in the maxillary central and lateral incisors. Teeth that have been devitalized can often be saved with a root canal filling. Luxated permanent incisors or cuspids can often be reimplanted with or without a root canal filling, but this should be done within three to four hours. These teeth are wired into place with an arch bar or a lacing wire.[13] A permanent tooth with a fractured crown, but intact roots, can be salvaged with endodontic treatment and a rebuilt crown. Teeth that are attached to the buccal plate or a large portion of the alveolus can be repositioned gently and held in place with various types of wire fixation. Often these teeth are displaced at the incisal edge, but moved little at the apical end, so often these teeth will remain vital. Even if these teeth do not maintain their vitality, they may serve to hold a large bone fragment in place, saving this portion of the alveolus even if dental treatment is not successful and the attached teeth are later extracted.

One must be well aware of the fact that a traumatized tooth can become discolored or abscessed months later. The parents should be forewarned of this possibility and there should be a dental examination of the patient two to three months after such an injury. The preceding points are emphasized to avoid possible needless malocclusion and unnecessary extractions or otherwise unnecessary dental treatment that can be prevented with proper initial care.

COMPLICATIONS OF MIDDLE THIRD FACIAL FRACTURES IN CHILDREN

Early complications in children are rare, particularly with antibiotics and prompt treatment. The rapid healing of tissues may result in malunion, malocclusion and facial deformity, which can be avoided by early reduction and fixation. Late complications include dishface deformity, malocclusion and delay in eruption or malformation of the teeth. Facial deformity may result from malunion or from interference with growth and development of the facial bones. Diplopia, saddle nose, and traumatic hypertelorism are not different from these complications in the adult. An unattended cerebrospinal fluid rhinorrhea may result in acute meningitis. The premature loss of teeth in the child results in the lack of normal development of the body and alveolar process of the maxillary and mandibular bones and malocclusion.

Complications are fewer when the fracture is attended to promptly and efficiently, and the great majority of complications are preventable. There are, however, certain unavoidable complications related to the severity of the injury rather than to neglect or ignorance. Posttraumatic headaches and epilepsy do occur, as well as CSF leaks. There may be a permanent impairment of the sense of smell with a cribriform plate injury.

Ocular palsies can occur by stretching the third and sixth cranial nerves with head trauma, and on occasion, this can be permanent. Retrobulbar neuritis and secondary optic atrophy can occur with severe damage to the orbital floor. A severe retrobulbar hemorrhage may occasionally be encountered.[14]

SUMMARY

Middle third facial fractures are less common in children than in adults, but they can produce serious and possibly lifetime deformities if proper consideration and treatment are not given to such injuries initially. Because of the mixed dentition in children and the presence of active growth centers in the various facial bones, special attention and care must be given in treatment of such fractures to keep complications to a minimum. With proper and prompt care, a great service may be rendered to young patients.

REFERENCES

1. Converse, J. M. (Ed.): *Reconstructive Plastic Surgery,* Vol. 2. Philadelphia, W. B. Saunders Co., 1964, pp. 542–547.
2. Cottle, M. H.: Nasal surgery in children; effect of early nasal injury on growth of the nose. *Ear, Nose, Throat Monthly,* 30:32, 1951.
3. Farrior, R. T., and Connolly, M. E.: Septo-rhinoplasty in children. *Otolaryn. Clin. N. Amer.,* 3:345, 1970.
4. Kirchner, J. A.: Traumatic nasal deformity in the newborn. *Arch. Otol.,* 62:139, 1955.
5. Heinberg, C. J.: In Farrior, R. T.: Corrective surgery of the nasal framework. *J. Florida Med. Assoc.,* 45:276, 1958.
6. Carter, W. W.: The relation of minor injuries to the nose to subsequent nasal deformities. *Trans. Amer. Laryngol. Rhinol. Otol. Soc.,* 344, 1926.

7. Hinderer, K. H.: Common causes of disturbed nasal function. *Postgrad. Med.,* 30:580, 1961.
8. Kazanjian, V. H., and Converse, J. M.: *The Surgical Treatment of Facial Injuires,* 2nd Ed. Baltimore, Williams & Wilkins, 1959.
9. Bloom, S.: Rhinoplasty in adolescence. Presented at the World Congress of Oto-rhino-laryngology, Vol. 88, August 1968, pp. 193–196.
10. Dingman, R. O., and Natvig, P.: *Surgery of Facial Fractures.* Philadelphia, W. B. Saunders Co., 1964, pp. 311–337.
11. Bernstein, L.: Maxillofacial injuries in children. *Otolaryng. Clin. N. Amer.,* 2:397, 1969.
12. Brown, M., and Alexander, F.: Improved intermaxillary wiring. *Arch. Otol.,* 88:193, 1968.
13. Archer, W. H.: *Oral Surgery.* Philadelphia, W. B. Saunders, 1966.
14. Rowe, N. L., and Killey, H. C.: *Fractures of the Facial Skeleton.* Baltimore, Williams & Wilkins, 1955, pp. 256–489.
15. Farrior, R. T.: The management of facial injuries. *J. Miss. State Med. Assoc.,* 2:431, 1961.

Chapter Seventy-Nine

NASAL POLYPS

WILLIAM E. LAUPUS, M.D.

Nasal polyps are benign tumors that are occasionally seen in children with chronic nasal disease of infectious or allergic or combined origin. Polyps have been known for more than twenty centuries. In recent years they have been most commonly seen in children with long-standing cystic fibrosis of the pancreas and other organs (muco-viscidosis). They are pedunculated, edematous mucosal swellings that present in the nasal cavity as pale, smooth, grape-like masses arising from the surfaces of the middle turbinates and the ostia of the ethmoid and maxillary sinuses. They may also be found within the maxillary sinus, but the frontal and sphenoid sinuses seldom give rise to polypi.

If they protrude anteriorly through the nares, they are usually yellow-gray or dense white in color due to squamous metaplasia from chronic irritation. They may prolapse through the posterior choanae to cause obstruction of one or both choanal orifices. They are freely movable because of the narrow stalk that connects them to the mucosa.

Symptoms associated with nasal polyps are predominantly obstructive; secondary infection is frequently present. These children are mouth breathers with the distorted facial features associated with chronic nasal obstruction, an "adenoid" facies, often with depression and widening of the bridge of the nose. Nasal secretions are increased and a chronic mucoid or mucopurulent nasal discharge is commonly seen. Ethmoid and maxillary sinusitis, confirmed by transillumination and x-ray, is usually present.

The pathogenesis of polyp formation is not fully understood. Histochemical and microscopic studies have excluded myxomatous and glandular origins. The nature of the defect that causes the respiratory mucosa in atopic individuals to react excessively to a variety of different stimuli is imperfectly defined, but it appears to be related to increased permeability of the mucous membrane to antigens and to transmucosal stimulation of antibody (IgE) production. Although many children with nasal polyps are atopically sensitized and have other forms of atopy, evidence supporting an etiological relationship to a single antigen is only occasionally demonstrable.

Regardless of the cause, chronic mucosal edema and inflammatory changes (hyperplastic rhinitis and sinusitis) are fundamental to polyp formation. These conditions predominate along the middle turbinates and within the maxillary and ethmoid sinuses, where the mucosal reaction may be more severe or the stroma may be less confining.

As the polyp develops and grows in size, its reticular connective-tissue stroma binds increasing amounts of edema in the amorphous gel of its ground substance. Continuing accumulation of fluid within the polyp contributes to its shape, which gradually becomes bulbous but retains its connection to the mucosal base via a narrow stalk. Fibroblasts, histiocytes, eosinophiles, lymphocytes, mast cells and polymorphonuclear leukocytes are found in varying numbers in the stroma. Inclusion glands originating from invaginations of the polyp's epithelium are numerous in the stroma. The surface of the polyp is covered by a single layer of pseudostratified columnar epithelium and its basement membrane.

Schwachman and his associates have reported on the frequent association between cystic fibrosis and nasal polyps. Children with cystic fibrosis have inborn abnormalities of the secretions of exocrine and eccrine glands that lead to pancreatic obstruction, chronic pulmonary disease and disturbances of sodium and chloride homeostasis. The pulmonary (and pancreatic) disease relates to increased viscosity of mucosal secretions, which both causes obstruction and promotes acute (and then, later, chronic) nasal and sinus infection.

H. staphylococcus is the most frequent original organism involved in the pulmonary and nasal infections, but Pseudomonas, Klebsiella or Aerobacter organisms may predominate after the respiratory flora is altered by administration of broad-spectrum antibiotics.

In Shwachman's series of 742 patients with cystic fibrosis, 50 (6.7 per cent) had nasal polyposis. In the majority of children, the polyps appeared between the ages of 4 and 13 years. Approximately half of the affected children had associated allergic rhinitis and other allergies; all showed sinus involvement on x-ray. The diagnosis of cystic fibrosis was confirmed both by abnormal sweat chloride determinations (sweat chloride < 60 mEq./L.) and by clinical course. The predominating microorganisms isolated from the nasopharynx of these patients were *H. staphylococcus aureus* and *Pseudomonas aeruginosa.* All patients had received antimicrobial therapy for long periods prior to the study for nasal polyps.

Evaluation of children with nasal polyps requires examination for allergic and infectious factors and for cystic fibrosis. Although the polyps are susceptible to local removal, simple excision by any technique is seldom of permanent value unless the underlying condition is treated simultaneously and after-treatment is provided.

When the causative factor is determined to be allergic, environmental control and immunotherapy (hyposensitization or desensitization injections) will frequently be helpful after careful evaluation and skin testing. Continuous administration of antihistamine is useful to control rhinorrhea and to lessen mucosal edema. Although there are individuals who are sensitive to aspirin (acetylsalicylic acid) and who have nasal rhinitis, polyposis, and bronchial asthma which may respond only to corticosteroid therapy, this condition is rarely seen in children, and administration of corticosteroids to children with nasal polyposis should be limited to otherwise intractable situations. When the cause is infectious, the obstruction must be relieved and prolonged administration of the appropriate antimicrobial agent in adequate dosage for three to six weeks or longer must be provided to effect a good result.

In the child with cystic fibrosis, therapeutic measures for polyposis should be as simple as is possible, and the suppressive effect of orally administered broad-spectrum antibiotics may be all that is needed to prevent regrowth of polyps.

For patients *other than those with cystic fibrosis,* extensive surgical procedures such as maxillary sinus antrostomy and ethmoid exenteration may be rarely indicated.

Very rarely, nasal polyps may be neoplastic. Benign fibroangiomata, neurofibromata and gliomas have been noted in young children but are easily differentiated by biopsy. Malignant polypi are solid, friable and hemorrhagic; on biopsy, they are either carcinomatous or sarcomatous.

REFERENCES

Dolowitz, D. A., and Dougherty, T. F.: Nasal polyposis. *Arch. Otolaryng.,* 74:63, 1961.
Lederer, F. L.: The problem of nasal polyps. *J. Allergy,* 30:420, 1959.
Samter, M. (Ed.): *Immunological Disease,* Volume II. Boston, Little, Brown and Co., 1971.
Taylor, M.: Histochemical studies on nasal polypi. *J. Laryngol.,* 77:326, 1963

Chapter Eighty

FOREIGN BODIES

WILLIAM E. LAUPUS, M.D.

Obstruction of one nostril by a small, solid object is a frequent occurrence in childhood. Usually the foreign body is introduced by the child, whose unskilled attempts at removal force the object deeper into the nostril, where it may lodge in the anterior vestibule or in the inferior meatus on the floor of the nose. Beads, buttons, stones, peas, beans, erasers, nuts, paper wads, marbles and cherry pits are the most common objects. Some foreign bodies are hygroscopic and increase in size as water is absorbed.

Rhinoliths are special varieties of foreign bodies composed of insoluble salts derived from the nasal secretions; these salts are incorporated into a calcareous mass about a core such as a blood clot, mucus crust, dried pus or a small foreign body. Larvae of flies have also acted as foreign bodies when deposited in the nasal passages (myiasis).

The initial symptom is local obstruction, with mild or no discomfort. Severe pain is unusual unless the object is large or irregular and sharp. Irritation from the foreign body leads to mucosal swelling and to greater obstruction. Infection often follows and is associated with a purulent or sero-purulent discharge with a putrid odor. The drainage may be blood-tinged or frankly bloody if local ulceration and necrosis ensue. Rarely, perforation of the nasal septum may be a late complication of a long-standing foreign body reaction.

The combination of unilateral nasal obstruction and discharge should lead one to suspect the presence of a foreign body; the suspicion can usually be confirmed by examination through a nasal speculum. The foreign body should be removed promptly to minimize the danger of its aspiration into the larynx or tracheobronchial passages and to prevent local infection and necrosis.

Removal of a foreign body is not always simple and the physician should carefully consider all possible obstacles to easy removal before undertaking the procedure. The considerations should include the following: Is the nature of the foreign body known? How large is it? Is its surface smooth or irregular? Is it impacted or imbedded? How long has it been in place? How much mucosal reaction or infection is present? Will the foreign body come out readily without lacerating the mucosa or otherwise making removal a traumatic and painful experience for the child? Will local or general anesthesia be preferable? Is the child anxious or fearful? Is he old enough to reasonably be expected to hold himself still? Will restraints be necessary? Will the presence of one or both parents during the procedure be helpful or be a hindrance?

In preparing the child for the operation, a brief and simple explanation of what is to be done and what is expected of him while it is underway is essential. If restraint of the child is needed, he should be restrained adequately *before* any attempt at removal is made. If the child is cooperative, topical anesthesia should suffice; general anesthesia is occasionally required for the frightened and anxious child who rebels when removal is attempted under local anesthesia.

Simple instruments such as "alligator" forceps or a probe with a curved, noncutting hook at the tip (crochet needle) and nasal suction apparatus suffice for the extraction of most foreign bodies. The forceps are used to grasp rough and irregular objects, which fit easily between the tips of the instrument. The curved probe is best adapted for smooth masses such as beads, marbles and dried beans. The tip of the probe is passed beyond the object, which should come out readily when the probe is pulled back through the anterior nose. Tilting the head forward assists the movement of a heavy object, such as a steel ball, toward the anterior naris.

Removal of rhinoliths, which are often impacted, is more difficult and may require general anesthesia for extraction. Nosebleeds commonly follow removal of a foreign body; most will subside spontaneously or will respond to local measures short of packing. The infection associated with a foreign body tends to become more widespread with packing; hence, packing should be reserved for instances in which simpler measures fail.

Saline (0.9 per cent) nose drops instilled four times daily for five days after removal will aid in cleansing the irritated mucous membranes. Most infections will subside spontaneously; if the discharge is persistent and a second foreign body is not identified, culture and appropriate systemic antimicrobial therapy are indicated.

Chapter Eighty-One

EPISTAXIS

WILLIAM E. LAUPUS, M.D.

Nosebleed is a distressingly common problem in childhood, reaching peak incidence in the age range of 4 to 10. Males are more affected until puberty; then it occurs more often in females. It is rarely seen in infancy except as the result of trauma; in the newborn sepsis and disorders of hemostasis should also be suspected as possible causes.

The anterior septal and turbinate areas are the most common sites of epistaxes that occur usually without warning, often while the child is asleep at night or following minor trauma. The source of the bleeding tends to be obscure; a tiny bleeding point may be the only visible abnormality. In the majority of instances the source of the hemorrhage is a small vessel of Kiesselbach's plexus in Little's area on the anterior portion of the nasal septum. This plexus is made up of tiny anastomotic vessels that are poorly protected by the thin overlying mucosal and the sparse surrounding submucosal tissues. By its location, Little's area is subjected to drying on inspiration and multiple minor injuries, often unnoticed. Picking the nose, forcible blowing, introduction of a foreign body, nasal instrumentation and external trauma are the usual predisposing causes.

Rhinitis, sinusitis, nasal allergy, polyps and adenoidal hypertrophy contribute to vascular congestion of the nasal mucosa and to increased frequency of epistaxis. Rheumatic fever, typhoid fever, scarlet fever, varicella, measles, influenza, pertussis, diphtheria and malaria are associated with heightened susceptibility to nosebleed. Adolescent females occasionally bleed from the nose during menstruation. Trauma, vascular abnormalities (telangiectasias, varicosities), arterial hypertension, venous congestion secondary to increased venous pressure, blood dyscrasias and disorders of hemostasis are causes of serious hemorrhage from the nose. Highly vascular tumors such as angiofibromas may be responsible for major and repeated epistaxes.

Treatment in most instances is directed toward local control of the hemorrhage, which can be accomplished by compression of the nares. If bleeding is persistent, an anterior nasal pack should be inserted. Selvage-edged petrolatum gauze packing (1/2 inch in width) is preferred. The gauze is inserted first into the upper posterior nasal cavity and then added anteriorly until the cavity is filled. The packing should be removed in 24 to 36 hours, and may be reinserted if significant bleeding recurs.

An aqueous epinephrine solution (1:1000), topical thrombin and other hemostatic agents, such as oxidized cellulose and thromboplastin, may be useful occasionally. Caution must be exercised in the use of topical anesthetic agents when bleeding is active. It is easy to give excessive amounts of these drugs in the trying circumstances of attempting to halt large hemorrhages, and it is prudent to use them sparingly to avoid toxicity, which may result when they are swallowed. Placing the patient in an erect or semi-erect position with the head tilted forward facilitates clot formation and eliminates the annoyance of blood trickling posteriorly into the pharynx. When the site of bleeding cannot be found or when the bleeding originates in the posterior nares, combined anterior and postnasal or postchoanal packing is indicated (see Chapter 95).

Posterior packing of the nose is a much more complicated procedure than anterior packing and should be delegated, whenever possible, to the experienced otorhinolaryngologist. The pack consists of a suitably-sized piece of cotton, to which a strong tape or silk ligature, 18 to 24 inches in length, has been firmly tied. After applying as much anesthesia locally as is possible, a small rubber or polyethylene catheter is introduced through the appropriate naris into the pharynx, where it is grasped by forceps and pulled out of the mouth. After the free (suture) end of the previously prepared pack has been attached to the end of the catheter protruding through the mouth, the catheter is pulled back from the nose, bringing the tape or suture through the nostril, where it can be freed from the catheter. Traction on the suture is then applied to position the tampon in the nasopharynx, using a finger in the oral cavity to guide the placement. The pack should be left in place for 24 to 36 hours before removal and should be replaced if bleeding recurs. When packs are inserted into both nasal passages, the sutures should not be joined and tied at the nasal orifices, for this may cut or otherwise damage the columella, unless tied over a sponge.

Obliteration of the bleeding site by cautery with silver nitrate or electrocoagulation is useful when bleeding has been controlled, but it is seldom helpful when hemorrhage is active. Therapy with estrogens (orally or parenterally, or both) has not been proved to be of value. Applying ice packs to the nasal area and to the back of the neck is a time-honored effort of dubious value in the control of serious hemorrhage. Sedation may be beneficial when anxiety contributes to the patient's discomfort.

Hospitalization is indicated when bleeding is severe or underlying disease requires special therapy. Blood transfusion may be required when blood loss has been severe. The use of blood derivatives (platelets, fresh plasma, stored plasma and the like) may be necessary to control bleeding in patients who have underlying disorders of hemostasis. Although estimation of acute blood loss from severe epistaxis will sometimes be difficult, the amount of blood lost in most childhood nosebleeds is usually insignificant. If the quantity of blood lost is large, repeated determinations of hemoglobin and hematocrit levels will be helpful in assessing the need for blood replacement after the hemorrhage has been controlled; in childhood epistaxis, however, blood replacement is seldom necessary except in disorders of hemostasis, severe nasal trauma, tumors and other complicated situations.

Comprehensive care of the patient with nontraumatic and persistent nosebleed means a careful search for underlying and contributing causes of epistaxis. The investigation should include complete history, physical examination and appropriate laboratory studies, followed by specific preventive or corrective therapy wherever applicable.

In the usual circumstances relating to childhood epistaxis, study of coagulation factors will be normal. If such study is warranted, platelet count, prothrombin time, partial thromboplastin time, bleeding time, clotting time (Lee-White method) and clot retraction will be most useful in screening the possible disorders of hemostasis, which will include thrombocytopenia, "pseudohemophilia" and hemophilia, among others. Primary (idiopathic thrombocytopenic purpura) and secondary thrombocytopenias (leukemia) should be accompanied by other signs of an underlying ecchymotic disorder. Von Willebrand's disease, formerly a "pseudohemophilia," an autosomal dominant hereditary disease occurring in both sexes, is now considered to result from deficiency of a plasma factor needed for platelet adhesiveness. In this condition the bleeding time may be prolonged and Factor VIII, the antihemophilic factor, may be variably deficient. Von Willebrand's disease is being recognized with increasing frequency as a cause for severe epistaxis, which may be its only clinical manifestation. Therapy combining packing and the administration, as appropriate, of fresh whole blood or plasma, fresh or fresh frozen, will usually be successful in stopping the hemorrhage.

Rarely will the physician need to consider the possibility of ligation of the arterial blood supply to the bleeding area when a severe, exsanguinating, chronic nosebleed is otherwise unmanageable. In such instances, which arise more frequently from extensive trauma in childhood than from other causes, blood dyscrasias and coagulopathies should first be excluded and treated with appropriate blood factors, and nasal packing should be given ample opportunity to produce hemostasis before operative intervention is made.

Chapter Eighty-Two

NASAL ALLERGY

HARRY LOUIS MUELLER, M.D.

One of the most common allergic manifestations in children is involvement of the nasal passages. It appears most frequently after the age of six, but it can occur in early infancy or at any time during childhood and adolescence. Nasal allergy may appear in different forms, depending on its causative allergens, its association with infection and its seasonal, perennial, diurnal or sporadic occurrence. Nasal allergy is correctly termed allergic rhinitis and may be perennial or seasonal. It must be differentiated from nasal infections and from so-called vasomotor rhinitis, which is attributed to a vasomotor disturbance of the nasal tissues, usually because allergy can not be established as a cause of the nasal symptoms. Differentiation from all the other possible causes of nasal blockage and discharge has been discussed in preceding chapters.

PATHOLOGY AND PHYSIOLOGY

The histopathological changes in patients with nasal allergy during the early stages consist of edema and marked eosinophilic infiltration of the epithelial and subepithelial structures. In the more advanced forms, the epithelial layers show thickening and hyperplasia. The subepithelial layer is edematous, with eosinophilic, mononuclear and lymphocytic infiltration. The periosteal layer may show connective tissue proliferation and round cell infiltration with hyperplastic changes in the bony structure itself. If the allergy is modified by infection, the most characteristic change consists of infiltration with polymorphonuclear leukocytes and diminution of the eosinophils.

The nasal obstruction of allergic rhinitis will eventually interfere with the normal ventilation and cleansing function of the nasal passages that is usually accomplished by the mucosa with its cilia and the mucosal glands. Continued obstruction leads to poor ventilation and drainage, resulting in drying of the nasal mucosa, injury to the cilia, and increased susceptibility to infection. When the mucosa becomes edematous and irritated, even minor temperature or humidity changes may cause tissue reactions. Sinus drainage is obstructed, accounting for the headaches that may accompany the condition. If the obstruction persists, infective nasopharyngitis can follow. Continued swelling of the mucosa leads to constant nasal obstruction, which, in turn, results in mouth breathing. Although deformities of the mouth and teeth found in some children with nasal allergy have been ascribed to the continuous nasal obstruction, recent dental studies have indicated that malocclusive abnormalities are more likely caused by genetic factors.

Allergic rhinitis is an important consideration in the etiologic diagnosis and treatment of serous otitis media. Eustachian tube malfunction is the major cause of accumulation of fluid in the middle ear with serous otitis media, and such malfunction may frequently result from the pathophysiology of allergic rhinitis. In addition to the allergic involvement of the eustachian tube, the tissues of the middle ear itself may be affected, with edema and more persistent accumulation of fluid.

ETIOLOGY

Nasal allergy is more prevalent in children than is generally believed because the nasal symptoms are often misinterpreted as persistent or frequent colds, particularly when they precede or accompany an attack of asthma. A careful history of children with asthma who have nasal symptoms that were regarded as colds will reveal that many of these colds were really allergic rhinitis, and that in some children, they antedated the asthma by months or years.

Allergic rhinitis occurs twice as often in males as females before the age of 10, but more females are affected between the ages of 10 and 20 years. A family history of allergy makes it more likely that nasal symptoms in the child are of allergic origin. Frequent or excessive contact with a specific allergen is a factor in the development of any allergy, and in the case of inhalant allergens it is an important predisposing cause of allergic rhinitis. However, contact alone does not necessarily induce nasal allergy, as indicated by the fact that although all atopic children in almost all parts of this country inhale large amounts of grass pollen every year, only a relatively small number of them will develop allergic rhinitis due to grass pollen.

Connell has shown that once clinical nasal sensitivity is established, repeated daily exposure to the allergen by controlled inhalation challenge increases the reactivity of the nasal tissue, so that equal or even smaller subsequent doses produce a more severe and prolonged clinical reaction of allergic rhinitis. This has been called the priming effect of antigen exposure. He has also shown that this is a local effect on the tissues and not a systemic antibody response, since when only one nostril is primed by continued allergen challenge, the other nostril fails to respond to the same dose of the allergen. So-called priming is apparently nonspecific, since challenge of the primed tissue with another allergen that normally does not cause symptoms in the primed patient will precipitate allergic rhinitis at that time.

This hyper-reactivity of the nasal membrane produced by repeated daily challenge is reversible. After being produced by four successive days of challenge, elimination of challenge for two days causes the nasal membrane to return to the resistant state it was in, on the first day of challenge. The longer the duration of challenge, the longer the period needed for recovery. The mechanism for the priming effect is unknown, but Connell has postulated that the allergen challenge causes a chemotactic response, so that antibody-containing cells or cells containing chemical mediators of the allergic reaction migrate into the nasal membranes. Thus, on subsequent challenges, cells required for the production of an allergic reaction are already available locally.

This may explain the great variability of the clinical response in allergic rhinitis. An allergen to which a patient has minimal sensitivity may cause severe symptoms at a time when the tissues have been primed. On the other hand, exposure to an allergen that usually causes symptoms may cause little or no trouble if the patient has been free of antigen exposure for some time. It could explain why simultaneous exposure to two or more allergens may cause clinical symptoms when exposure to only one would produce no difficulty, the so-called summation effect of Rackemann.

Emotional and psychic factors may aggravate an already established allergic rhinitis, but rarely, if ever, are they the primary causes. Environmental conditions near the home, such as organic dusts, smoke, and chemical fumes from air pollution, or weather changes in temperature, humidity, and barometric pressures may predispose children to develop allergic rhinitis or may aggravate it after it has become established.

Etiologic Factors

The excitants most commonly responsible for allergic rhinitis, in order of frequency, are seasonal and environmental inhalant allergens, ingestant allergens, and possibly bacterial organisms and their products.

SEASONAL INHALANTS. The most

important excitants of seasonal allergic rhinitis are plant pollen and seasonal molds. Plant pollen is a cellular structure corresponding in the plant to the male sperm cell of the animal. Fertilization is the transfer of the pollen from the male element (stamen) to the female element (pistil). This is accomplished in several ways, and only those plants whose pollen is transferred by wind are likely to cause allergic rhinitis. Such plants produce huge amounts of pollen that is light and buoyant. (It has been estimated that during the pollinating season in some areas, there may be as much as three tons of ragweed pollen in a cubic mile of air.) Although many wind pollinated plants exist, only a relatively few possess the characteristics of wide distribution—small, light, buoyant grains and active antigenicity—necessary to induce clinical sensitivity. In this country, the most important pollens are from deciduous trees, grasses and weeds; specific species, dates, and length of season vary in different areas. The physician must acquaint himself with the important pollens of his own region before attempting to diagnose or to treat seasonal allergic rhinitis.*

Inhalant Environmental Allergens. These allergens are the most common causes of perennial allergic rhinitis in children. House dust and animal danders are the most frequent offenders, probably because children of all ages are down on the floor where these allergens abound and also because children usually have more intimate contact with animals than adults. Animal danders are particularly potent excitants of allergic rhinitis, and once sensitization has developed, even minute amounts of dander on the clothing of others may induce an allergic response. Cattle, hog, and horse hair with jute are used in felt rug pads, and children who habitually lie or play on the floor may develop symptoms from such exposure. House dust is believed to be a specific allergen, possibly a breakdown product of various textile fibers, but it may also contain other excitants, such as mites, fungi, and bacterial substances that are specific allergens causing allergic rhinitis. Other environmental inhalant allergens, such as feathers, wool, kapok, cotton linters, and even synthetic fibers, are less common excitants in allergic rhinitis. Very detailed environmental histories are necessary to discover the etiologic factors in obscure cases.

Food Allergens. As a cause of perennial allergic rhinitis, food is probably more important than is generally appreciated, especially in younger children. Common food sensitivities, i.e., to egg, wheat, corn, and milk, are difficult to detect because these foods are ingested in many forms daily in an ordinary diet, and with day-to-day symptoms a relationship can not be established. Furthermore, one can not rely upon skin test evidence for such determination, since the sensitivity may be due to a digestive break-down product of the ingested food rather than to the food from which the testing extract is made. Trial with elimination diets may be utilized to help uncover causative food factors.

Drugs. Drugs are infrequent causes of allergic rhinitis in children, but drugs instilled into nasal cavities may be responsible for initiation or aggravation of nasal symptoms because of local irritation (rhinitis medicamentosa mimics allergic rhinitis). Rarely, allergic rhinitis may be due to sensitivity to the topically-applied drug acquired through repeated use. It is inadvisable to use such potent sensitizers as the sulfones and antibiotics for local application to the nasal mucosa. Bacterial agents are regarded as factors in allergic rhinitis, but it is difficult to prove bacterial sensitization, and such a diagnosis usually must be made by the process of exclusion. The presence of infection is more frequently the result than the cause of allergic rhinitis.

Physical Agents. These are less frequent but still important excitants of allergic rhinitis. Whether the symptoms are caused by physical allergy or by non-

*This information is readily available either in standard texts on allergy or from pharmaceutical companies that produce extracts of allergens for diagnosis and treatment.

specific irritating factors has not been clearly established, but some children are particularly sensitive to temperature and climatic changes. They may have attacks with changes of season, particularly summer to fall and winter to spring. Some children do poorly at the seashore; others improve markedly. The same results can be found with almost every climatic or geographic change. However, the development or accentuation of allergic rhinitis in children from what are considered physical or climatic factors may really be caused by exposure to changes in environmental allergens at these times. There may be changes in house furniture and bedding as well as absence of pets in a summer cottage. Changes of season, in addition to being accompanied by increased incidence of respiratory infections, are also associated with turning the heat on or off, thus altering the concentration of environmental allergens in the home.

PSYCHOSOMATIC FACTORS. Finally, there is the possibility that allergic rhinitis symptoms are initiated by psychosomatic factors. When a symptom complex or complaining organ defies analysis by the usual methods, the baffled and irritated physician turns with increasing frequency to the psychosomatic to explain the unexplainable rather than spend further time attempting to unravel the obscure etiologic problem. There is no question that allergic nasal symptoms can be precipitated or accentuated by emotional factors, but there is no documented evidence or controlled study indicating that they are more than secondary, as emotional overlay on an underlying primary allergic etiology.

DIAGNOSIS

Clinical Diagnosis

The most characteristic symptom of nasal allergy is some degree of obstruction accompanied by a discharge that is usually profuse and watery. If the discharge becomes thickened and colored, superimposed infection should be suspected. Allergic nasal obstruction may be a very unpleasant symptom for both the patient and the parent, because it frequently leads to constant sniffling, mouth breathing, snoring, and nasal voice. Annoying postnasal discharge associated with cough, dryness, and irritation of the throat plus auditory disturbances of blocking and popping sensations are all common secondary symptoms of allergic rhinitis (Table 1).

There may be loss of the senses of smell and taste, frontal headaches, and lassitude. Other common symptoms are itching of the nose, sneezing, and itching and watering of the eyes, particularly in seasonal allergic rhinitis due to pollen sensitivity. These symptoms lead to nasal twitching and rubbing of the tip of the nose in a characteristic transverse or upward motion, commonly described as "the allergic salute" (Fig. 1). If this is done repeatedly over several years, it may result in a transverse nasal crease across the lower third of the nose at the junction of the bulbous soft portion and the more rigid bridge (Fig. 2). Persistence of the obstruction may bring about a broadening of the bridge of the nose because of edema and swelling of surrounding tissues. The associated irritation of mucous membranes, marked sneezing, forceful blowing, and mechanical picking or rubbing are all probable contributing causes to the increased frequency of epistaxis in children with nasal allergy. About one-third of children with untreated allergic rhinitis will develop asthma. Persistent dry cough with allergic rhinitis is an early warning signal of the probable onset of a complicating asthma. Another physical sign of nasal allergy in children is the dark circles or discoloration in the lower orbitopalpebral grooves, possibly caused by venous stasis in this area, known as the "allergy shiner" (Fig. 3).

On examination of the child with active allergic rhinitis, the turbinates usually appear pale or purplish, boggy and covered with glistening mucus, but allergic changes are rapidly reversible

TABLE 1. DIFFERENTIAL FEATURES OF ALLERGIC AND INFECTIOUS RHINITIS

Characteristics	Perennial Allergic Rhinitis	Infectious Rhinitis (Common Cold)
Onset of acute attack	Often sudden	Gradual with stuffy and runny nose and fever
Sneezing	Often prominent	Slight or absent
Nasal discharge	Thin, watery and profuse, particularly at the onset; later thicker, but usually colorless throughout and nonirritating	Thick and mucoid, becoming increasingly so. Colorless at outset, but quickly becomes yellowish or grayish. Irritating to skin of external nares and upper lip
Nasal obstruction	Present and variable	Rather marked; subsides gradually
Eye symptoms (e.g., itching, lacrimation, and conjunctivitis)	Often present, particularly in older children	Usually absent
Constitutional symptoms (e.g., fever and malaise)	Usually absent	Often present
Contagion	None	Marked
Duration of symptoms	A few hours to two to three days, with rapid clearing and frequent recurrences. Mild rhinorrhea in between	Four to seven days or longer. Usually clears completely, with infrequent recurrences
Hereditary factor or other evidence of allergy	Often present	Usually absent, unless it occurs in child with allergic rhinitis
Nasal smear	Shows predominance of eosinophils	Predominance of neutrophils, with few or no eosinophils
Response to antihistaminics	Usually prompt with temporary relief	Little or none

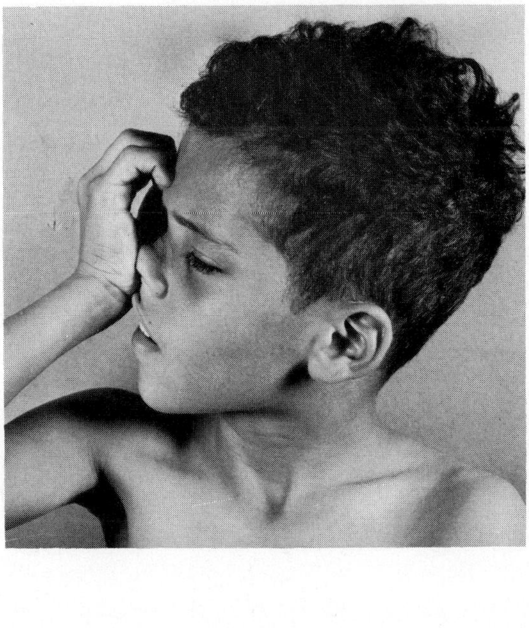

Figure 1. Allergic salute in child, aged 9 years, who has had perennial allergic rhinitis since infancy and bronchial asthma since age 2. (From Marks, M. B.: *Physical Signs of Allergy of the Respiratory Tract in Children.* The Upjohn Company, 1967.)

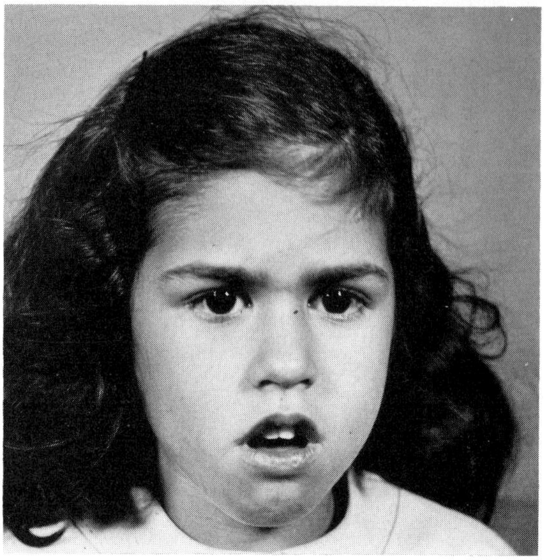

Figure 2. Typical gaping appearance in child, aged 4 years, with perennial allergic rhinitis since 1 year of age. This child has been a mouth breather since birth. V-shaped palate is present with over-riding maxillary incisor teeth. (From Marks, M. B.: *Physical Signs of Allergy of the Respiratory Tract in Children.* The Upjohn Company, 1967.)

and at times the turbinates in these patients may be pink, moist and normal in appearance. Long-standing allergic rhinitis is usually associated with hypertrophied lymphoid follicles on the pharyngeal wall, which is thought to be a part of the immune response in allergic children, since this hypertrophic tissue, including adenoids, may recede following specific treatment of the allergy. True nasal polyps or polypoid changes in the turbinates are rare in children. If found, they indicate the probable presence of cystic fibrosis.

Laboratory aids in diagnosis include smears of nasal secretions stained with Wright's or Hansel's stain to identify eosinophils and Papanicolaou stains of nasal smears of mucosal cellular elements to identify changes in the epithelial cells as well as the presence of eosinophils. If a large number of eosinophils are present repeatedly, or if the epithelial cells are swollen and distorted, it

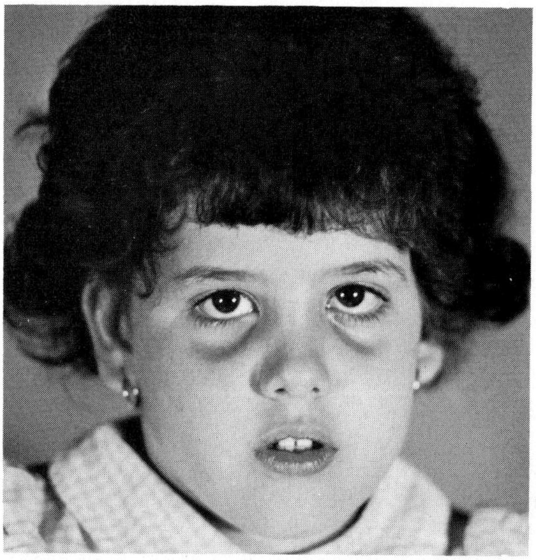

Figure 3. Allergic shiners in child, aged 4 years, with pronounced perennial allergic rhinitis due chiefly to foods and inhalants. (From Marks, M. B.: *Physical Signs of Allergy of the Respiratory Tract in Children.* The Upjohn Company, 1967.)

suggests the presence of an allergic reaction. If neutrophils predominate, or if the epithelial cells are pyknotic with shrunken nuclei, the presence of infection is likely. Of course, if infection is superimposed upon an allergic reaction, then all of these changes may be present. A blood eosinophilia above 5 per cent or a total eosinophil count above 400 suggests that the condition is allergic in origin. X-ray studies of the sinuses in older children and adolescents with allergic rhinitis may reveal large swollen turbinates and swelling of the lining membranes of the sinuses without evidence of retained secretions or fluid levels and be helpful in differential diagnosis.

In those patients who have marked nasal obstruction with hypertrophic turbinates but who have little or no sneezing or rhinorrhea and in whom repeated examination of the nasal smear shows few or no eosinophils, the condition is more likely to be of the nonsensitive type, which is designated as vasomotor rhinitis. In such patients, determination of a specific cause for the nasal symptoms is unlikely to be successful, and treatment with antihistaminic drugs usually is ineffective.

Etiologic Diagnosis

The methods employed in determining the specific excitants in allergic rhinitis are history taking, allergy testing, therapeutic elimination and challenge, and diary records. A detailed description of these procedures is beyond the scope of this chapter and the reader is referred to standard texts on pediatric allergy for such specific diagnostic procedures. Suffice it to say that the most important diagnostic tool in most cases is a careful detailed history with all the relationships of time, place, contacts, ingestants and environment.

It must be remembered that skin tests are *aids* to diagnosis, require experience for interpretation, may give false positive reactions, and must be placed in their proper perspective. A true positive skin test indicates that the patient has developed a measurable skin sensitizing antibody, probably of the gamma E class of immunoglobulins, to the allergen used for that test. It means that the patient may have been clinically sensitive to that allergen in the past, may be sensitive to it at the present, or is potentially, clinically sensitive to it in the future.

In the author's opinion, skin testing should be done by the scratch method first. In children, such tests are easier to perform, less painful, more specific, safe and less expensive. In many instances, all the indicated testing can be done at one visit, which is a distinct advantage in children who build up emotional tensions over repeated visits involving unpleasant procedures. Intracutaneous testing is more sensitive, but it also gives many more nonspecific false positive reactions, and in the exquisitely sensitive patient, it can cause serious and even fatal reactions. *An intracutaneous test should not be done with any allergen until the patient has first been tested with that allergen by the scratch method.* If the scratch test is positive, no further skin testing information is needed. If the scratch test is negative and the history indicates that that allergen is suspected, then an intracutaneous test can be done without fear of a severe or dangerous reaction. In most instances, this limits painful and time-consuming intracutaneous testing to a relatively few selected allergens.

A detailed description of skin testing methods and their interpretation is not within the scope of this chapter, but certain points will bear emphasis. The routine use of large numbers of allergens in testing should be avoided. The choice of allergens used should depend upon the history and, to some extent, upon age. It is not ncessary to test an infant or young child with all kinds of food allergens when his diet is limited. Since a child can be allergic to the odor of a food being cooked, particularly seafood and egg, this must be taken into consideration in the selection of foods for testing. If the history reveals the symptoms to be limited to pollen seasons, then testing can be limited to pollens and seasonal molds. If the diagnosis is in doubt by history and skin testing, then inhalation challenge or ophthalmic testing can be performed to confirm the clinical sensitivity by actually producing the allergic reaction in the offending tissue.

TREATMENT

Treatment depends upon the results of the diagnostic procedures. If the specific cause can be determined, treatment is directed toward eliminating those allergens or toward hyposensitization with them. Hyposensitization treatment lessens the patient's sensitivity by blocking the interaction of antigen with antibody that ordinarily releases the chemical mediators causing the clinical allergic reaction. If a specific cause cannot be found, then treatment must be symptomatic.

The best way to treat any allergy is to remove the allergen. Not only does the allergic reaction stop, but with continued elimination there is a tendency for the sensitivity to lessen or subside, as there is no antigen present to stimulate the production of specific antibody. In food allergy, elimination is the only successful method of treatment. Most environmental allergens, such as animal danders, fibers, feathers, textiles, molds, and even house dust to a variable extent, can be eliminated well enough to effectively reduce exposure to them. Contact with such nonspecific irritants as paint, insecticides, powders, highly scented materials and tobacco smoke should also be avoided.

When it is impossible or impractical to eliminate the causative allergen, then hyposensitization injection treatment should be tried. Pollens, molds, house dust and, in certain instances, animal danders, are used for this treatment. These should be employed individually to attain the maximum tolerated dose of each specific allergen involved. Using mixtures of extracts of allergens that happen to give positive skin tests in the patient, regardless of correlation with history, is the worst kind of blind shotgun therapy and has no place in treatment that is presumably based on specific immunological reactions.

The principle utilized in hyposensitization treatment consists of the subcutaneous introduction of gradually increasing amounts of the specific allergen until the maximum tolerated dose is reached, resulting in lessened sensitivity, and then maintaining that protection by boosters of that maximum tolerated dose at the greatest interval possible. The dose of the initial injection must be judged by history and results of skin testing. Children tolerate relatively larger doses of allergens than adults and are less likely to have constitutional reactions, but the treatment must be individualized for each patient. Increases depend upon the size or degree of the local reaction following each injection and upon the presence or absence of any systemic symptoms.

The interval between injections depends on the patient's reactions and on the speed with which it is necessary to obtain the desired protection. Using aqueous extracts of allergens, the average patient requires approximately 12 to 16 injections to reach the maximum tolerated dose. For example, if a patient whose symptoms occur each year from August 15 to frost presents for treatment in June, the injections must be given twice a week for the build-up period to reach the maximum tolerated or protective dose before the beginning of the ragweed season. If the same patient presents for treatment in November, then the build-up injections can be given at two- to four-week intervals and still reach the protective dose by the next pollen season. After the protective dose is reached, the interval between booster doses should be increased to four weeks, or even longer if there is no excessive reaction and the patient is improved. Once the protective dose is determined, the individual allergens can be combined in mixtures specially prepared for the indicated dosage or can be given in one syringe if the total amount does not exceed 1.0 ml. (the capacity of a tuberculin syringe).

Failure to obtain clinical improvement with hyposensitization treatment may mean that the dosage was incorrect (too small or too large), that the allergen being given was not etiologically significant, or that it was not antigenic because of either preparation or deterioration.

If clinical improvement has resulted, treatment is maintained on a perennial schedule for a minimum of three years, and then the patient should be given a year of observation without injection treatment. If the patient does as well without treatment as he had done with it, then it seems obvious that injections are no longer necessary. If the patient does not do as well without treatment, injections should be resumed to get the desired effect again. In the author's experience, approximately four out of five children will retain the protection when injections are stopped after three years with satisfactory improvement. Only a few of these patients will have a relapse more than one year after stopping treatment.

There are two types of allergenic extracts commercially available. These are conventional aqueous extracts and alum-precipitated pyridine extracts.* If alum-precipitated pyridine extracts are employed, the treatment requires fewer injections at longer intervals and will have fewer side reactions. These extracts, introduced in 1959, presumably have the active undefatted allergen in precipitated form, resulting in slower absorption and less likelihood of systemic reactions. Larger doses can be given to highly reactive patients. In the author's experience, this is advantageous in some patients, and children doing poorly on aqueous extracts may do well on Allpyral extracts. However, the reverse also seems to be true; that is, children doing poorly on Allpyral may do better when given aqueous extracts. There have been conflicting reports concerning Allpyral extracts, and controlled comparative studies are needed to confirm the clinical reports of its effectiveness. The choice of extracts will depend on the patient, the allergens involved and the physician's personal experience with them.

Repository or emulsion extracts for treatment have been used in an attempt to eliminate the necessity for multiple injections and perhaps to induce a better immune response, based upon the principle of Freund's adjuvant. Emulsion therapy is in the experimental phase, but it has not been approved by the Food and Drug Administration for commercial distribution, and it should not be used in treating children until its safety and effectiveness have been established.

Symptomatic treatment is frequently necessary to relieve the annoying symptoms of nasal allergy, and it may be the sole method of treatment if specific etiologic allergens cannot be determined. Medications include those drugs given internally and those applied locally to the nasal mucosa. Internally, antihistamines of the various groups may be useful in combating the histamine effect of edema and excessive secretions. Because of their vasoconstricting decongestant effect on nasal mucosa, drugs in the ephedrine group will reduce the obstruction but may increase the rhinorrhea. When they are combined with antihistamines, more effective symptomatic relief is usually obtained. Since patients show variable responses to such combinations, it may be necessary to try several different ones before finding an effective medication for the individual patient.

The application of shrinking agents directly to the nasal mucosa by dropper or spray often provides temporary symptomatic relief. Brief discussions of these drugs and their usage are given in earlier chapters. Shrinking agents that contain an ephedrine type of drug in combination with a corticosteroid may be very beneficial in allergic rhinitis if they are used with discretion. It must be remembered that persistent or too frequent use of local medications may create a vicious cycle in which the primary shrinking effect is followed by a secondary obstructive reaction, and it may develop into a full-blown rhinitis

---

*Allpyral, Dome Laboratories, West Haven, Conn.

medicamentosa that is mistaken for the original allergic rhinitis. Often, patients are referred for diagnosis and treatment of rhinitis, and elimination of medications results in clearing of the symptom complex. Withdrawal of medications in these patients may temporarily result in such severe obstruction that the patient and parent will not continue the elimination program long enough for the inflammatory reaction to subside. It is useful to put patients suspected of having rhinitis medicamentosa on full doses of corticosteroids (20 to 30 mg. daily) for the first week during withdrawal of local medication. This usually clears the inflammatory reaction long enough to allow it to subside without that initial period of severe withdrawal obstruction.

Oral corticosteroids are frequently very helpful in relieving the symptoms of allergic rhinitis and may be used for short periods when other medications are not effective. They are particularly useful in pollen seasons when heavy pollen counts produce severe symptoms. When corticosteroids are discontinued, the nasal allergy recurs if the etiologic allergen is still present. Long-continued use of corticosteroids is inadvisable because of their well-known adverse side effects.

Antibiotics should be given in allergic rhinitis only when there is associated infection. The possibility that allergic rhinitis is secondary to bacterial allergy has never been clearly established, and if such a thing occurs, it must be quite rare. In patients with nasal symptoms that are impossible to determine as infectious or allergic rhinitis, the use of an antibiotic may be helpful in making this differentiation.

Nasal surgery should not be attempted in patients with allergic rhinitis until the results of adequate allergic management have been evaluated. Close cooperation between the rhinologist and allergist is essential for that evaluation.

REFERENCES

Brown, E. A.: Treatment of pollinosis by means of a single annual injection of emulsified extract. *Ann. Allergy,* 17:34, 1959.

Connell, J. T.: Quantitative intranasal pollen challenges. III. The priming effect in allergic rhinitis. *J. Allergy,* 43:33, 1969.

Davison, F. W.: Middle ear problems in childhood. *J.A.M.A.,* 10:126, 1966.

Ferguson, C. F.: Changing concepts in otolaryngology for the pediatrician. *Pediatrics,* 25:1043, 1960.

Marks, M.: Physical signs of allergy of the respiratory tract in children. *Ann. Allergy,* 25:310, 1967.

Mueller, H. L.: Dosage in the treatment of pollinosis. *Pediat. Clin. N. Amer.,* 1:4, 1954.

Shirkey, H. C.: *Pediatric Therapy.* St. Louis, C. V. Mosby, 1969, pp.817–819.

Shwachman, H., Kulczyki, L. L., Mueller, H. L., and Flake, C. G.: Nasal polyposis in patients with cystic fibrosis. *Pediatrics,* 30:3389, 1962.

Tuft, L.: Treatment of allergic conditions with alum-precipitated pyridine extracts of allergens other than ragweed. *Acta Allergol.,* 21:414, 1966.

Tuft, L., and Mueller, H. L.: *Allergy in Children.* Philadelphia, W. B. Saunders Co., 1970.

Whitcomb, N. J.: Allergy therapy in serous otitis media associated with allergic rhinitis. *Ann. Allergy,* 23:232, 1965.

Chapter Eighty-Three

ACUTE RHINITIS (ACUTE NASOPHARYNGITIS; COMMON COLD; CORYZA)

HENRY G. CRAMBLETT, M.D.

Acute rhinitis is the most common respiratory illness of infants and children. Almost by definition, this is a disease of viral etiology (Table 1).

Incidence

It is estimated that each child has an average of three to six episodes of acute rhinitis, common cold or undifferentiated upper respiratory tract disease each year.

Etiology

Bacteria rarely, if ever, cause primary rhinitis. A wide variety of viruses, including the rhinoviruses, adenoviruses, enteroviruses, influenza viruses, parainfluenza viruses and respiratory syncytial virus, have been shown to cause this anatomic syndrome. The importance of the recently described coronaviruses in childhood infections is not known. To date, in studies of adults, the rhinoviruses have proved to be the most important agents in the causation of acute rhinitis. They play a less important etiologic role in upper respiratory tract disease in infants and children. There is nothing in the clinical picture that would help one to differentiate the common cold due to one virus from that due to another.

TABLE 1. ETIOLOGIC CLASSIFICATION OF ACUTE RHINITIS

A. Bacterial (rare if ever)

B. Viral
  1. Adenoviruses
  2. Coronaviruses
  3. Enteroviruses
  4. Influenza viruses
  5. Parainfluenza viruses
  6. Respiratory syncytial virus
  7. Rhinoviruses

C. Mycoplasma
  1. *Mycoplasma pneumoniae*

Pathogenesis

The primary focus of infection in this disease is in the mucosa of the nose. Initially there is mononuclear infiltration, which later may be followed by a polymorphonuclear infiltrate. Ordinarily other portions of the respiratory tract, including the pharynx, larynx, the tracheobronchial tree and occasionally the accessory sinuses, are involved in the infection.

Clinical Manifestations

The child with acute nasopharyngitis differs from the adult with the same disease in that the child usually has accompanying fever, whereas the adult is usually afebrile. In infancy, a frequent presenting sign of acute nasopharyngitis is fever which may precede by several hours the onset of a serous or seromucoid nasal discharge and other signs of

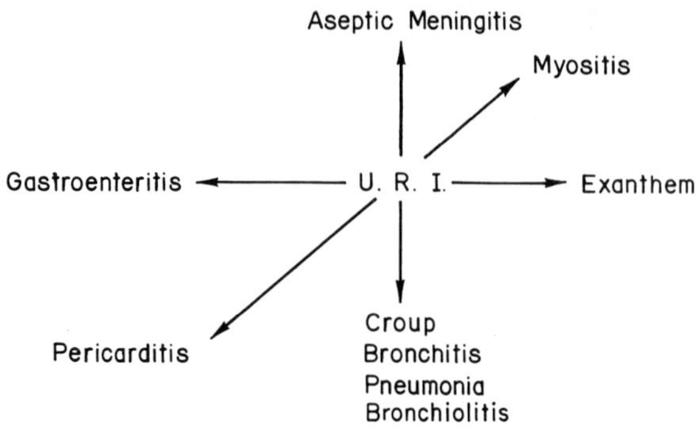

Figure 1. Schematic representation of biphasic viral illnesses in which the initial disease is an upper respiratory illness. (From Cramblett, H. G.: Viral respiratory illnesses of infants and children. *Bacteriol. Rev.*, 28:431, 1964.)

coryza, including cough and sneeze. In older children, fever may not be as prominent, and the initial complaint may be a feeling of dryness of the nose or the nasopharynx followed by a profuse watery, serous or seromucoid nasal discharge. Cough may occur because of postnasal drainage or because of actual involvement of the tracheobronchial tree. In infancy, vomiting and diarrhea, usually not severe, may accompany the respiratory symptoms.

Diagnosis

In considering the diagnosis of primary acute rhinitis, one must rule out the existence of other diseases that are viral and biphasic in nature and in which the minor illness may be rhinitis. These diseases with more major manifestations include exanthematous disease, aseptic meningitis, pneumonia and croup (Fig. 1). There is nothing distinctive about nasopharyngitis caused by one virus as opposed to that caused by another virus. Etiologic diagnosis depends upon recovery of virus from nasopharyngeal secretions or upon serologic testing. Since these procedures are time-consuming and expensive, they are not indicated, other than for epidemiologic purposes.

Complications

The most frequent complication of acute rhinitis in infancy and childhood is the development of otitis media. Although this may begin as a serous otitis media, it frequently develops into purulent otitis media with inflamed, bulging ear drums. In addition, either primary or secondary pneumonia may occur. Moreover, secondary purulent bacterial rhinitis may follow a primary viral rhinitis.

Treatment

Since nasopharyngitis is due entirely to viruses, there is no specific therapy. Symptomatic therapy of infants with this disease includes the judicious use of phenylephrine hydrochloride (0.25 or 0.125 per cent) nose drops or spray, adequate hygiene to the nose, and the use of a vaporizer. In infants in whom the nasal discharge becomes so thick and profuse that it interferes with feeding, it may be necessary to irrigate the nasal passages gently with normal saline solution by means of an ear-bulb syringe. In case of secondary purulent rhinitis, the use of a nasal spray with neomycin or bacitracin, after careful cleansing of the nose, may be helpful.

Other symptomatic measures that may be of value include the use of acetylsalicylic acid and one of the antihistamines.

REFERENCES

Cramblett, H. G.: Viral respiratory illnesses of infants and children. *Bacteriol. Rev.*, 28:431, 1964.

Hamparian, V. V., Leagus, M. B., and Hilleman, M. R.: Additional rhinovirus serotypes. *Proc. Soc. Exp. Biol. & Med.*, 1116:976, 1964.

Chapter Eighty-Four

ACUTE SINUSITIS

WILLIAM E. LAUPUS, M.D., and PETER N. PASTORE, M.D.

Although the nasal accessory sinuses are present in a rudimentary form at birth, only the maxillary antra and the anterior and posterior ethmoidal cells are sufficiently well differentiated and pneumatized to be involved in nasal infection in young infants and children. The frontal sinuses, derived from anterior ethmoidal cells, are incorporated into the growing frontal bone after the second year of life; they become pneumatized slowly and are of clinical importance after the sixth year. Ethmoidal infection early in life may prevent or impair the development of the frontal sinuses, which may then be small, unilateral or even absent. Variations in size, shape, position, and number of sinuses are common, especially in the ethmoid and frontal groups. The sphenoid sinus is intranasal until about the third year, when, through growth and absorption of intervening cartilage, it becomes surrounded by the sphenoid bone; it is rarely of clinical significance in childhood and then only after the fourth or fifth year of life.

The ciliated pseudocolumnar epithelial mucosal lining of the sinuses is continuous with that of the nasal passages; it is covered by an intact layer of mucus that is propelled toward and through the sinal ostium by ciliary action, providing for drainage of the sinus without mucus accumulation within its cavity and for constant replenishing of the mucus "blanket," two of the most important factors in maintaining the regional immunity of the respiratory tract.

The nose and accessory sinuses harbor a "normal" flora, consisting of poorly defined numbers of nonpathogenic bacteria (*N. catarrhalis,* diphtheroids, *Staphylococcus epidermidis*) and viruses, in addition to potentially pathogenic organisms that colonize for a short time or for longer periods, sometimes maintaining a semipermanent "carrier" state. Knowledge pertaining to resistance to infection is far from complete, but anatomic deviations that interfere with the flow of the mucus blanket, noxious inhalants that decrease ciliary activity or give rise to mucosal edema and allergic changes, and the number of pathogenic organisms in the inoculum are important contributing factors to reduction in local immunity and the subsequent development of infection. The mucous membranes of the nose are in constant contact with the external environment; the variations in pH, electrolyte, carbohydrate and protein content of mucosal secretions in response to inhalation of irritants, smoke, pollutants, and allergens reflect the sensitivity and reactivity of the mucosa to environmental conditions.

Secretory IgA antibodies, 11S immunoglobulins synthesized in the plasma cells present in the lamina propria of the mucous membrane and in secretory glands, have assumed increasing importance in specific immunity to most respiratory viruses; they appear to play no role in mycoplasma and bacterial infections. Secretory enzymes, characterized earlier as lysozymes, probably exert a significant nonspecific antimicrobial effect on invasive organisms. Cellular immunity, phagocytosis, other secretory substances and nonspecific humoral factors probably contribute substantially to immunity, but their roles have not been studied as thoroughly as the more readily measurable antibodies. These modalities of resistance to infection are presumably shared by the nasal accessory sinuses.

Acute Catarrhal Sinusitis

Acute nasal infections of the "common cold" type involve the sinuses as well as the nose. The nasal secretions are thin and increase in amount; nasal obstruction is frequently present; headache, usually localized to the face and forehead, is common; pain in the posterior upper teeth and maxillary areas is occasionally present. The mucosa becomes hyperemic and edematous; ostia of the sinuses may become partially or completely occluded, predisposing to acute bacterial sinusitis if the obstruction is prolonged more than two to three days and organisms capable of mucosal invasion are present. Such infections are short-lived and subside concomitantly with the nasal infection, at most, requiring conservative management.

Acute Suppurative Sinusitis

This pyogenic bacterial infection is most commonly seen as a complication of an acute viral rhinitis. Viral infections appear to upset the balance between inactive pathogenic organisms present in the "carrier" state and host resistance in two ways: first, by lessening physical properties of immunity, such as ciliary action and integrity of the mucus blanket, thereby creating stasis and facilitating bacterial invasion; and second, by in some way (perhaps through alterations in the physical properties of the mucus) encouraging rapid multiplication of the pathogenic organisms. Pre-existing adenoidal obstruction of the nasal airways, chronic allergic rhinitis, severe deflection of the nasal septum, nasal polyp or other tumor, or nasal foreign body may provide additional contributory local factors in children.

Once the normal defense mechanism is overcome, the organism gains entrance to the mucosal cells of the nose and sinus and bacterial infection takes place. When the sinal mucous membrane becomes infected, narrowing of the ostium of the involved sinus may interfere with the movement of mucopurulent secretions from the sinus, leading to further stasis and, if the ostium is obstructed, producing an empyema in which none of the purulent material drains into the nose. Usually, the sinus orifice is partially open and the purulent discharge drains into the nasal cavity. Pus seen superior to the middle turbinate usually originates from the sphenoid or posterior ethmoid sinuses, whereas secretions found in the region of the middle meatus arise in the anterior sinuses (maxillary, frontal or anterior ethmoid). In infants and small children, periorbital edema may be seen with infection in the ethmoid cells.

Fever, nasal congestion, sensation of fullness or pain, tenderness over the sinus, disturbances of smell and facial paresthesias are common complaints in acute sinus infections. Older children with acute sinusitis complain of pain (headache) in the temporal region or above or between the eyes (with anterior ethmoiditis), in the postauricular (mastoid) region (with posterior ethmoiditis), in the face or upper teeth (with maxillary antritis), in the forehead (with either frontal or maxillary disease, alone or in combination) and in the suboccipital area (with sphenoiditis).

The diagnosis should be suspected when the preceding signs and symptoms appear three to five days following a viral upper respiratory infection. Rhinoscopy will usually reveal purulent discharge in the nasal passages with a red, thickened, edematous nasal mucosal surface, findings consistent with rhinosinusitis. Tenderness may be elicited over the frontal, anterior ethmoid or maxillary sinuses. Transillumination in older children may be helpful in delineating frontal and maxillary disease. X-ray films are not usually necessary to establish the diagnosis of acute sinusitis, but may show opacification of the involved sinus or sinuses.

Pneumococci and group A hemolytic streptococci (beta) are the predominating bacterial organisms; alpha streptococci, *H. staphylococcus* (coagulase-positive) and *Hemophilus influenzae* are less common offenders. Other organisms, including *E. coli* and those generally considered to be nonpathogens, may occasionally be involved.

Conservative, nonoperative therapy is usually successful and is directed to promoting drainage of the infected sinus and to specific antimicrobial therapy of the infection. Instillations of nasal vasoconstrictors at regular intervals by dropper, or preferably by spray and gentle aspiration are helpful in shrinking the nasal mucosa, opening the sinal ostia and keeping the airways clear; prolonged use, more than seven to ten days, is not recommended. Nasal aspirations may be helpful. Blowing of the nose should be avoided. Preferred nasal vasoconstrictors include 1 per cent ephedrine and 0.25 per cent phenylephrine (Neo-Synephrine) solutions every three to four hours or 0.05 per cent oxymetazoline hydrochloride (Afrin) solution every 12 hours in children 6 years of age and older. The vasodilatory rebound phenomenon seen commonly with all vasoconstrictors should not be troublesome in short-term therapy. Use of combination nasal drops and sprays containing vasoconstrictors, antihistamines, steroids, and antibiotics in low dosage should be firmly discouraged.

Effective use of nose drops and nasal sprays requires careful instruction by the physician. For best results with drops, the child should be positioned on his right side with his head tilted downward slightly (at a 30-degree angle) over the edge of a bed or couch. Two to four drops are instilled into the right nostril and allowed to spread over the mucosa for 30 to 60 seconds. Sniffing gently will assist in the distribution of the medication. The patient is then similarly positioned on his left side and the drops are instilled into the left nostril. When sprays are used, the child should be sitting upright. Each nostril should be sprayed once (single spraying) to bring about vasoconstriction of the anterior portion of the nose. One to two minutes later the spraying is repeated to reach the upper and posterior parts of the nose, especially the regions between the turbinates near the sinal ostia.

Although therapy with antihistamines in acute sinusitis is somewhat controversial, it may be helpful in sustaining the vasoconstriction and decongestion brought about by the nasal vasoconstrictor applications. Antihistamines may also be useful in controlling the allergic rhinitis that frequently underlies instances of recurrent acute sinus infections. Whenever used, these agents should be administered orally in appropriate dosage. Preferred antihistamines include pyrrobutamine compound (Co-Pyronil), administered every twelve hours, brompheniramine maleate (Dimetane) every six hours and chlorpheniramine maleate (Chlor-Trimeton) every six hours.

Local heat has long been utilized to provide comfort to the patient and to combat local infection, although its usefulness in this latter capacity is questionable. Dry heat from a 60 to 75 watt bulb in a reading lamp with a metal reflector at a distance of 30 inches from the face is suitable for this purpose when used for 10- to 15-minute periods, three or four times per day. Pain and fever may also be lessened by age-related doses of acetylsalicylic acid. Narcotics are rarely needed for the relief of sinus headaches in children and may obscure signs of local or systemic spread of infection in frontal or ethmoidal disease.

Although most acute sinusitis will resolve without antimicrobial therapy, appropriate antibiotic treatment will shorten the course of the acute disease and reduce both the course of the illness and its complications, particularly *chronic* sinusitis. Culture of the nasopharynx aids in the selection of the proper antimicrobial agent, which should be given in full therapeutic dosage until the nasal symptoms have cleared, which usually takes seven to 10 days. Undertreatment in terms of dosage and duration of therapy is common and may lead to recrudescence of the infection or to subacute or chronic sinusitis.

Penicillin, orally or parenterally, is effective in streptococcal and pneumococcal infections and in those staphylococcal infections in which the organism does not produce penicillinase. For staphylococci resistant to penicillin, cloxacillin (Tegopen), dicloxacillin (Dynapen), erythromycin (several brands), lincomycin (Lincocin), clindamycin (Cleodin) and cephalexin (Keflex) may be given orally. Similarly, parenteral agents such as methicillin (Staphcillin), nafcillin (Unipen) and cephalothin (Keflin) may be used intravenously as appropriate and as required. Ampicillin, orally or parenterally, is advocated for *H. influenzae* infections.

Virtually all acute sinus infections will respond satisfactorily to the combination of vasoconstrictive nasal solutions and appropriate antibiotic therapy. Patients with true empyema of the maxillary may benefit from surgical drainage, either by cannulation of the natural orifice or, less preferably, by puncture of the nasoantral wall. Irrigation is commonly used in conjunction with drainage procedures. Instillation of antibiotic solutions into the sinus cavity is often practiced, but it is of questionable value, and it may increase the degree of inflammatory reaction in the mucosa. The sphenoids and frontal sinus orifices can also be cannulated, but these measures should be reserved for the skilled rhinologist, who will make use of them in unusual situations when drainage cannot otherwise be established or when serious complications threaten (see Chapter 85).

Complications of acute sinusitis include meningitis, subdural, epidural, and brain abscess, osteomyelitis (especially of the frontal bone), otitis, cavernous sinus thrombosis; osteomyelitis, oroantral fistula formation, and nephritis. Aspiration of infected purulent drainage may cause lung abscesses. In infants and young children, an acute ethmoidal infection may perforate through the bony wall of the ethmoid cell into the surrounding periorbital soft tissue, leading to orbital edema and cellulitis and thence to bacteremia and remote metastatic infections in the meninges, bones, joints, kidneys, lungs and endocardium. Such infections are amazingly virulent and life-threatening, calling for prompt diagnosis and intravenous administration of a suitable antibiotic to arrest the progress of the disease.

Chapter Eighty-Five

CHRONIC SINUSITIS

JOHN P. FRAZER, M.D.

Sinus disease, both acute and chronic, is similar in some respects in both children and adults, yet there are important differences. Since the present and future generations of pediatricians and otolaryngologists have largely trained during an antibiotic era, they may have missed seeing sufficient cases and complications to maintain an adequate suspicion of the prevalence of sinusitis.

Bernstein reiterates the variations from adult sinus disease that characterize childhood sinusitis: (1) The development and anatomy of the sinuses with progressing age must be considered; (2) sinus disease in the young tends to be of short duration, the process reversible with conservative treatment, and chronicity is less common than in adults; (3) allergy is frequently associated with sinus disease, especially those cases of chronic or recurrent nature; and (4) complications must be kept in mind during the course and management.

INCIDENCE

Although it is less common now than in preantibiotic years, chronic sinusitis in children still exists with significant frequency to warrant a high degree of suspicion when other respiratory tract and certain systemic manifestations are present. Chronic sinusitis may be the underlying cause of many recurrent upper and lower respiratory tract diseases. In an acute or chronic form, it may be present as commonly as respiratory tract infections in general. Although the true incidence may vary, Ebbs reported in a preantibiotic era that he found pathogenic organisms in one or more sinuses in 32.6 per cent of 496 routine autopsies. The antrum was most frequently involved. The incidence of pathogenic cultures increased from 21 per cent at 2 years of age to 50 per cent at 10 years. Wilson reported studies done on 580 children admitted for tonsilloadenoidectomy in the National Children's Hospital in Dublin. Puncturing the maxillary sinus at surgery revealed that pus or mucopurulent secretions were present in 27 per cent. Court reported that chronic nasal infection is part of respiratory infection in general. Respiratory infection causes two-thirds of all infective childhood disease under age 5.

The treatment of sinusitis accompanying bronchitis is discussed by Price. He reports on 384 admissions to the medical service of the Children's Hospital of Pittsburgh between September 1946 and September 1949. Of those in which an x-ray diagnosis of pulmonary disease was verified, 38 per cent also had x-ray evidence of sinus disease. A controlled group representing 26 out of the 384 cases revealed no symptoms of respiratory tract disease, and only 7.7 per cent revealed sinobronchitis on roentgen study.

Wilson reports on 735 cases of children referred to the x-ray department of the National Children's Hospital in Dublin for x-ray examination of the sinuses. A total of 571 patients (75 per cent) were diagnosed as having evidence of infection. This obviously is a weighted series, since upper respiratory tract disease must have been suspected to indicate the need for sinus x-rays.

ETIOLOGY

Wilson has written a rather extensive review of the etiology of chronic sinusitis in children. In considering the etiology of chronic sinus disease, we must consider the sinuses as part of the respiratory tract. The epithelium, basement membrane, glandular structures, secretions and functions have much in common with those of the remainder of the respiratory tract, both upper and lower. Chronic sinus disease is most commonly caused by acute rhinitis and sinusitis that has developed chronicity through one of several factors. The primary defense of the respiratory tract lies in an intact mucus blanket, functioning cilia, and a healthy mucous membrane. Factors which alter the integrity of this mucous membrane and of the moving mucus blanket lying thereon and affect the aeration of the sinuses may predispose to chronicity and irreversible disease. Normal nasal mucus contains lysozymes and antibodies. These are bacteriostatic and viricidal. Interference with the flow of mucus favors a chronic infection, since static mucus loses its bactericidal and beneficial properties and becomes a culture medium. Among factors that promote chronicity, Wilson includes environment, systemic factors, allergy, antibody deficiency, endocrine factors, mucoviscidosis (fibrocystic disease), heredity and infection (intranasal, neonatal).

Allergy is commonly manifested in childhood as allergic rhinitis. Many patients with allergic rhinitis later develop asthma. Specific allergens in children with allergic rhinitis are difficult to isolate. Food allergies are common, especially in the younger age group. Clinically, the importance of positive skin reactions is small. Infections may increase the permeability of tissues to allergens and infection may be the precursor of nasal allergy. The swollen and polypoid mucosa of the allergic nose interferes with ventilation. The progression of the mucus blanket is altered by allergic swelling, thus creating stasis and favoring secondary infection.

The *mechanical barrier* of the respiratory mucosa is not perfect. Some viruses, such as measles, create epithelial destruction that allows chronic mixed infections to become established. Meningococcus organisms, adenoviruses, rhinoviruses, whooping cough, and influenza viruses all penetrate the mucosa. Chilling, toxic gases, irritating medication, and anesthetic agents may inhibit ciliary action and allow an infection to become established in the mucosa.

Deficiency of antibody may be present in hypogammaglobulinemia or dysgammaglobulinemia; leukemia, advanced malignant disease and radiation all reduce the number of circulating globulins. Steroid or cortisone therapy and ACTH administration are possible iatrogenic causes of lowered resistance. The presence of these factors will be apparent from appropriate history or tests. Burton and Squire discuss and classify these hypogammaglobulinemia syndromes. The reader is also referred to standard texts on these subjects. Although these deficiency states are rare, they must be kept in mind, especially if the otolaryngologist is seeing the patient before the child has been completely evaluated by the pediatrician. Squire reports the mortality in these syndromes as 15 per cent for boys and 56 per cent for girls.

Endocrine factors influencing the mucosa of the nose predisposing to chronicity are rare in children. Myxedema is associated with increased ground substance. The increased incidence of epistaxis at puberty and during menses is recognized. Nasal congestion during pregnancy and when using contraceptive medication is also recognized. This increased vascularity or congestion predisposes to mucus stagnation, but fortunately it is not a common problem in pediatric rhinology. Cretinism is rare in most western nations thanks to early recognition and therapy.

Heredity plays a role as a recessive characteristic in congenital hypogammaglobulinemia. Other chronic sinus disease may be due to congenital or hereditary situations. Congenital luetic infections in the nasal cavity predispose to chronicity and permanently damaged membranes. Choanal atresia creates stasis of mucus. Gargoylism (Hurler's disease) and mongolism (Down's syndrome) also result in chronic nasal infection. The gargoylism may predispose to altered polysaccharide and mucopolysaccharide metabolism.

Mucoviscidosis (cystic fibrosis) is marked by chronic rhinosinusitis and nasal polyposis. This is inherited as a mendelian recessive and occurs in about 1 in 1000 live births. The bronchiectasis accompanying cystic fibrosis also tends to create chronicity of the nasal and sinus infections.

Bilateral choanal atresia is rarely missed in evaluating the newborn. Unilateral atresias, however, may persist undiscovered into early childhood, and must be suspected when unilateral nasal discharge is noted.

Kartagener's syndrome, a congenital malformation, is marked by chronic sinusitis, situs inversus and bronchiectasis. There is evidence that the bronchiectasis perpetuates the infection of the sinuses. We also know that lymphatics from the nose and pharynx can contaminate hilar and mediastinal lymphoid tissues, and thus sinusitis may maintain reinfection in congenitally altered bronchioles.

Local Causes

Intranasal infections may occur during prolonged labor or early membrane rupture. Gonococcal rhinitis is no longer common, but *E. coli* has been cultured from the pharynx in newborns, as reported by Wilson in studies at the Rotunda Hospital in Dublin. The same author proposes that sinusitis and bronchiectasis may occur if the newborn has inhaled meconium or amniotic fluid or if vigorous resuscitation has been used.

A significant number of newborns, especially after difficult delivery through a small birth canal, present nasal septal deviations. The anterior or caudal aspect of the septal cartilage can be dislocated from the maxillary ridge and premaxilla as well as from the vomer. These birth injuries may present as nasal septal obstructions. The deformity of the airway and sinus ostia obstruction foster abnormal nasal physiology and handicap aeration and drainage. Asymmetry of the cartilaginous nasal pyramid may create mouth breathing. Mouth breathing is abnormal, and with it the normal resistance of the nasal airways, which is essential to normal respiratory function, is lost.

Wasson concluded from radiologic studies that amniotic fluid was not cleared from the sinuses by complete aeration of these cavities for several months. This persisting presence of a protein medium plus the physiologic hypogammaglobulinemia may enhance the risk of infection being established early in the neonatal period. He also proposed that cleaning of infant nostrils with cotton applicators might infect the remaining amniotic fluid before immunity had developed.

As older children leave the familiar bacteriologic environment of the home and neighborhood, respiratory infection increases in frequency. Children encounter new strains of organisms against which they have developed no immunity. It is also during these early years that the lymphoid tissue of Waldeyer's ring is in its most active and physiologically hyperplastic stage. The stimulus of infection increases the normal hypertrophy and hyperplasia and may lead to obstructive adenoid enlargement. The stasis of nasal secretions thus created perpetuates the infection of the nasal mucosa and interferes with the progress of mucus into the pharynx and stomach as is normal. Vigorous nose-blowing is often taught at this stage of life by uninformed parents. This may force infected material into sinus orifices and the eustachian tubes. During this same period, children are exposed to exanthemata, which reduce the resistance of the nasal mucosa.

The lowered relative humidity of the typical centrally heated home and school creates drying and stasis of the mucus blanket, favoring ciliary insufficiency.

In the active childhood years, nasal trauma becomes an increasingly significant factor. An apparently minor injury to nasal septum and cartilaginous pyramid, often without bony fracture, can lead to intranasal deformity. Hinderer has elaborated on the deformities resulting from childhood nasal injuries. Septal abscesses, which may follow hematomata, with subsequent loss of quadrilateral cartilage, may result in contracture, loss of support offered by the septum, and eventual saddle deformity. Such abscesses and hematomata are often unrecognized except by the wary and informed rhinologist. The deformities, both intranasal and those of the external pyramid as sequelae of nasal injuries, create a situation that the rhinologist must consider as a cause of chronic rhinosinusitis. The hematoma involving lateral nasal walls with submucosal collections of blood may create obstruction of the sinus ostia, which in itself predisposes to infection of the sinus cavity, even without septal problems.

Children insert foreign bodies in the nose as they explore natural body orifices. Unilateral nasal obstruction is often a clue to the presence of foreign bodies or rhinoliths. Bleeding and ulceration from foreign bodies may accompany deep mucosal disease.

With increased leisure and affluence in much of our society, travel by land and air affords an opportunity for barometric trauma. The pressure changes, unequalized as a result of allergy or infection about the ostia, can create edema and even hemorrhage in the sinus mucosa. Even though jet aircraft are pressurized, the changes in cabin pressures, especially during ascent and descent, may cause pain and hemorrhage, especially in the young child or infant unable to express his symptoms or carry out inflation techniques.

Another effect of a sports- and leisure-oriented society is increased participation in swimming, scuba diving and other aquatic sports. Man is the only mammal who dives voluntarily who is unable to close a valve in the respiratory apparatus to exclude water. Whales, porpoises, seals, sea lions, and even the hippopotamus have valves for closure of the nasal orifice or trachea. The tell-tale sign of a whale "blowing" upon surfacing is an exhalation of warm air from the external tracheal opening.

Introduction of water into the nose and even into the sinuses may occur, especially when the person jumps in the water feet-first. Salt water is hypertonic, and hence irritating. Fresh water is hypotonic and may contain halogen compounds (used to purify swimming pools) or may be contaminated by viruses or bacteria (a problem in lakes and streams as population growth creates an overload on sewage systems). Inadequately treated wastes may contaminate streams and lakes that were previously safe. *E. coli* is the principal offender and is the basis for measuring the extent of contamination. Other pathogens and saprophytes are also present in water and can infect sinuses already irritated by the hypo- or hypertonicity of the water. Introduction of contaminated water into nasal and sinus cavities may establish fulminating sinus infection, since no pre-existing hyperemia or edema is present from pre-existing disease to act as a deterrent to access of contaminants to the sinuses. Osteomyelitis and bony wall involvement follow infection introduced during water sports.

In summary, the role of trauma must be considered as it pertains to hematoma, ostia edema, deformed airways and poor drainage. Chronic insult to specialized mucous membrane interferes with ciliary action, the protective flow of mucus and aeration of the sinuses. Any situation that encourages stasis of mucus may lead to chronic inflammatory changes.

PATHOLOGY

In general, the pathological picture is not caused by specific infectious agents in childhood. Tuberculosis has been reported but is rare. Leprosy of the sinuses is never primary, but purulent sinusitis may follow nasal leprosy, with destruction and membranous involvement of the lepromatous type extending from the face. Aspergillosis can occur, especially in patients who are being vigorously treated with antibiotics. (It has been reported in adults in the maxillary sinuses but not in children.)

Eggston offers a classification of chronic sinus disease according to the histologic picture, as follows.

HYPERTROPHIC OR POLYPOID. Here the inflammatory change starts about the efferent vessels and lymphatics. Periphlebitis and perilymphangitis occur with lymphocytic perivascular (venous) infiltration. The arteries remain normal. Eventual fibrotic changes create edema and polypoid changes secondary to fibrosis about the venous and lymphatic channels. Polypi and (rarely) infection of bone may occur.

ATROPHIC OR SCLEROSING. This sinusitis reveals changes in the afferent vessels. First there is reaction around the arterioles and arteries. Later, thickened vascular walls and luminal narrowing ensue. Endarteritis and thrombosis may occur. In atrophic or sclerosing chronic sinusitis there is less increase in depth of tissue, and such increase is due more to the increased submucous fibrosis than to stromal edema. It is important to realize that these two types may coexist, even in the same sinus, with atrophy in one area and polyposis adjacent to it.

PAPILLARY HYPERTROPHIC. Eggston believes that there is a third, rare type, which he calls "papillary hypertrophic." He believes that it is caused by a virus. This type of sinus mucosal reaction may raise the suspicion of neoplasia. The ciliated epithelium undergoes metaplasia to a squamous form. Papillary hyperplasia of the epithelium occurs and inflammatory cells infiltrate the epithelial and stromal layers. These lesions may resemble tumors of transitional cell origin, but in sinusitis the inflammatory cells are more numerous than they are in papillary neoplasms.

The chronic inflammatory picture in the sinus mucosa may show, in addition to the lesions just described, metaplasia of ciliated columnar epithelium. Mucous glands and goblet cells may diminish as fibrosis, vascular narrowing, and infiltration with inflammatory cells occur. Stasis of secretions can precede sloughing and ulceration of the specialized epithelium. Fibrosis and scarring may obstruct mucous glands and create cysts. Hyperplastic mucosa creating polypoid thickening often blocks egress of secretions from sinus cavities. The stasis further predisposes to perpetuating the chronic infected state, with subsequent metaplasia and loss of specialized function. Intramural microabscesses may occur.

Recent investigations using electron microscopy have given us new insight into the ultrastructure of the cells. The nature of the ciliated epithelium of the respiratory tract is better understood. The potential for reversible pathological states is now recognized. The ability of the mucosa to revert to a functioning ciliated membrane is the basis for the success of the conservative therapy. The older practice of extensive removal of nasal and sinus tissue gave deleterious end results. Present appreciation of the recuperative powers of the nasal and sinus mucous membrane forms the pathological and physiological basis for treatment, especially in children.

BACTERIOLOGY

In chronic sinusitis, the cultures from properly taken specimens reveal streptococci or pneumococci, or both in over 90 per cent of the cases. These generally exist in a mixed distribution in the same specimen. To accurately determine the organisms present, a small swab must be taken from near the sinus ostium. This avoids contamination from the vestibule and anterior nasal wall, sites in which normal flora may exist even though pathogens and chronic inflammation are present elsewhere. A postnasal swab may be more accurate than an anterior specimen. When possible, the specimen secured by puncture or irrigation of the cavity involved is preferred.

Chronic sinusitis rarely reveals the pure cultures seen in acute cases. *M. catarrhalis, B. pfeiffer, B. friedlander,* pneumococci and staphylococci are commonly present in the mixed flora of chronic cases. Although maxillary sinusitis of dental origin is uncommon in childhood, the fetid odor must arouse suspicion of such disease. Anaerobic streptococci, coliform bacilli, and organisms characteristically present in the mouth may be cultured on special media.

DIAGNOSIS

The diagnosis of chronic sinusitis in pediatric practice depends on a high degree of suspicion in respiratory tract and systemic diseases even though the sinus and nasal areas may be relatively symptom-free.

The history is often sufficient in itself to raise a strong suspicion of the diagnosis. The following symptoms are common in patients with chronic disease of the nasal sinuses.

Frequent Colds. Colds may be exacerbations of chronic sinus disease. Chilling, fatigue, viral infection, superimposed allergy and exposure to irritant water from aquatic activity may reactivate chronic sinusitis.

Nasal Obstruction. This is a common complaint. Allergy, nasal deformities and adenoidal hypertrophy can account for obstruction and predispose to chronic rhinitis and sinusitis.

Cough. Cough is present in a large percentage of children with chronic sinusitis. It may be nocturnal, for in lying down the posterior pharyngeal secretions irritate the laryngeal area. The cough in sinus disease is not "croupy" as it is in laryngitis.

RHINORRHEA. Although this may be present in other conditions it must also be considered as a frequent symptom.

PAIN. Pain is not common. It was present, however, in 14 out of 84 cases reported by Birdsall. Nasal obstruction, frequent colds, and cough were twice as frequent as pain. The complaint is often of a dull ache or fullness rather than sharp pain. When present, pain may be referred to the frontal, the vertex or parietal area, but generally localization is difficult. Pain from maxillary disease is rare. Headache is more common in sinusitis in older children and is rarely expressed as a complaint under age 6.

PHARYNGEAL SYMPTOMS. A sore throat is common. Tonsillectomy may seem indicated if investigation of the sinuses is not pursued. If throat discomfort persists after tonsil surgery, it may indicate that sinus disease is present.

OTALGIA AND OTORRHEA. Although this is not as common as other symptoms, any chronic ear complaint must indicate the need for an evaluation of the nasopharyngeal and sinus areas.

ANOREXIA, LASSITUDE AND MALAISE. These must raise the suspicion of sinus disease, especially when no other etiology is apparent. Obviously, systemic disease, anemia, chronic pulmonary disease, urological problems, malignancies and dietary or gastrointestinal disease must be ruled out even though sinusitis is proven present.

BRONCHITIS. Bronchitis with cough, sputum, fever and recurrent pneumonitis may coexist with sinus disease. The incidence of sinusitis in patients with bronchiectasis may be as high as 70 per cent.

FEVERS OF UNKNOWN ETIOLOGY. Unfortunately, a careful intranasal examination in childhood is not always easily performed. A thorough evaluation by inspection, culture, and x-ray of the sinus areas is indicated in cases of undiagnosed pyrexia. When other more obvious sources of infection have been ruled out, examination of the nose, perhaps including puncture of the antrum when its development makes it suspect, should be carried out (under anesthesia if necessary).

EPISTAXIS. The chronic nasal mucosal hyperemia that may accompany chronic rhinosinusitis predisposes to epistaxis and warrants diagnostic studies.

POSTNASAL DRIP AND PHARYNGEAL LYMPHOID HYPERPLASIA. These may be present in the oral pharynx in chronic sinus infections. Adenoiditis and Thornwald's disease must also be considered as causative of such complaints.

ANOSMIA. This may be almost pathognomonic of ethmoiditis, generally bilateral. Septal deviation with obstruction of the olfactory area and contralateral ethmoiditis can cause anosmia, as can injudicious use of irritant nasal medications that can destroy the neurosensory epithelium in the olfactory area.

EXTERNAL NASAL DEFORMITIES. Deformities of the external nasal pyramid, either bony or cartilaginous, especially those which cause widening of the nasal pyramid below the inner canthi, may indicate ethmoiditis and polypi. Pyramid deformities following trauma may be etiological in establishing sinusitis, with polyposis following secondarily.

TONSILLAR HYPERTROPHY. Chronic or recurrent tonsillitis with tonsillar hypertrophy may not be primary tonsillar disease. Tonsillar hypertrophy may be secondary to sinusitis, and the tonsils may return to an asymptomatic and functional state after successful resolution of sinus problems.

Other Diagnostic Signs

The diagnosis of chronic sinus disease may also be substantiated by certain other rhinologic fndings, as follows.

ANTERIOR NASAL MUCOPURULENT SECRETIONS. Depending on the age of the patient and the degree of sinus development, the secretions in the middle meatus and nasal floor anteriorly may come from the antrum, the anterior ethmoids or the frontal sinuses. It is commonplace to find radiologic evidence confirming the diagnosis of sinus disease when anterior nasal purulence is present.

NASAL VESTIBULITIS. Crusting, fissures, dermatitis and even pustules may occur in the anterior nares in chronic disease. These findings are secondary to the stasis of infected secretions and generally disappear when nasal drainage and aeration are restored.

ADENOIDAL HYPERTROPHY. The enlarged adenoids may represent a response to chronic sinus disease or physiological hypertrophy of the adenoids may have established stasis in the nose and sinuses. Adenoidal examination by palpation or inspection with a mirror or nasopharyngoscope should be part of a thorough rhinological examination. If palpation, a mirror examination and a telescopic view are not successful, a lateral film of the nasopharynx may show the soft tissue mass.

MUCOSAL CHANGES. Mucosal changes in the nose may corroborate the suspicion of chronic sinusitis. One must keep in mind that nasal mucosa undergoes cyclic engorgement and constriction even in a normal state. Persistent hyperemia, especially when associated with secretions, crusts and other signs, adds to the diagnostic certainty. However, as chronicity persists, mucosal changes with pallor, atrophy and crusting may take place. The mucosal status in one nasal passage may not necessarily correspond to the findings in the opposite side.

TRANSILLUMINATION. When antral and frontal sinuses are sufficiently developed, transillumination may be of diagnostic importance. If a significant difference in illumination between the right and left occurs, it should favor the diagnosis of infection on the darker side. If illumination is equivocal, roentgen studies may clarify the status. The transillumination may augment other findings to obviate the need for x-ray studies.

Radiologic Evaluation

Radiologic evaluation of the sinuses may solve or confirm a diagnostic suspicion. Standard views will generally suffice to establish the roentgen diagnosis of sinusitis. One must keep in mind the aforementioned reversibility of nasal and sinus mucosal disease. Edema of the mucosa with x-ray evidence of sinus disease may exist in any acute or allergic process. It is only when such changes are persistent or accompanied by other criteria of chronicity that roentgen evidence can corroborate the diagnosis of a chronic state. The use of contrast media in older children with more mature sinus development may be necessary to outline thickened mucosa, polypi and cysts in roentgen studies if routine views are equivocal.

In radiologic evaluation of sinus disease in children, one must keep in mind the development of the sinuses. The ethmoid complex may be almost completely developed at birth, enlarging thereafter but not involving new areas of bone. Great variability is present in the number and shape of the ethmoid cells. There may be as many as 12 or more separate cells in the complex or as few as four or five. The maxillary sinus, on the other hand, is merely a tubular outpouching of the middle meatus or a dimple at birth. The maxillary sinuses do not attain full adult size and proportion until adult dentition has erupted.

The sphenoid is of no clinical significance at birth. It enlarges slowly for four to five years, and then grows more rapidly to reach adult size by adolescence. The frontal sinuses have the least consistent development pattern. They are rarely present at birth, and may not appear until age 2 or 3. Growth may be asymmetric. One frontal sinus may never develop at all. The frontals do not reach the adult level until age 16. For more detailed description and measurement of the sinuses as development occurs, the student is referred to the works of Davis and Schaeffer.

Radiologic diagnosis depends on the detail and clarity of the film as well as the familiarity of the radiologist and otolaryngologist with the appearance of normal and diseased sinuses. The radiologic interpretation may be inconsistent with the clinical picture. A maxillary sinus that is clear on x-ray is rarely diseased, but two antral cavities that are equally hazy or opaque may not have comparable clinical findings. The film must not be distorted by motion. Occasionally sedation may be necessary to ensure that the patient does not move during the exposure. It may be advisable to have the parent stand with the child during the exposure.

A posteroanterior view that projects petrous ridges below the floor of the maxillary sinus may be taken as the first film if the child is restless. Then, if only one film is available, this view may prove adequate.

Contrast radiography may occasionally be necessary to outline possible masses and determine the extent of mucosal thickening. The puncture of an antrum that is sufficiently developed can be performed through the inferior meatus. Thus, aspiration to determine the nature of antral fluid, if any, and allow instillation of opaque media can be accomplished at one procedure. Topical anesthesia to the nasal walls must be thorough to assure a cooperative patient.

Opaque or contrast studies of the antrum can also be obtained by puncture done under brief general anesthesia. The opaque medium, preferably a water-soluble type, can be introduced and the child moved immediately to a nearby x-ray diagnostic area for the exposure before the contrast material drains away. One must keep the child's head in such a posture that the medium tends to remain away from the ostium until the exposure is made. The radiologist should cooperate in positioning to properly outline the lesion suspected. The antral puncture needle can be used as a cannula and a suitable size plastic tube inserted through it into the sinus. The needle may then be withdrawn over the plastic tube, leaving the tube in place, secured with tape. At a convenient time thereafter, the contrast medium can be instilled. Several positionings can be achieved in this fashion for better delineation of sinus walls. With tubing in place, films can be repeated if a satisfactory outline is not achieved. Similar indwelling tubes have been used for instilling therapeutic solutions into the antral cavities.

The displacement method of Proetz for instilling radiopaque media is difficult when working with young children. The technique is described in standard otolaryngologic texts. A further disadvantage with this technique is that the opaque medium may fill more than one sinus cavity on the same side, even though each cavity may be only partially filled. Interpretation of such films is difficult. At present, tomography may offer the best detailed picture of masses, polypi and cysts; however, the moving tube and film cassette may upset an apprehensive child.

In the diagnosis of chronic sinusitis, one must strongly consider the presence of allergy. Allergic rhinitis may simulate some manifestations of chronic sinusitis both by x-ray and by clinical picture. Allergy and infection may each account for part of the radiologic picture and both will need therapy.

THERAPY

Because the child's nasal and sinus spaces are small and not fully developed. therapy must be gentle and nontraumatic. The apprehension that children may display indicates the need for a painless approach whenever possible. Over recent years, the great potential of the nasal mucosa to revert to normal has been recognized. Our therapy must be directed to preserving and protecting normal relationships, respecting the physiological status, and avoiding noxious, irritating or destructive drugs or procedures. The pH of the nasal mucosa is slightly acid, varying with environmental and therapeutic factors.

Nasal mucus is bacteriostatic for about 24 hours after it is secreted. Thereafter it becomes a culture medium. Its presence may actually increase the virulence of an infection. Hence, therapy must be directed toward liquefying and improving ciliary removal of mucus. All therapy must be directed toward improving the drainage of nasal secretions, establishing a normal airway, restoring or maintaining a proper pH, and avoiding any noxious therapy or drug that could paralyze or destroy cilia or mucosa. Tissue destruction or removal must be avoided when possible. Indiscriminate destruction of turbinate tissue has created more problems than it solves, and cautery and chemical destruction of redundant tissues may jeopardize their ability to return to a normal functional state. With certain general premises in mind, we can consider therapy as either conservative or operative (radical).

A conservative regime of sinus therapy is frequently all that is needed in the pediatric patient. To pursue the physiological therapy mentioned, several local and general routines are useful. It must be recognized that the best treatment of chronic sinusitis lies in adequate therapy of the acute conditions that predispose to chronicity. In this phase of acute therapy, the appropriate use of antibiotics and measures to liquefy and remove secretions are indicated. Establishing drainage by the use of liquefying techniques, control of allergies, avoidance of irritants (swimming, faulty nasal medications, and so forth) and antibiotics are all of importance to treat the sinus disease in its acute stage, and thus avoid progression to the chronic stage.

The mucosa has been mentioned as having marked powers of recovery and resumption of its secretory and ciliary action. In the chronically infected sinus, the membrane is diseased and secretions are not moved out. These retained secretions perpetuate the mucosal disease and further promote ciliary stasis. Aeration of the sinuses, creation of patent ostia, liquefaction of secretions, and removal of obstruction would in many cases suffice to relieve chronic disease and allow function and microanatomy to revert to normal.

Therapeutic Techniques

LIQUEFACTION OF SECRETIONS. Particularly in the winter months in centrally heated homes, the relative humidity is too low for effective ciliary action. Dry secretions with increased viscosity inhibit the cilia and promote chronicity. These circumstances may exist year around, indoors or out, in certain high-altitude or desert areas. A humidifier should be recommended for use in the home or school environment. A relative humidity of 40 per cent is desirable. The patient should be encouraged to force fluids. The use of expectorants is recommended. For children, these may be given in flavored proprietary mixtures, or a saturated solution of potassium iodide may be mixed in fruit juice in appropriate dosage. One must be sure that the potassium metabolism will not be jeopardized and that any coexisting renal, vascular or cardiac conditions do not create a contraindication.

LOCAL THERAPY. Along with systemic or oral use of expectorants, the local use of liquefying techniques will expedite drainage and improve ciliary efficiency. Alkaline washes, sprays and douches are unphysiologic. Irrigation with warm normal saline or Ringer's solution is a helpful procedure in chronic sinus disease. It is preferably done with the head bent forward and the mouth open. The patient breathes through his mouth while holding his head over a sink or receptacle. After gentle irrigation, nose blowing to clear one side at a time can be taught. Such irrigation should be repeated three to four times daily. The irrigation can be carried out from a douche bag or irrigating can suspended 2 feet above the head level. An olive-tipped nasal irrigating device can be secured to the tubing, and with practice and encouragement children will tolerate the therapy, especially in view of the relief it brings.

If irrigation is impossible, simple use of a nasal atomizer or plastic spray bottle dispenser to spray saline or Ringer's into the nose four times a day will be helpful. Holding the face low after the irrigation or spray will encourage flow of the liquefied mucus. Crying in this position will often further clear the nasal passages. Several rhinologists have suggested holding very young infants and children prone, with their heads low, to encourage drainage. This position may institute crying to increase nasal secretions.

CHEMOTHERAPY. In the past, oily

solutions of vasoconstrictor or sympathicomimetic drugs have been used. Aqueous solutions of silver protein products, aromatic compounds and deleterious substances were not uncommon. Our new knowledge of the physiology of the membrane contradicts the use of such preparations. However, in normal saline, mild vasoconstrictors are a useful adjunct to liquefy secretions and improve aeration. The widely available plastic nasal spray dispensers distribute only small but effective amounts of the vasoconstrictor and thus avoid systemic absorption. In such sprayers, the solution is dispersed in a fine mist, which tends to cover all mucosal surfaces. The brief use of the spray with one or two quick applications can be repeated after five minutes or so. This technique allows the first spray to create a preliminary vasoconstriction so that the second application is more effective in reaching sinus ostia and meati closed by edema and hyperemia. Ephedrine, 0.25 to 0.50 per cent in saline, is a safe drug. Phenylephrine is likewise effective in similar concentrations in isotonic saline or Ringer's solution. Some of the newer sympathicomimetic drugs are less likely to give vasopressor or central nervous system side effects. Oxymetazoline is a mild and useful drug of this type.

Vasoconstrictors. Some rhinologists recommend the use of the head-low position for the application of local vasoconstrictors by dropper rather than by spray applicator. The head must be in a lateral position. Supporting the neck with a pillow or rolled sheet will help hold the head so that the midline plane lies horizontally. This allows the medication to distribute itself over the lateral nasal wall without running rapidly into the nasopharynx or out the nose. Mouth breathing is encouraged while the warmed nasal solution is instilled. The head should be maintained in this position for five minutes, if possible. After this treatment, a gentle snorting or blowing of one nostril at a time may help to expel secretions.

The displacement method of Proetz, referred to in the discussion on contrast radiography, can also be used to instill vasoconstrictor medications into nasal meati so that multiple sinus ostia are exposed to the decongestant action of the topical vasoconstrictors. Proponents of this therapy believe that its advantages in chronic disease are considerable. The opposition maintains that with the head in the Proetz position, secretions and medication bathe the olfactory recess and create irritation and neuroepithelial damage.

IRRIGATION. The controversy is not yet settled as to whether irrigations are harmful or beneficial. There are those who maintain that such irrigations, especially after vasoconstrictors have been given, merely spread contaminated secretions into a sinus that is not yet involved. Others admit this, but state that the benefit obtained in removing secretions outweighs the occasional disadvantage of spreading infection. Some rhinologists maintain that this spread to uninvolved areas occurs in acute sinusitis, but that in chronic cases involvement may already be diffuse, and the good effect of irrigation outweighs the disadvantages.

Decongestants. The use of systemic decongestants has many supporters. Ephedrine to be taken by mouth is available in several pleasant-tasting proprietary preparations. When used as directed, these may be effective in improving aeration. Several other synthetic compounds are available in suitable liquid or solid form. In cases in which abuse of nasal sprays and topical medication has already resulted in rhinitis medicamentosa, systemic vasoconstrictors may be an effective substitute, and may be augmented by local irrigation, expectorant mixtures and humidification.

In children too young to learn snorting or gentle nose blowing techniques, the use of soft rubber aspirating bulbs may be helpful. The child's head should be hyperextended and held on the lap or on a treatment table. Medication, saline solution or Ringer's solution may be instilled into the nares. This act in itself may establish crying and snorting, which tends to clear the nasal passages. After instillation of medication or saline, the nasal vestibules can be suctioned with the tip of a soft rubber, pear-shaped syringe that is available in most pharmacies. As secretions are aspirated, more saline solution or mild vasoconstrictors may be introduced and the process repeated until the nasal airway is open.

Antibiotics. In chronic sinusitis, the use of antibiotics is advised only if a susceptible organism is present by culture and by sensitivity studies of properly obtained secretions. The isolation of a pathogenic organism probably indicates that an acute infection is superimposed on a chronically diseased membrane. An adequate trial of an appropriate antibiotic in proper dosage is justified in these cases. It should be used in conjunction with the other therapies already mentioned. The use of antibiotics without proper culture and sensitivity studies is rarely indicated except to treat complications. We have mentioned that the usual flora in chronic disease is not necessarily pathogenic. The chronically inflamed membrane with diminished vascularity may be a poor means of carrying an adequate antibiotic level to the infected tissues, even though the blood level may be therapeutic.

ALLERGIC MANAGEMENT. In sinusitis complicated or preceded by allergic rhinitis, with or without polyps, the allergic management is of the utmost importance. It is not possible in this section to deal with the allergic management, but a cooperative effort must be sought and followed if success is to be achieved. Occasionally the allergy may appear to be secondary to an infected focus and will respond to the elimination by drainage or removal of the septic focus. The status of bacterial allergy is controversial, yet clinical experiences are cited frequently enough to indicate that the removal or resolution of a chronically infected focus has beneficially altered an allergic response (see Chapter 83).

Surgical Therapy

In chronic sinusitis in children, the surgical procedures that are useful in adults are infrequently indicated. Relatively simple procedures are generally successful if the conservative methods already described fail to cause resolution. Several such procedures constitute the usual surgical armamentarium of the rhinologist, the pediatrician and the allergist.

ADENOIDECTOMY. The removal of an enlarged obstructing adenoidal mass frequently affords the relief from stasis that allows natural defenses to produce complete resolution. Under proper general anesthesia, careful removal of nasopharyngeal lymphoid tissue may allow such improved nasal physiology that the infectious stimulus to hyperplasia of the remainder of Waldeyer's ring is no longer present. In such cases, the tonsillitis and cervical adenitis may undergo significant resolution. The mouth breathing created by adenoid hypertrophy is often relieved, and with the resumption of nasal breathing the normal negative pressures in the sinuses and meati during inspiration benefit drainage and mobilization of secretions. The resumption of ciliary function may follow when secretions can move posteriorly to the nasopharynx and pass to the stomach.

POLYPECTOMY. If polypi exist, secondary to allergy, infection, or especially cystic fibrosis (mucoviscidosis), their removal is indicated if they do not respond to shrinking, vasoconstrictors or the judicious use of steroids in appropriate cases. The cooperation of the allergist or pediatrician in the use of steroids, desensitization routines and other allergic management must be sought in the presence of nasal allergy with polyps.

ANTRAL LAVAGE. Most rhinologists reporting large and well-controlled series indicate that one or two carefully performed antral irrigations are effective in reversing chronic maxillary disease. Careful radiologic evaluation of the size and relationship of the antrum is necessary before antrum puncture can be done safely in children. Antral lavage is advised only if conservative measures have failed.

When the antral floor is below the attachment of the inferior turbinate, the trocar can be inserted through the inferior meatus. Evaluation of progression of the second dentition and the x-ray evaluation of the extent and location of the pneumatization will give the operator information as to the safety of this technique. Such irrigation often reveals thick secretions. Specimens should be taken for culture; and then sensitivity studies and thereafter irrigation with saline or Ringer's solution should be carried out.

If x-rays reveal that the maxillary sinus is in such an early stage of development that its floor is above the inferior turbinate attachment, irrigation can be carried out through the middle meatus. Care must be exercised in such middle meatus irrigations because trauma to the natural ostium can promote chronicity by damage to the specialized ciliated membrane in this vital area. During any antral lavage, the position of the trochar tip must be known. Penetration into the orbital floor, the orbit, or the lateral antral wall is possible. Withdrawal of secretions or air indicates a safe position of the tip, this should be established before irrigation begins.

Several irrigations generally clear up maxillary sinusitis in children. Local instillation of antibiotics has proved disappointing, and when pathogenic organisms are proved present by adequate specimens, parenteral or oral use of the antibiotics is preferred.

ANTROSTOMY. This is rarely indicated in children, since the preceding measures are generally sufficient to cause reversal of the disease. Two methods are available. The *intranasal* antrostomy is difficult because the space available to the operator in the inferior meatus is limited and the inferior turbinate lies closely adjacent to the nasal floor at its free border. Intranasal antrostomies frequently close in children; hence their efficacy may be little greater than several well-performed antral lavages. In a child younger than 10 years whose second maxillary bicuspid has not erupted, the *Caldwell-Luc* operation is not recommended. When surgery of the Caldwell-Luc type is attempted, the bony approach into the cavity must be high on the anterior maxillary wall, just beneath the infraorbital foramen. The root length of a permanent tooth is twice the height of its crown. This measurement should guide the point at which the burr or chisel enters the antral wall. One must proceed higher toward the infraorbital foramen and rim than in an adult.

OTHER SURGICAL PROCEDURES. *Submucous resection* may be necessary if impaction or spurs interfere with drainage. Simple deviations or "bends" rarely interfere with sinus drainage. However, a spur or fracture of cartilage or vomer encroaching on a meatus may be one of the factors perpetuating the disease. Most rhinologists now accept that a conservative removal of only the obstructing spur can be done in children. The idea that all septal surgery must wait until adolescence is no longer widely held. In must be stressed, however, that wide removal of bone and cartilage in the classic septal resection is unwise in children. If removal of a severely fractured and obstructing septum is necessary to restore airway symmetry, reconstruction by replacing straightened or crushed fragments into the septal pocket is important. The least extensive septal surgery that will restore a straight septum is the operation of choice.

Often an anterior or caudal septal dislocation existing since birth or early nasal trauma can be corrected to remove a vestibular obstruction that interferes with normal breathing. Anterior nasal airway obstruction also alters the negative pressures established during respiration, as well as obstructing the rhinologist's view and hindering examination and treatment of the nose. In such cases, simple removal of a strip of cartilage along the maxillary ridge by a septal approach may allow the septum to assume a midline position. When a single spur impacts into the middle meatus, it can often be removed without separating mucosa elsewhere. If surgery is limited only to the deviated portion, sparing all other areas, the growth and support of the septum and pyramid will not be jeopardized. Badly fractured nasal pyramids and septa should be worked on as little as possible, since eventual rhinoplastic correction may be desirable after growth is completed.

In discussing surgery with parents, it must be stressed that the procedure is perhaps preliminary and is intended to help the child at present, but that later surgery may be essential to good appearance or function. A child should not be denied septal surgery because of his age if the septal deformity is perpetuating chronicity by interfering with drainage or aeration.

General, local and topical anesthesia and vasoconstrictors will be needed in the young. Sedation rather than general anesthesia may be sufficient with the foregoing measures in children of 12 years and older.

Ethmoidectomy in children is mentioned only to decry its use. The sinuses in childhood and adolescence have ostia that are larger in proportion to the cavity size than those in adults; hence, the conservative measures mentioned and the simple intranasal and external surgical procedures generally suffice to restore normal function and permit drainage and aeration without extensive removal of tissue.

Surgery of the Inferior Turbinate. In the past, various destructive surgeries, electrical coagulation and chemical cautery of the inferior turbinates have been practiced. Although there are some who still feel that a small portion of the anterior tip of the inferior turbinate can be removed, the present attitude toward altering turbinate size or position is more conservative. This type of surgery was performed before newer knowledge of physiology was available or accepted. Turbinate hypertrophy is almost never primary. The physiologic importance of the inferior turbinate in nasal function and airway resistance must be respected. When infections, allergic conditions and occasionally endocrine factors are corrected, the turbinate will return to normal.

COMPLICATIONS

Lower respiratory tract diseases, such as bronchopneumonia, bronchiectasis and chronic bronchitis, may accompany or be exacerbated by sinusitis. It is also recognized that lower respiratory tract disease maintains infection in the sinuses or reinfects them after sinusitis has resolved. The sinuses must be treated as discussed previously while the lower tract is also treated appropriately. However, persisting bronchiectasis, bronchitis and recurrent pneumonitis jeopardize the success of sinus treatment. Secretions expelled from the tracheobronchial tree during coughing are projected into the posterior nasopharynx and create a chronic infection in this area. Sinus surgery or treatment may be unsuccessful until lower respiratory tract infection has been resolved medically or surgically.

Otitis media, either suppurative or serous, may result from constant drainage of infected secretions past the pharyngeal orifice of the eustachian tube. In the presence of recurrent acute or chronic middle ear or tubal disease, the sinuses must be evaluated and treated appropriately to insure maximum benefit from therapy to the middle ear cleft and mastoid.

Tonsillitis may be secondary to chronic sinus suppuration. Tonsillectomy will prove fruitless, the pharyngeal lymphoid tissues will hypertrophy and sore throats and other symptoms will persist if the sinusitis is not controlled first.

Intracranial Complications

Fortunately, these are rare, especially since antibiotics are generally used early for febrile and severe respiratory infections. In the presence of meningitis, intracranial abscesses (subdural, extradural or cerebral) and cavernous sinus thrombosis, the sinuses must be considered as a possible etiologic focus. Chronic sinus disease is less apt to lead to intracranial complications than are acute fulminating infections. The ethmoids, the frontals and the sphenoids are more apt to create intracranial problems by their anatomic location than the maxillary sinuses. Ill-timed surgical intervention in acute sinus disease is more likely to cause intracranial extension of infection than the simple presence of chronic sinusitis.

In chronic disease, the inflammatory barrier has been well established. In the acute stages, perilymphatic and thrombophlebitic channels may still be open, and surgical intervention may spread or activate a septic focus. A frontal sinusitis with an acute exacerbation superimposed on a chronic infection may occasionally need drainage in the presence of threatened or established intracranial extension. In such a case, the simplest possible drainage by trephine through the floor is all that is indicated in the early stage. Such trephine is carried out medial to the supraorbital foramen through the floor of the sinus after incision through the brow. The use of vasoconstrictors, humidity and liquefying agents must supplement surgery to re-establish drainage through the nasofrontal duct. *The integrity of the nasofrontal duct must be respected.* In the past, ill-advised manipulations of this duct have lead to chronicity.

Orbital Cellulitis and Abscess

The ethmoidal veins traverse the orbital soft tissues to enter the nose. The orbit is separated from the nasal cavity and ethmoidal labyrinth by the thin bony lamina papyracea. Orbital infection may occur by direct spread through bony dehiscence in this plate or by septic thrombophlebitis propagated along venous channels. Palpebral edema is the sign first apparent in such orbital infections. The inner canthus is the site of abscess formation. Motion of the globe is generally not restricted and disc changes are not common in the early stage.

Conservative measures to improve nasal aeration and secretions are indicated. Irrigation, the use of vasoconstrictors and aspiration are useful in orbital cellulitis and abscess in infants. Culture from the middle meatus may give the best clue as to the organism responsible and antibiotics should be used in effective dosage. If periostitis and abscess have occurred, incision and drainage is indicated. At that time, adenoids should be removed if they are enlarged or obstructing and thorough vasoconstriction of the nasal passages, under careful inspection and spot suction should be carried out. If orbital abscess has not occurred but cellulitis persists, adenoidectomy and the intranasal shrinking and suction may be adequate.

Osteomyelitis

Suppurative complications of sinus disease may occur in the maxilla or frontal bones. In the maxilla it may not represent a complication of chronic sinus disease, since most osteomyelitis occurs under two months of age. In frontal sinus disease, it arises as a complication most frequently as a new infection, and only rarely as a complication of chronic disease. It can, however, complicate an acute exacerbation of chronic disease.

Maxillary osteomyelitis is generally due to staphylococci. Pathogenesis is uncertain. Cracked nipples, skin lesions or breast abscesses in the infant's mother, skin infection, styes and boils may be responsible for a hematogenous spread to the maxilla. These etiologies have all been recorded. Some believe that an infected lacrimal sac or dental sac on the deciduous first molar is the site of origin. Others suggest that it is hematogenous from an unknown source and that the maxillary sinus may be the first locus of infection, even though the infant maxillary sinus is only a small pit in the lateral nasal wall.

The onset is marked by fever, anorexia, swollen red cheek, lid edema and areas of abscess in the canthi, the nose or the palate. Pressure on the swollen cheek may create visible purulent discharge in the nose or in any fistulae. Unilateral nasal purulence in the very young must alert us to consider this disease.

Therapy of osteomyelitis of the maxilla must begin early to avert complications. Parenteral use of the proper antibiotic in high dosage may avoid sequestration, fistulae, scarring, ectropion and later asymmetry and faulty dental development. The therapy of maxillary osteomyelitis should be conservative until an obvious drainage site for incision is apparent. The presence of the buds of the permanent teeth in the maxilla makes surgical intervention unwise if it can be avoided. Heavy antibiotic dosage by parenteral route is indicated. If therapy is delayed, abscess and fistulae formation may occur. Fistulae have been reported draining into the palate, under the lip and below the inner canthus. When drainage first occurs, cultures should be taken and antibiotic sensitivities established. The therapy of choice may need to be altered. Staphylococcal etiology is most common, but streptococci have been isolated. Drainage and fistulae persisting may indicate that sequestration will follow. Sequestra must be removed as gently as possible.

The prognosis is good if adequate antibiotic therapy is established early, and maxillary and dental development may proceed normally. When therapy is late, and where fistulae and sequestrum have developed, the second dentition may be faulty or even absent, and scars, fistulae, ectropion and maxillary asymmetry may ensue as growth develops.

Since the predominant pathology is a central softening and abscess in the maxilla, early nasal purulence is the rule. This central abscess commonly communicates with the sinus cavity. Cavanaugh recommends insertion of a plastic tube into the central necrotic cavity or sinus of the infant through an antral cannula or into the cavity directly on nasal examination. The tube can be sutured to the cheek or nose to allow irrigation of this necrotic area.

Administration of topical antibiotics through this tube is advocated by some to augment parenteral dosage. Incisions in the alveolus should be avoided if at all possible and therapy should be maintained until two to three days after all purulence has stopped.

Frontal osteomyelitis is rare but may follow sudden fulminating acute sinusitis or an acute exacerbation of a pre-existing chronically infected membrane. Although the latter is less common, since a barrier has already been established by the infection, the sudden introduction of infected water during aquatic sports may initiate the process. Fever, pain and edema over the sinus and lids may be present. Fluctuation appears later. Displacement of the globe may follow cellulitis extending from the frontal floor. Since the sinus floor is the thinnest area, it is here that abscesses may point into the orbit. Incision in the brow and trephine of the floor of the sinus anteriorly and medial to the supraorbital notch are the conservative measures to initiate drainage. Parenteral antibiotics and local instillation through a small plastic tube inserted through the trephine are concomitant therapy. Institution of saline irrigation through the plastic tube as well as topical instillation of vasoconstrictors helps to remove secretions and open the nasal frontal duct that may be closed by edema. Nasofrontal duct patency can be evaluated by instilling dye through the drainage tube after acute inflammation has subsided. Dye instilled through the drainage tube appearing in the nose indicates patency of the nasofrontal duct, and at this point the tube, sutured in place, can be removed. It is essential to suspect the presence of frontal osteomyelitis on the early signs. To wait for radiographic findings is to create a potentially hazardous delay.

REFERENCES

Bernstein, L.: Pediatric sinus problems. *Otolaryngol. Clin. N. Amer.*, 4:127, 1971.

Birdsall, S. E.: Symptoms, signs and treatment of nasal sinusitis in children. *J. Laryngol. Otol.*, 54:549, 1939.

Bruton, O. C.: Agammaglobulinemia. *Pediatrics*, 9:722, 1952.

Bruton, O. C.: Absence of serous gamma globulins. *Amer. J. Dis. Child.*, 84:632, 1952.

Cavanagh, F.: Osteomyelitis of the superior maxilla in infants. *Brit. Med. J.*, 5171:468, 1960.

Court, S. D. M.: The origins of chronic sinusitis in childhood. *Proc. Roy. Soc. Med.*, 54:663, 1961.

Davis, W. D.: Anatomy of the nasal accessory sinuses in infancy and childhood. *Ann. Otol., Rhinol. Laryngol.*, 28:940, 1918.

Ebbs, J. H.: A note on the incidence of sinusitis in children. *Brit. Med. J.*, 1:385, 1938.

Eggston, A. A., and Wolff, D.: *Histopathology of the Ear, Nose and Throat.* Baltimore, Williams & Wilkins, 1947.

Hinderer, K.: *Fundamentals of Anatomy and Surgery of the Nose.* Birmingham, Ala., Aesculapius Publishing Co., 1971.
Nowak, R.: Diagnostic, therapeutic and pathogenic problems of chronic maxillary sinusitis in children. *Deutsche Gesundheitswesen,* 124:103; 124:156, 1969.
Price, W. C.: Sinobronchitis in infancy and childhood. *J. Pediatrics,* 38:590, 1951.
Proctor, D. F.: *The Nose, Paranasal Sinuses and Ears in Childhood.* Springfield, Ill., Charles C Thomas, 1963.
Schaeffer, J. P.: *The Nose, Paranasal Sinuses, Nasolacrimal Passageways and Olfactory Organ in Man.* Philadelphia, P. Blakiston's Son & Co., 1920.
Schaeffer, J. P.: Various types of congenital atresia of the nose and their genetic interpretation. *Trans. Amer. Laryngol. Assoc.,* 56:126, 1934.
Squire, J. R.: Hypogammaglobulinemia. *Proc. Roy. Soc. Med.,* 55:393, 1962.
Walter, J. B., and Israel, M. S.: *General Pathology,* 3rd ed. Baltimore, Williams & Wilkins, 1970.
Wasson, W. A.: Changes in the nasal accessory sinuses after birth. *Arch. Otolaryngol.,* 17:197, 1933.
Wilson, T. G.: Etiology of chronic rhinitis and sinusitis in children. *J. Laryngol. Otol.,* 79:365, 1965.
Wishart, D. E. S.: Diagnosis and treatment of sinusitis in children. *Laryngoscope,* 54:97, 1944.

Chapter Eighty-Six

CONGENITAL CHOANAL ATRESIA

CHARLES F. FERGUSON, M.D., F.A.C.S.

Although congenital bilateral choanal atresia is an anomaly often fraught with disaster, and even death, satisfactory life-saving treatments have been developed and can easily be employed, provided only that the condition is promptly recognized. Today there is no excuse for missing one single case if a soft #8 feeding catheter is routinely passed into the nasopharynx through each nostril of every newborn infant while still in the delivery room. This, moreover, should be one of the most important parts of every immediate postnatal evaluation. If the catheter does not pass through *both* sides of the nose, then an adequate airway can immediately be established by some means or other. If the obstruction is unilateral, nothing of an emergency nature usually need be done. It should, however, be recognized that a newborn infant with complete bilateral nasal obstruction will often die before he will open his mouth to establish air exchange. Vigorous attempts at respiration will be made if the infant is otherwise normal, but cyanosis, pallor and severe retractions rapidly develop and death may ensue unless an airway is established. The harder the infant attempts to breathe, the tighter his mouth and jaws close. Only if he cries is he able to effect a momentary inspiration. This tendency to keep the mouth closed, forcing air up over the olfactory area, goes back to earlier evolutionary stages when, in order to protect his own life, the animal needed to be able to sniff out potential sources of danger.

Choanal atresia is a very important cause of neonatal mortality. Yet many cases are lost to records or reporting, as they have been tabulated merely as "stillbirths." Statistical studies, therefore, are invalid.

HISTORY AND INCIDENCE

The earliest record of this anomaly is found in an article by Johann Georg

Roederer published in Göttingen, Germany around 1755. Otto, in 1830, in discussing choanal atresia, quotes from Roederer: "Sometimes the posterior nasal openings are lacking due to a congenital anomaly." Thus, the condition was recognized well over 200 years ago. It was not until 1851 that Emmert described the first operation, which consisted of puncturing a bony obstruction in a 7-year-old boy with a curved trocar inserted through the nose. In recent years various techniques for repair of this anomaly have been described utilizing intranasal, transeptal, transantral and transpalatal approaches. Today most of the definitive surgery is done by the transpalatal method. Many of the other approaches are applicable only to the older child or the adult.

In the literature the incidence has been quoted to be around 1 to every 8000 births, but in all probability this is much too low, since countless cases have gone unrecognized and, therefore, unreported. The largest series of cases up to 1959 was published by Craig and Simpson from The Hospital for Sick Children in Edinborough, and in 1965 Flake and Ferguson reported 30 operations performed in a series of 40 infants and children from Children's Hospital Medical Center in Boston.

EMBRYOLOGY

Around the third to fourth week of embryonic life, primitive nasal pits lined with ectoderm burrow into the mesodermal bed on both sides of the developing face and extend posteriorly to the region of Rathke's pouch. These primitive nasal pouches (olfactory cavities) come to overlie the primitive mouth (buccal cavity). The floor of the olfactory cavities (i.e., the roof of the buccal cavity) thins out, the intervening mesoderm disappears and the nasal and oral cavities then remain separated by only a thin partition (Fig. 1). This diaphragm (or bucconasal membrane of Hochstetter) normally ruptures between the thirty-fifth and thirty-eighth day of fetal life, producing the primitive choanae,

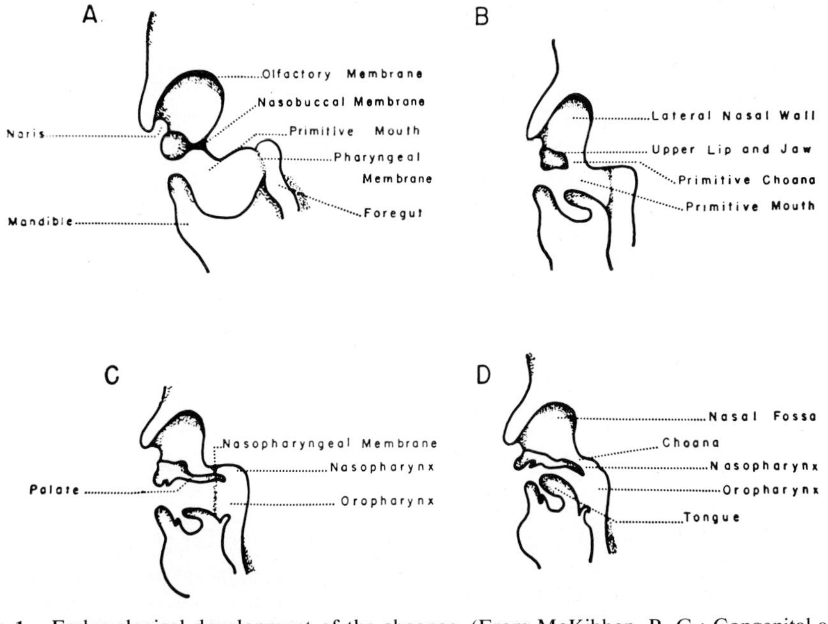

Figure 1. Embryological development of the choanae. (From McKibben, B. G.: Congenital atresia of the nasal choanae. *Laryngoscope,* 67:731, 1957.)

thereby establishing direct continuity between the nose and the mouth. Failure of rupture could produce atresia, but such an atresia should be considerably anterior and more superior to the definitive choanae. If mesodermal remnants persist between the nasal and buccal epithelial surfaces, the atresia could be bony. The anomaly cannot necessarily be described as failure of perforation of the bucconasal membrane, since development may never have progressed to the thin membranous stage. Less than 10 per cent of choanal atresias are membranous, and over 90 per cent are bony.

The primitive choanae enlarge, and the primitive palate is left as a wedge of bone between the nasal pits externally and the primitive choanae internally. As the face develops, the lateral palatal processes and nasal septum grow backward, and these two palatal processes unite immediately to form the secondary palate. As the palate grows posteriorly as a horizontal shelf, it divides the primitive buccal cavity into the mouth inferiorly and a small portion of the nasal cavity superiorly. Thus, the definitive choanae are a backward extension of the primitive choanae and are located considerably more posterior (Fig. 2). Persistence of another membrane (the buccopharyngeal membrane from the foregut) in this narrow posterior position could result in an atresia. This may be the cause of the more posterior *membranous* atresias (5 to 10 per cent). Bone in this region would be hard to explain embryologically. Craig and Simpson have postulated a theory of congenital adhesions, but C. M. Hopmann suggested that a choanal stenosis occurs first, followed by reocclusion of the stenosis. Because cartilaginous elements have been found in the atretic bony partitions, it has been postulated that choanal atresia may be due to medial overgrowth of the vertical and horizontal processes of the palatal bone. Cartilage, however, should not be present in truly membranous bone. In the literature the generally accepted cause is failure of the bucconasal membrane (or on occasions the buccopharyngeal membrane) to rupture, leaving

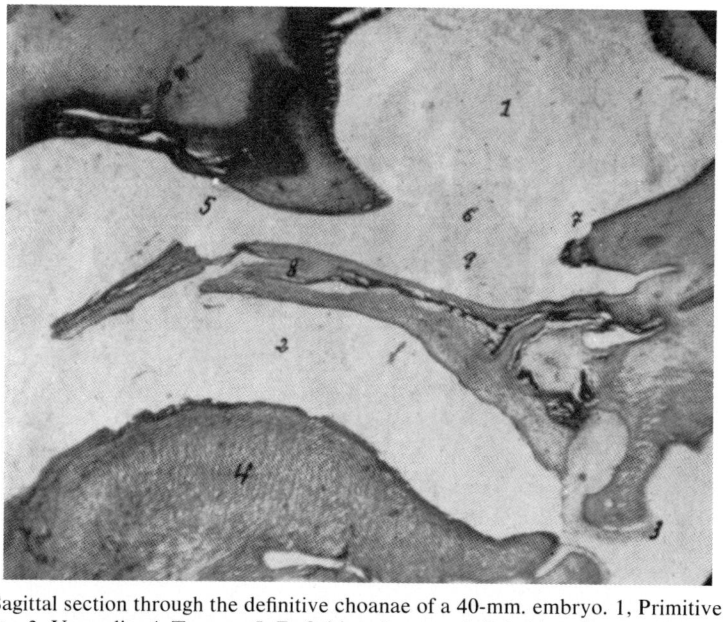

Figure 2. Sagittal section through the definitive choanae of a 40-mm. embryo. 1, Primitive nasal cavity. 2, Buccal cavity. 3, Upper lip. 4, Tongue. 5, Definitive choanae. 6, Primitive choanae. 7, Inferior turbinate. 8, Secondary palate. 9, Secondary nasal cavity. (From Poch-Vinals, R., and Calvo, R. R.: Choanal atresia: embryological, clinical and therapeutic study. *Arch. Otol.,* 63:559, 1956.)

some type of partition (bony or membranous) separating the nose from the nasopharynx.

SYMPTOMS AND DIAGNOSIS

A strong familial tendency is well recognized in congenital choanal atresia, and several reports have included two or three siblings in one family or a parent-child relationship. It has been reported that about 50 per cent of infants born with choanal atresia have other, often more serious, anomalies. Congenital heart disease is one of the most common; others which are often present are facial, nasal and palatal abnormalities, congenital coloboma of the iris or retina, malformations of the external ear, and polydactylism. Esophageal atresia, tracheo-esophageal fistula, meningocele and craniosynostosis have also been reported. The sex incidence is equivocal. Craig and Simpson have reported seven males and three females in their series of ten patients; Flake and Ferguson discovered twenty-seven females and thirteen males; and Fearon's report from The Hospital for Sick Children in Toronto includes thirty-four males and twenty-nine females. Bales, from Rochester, New York reported three cases of choanal atresia in premature infants and stated that there were only two others in the literature. A high index of suspicion is the most important factor in the diagnosis of this malformation. Symptoms of bilateral nasal obstruction should be noticed immediately after birth because the infant has marked difficulty in attempting to breathe. Although he makes vigorous respiratory efforts, his mouth closes even tighter and asphyxia results. Mouth-breathing is definitely an acquired habit and is usually not learned for several days or even weeks. The dyspnea and cyanosis in choanal atresia are characteristically cyclic, with recurring phases of cyanosis and asphyxia, followed by a cry, then an open mouth and then temporary mouth-breathing. For a moment there is no noise, and the color improves; then, as the mouth closes and cyanosis and asphyxia recur, the whole cycle is resumed. Retractions of the chest indicate main airway obstruction. Inability to coordinate breathing with swallowing makes feeding difficult and dangerous. Aspiration of feedings with secondary pneumonitis is relatively frequent. As the patient grows older a thick, glairy, mucoid discharge drains constantly from the affected side of the nose. There is no "bubbling" of this mucus, and the patient is unable to blow his nose on the obstructed side. Voice sounds are nasal and flat, and anosmia is present if the atresia is bilateral.

On *physical examination* the mucous membrane of the nose appears pale or slightly bluish, and the turbinates are boggy and edematous. In the older patient the nares and upper lip are often excoriated from the constant irritation of secretions. If the atresia is unilateral, the patient may grow into adult life before it is ever discovered. Unilateral atresia is somewhat more common than bilateral, and the right side is much more often affected than the left.

Diagnosis should be simple if a soft catheter is merely passed through the nares into the nasopharynx of every infant at the time of delivery. Care, however, must be taken that the catheter does not become caught in the turbinates or against the nasopharyngeal vault. Beinfield has determined measurements on many newborns and feels that if a metal probe cannot be passed beyond 32 mm. from the edge of the nostril, atresia is present. If the probe is passed the entire length of 44 mm. (or more), patency is apparent. In general, these figures have been found to be accurate. If there is any doubt, a few drops of methylene blue may be dropped into the nostril while the infant is recumbent, and the dye will appear in the pharynx if the choana is patent. The use of a Politzer bag with a small nasal tip to seal the nostril will also give a quick determination of patency. Movement of a wisp of cotton held in front of each nostril is seen if the airways are patent. A Toynbee auscultation tube or the open end of the stethoscope can

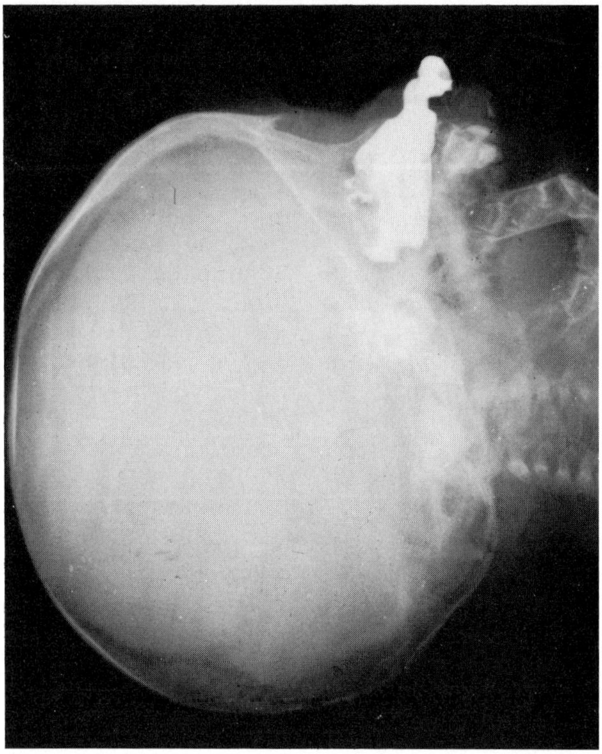

Figure 3. Lipiodol nasogram in a 4-month-old infant, showing atresia. (From Flake, C. G., and Ferguson, C. F.: Congenital choanal atresia in infants and children. *Ann. Otol.,* 73:458, 1964.)

be applied to the nostril and the air exchange detected audibly. If necessary, Lipiodol or Dionosil may be dropped into the nasal cavity while the patient is supine, and a lateral x-ray is then taken to determine whether or not the dye has trickled down into the nasopharynx (Fig. 3). Usually, however, the nasogram is not necessary, since the diagnosis can be made from the more simple above mentioned clinical tests. In infants and very young children, the postnasal mirror is practically useless.

McGovern has shown that, contrary to expectation, untreated atresia of the posterior choana does not necessarily lead to underdevelopment of the nose or sinuses or to persistent disturbance of nasal physiology.

TREATMENT

The successful initial management of bilateral choanal atresia postulates a proper diagnosis as soon after birth as possible and requires merely the prompt establishment of an adequate artificial airway. If such procedure is accomplished, *emergency* surgery is not necessary. Various means have been used to effect such an airway, including metal, rubber or plastic pharyngeal airways or tubes taped in the mouth or even sutures through the tongue to hold both tongue and jaw forward. An indwelling gavage tube passed through the mouth and into the stomach breaks the tight seal of the tongue against the palate and allows at least a fair airway, at the same time decompressing the upper gastrointestinal tract of engulfed air.

A more satisfactory and ingenious method which has stood the test of the past ten years was described by McGovern. It consists of the use of a large-flanged, old-fashioned rubber nipple, strapped in the mouth by tapes adjusted around the ears (Fig. 4). Through this nipple, which has one or two large holes, an adequate oral airway is thereby

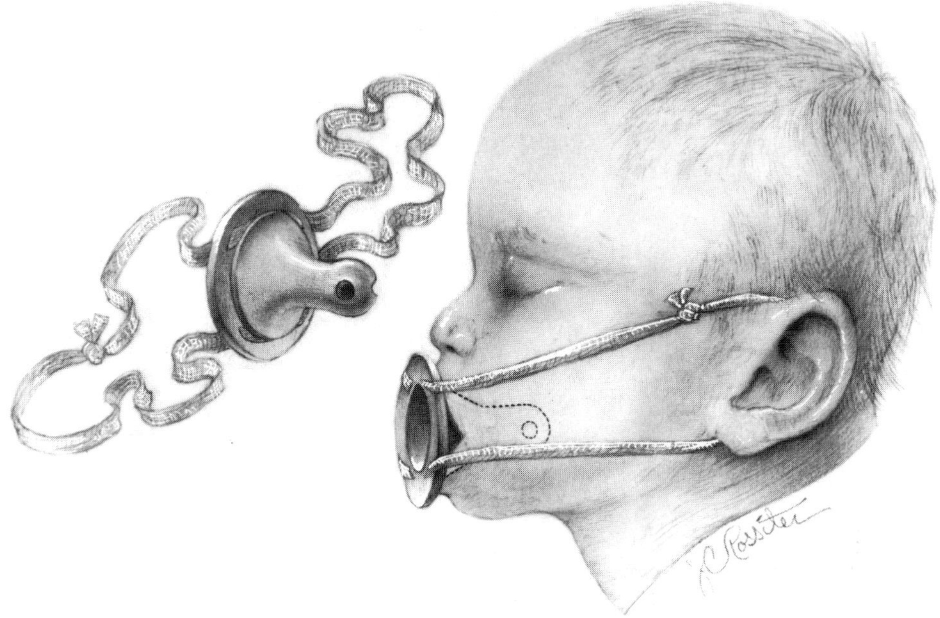

Figure 4. Nipple technique for temporary medical management. (From McGovern, F. H.: Bilateral choanal atresia in the newborn: a new method of medical management. *Laryngoscope,* 71:480, 1961.)

established, as well as a means of receiving periodic feedings. Within several days, or two or three weeks at the most, the infant learns to coordinate and alternate breathing and swallowing. Thereafter, he is "on his own," and the device can be abandoned. Good nutrition can be satisfactorily maintained as well as an adequate airway at the same time. Within a year, the operative field has practically doubled in size, and at that time a definitive surgical procedure will obviously be technically much easier, especially for a surgeon not accustomed to working on small infants. Since more serious congenital malformations are frequently found in the same patient, further valuable time can thereby be obtained for better evaluation, observation and other necessary treatments. No matter which method is used, however, there is no substitute for constant, intelligent nursing care until mouth-breathing has been safely and satisfactorily mastered. It must be stressed that mouth-breathing is not innate, but has to be learned, although an occasional infant may be able to alternate swallowing and breathing satisfactorily within only a few hours after birth.

Tracheotomy is not indicated in the management of choanal atresia, except under very rare circumstances when other complicating conditions such as laryngeal or tracheal stenosis or the Pierre Robin syndrome compromise the airway. It is generally accepted that tracheotomy is a procedure to be avoided if at all possible, since extubation of the small infant may pose a problem and because there are possible complications. Other methods of handling the airway problem give better results with fewer complications. Endotracheal intubation also is ordinarily not necessary.

In the 5 to 10 per cent of cases in which the obstruction is simply membranous or in which there is merely a very thin plate of bone, simple intranasal perforation produces a good airway; this airway can usually be satisfactorily maintained without indwelling tubes, although followup dilatation on occasions may be necessary. In 90 to 95 per cent of

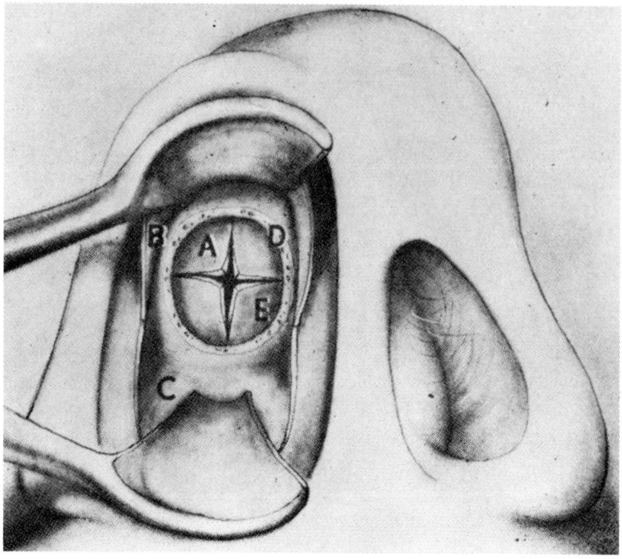

Figure 5. Intranasal operation. A, Crucial incision in the pharyngeal mucosa (raw surface showing). B, Raw surface of the elevated nasal mucosa. C, Bony floor of the nose. D, Bare bony rim of the newly created opening. E, Overhang of the pharyngeal mucosa created by the incision at A. (From Beinfield, H. H.: Bilateral choanal atresia in the newborn. *Arch. Otol.,* 73:659, 1961.)

choanal atresias, however, the occlusion is due to solid bone, and a more definitive surgical procedure is necessary.

The earliest surgical procedures were blind transnasal punctures which, unfortunately, are still used in some quarters as an emergency treatment. If much bone is present in the atretic partition, such openings frequently close, and more definitive surgery is necessary later to enlarge the passageway or to create an entirely new one. A more important consideration is the risk of perforation into the spinal canal. (A newborn with such a complication after an intranasal procedure was recently admitted to Children's Hospital Medical Center in Boston. A radiopaque catheter could be passed through the nares directly into the lateral venous sinus of the skull!)

Over the years Beinfield has been a strong advocate of early intranasal operations and deserves great credit for warning of the dangers of this route. His present technique for the newborn consists of perforation of the atresia intranasally by the use of a #2 Lempert mastoid curette, sacrificing the nasal mucosa, but temporarily preserving the pharyngeal mucous membrane layer. He starts to remove the bone from the floor of the nose, rotating the curette until perforation of the vertical partition is accomplished. The opening is then gradually enlarged. Markings on the curette at 3.5 cm. and 4.5 cm. from its tip act as a guide for a safe working distance. If the curette is not pushed in farther than the markers, danger of perforation of the posterior pharyngeal wall or of other even more vital structures should be avoided. The surgeon's finger in the nasopharynx is also another safeguard. A #11 blade is then used to make a stellate incision in the pharyngeal mucosa after the atretic bone has been peeled from it (Fig. 5). Flaps so created are then pushed forward into the nasal cavity to cover the raw bony surfaces, by pulling a polyvinyl tube from the nasopharynx up through each side of the nasal cavity in retrograde fashion (Fig. 6). These tubes are fixed in place and remain for four weeks. Later dilatations, if necessary, can be then carried out.

In 1968 Fearon devised an emergency intranasal technique, not necessarily to replace the more definitive transpalatal procedure, but to offer a method for immediate relief of bilateral atresia in the newborn. Because the floor of the nose of the infant is not straight but runs along the curve of the hard palate, he developed four curved, hollow tubes with

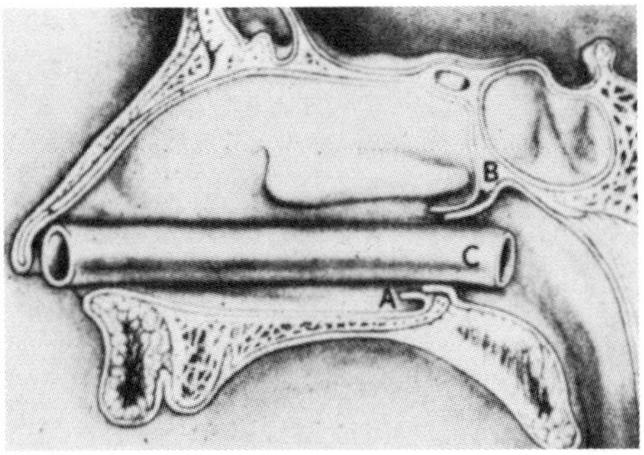

Figure 6. Lateral view of same intranasal operation shown in Figure 5. A, Overhang of the raw mucosal surfaces. B, Newly created bare bony rim. C, Catheter pulled up from the nasopharynx and anchored in the nose. (From Beinfield, H. H.: Bilateral choanal atresia in the newborn. *Arch. Otol.,* 73:659, 1961.)

solid blunt tips, varying in size from #10 to #16 French (Fig. 7). Near the tip is a double-edged cutting blade which enlarges the opening by rotation back and forth once perforation has been accomplished. By using increasingly larger sizes, an adequate airway is established. These hollow tubes have fenestrae near the tip to aid in determining whether the dilator is in the nasopharynx. The surgeon listens for air passing up the tube and is able to aspirate secretions through it. Repeat use of this "perforator-dilator" may be indicated in two or three days. Although it is stressed that this procedure is advocated only as a temporary measure, later surgery in many cases has not been necessary, as the airway has frequently remained open. Fearon's intranasal technique for more definitive surgery later on consists of the use of the Hall air drill, with a long-shafted, small cutting burr, visualized directly by a Wolff retrograde nasopharyngoscope previously passed through the mouth into the nasopharynx, removing the adenoid if necessary (Fig. 8). One to 2 cm. of the posterior portion of the vomer is also resected.

The intranasal procedures, which in the past were generally superseded by the transpalatal operation, are now coming back into favor again with some surgeons. This renewed interest has been due to the development of microsurgical techniques in otology which employ magnification. Morrow, Singleton

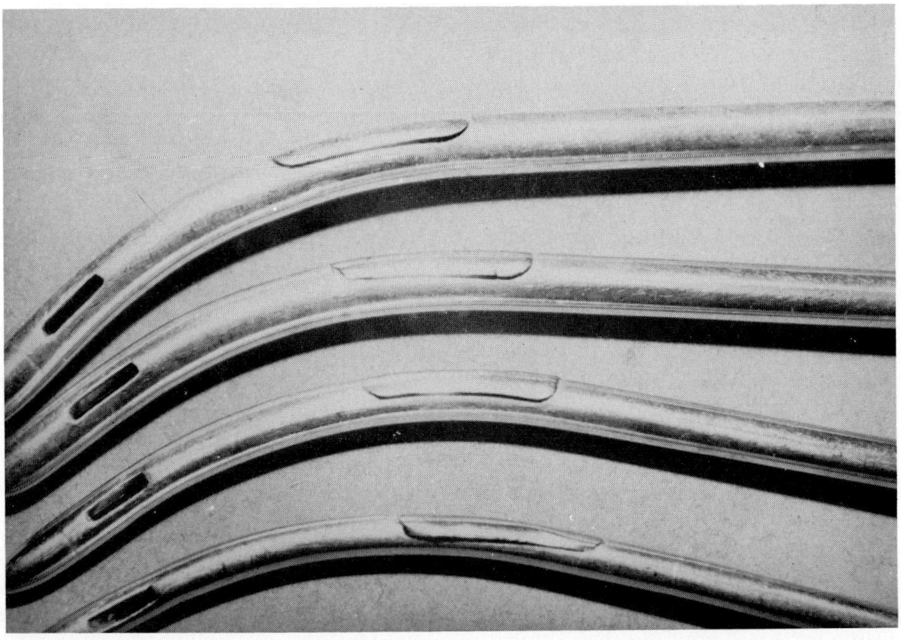

Figure 7. Fearon's set of four "perforator-dilators." (From Fearon, B., and Dickson, J.: Bilateral choanal atresia in the newborn: a plan of action. *Laryngoscope,* 78:1487, 1968.)

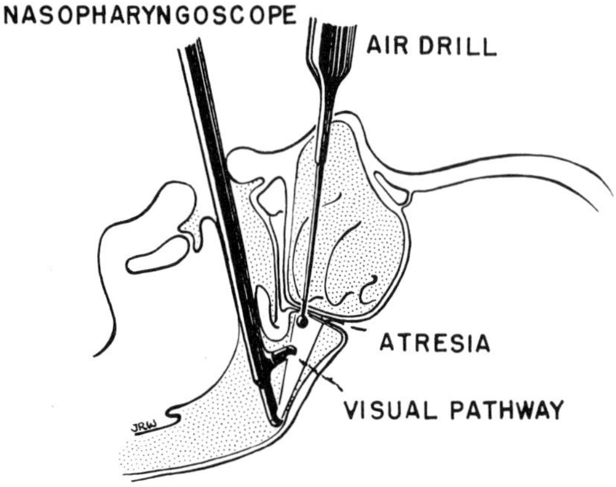

Figure 8. Wolff retrograde nasopharyngoscope (left) in mouth and air-drill burr (right) just distal to the atresia. Note the cone of light illuminating the atretic area. (From Fearon, B., and Dickson, J.: Bilateral choanal atresia in the newborn: a plan of action. *Laryngoscope,* 78:1487, 1968.)

and others use the operating microscope with a large aural speculum and holder and perform the operation using a technique similar to that of Beinfield.

The first successful transpalatal procedure performed in an adult was described in 1931 by Blair, and the first performed on a child (3 years old) was in 1945 by Ruddy. Owens in 1951 modified Ruddy's technique. The transpalatal approach has many advantages in that the exposure is direct, giving excellent visualization even in the small nasopharynx with a high-arched palate and a deviated septum. The largest possible opening can be created very simply. It is feasible even in the very young, and in a series of 40 infants and young children with congenital choanal atresia reported by Flake and Ferguson, thirty were operated on successfully by this method. In this series, nearly 50 per cent of those operated upon by the transpalatal approach were under 6 months of age at the time—the youngest was only 15 days old. If the infant has learned by the McGovern nipple technique to alternate breathing and swallowing, continues to develop properly, and is doing well nutritionally, there is no reason to carry out surgery for some time. Within a year the operative field will have doubled in size, and definitive surgery will be even easier. Fear has been expressed in some quarters that the transpalatal procedure may interfere with growth and development of the palate or may interfere with the speech process. However, over 30 years of experience with transpalatal techniques performed in very young children has convinced us that such fears are groundless if the procedure is properly performed.

Various techniques using the transpalatal approach have been employed over the years, and have been well documented by Ruddy, Owens, McGovern, Fitz-Hugh and others. The technique employed at The Children's Hospital Medical Center in Boston for the past 30 years, with only slight modification from time to time, will be described in the following paragraphs.

Intratracheal halothane anesthesia is used, and the patient should lie flat on the table with the head extended. A suitably bent malleable retractor placed over the tongue and lower jaw gives excellent exposure of the palate. The initial incision is made through the mucous membrane and periosteum in the midline of the hard palate and is carried from its edge anteriorly over halfway to the gingiva. A second incision is made at right angles to the first along the normal curve of the hard palate, exposing its edge, but not going through the soft palate. The lateral extent of this incision in patients who have bilateral atresia may be as far as the pterygomandibular ligament, but if the obstruction is unilateral, this incision is short on the side of the normal opening.

Care must be taken not to injure the greater palatine arteries which are situated laterally. The mucoperiosteal flaps of the hard palate are stripped back with a right-angled elevator, and a silk suture placed through the tip of each flap everts and retracts them laterally. After bleeding is controlled, the soft palate is then detached from the edge of the hard palate and falls back into the pharynx, now giving excellent exposure of the entire field. A small laryngeal mirror helps in orientation. A sphenoid rongeur removes the edge of the hard palate on

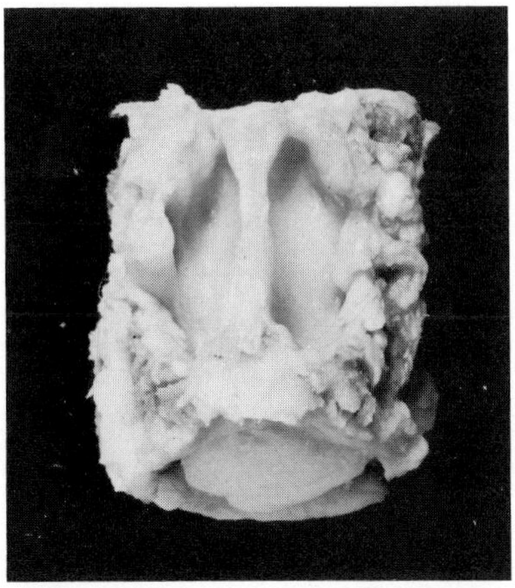

Figure 9. Frontal view of bilateral bony atresia in a 3-month-old infant who died of pneumonia. (From Flake, C. G., and Ferguson, C. F.: Congenital choanal atresia in infants and children. *Ann. Otol.,* 73:458, 1964.)

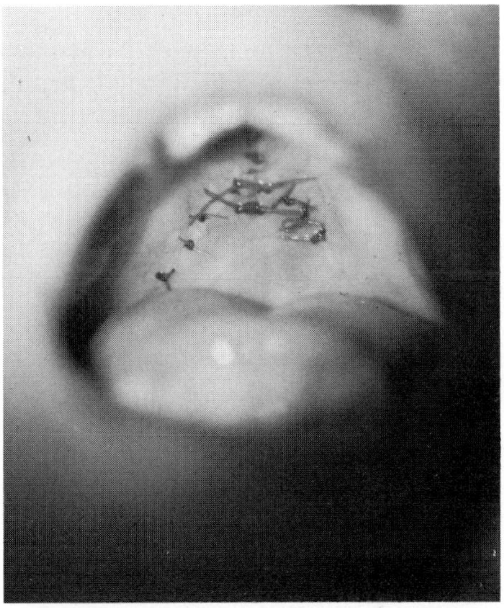

Figure 10. Intraoral view of sutured incision. (From Flake, C. G., and Ferguson, C. F.: Bilateral choanal atresia in infants and children. *Ann. Otol.,* 73:458, 1964.)

each side of the septum anteriorly up to the obstruction. (The atresia is usually 1 or 2 mm. anterior to the border of the hard palate.) The bony partition may be anywhere from 1 to 10 mm. thick (Fig. 9). It is perforated through the nose, and a small rongeur is then used to enlarge the opening as completely as possible in all directions. The bone is usually thin in the center and on the lateral margins but is thicker near the septum.

The boundaries of the atretic area are the body of the sphenoid and ala of the vomer superiorly, the horizontal plate of the palatine bone inferiorly, the posterior border of the vomer and nasal crest of the palatine bone medially, and the medial pterygoid plate of the sphenoid bone and perpendicular portion of the palatal bone laterally. The entire posterior end of the septum, including the remaining area of atresia (in an infant), is cut with heavy scissors (in an older patient it is done with a gouge) and detached from the base of the skull. An incision around the upper end of the septum leaves a flap. By freeing the mucous membrane from one side of the septum anterior to the atresia, this flap will cover the posterior end of the septum when the atresia has been removed. Flaps, however, are not practical in the very small infant, are very difficult to mobilize, and fortunately are not too important in the process of healing.

The choana on each side should now be wide open, and the only significant area not covered by mucous membrane is on the floor of the nose. The nasal chambers are cleaned of any debris by suction and irrigation. Beinfield maintains that regrowth of the atresia is due to bone chips attached to the two mucous membrane surfaces which are left in place. Owens and Flake and Ferguson feel that if the posterior portion of the septum is not sufficiently removed, more frequent recurrences will develop. The palatal incision is then approximated with #0000 chromic catgut on a malleable cutting needle (Fig. 10). If bleeding has been slight, no packing or tube of any kind is used. If a pack is necessary, it is usually removed on the following day. A portex tube may be passed through the nose to provide an airway during recovery from anesthesia. The patient is kept on full doses of broad-spectrum antibiotics postoperatively for several days until the palate has completely healed. Diet is limited to liquids for four or five days. If the palate is carefully resutured, and the sutures are not too tight, the danger of perforation is negligible, and healing in almost every case takes place by primary intention.

REFERENCES

Bales, G. A.: Choanal Atresia in the Premature Infant. *Laryngoscope,* 76:122, 1966.

Beinfield, H. H.: Bilateral Choanal Atresia in the Newborn. *Arch. Otol.,* 73:659, 1961.

Beinfield, H. H.: Closure of Choanal Atresia Opening Explained. *Arch. Otol.,* 83:480, 1966.

Blair, V. P.: Congenital Atresia or Obstruction of the Nasal Air Passages. *Ann. Otol. Rhinol. Laryng.,* 40:1021, 1931.

Craig, D. H., and Simpson, N. M.: Posterior Choanal Atresia with a Report of Ten Cases. *J. Laryngol. Otol.,* 73:603, 1959.

Emmert, C. F.: *Lehrbach der Chirurgie.* Stuttgart, F. V. R. Dann, 1853.

Fearon, B., and Dickson, J.: Bilateral Choanal Atresia in the Newborn: a plan of action. *Laryngoscope,* 78:1487, 1968.

Flake, C. G., and Ferguson, C. F.: Congenital Choanal Atresia in Infants and Children. *Ann. Otol.,* 73:458, 1964.

McGovern, F. H.: Bilateral Choanal Atresia in the Newborn: a new method of medical management. *Laryngoscope,* 71:480, 1961.

McGovern, F. H., and Fitz-Hugh, G. S.: Surgical Management of Congenital Choanal Atresia. *Arch. Otol.,* 73:627, 1961.

McGovern, F. H., and Fitz-Hugh, G. S.: Congenital Choanal Atresia. *EENT Digest,* pp. 85–95, 1965.

McKibbin, B. G.: Congenital Atresia of the Nasal Choanae. *Laryngoscope,* 67:731, 1957.

Otto, A. W.: *Lehrbach der Pathologischen Anatomie der Menschen und die Tiere.* Berlin, A. Bucker, 1830.

Owens, H.: Observations in Treating 25 Cases of Choanal Atresia by the Transpalatine Approach. *Laryngoscope,* 75:84, 1965.

Poch-Vinals, R., and Calvo, R. R.: Choanal Atresia: embryological, clinical and therapeutic study. *Arch. Otol.,* 63:559, 1956.

Ruddy, L. W.: A Transpalatine Operation for Congenital Atresia of the Choana in the Small Child or Infant. *Arch. Otol.,* 41:432, 1945.

Singleton, G. T., and Hardcastle, B.: Congenital Choanal Atresia. *Arch. Otol.,* 87:620, 1961.

Tschopp, C. F., and Morrow, R. C.: Transnasal Correction of Choanal Atresia. *Arch. Otol.,* 83:607, 1966.

SECTION XIV

THE MOUTH

Chapter Eighty-Seven

EMBRYOLOGY, APPLIED ANATOMY, AND PHYSIOLOGY

LEROY SMITH, M.D., and J. LATANE WARE, M.D.

An adequate evaluation and interpretation of abnormal conditions of the oral cavity occurring in infancy and childhood must be based on an understanding of the embryology, anatomy and physiology of the area. In addition, an understanding of the predictable postnatal development of the oral and facial structures is helpful in planning and timing treatment. This chapter will discuss these essential concepts.

EMBRYOLOGY

The earliest period of embryonic development is the period of the ovum and extends from fertilization through the first week. The second through the eighth week is the period of the embryo and is subdivided into the period of the two-layered embryo (second week), the period of the three-layered embryo (third week), the period of the embryo with somites (fourth week) and the period of embryo completion (fifth through the eighth weeks). The period of the fetus extends from the third through the tenth month. Facial growth and development takes place from early in the fourth week through the eighth week (Fig. 1).

From the thirtieth day of embryonic life, the age of the embryo is estimated by crown-rump length, which is measured from the vertex of the skull to the midpoint between the apices of the buttocks. At 32 days, the crown-rump length is approximately 5 mm. Thereafter, it increases by approximately 1 mm. per day until the fifty-fifth day and then by 1.5 mm. per day. The embryo increases in length during the fourth week from approximately 1.4 to 3.6 mm.

The branchial arches appear at the cephalic end of the embryo and are separated from one another by the branchial grooves. Five arches and four grooves develop—the upper three arches during the fourth week and the remainder during the fifth. Above the first arch on the ventral surface, the stomodeum (primitive oral cavity) appears as a shallow depression. The primitive gut within the embryo ends as a blind tube just beneath the stomodeum. The stomodeum and the gut are separated by the oropharyngeal membrane, formed by the fusion of stomodeal ectoderm with gut entoderm. Toward the end of the fourth week, this membrane ruptures, forming the oral cavity. Lateral expansion of the pharyngeal portion of the gut leads to the formation of pharyngeal pouches, which lie adjacent to branchial grooves. The ectoderm of the branchial grooves and the entoderm of the pharyngeal pouches fuse. The branchial arches become more prominent laterally and extend to the midline on the ventral surface to meet the corresponding arch from the other side. Early in the fourth week, the first arch bifurcates to form the maxillary and mandibular processes. The maxillary processes lie on either side of the stomodeum and the mandibular process forms the inferior border of the stomodeum. The superior boundary is formed by the frontonasal prominence and the projecting forebrain. Nasal placodes near the

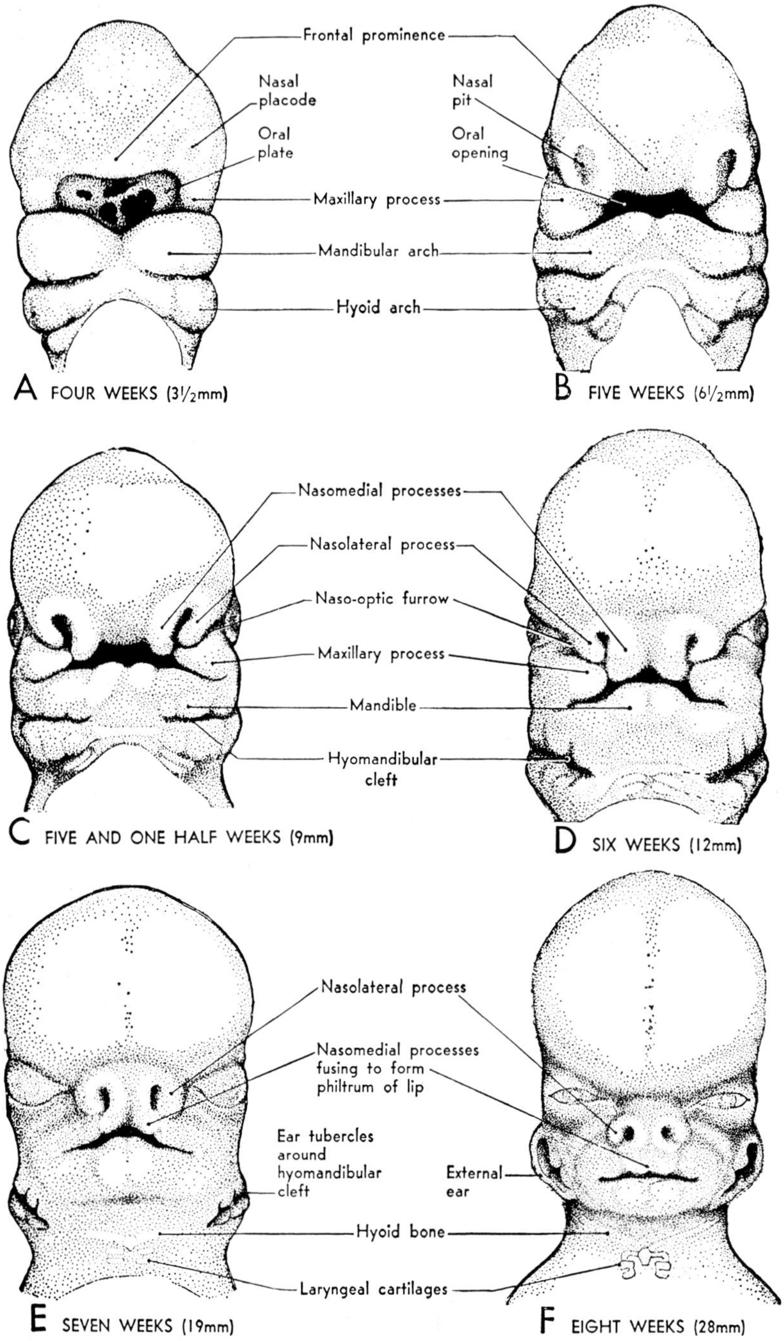

Figure 1. Drawings, in frontal aspect, showing the important steps in the formation of the face. (From *Human Anatomy* by Morris as it appears in *Human Embryology* by Patten, B. M. Copyright 1968, McGraw-Hill, Inc. Used with permission of McGraw-Hill Book Company.)

lateral borders of the frontal prominence and the optic sulcus somewhat more lateral appear during this period.

During the fifth week, the crown-rump length of the embryo increases from approximately 3.6 mm. to 8 mm. It is during this period that two paired lateral swellings (lateral tubercles) and an unpaired medial swelling (tuberculum impar) arise on the stomodeal wall formed by the mandibular arch. The swellings, which lead to formation of the body of the tongue, are covered with ectoderm, since they lie in the stomodeum anterior to the oral membrane. Beginning at approximately the same time, and continuing into the seventh week, the second, third, and possibly the fourth branchial arches from either side, which lie behind the oral membrane area, fuse in the ventral midline and are united by a median elevation, the copula. The thyroid diverticulum arises between the copula and the tuberculum impar, and this is the area of the foramen cecum on the adult tongue. Fusion of the lateral tubercles, tuberculum impar, and the posterior elements is completed during the seventh week. The maxillary processes and mandibular arches continue to enlarge. Likewise, the second branchial arches (hyoid arches) enlarge and merge in the midline. This arch extends caudally and forms an apron (operculum) over the third and fourth arches, which thus lie in a depression (cervical sinus).

The sixth week is characterized by vigorous growth of the maxillary and medial nasal processes. The crown-rump length increases from 9 to 15 mm. The border between the maxillary process and the lateral nasal process exists as a deep groove (the nasomaxillary groove) extending from the stomodeum to the inner canthus of the eye. Merging of the mandibular prominences is completed. The first evidence of the formation of the external ear between the mandibular and hyoid arches appears. Growth of the lateral tubercles forming the tongue leads to formation of a trough in front and on either side so that the anterior body of the tongue becomes free and mobile. Late in the sixth week, or early in the seventh, tissue develops that separates the jaws into lip and developing gum.

During the sixth week, we see the beginning of the formation of the three paired major salivary glands. The primordium of the parotid glands appears at this time as an epithelial flange near the angle of the mouth on either side. During the seventh week, this flange elongates and separates from the parent epithelium. Somewhat later in the sixth week, the submandibular glands begin on either side as a ridge near the junction of the forming tongue and jaw. Still later, in the eighth week, the sublingual glands appear as a series of solid epithelial buds. The development of each of these glands is similar after formation of the epithelial bud. The bud grows and elongates with branching into a system of solid cords with ends that round out to form acini. This is completed in the sixth month.

Crown-rump growth during the seventh week is from 16 to 22 mm. The foundation for the upper lip and jaw is completed by fusion of the maxillary processes and the merged medial nasal–frontonasal processes.* The fusion of the maxillary process to the medial nasal process begins as an epithelial fusion followed by a breakdown of the contacting epithelial surfaces. Mesodermal fusion then progresses by proliferation and crossing over of capillaries and fibroblasts. If there is insufficient mesodermal progression, the epithelial junction may tear apart, leading to the formation of a cleft lip.

The lateral palatine processes arise from the maxillary processes in the oral cavity. They are forced to grow downward and are prevented from fusing because of the elevation of the posterior portion of the developing tongue. When fused, these shelves will form the secondary palate. (The secondary palate

---

*The area formed by the merging of the frontonasal and medial nasal processes has been termed the primary palate. It comprises the central portion of the upper lip, premaxilla, upper incisors and anterior nasal septum.

consists of that part of the hard palate behind the incisive foramen and the soft palate.)

The formation of the cranial and facial bones begins in the sixth week, but their cartilaginous origin is more obvious in the seventh week. Dense mesenchyme that envelops the cranial end of the primitive notochord and extends cephalad into the nasal region appears in the fifth and sixth weeks. Development of this mesenchyme leads to formation of Meckel's cartilage, the thyroid and hyoid cartilages, and the parachordal cartilages, which form the basal plate of the cranium. Thus, the bones of the base of the skull arise primarily from cartilage, with a significant membranous contribution. The remainder of the sides and the roof of the cranium are entirely of intermembranous origin. The ossification centers in the intermembranous portion do not appear until the eighth to tenth weeks.

The upper jaw (premaxilla, maxilla, palate and zygoma) forms from the maxillary process by undergoing ossification directly within mesenchymal tissue. These centers appear in the seventh week. As noted, the mesenchymal core of the mandibular process transforms into a cartilaginous bar (Meckel's cartilage). This cartilaginous mass does not, however, convert directly into the definitive mandible. It is replaced by membranous bone forming directly in the ventral body of the future jaw and enveloping Meckel's cartilage, except in the more dorsal area of the future ramus, where it forms a lateral plate. The invested portion of Meckel's cartilage disappears and contributes only the tip of the chin in the adult mandible. The ossification centers in this primitive mandible appear during the seventh week.

Oral development during the eighth week is characterized by differentiation of the muscles of the tongue and the appearance of taste buds. The embryo increases in length from 23 to 30 mm. The opening of the cervical sinus becomes obliterated. Failure of the ectoderm lining the cervical sinus to disappear may give rise to branchial cysts. Thus, by the end of the eighth week of embryonic development, most of the developing features of the face, skull, and neck have begun to form.

By custom, the embryonic period ends with the eighth week, and from the ninth week on we use the term fetus. During the ninth and tenth weeks, growth of the lower jaw allows the tongue to drop down. The palatal shelves rotate upward to lie above the tongue. This rotation begins posteriorly and progresses anteriorly. Once close approximation has taken place by this rotation of the shelves, fusion proceeds from an anterior to posterior direction. At the same time, fusion with the septum takes place. Fusion is completed during the twelfth week. Clefts of the secondary palate may be caused by a deficiency of mesoderm or by anything preventing the shelves from rotating or fusing.

Narrowing of the broad mouth opening progresses during the third month and cheeks are thus formed. By the end of the twelfth week, all the facial components have been formed, and in the following weeks of pregnancy they grow. Facial malformations do not normally develop after the twelfth week.

The growth of the facial bones is a composite process of remodeling growth in coordination with other growth, such as sutural growth, condylar growth and growth at synchondroses. It is not a process of uniform surface addition following pre-established surface contours. Growth occurs at several major growth sites and from the periosteal (outer) and endosteal (inner) surfaces. In the calvarium, the expanding brain is the displacing force leading to sutural separation. In the face, the enlarging nasal septum is believed to be the force pacing sutural separation.

Though the midface appears to grow forward and downward, the main thrusts of the multidirectional growth of the maxilla are posterior, with displacement occurring anteriorly and superior growth with inferior displacement. Growth sites are present in the sutures, the posterior maxillary tuberosity, the alveolar margins, and many other surfaces of the bone. The zygomatic bones enlarge in their overall dimensions, show widening of the arches, and move the anterior malar region and lateral orbital rim posteriorly because of resorptive and regressive growth. Surface addition to the nasal bones leads to lengthening and anterior movement, widening and lateral movement, elevation, and downward extension.

The mandible appears to grow forward and downward in the developing child's face. The forward projection results from displacement anteriorly following posterior growth at the condyle and along the posterior border of the ramus. In addition, all parts of the bone are involved in enlargement and remodeling.

ANATOMY

The bony facial structure is formed by the frontal, nasal, maxillary, mandibular, zygomatic and palatine bones. The facial muscles are divided into five groups, according to whether they move the mouth, the nose, the orbit, the ear, or the scalp. The platysma muscle in the neck is also a member of the facial muscle group. All of these muscles are innervated by the facial nerve.

The facial muscles affecting the mouth (Fig. 2) are subdivided into a lower group (depressor anguli oris, depressor labii inferioris and mentalis), an upper group (risorius, zygomaticus major, zygomaticus minor, levator labii superioris, levator labii superioris alaque nasi and levator anguli oris), the orbicularis oris, and the buccinator. These muscles arise from bone (except the risorius) and insert into skin, mucosa and other oral muscles.

The maxillary bone is the chief bony component of the upper jaw. The alveolar process of the maxilla is the tooth-bearing portion. There are 10 deciduous teeth (four incisors, two canines and four molars) and 16 permanent teeth (four incisors, two canines, four premolars and six molars) in the upper jaw. A corresponding number of teeth are present in the lower jaw. The suture line between the premaxilla and the maxilla in the fetus and infant extends between the lateral incisor and the canine. Thus, the bony segment bearing the four incisor teeth is referred to as the premaxilla. The gum (gingiva) is composed of mucosa with underlying fibrous tissue that is closely attached to the periosteum of the alveolar processes. The bony palate (hard palate) is covered by a dense structure of oral mucous membrane intimately adherent to periosteum. The soft palate is a mobile structure suspended from the posterior border of the hard palate, covered on its oral and nasal surfaces by mucosa, and formed by the palatine aponeurosis and palatine mus-

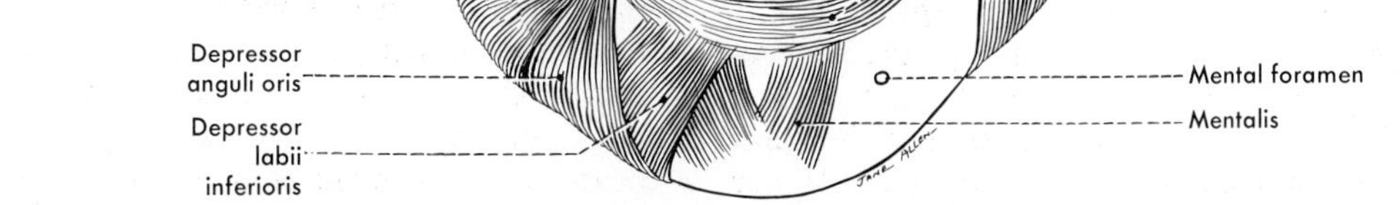

Figure 2. Facial muscles affecting the mouth. The superficial muscles are seen on the right side of the face and have been removed on the left side of the face. (After Hollinshead, W. H.: *Anatomy for Surgeons*, Hoeber, 1968.)

cles (tensor veli palatini, levator veli palatini, palatopharyngeus, palatoglossus and musculus uvulae).

The sensory innervation of the upper jaw is through the maxillary division of the trigeminal nerve, except for a portion of the buccal gingival mucosa, which receives its innervation over the mandibular division. In addition, the soft palate probably receives some sensory innervation from the facial and glossopharyngeal nerves. The major blood supply of the upper jaw is from the maxillary artery. The motor innervation of the soft palate muscles (except the tensor palatini) is by an ascending branch of the pharyngeal plexus carrying fibers from the accessory root of the vagus. The tensor is innervated by the mandibular branch of the trigeminal nerve.

The mandible is the only bony component of the lower jaw. The condylar portion of the mandible articulates with the temporal bone at the glenoid fossa. The temporomandibular joint is a hinge joint. The dentition is similar to that in the upper jaw. The sensory innervation of the mandibular teeth and gingiva and the buccal mucosa is from the mandibular division of the trigeminal nerve. The maxillary artery is the chief blood supply of the mandible.

Mandibular motion is chiefly affected by four muscles—the masseter, temporal, lateral (external) pterygoid and medial (internal) pterygoid—that are innervated by the mandibular division of the trigeminal nerve. The digastric (innervated by the mandibular and facial nerves) and the geniohyoid (innervated over the hypoglossal) are assistors. Closure of the jaw results from the combined action of the masseter, temporal and medial pterygoid muscles. Opening of the mandible is achieved by the pull of the geniohyoid and the digastric muscles along with relaxation of the elevator group and protraction by the lateral pterygoid. Retraction of the jaw is carried out by the posterior part of the temporal muscle and the deep part of the masseter. Deviation of the jaw to the side (as in the grinding movement of chewing) results from abduction by the temporal and masseter muscles of the same side and the medial pterygoid of the opposite side.

The tongue is a mobile mass of striated muscle covered by mucous membrane. On the dorsum, the mucosa presents with several types of papillae (Fig. 3). The circumvallate papillae, which contain numerous tastebuds, are arranged in a V at the junction of the anterior two-thirds and the posterior third of the tongue. Behind this group of papillae on each side is the sulcus terminalis. The sulcus separates the tongue surface facing anteriorly from that facing the pharynx and the portions of the sulcus from each side terminate in the midline at the foramen cecum. Posterior to the sulcus, the tongue surface is covered by lymphoid tissue. Over the anterior dorsal surface, the mucous membrane is moist, pink, and thickly studded with papillae, mostly of the filiform type. On the tongue margins and on the inferior surface, the membrane becomes thin, smooth, and without papillae, except for vertical folds at the posterior part of each margin called foliate papillae. The fungiform and foliate papillae contain a few taste buds.

The intrinsic muscles of the tongue are the genioglossus, hyoglossus and styloglossus. The intrinsic tongue muscles are named according to the spatial dimension of their fascicles. Thus, superior and inferior longitudinal lingual muscles and vertical and transverse lingual muscles are described. The intrinsic muscles are primarily responsible for changes in tongue shape; the extrinsic muscles elevate, depress, project, and retract the tongue.

The blood supply to the tongue is from the lingual artery (second branch of the external carotid) and the major venous return is through the accompanying lingual vein. Motor innervation of the intrinsic and extrinsic tongue musculature is from the hypoglossal nerve. The sensory innervation of the anterior two-thirds of the tongue is over the lingual nerve, which is a branch of the mandibular division of the trigeminal nerve. The taste fibers in the lingual nerve are

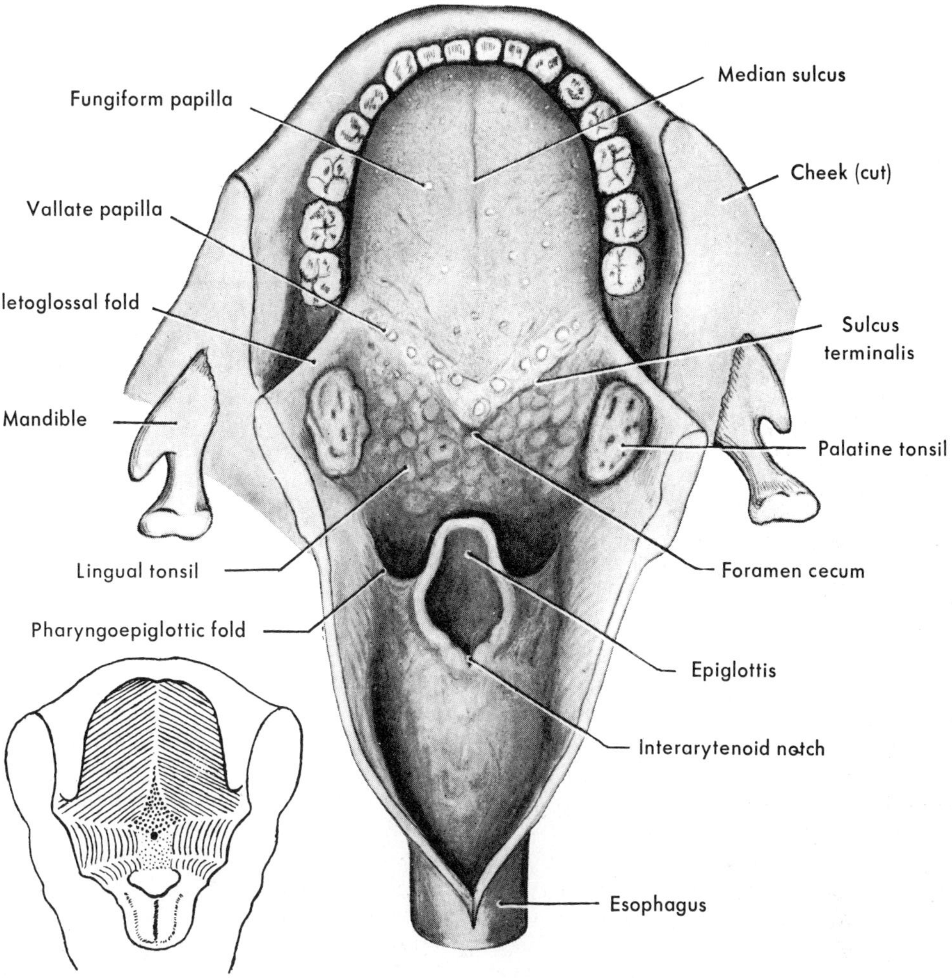

Figure 3. The tongue, the floor of the mouth and the pharyngeal region as seen from behind. In the lower left is a sketch depicting the embryologic origin of the parts of the tongue. (From *Human Embryology,* by Patten, B. M. Copyright, 1968, McGraw-Hill, Inc. Used with permission of McGraw-Hill Book Company.)

derived from the geniculate ganglion of the facial nerve and pass by way of the chorda tympani nerve. The sensory innervation of the posterior one-third of the tongue is from the glossopharyngeal nerve and the taste fibers arise from the inferior petrosal ganglion of that nerve.

The floor of the mouth is formed by the muscular structures and others that fill the area between the mandible and hyoid bone. The mylohyoid muscles form a diaphragm between the mandible and the hyoid bone. The right and left mylohyoid muscles meet in a midline raphe. The mylohyoid muscle is innervated by the mandibular division of the trigeminal nerve by a mylohyoid branch of the inferior alveolar nerve. The anterior belly of the digastric muscle lies against the inferior surface of the mylohyoid muscle. Anteriorly, it attaches to the mandible, and posteriorly it ends in a tendon which is continuous with the posterior belly and attaches to the hyoid bone. The posterior belly arises from the mastoid process. The anterior belly is innervated by the mylohyoid nerve and the posterior belly by the facial nerve. The stylohyoid muscle arises from the styloid process and descends anterior to the posterior belly of the digastric to insert on the hyoid bone. It is innervated by the facial nerve. The geniohyoid muscles lie on the superior surface of the mylohyoid muscles and arise from the mental spine of the mandible and insert on the hyoid bone. They are innervated by fibers of the first cervical nerve accompanying the hypoglossal nerve. The mucosal boundary of the floor of the mouth is the mucous membrane which is reflected from the side of the tongue to the mandible. The sublingual glands and a portion of the submaxillary gland also lie within this area.

The submandibular space is limited above by oral mucous membrane and the tongue. The floor of this space is the superficial layer of cervical fascia extending from the hyoid bone to the mandible. The mylohyoid muscle divides this space into the submaxillary space below the muscle and the sublingual space above the muscle. These subdivisions communicate posteriorly where the submaxillary gland lies partly above and partly below the mylohyoid muscle.

The lymphatic drainage of the oral cavity and associated structures is complex. The lymphatics of the upper face empty into parotid nodes, those of the midface empty into submandibular nodes, and those of the lower lip empty into submental nodes. The parotid nodes drain into the upper deep cervical chain of nodes and the submental and submaxillary nodes empty into the superficial cervical and upper deep cervical chains. The lymphatics of the hard palate and a portion of the soft palate empty into the upper deep cervical nodes. The remainder of the soft palate drainage is with the pharyngeal lymphatics to the retropharyngeal nodes. All the tongue lymphatics eventually drain into the deep cervical nodes. Those of the posterior tongue empty into the upper part of the chain. The lymphatics of the anterior two-thirds either pass directly to the deep cervical chain or drain first to the submandibular or submental nodes, which then empty into the deep chain. The buccal and labial surfaces of the upper and lower gum are drained by lymph channels terminating in the submental and submandibular nodes; the lingual surface lymphatics drain to the superficial cervical, the upper deep cervical and the lateral pharyngeal nodes. The submandibular nodes drain the anterior floor of the mouth and the upper deep cervical nodes drain the posterior floor of the mouth.

Major and minor salivary glands are described. The major salivary glands are the two parotids, the submaxillary and the sublingual glands. The parotid gland lies on the side of the face below and in front of the external ear. Its boundaries overlap the ramus of the mandible anteriorly, the mastoid process and sternomastoid muscle posteriorly, the zygomatic arch superiorly and the angle of the mandible inferiorly. Medially, the parotid gland is separated from the pharynx by a small amount of connective tissue. The facial nerve traverses the parotid gland. Approximately 1.5 cm. in front of the stylomastoid foramen, the nerve divides into temporofacial and cervicofacial trunks. The parotid duct (Stenson's duct) is 5 to 7 cm. in length and opens in the oral cavity opposite the upper second molar.

The submaxillary gland is about one-fourth the size of the parotid. For the most part, this gland is in the submaxillary triangle. It drains into the oral cavity through a 5 cm. duct (Wharton's duct) that opens in the oral cavity at the side of the frenulum linguae. The sublingual glands are one-third the size of the submaxillary glands and are located beneath the mucosa of the floor of the mouth. These glands have multiple ducts opening into Wharton's ducts and directly in the mouth at the plica sublingualis. The minor salivary glands are that salivary tissue present other than in the parotid, submaxillary, and sublingual glands. This tissue is found in the lips, buccal mucosa, gums, floor of the mouth, palate, tonsillar area, tongue and eyelids.

PHYSIOLOGY

The major physiologic functions of the oral cavity are speech, respiration, taste, mastication and initiation of deglutition. The function in respiration as an air passage is in association with the nasal cavity.

Taste is mediated through the previously described taste buds over the chorda tympani and glossopharyngeal nerves. The taste buds in the circumvallate papillae are more important and more numerous than those located in the anterior portion of the tongue. Though lesser in number, taste buds are found on the soft palate and in the pharynx. Smell mediated over the olfactory nerves is also important in taste.

Mastication is the first step in digestion. The up-and-down movement of the mandible results in biting by the incisors, and when this movement is combined with side-to-side movement, it enables the molar teeth to make particles of food small for swallowing. During mastication the taste buds are stimulated and odors are released to stimulate the olfactory epithelium. The secretion of the salivary glands assists by dissolving readily soluble foodstuffs, partly digesting starch, softening the mass of food, and covering the food bolus with mucus. The salivary secretions are controlled by neural stimulation. Parasympathetic stimulation produces secretion of water and salts and sympathetic stimulation produces a viscid secretion containing mucus and enzymes. Amylase is the only enzyme in saliva of importance to digestion. Mucin is the glycoprotein that gives saliva its slippery character.

Deglutition requires a complex synchronization of movement by the tongue, palate and pharynx. The food bolus is moved from the oral cavity into the pharynx by pressure of the tongue against the hard and then the soft palate. It is pushed toward the epiglottis by the palate, which had been tensed and elevated, being drawn down toward the tongue by the palatopharyngeus muscles. The soft palate is again elevated, as is the pharynx, and they meet to block off the nasopharynx. Contraction of the pharyngeal constrictors from above downward pushes the remaining bolus into the lower relaxed portion of the pharynx and then into the esophagus.

REFERENCES

Avery, L. B.: *Developmental Anatomy,* 7th Ed. Philadelphia, W. B. Saunders, 1965.

Enlow, D. H.: *The Human Face.* New York, Hoeber, 1968.

Grant, J. C. B.: *An Atlas of Anatomy,* 3rd Ed. Baltimore, Williams & Wilkins Company, 1951.

Holdsworth, W. G.: *Cleft Lip and Palate,* 3rd Ed. New York, Grune & Stratton, 1963.

Hollinshead, W. H.: *Anatomy for Surgeons,* Vol. I, 2nd Ed. New York, Hoeber, 1968.

Mountcastle, V. B.: *Medical Physiology,* 12th Ed. St. Louis, C. V. Mosby, 1968.

Patten, B. M.: *Human Embryology,* 3rd Ed. New York, McGraw-Hill Book Company, 1968.

Rogers, B. O.: Rare craniofacial deformities. In Converse, J. M.: *Reconstructive Plastic Surgery.* Philadelphia, W. B. Saunders Company, 1964.

Stark, R. B.: *Cleft Palate.* New York, Hoeber, 1968.

Chapter Eighty-Eight

CONGENITAL MALFORMATIONS OF THE MOUTH AND FACE

LESLIE BERNSTEIN, M.D., D.D.S.

There are numerous congenital defects of the oral cavity and of the face.[1,2,4] Some are gross and relatively common—such as cleft lip and palate—and others are minor and rare—such as lateral fistulas of the soft palate. Not all of these deformities can be explained by our present knowledge of embryology. On the contrary, some of our accepted concepts of embryonic development may readily be challenged on the basis of some of these congenital deformities.

Because maxillofacial clefts constitute the most common of the gross congenital deformities of the mouth and face, only these will be described in some detail in this chapter. Some of the less common deformities also need to be mentioned, if only for completeness, but only those of particular interest to the otolaryngologist are described.

INDIVIDUAL CONGENITAL LESIONS

Following is a classification, by no means complete, of various congenital lesions of the mouth and face according to their anatomic distribution.

Lips

CLEFTS. Lip clefts may be median (Fig. 1), paramedian (oro-nasal), oblique (oro-ocular and naso-ocular [Fig. 2]), or

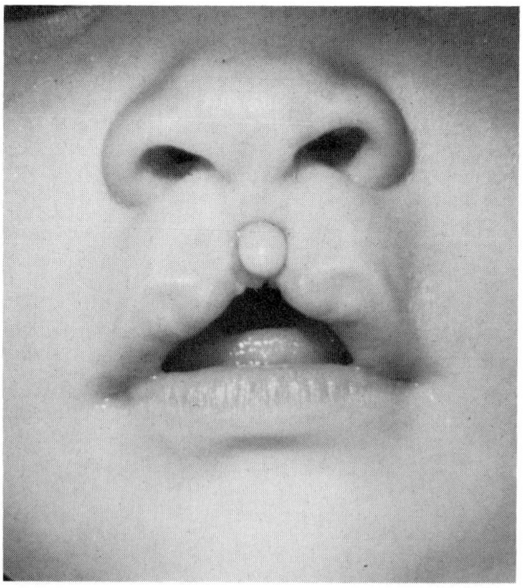

Figure 1. A rare example of a median cleft lip.

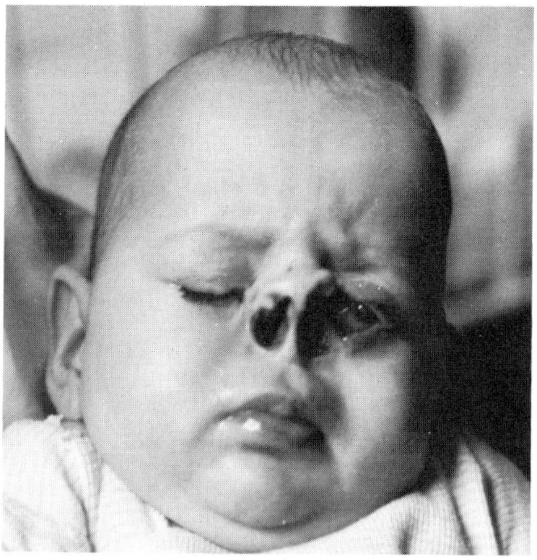

Figure 2. Bilateral naso-ocular clefts, complete on the left and partial on the right.

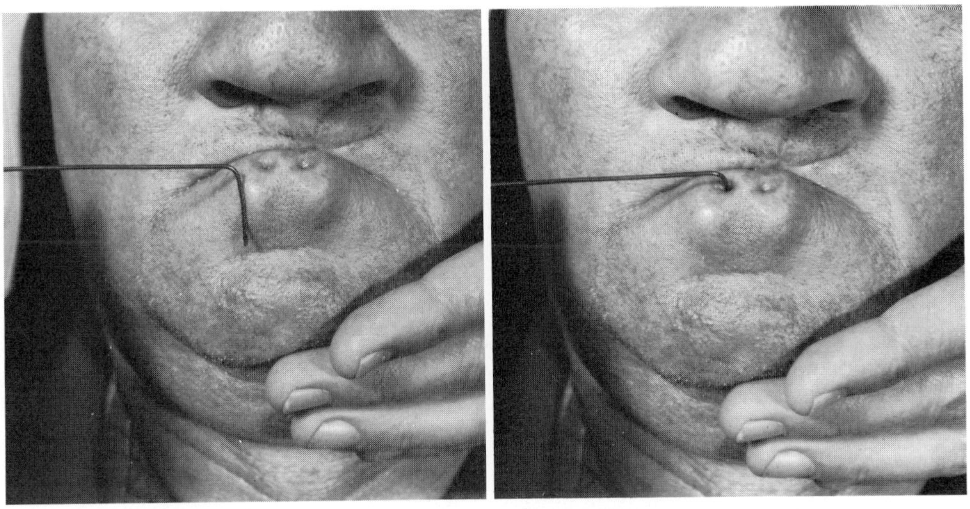

Figure 3. Labial pits in a subject with bilateral cleft lip and palate.

transverse (oro-aural). The oro-nasal varieties are the commonest and are described at the end of this chapter.

MACROSTOMIA. Oroaural clefts, or macrostomia, may present on one or both sides and vary greatly in their extent. They occur along the line of fusion of the maxillary and mandibular processes of the face and are commonly seen in mandibulofacial dysostosis.

MICROSTOMIA

PITS. These mucosal-lined sinus tracts usually present as symmetrical pits in the vermilion of the lower lip, and are invariably associated with maxillofacial clefts (Fig. 3). They extend vertically down the substance of the lip for a depth of up to 2.5 cm. and communicate with the underlying minor salivary glands. They may, therefore, transmit a mucoid secretion to the surface. When it is situated anteriorly, the vermilion-cutaneous border may bulge forward in relation to the openings of the pits. They are usually excised for cosmetic reasons. Similar pits may also be present in the vermilion at the oral commissure of cleft lip subjects.

"DOUBLE LIP." This is produced by an apparent horizontal duplication of the vermilion of the upper lip and can only be seen when the lips are parted, especially in smiling (Fig. 4). Actually it is due to redundant mucous lining of the lip, and this redundancy may be excised for esthetic reasons. At times this condition may be associated with blepharochalasis and a nontoxic goiter, as in Ascher's syndrome.

NEUROMUSCULAR AGENESIS. This is very readily diagnosed at birth when the infant cries. The lesion corresponds to a particular somatic branch distribution of the facial nerve.

Labial Sulci

The premaxillary labial sulcus is frequently absent, or very shallow, in bilateral clefts of the lip. Absence of the labial sulcus may also be encountered in chondroectodermal dysplasia, in which multiple frenula may also be present.

Hyperplastic frenula are invariably as-

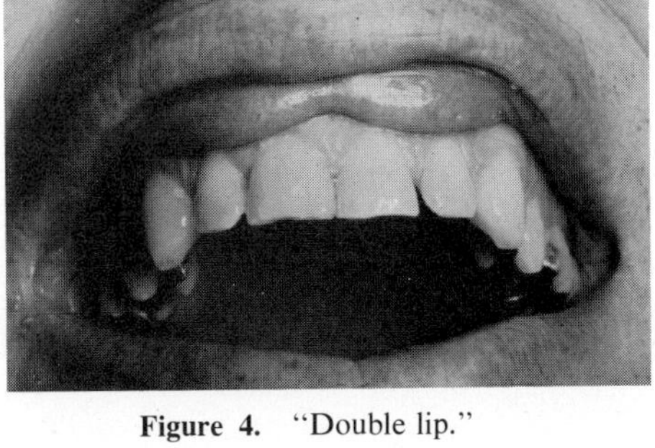

Figure 4. "Double lip."

sociated with a diastema of the teeth at the site of origin of the frenulum. Prior to undertaking orthodontic closure of such a diastema, the attachment of the frenulum at the crest of the alveolus may need to be resected.

Teeth

There may be partial or complete *agenesis* of the deciduous and/or the permanent dentition. On the other hand, *supernumerary teeth* may be found—additional teeth in the series.

Malformation of individual teeth is rather common, such as peg-shaped incisors, gemination (the crown appears bifid; the root is single), fusion (two teeth fused together), and a host of cellular malformations known as odontomas.

The stigmata of congenital syphilis may also be encountered in the form of notched (Hutchinson's) incisors as well as domed (Moon's) and mulberry molars.

Stained or mottled enamel may result from the ingestion of tetracycline, or of fluorides in excess of one part per million in the drinking water, during the antenatal and postnatal amelogenesis periods. Tooth enamel may also be hypoplastic (*amelogenesis imperfecta*).

Jaws

MICROGNATHIA. Micrognathia, or brachygnathia, of the mandible is found in the so-called Robin syndrome at birth. It also constitutes a characteristic feature of one of the types of Class II occlusion (malocclusion).

DYSOSTOSIS. This is seen in mandibulofacial dysostosis (Collins' syndrome).

CYSTS. Most, if not all, congenital cysts of the jaws occur at the anterior fusion planes. They usually present only after the first decade of life. Their names are derived from the embryonic segments between which they form. Thus, they may be median, incisive canal, globulomaxillary or naso-alveolar in the maxilla and median in the mandible.

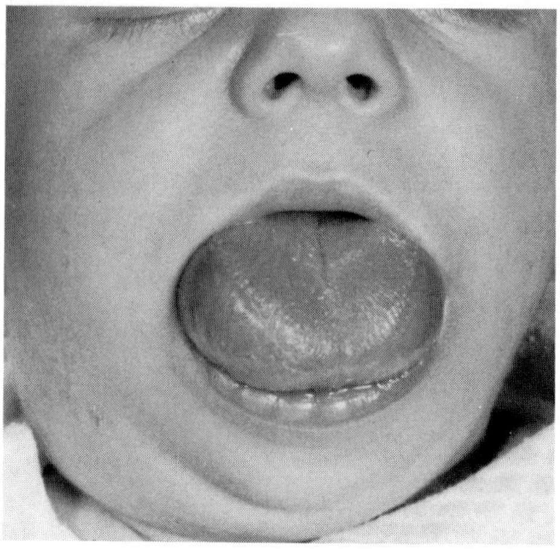

Figure 5. Macroglossia caused by lymphangioma. The tongue is in a resting position.

Tongue

UNDERDEVELOPMENT. This may range from a bifid tongue to microglossia and aglossia.

MACROGLOSSIA. Macroglossia may be idiopathic, or it may be due to lymphangioma (Fig. 5) or hemangioma. It is also a fairly common feature of mongolism.

ANKYLOGLOSSIA. Mandibular ankyloglossia is caused by varying degrees of underdevelopment of the lingual frenum. If it interferes with lingual function, as in speech, it is best corrected with a Z-plasty (Fig. 6).

LINGUAL THYROID (Fig. 7). This may be the only thyroid tissue in the body.

FISSURED TONGUE. This condition, also commonly known as "scrotal" tongue, is rarely congenital, but may appear in childhood.

MEDIAN RHOMBOID "GLOSSITIS." As a result of faulty development, the tuberculum impar appears on the surface of the tongue in front of the foramen cecum as a rhomboid wedge between the lateral halves of the tongue. It is devoid of papillae, appearing red in color; hence the erroneous "glossitis" (Fig. 8).

HYPERTROPHIC PAPILLAE. This is a common finding in mongolism.

INCLUSION DERMOID. Usually found

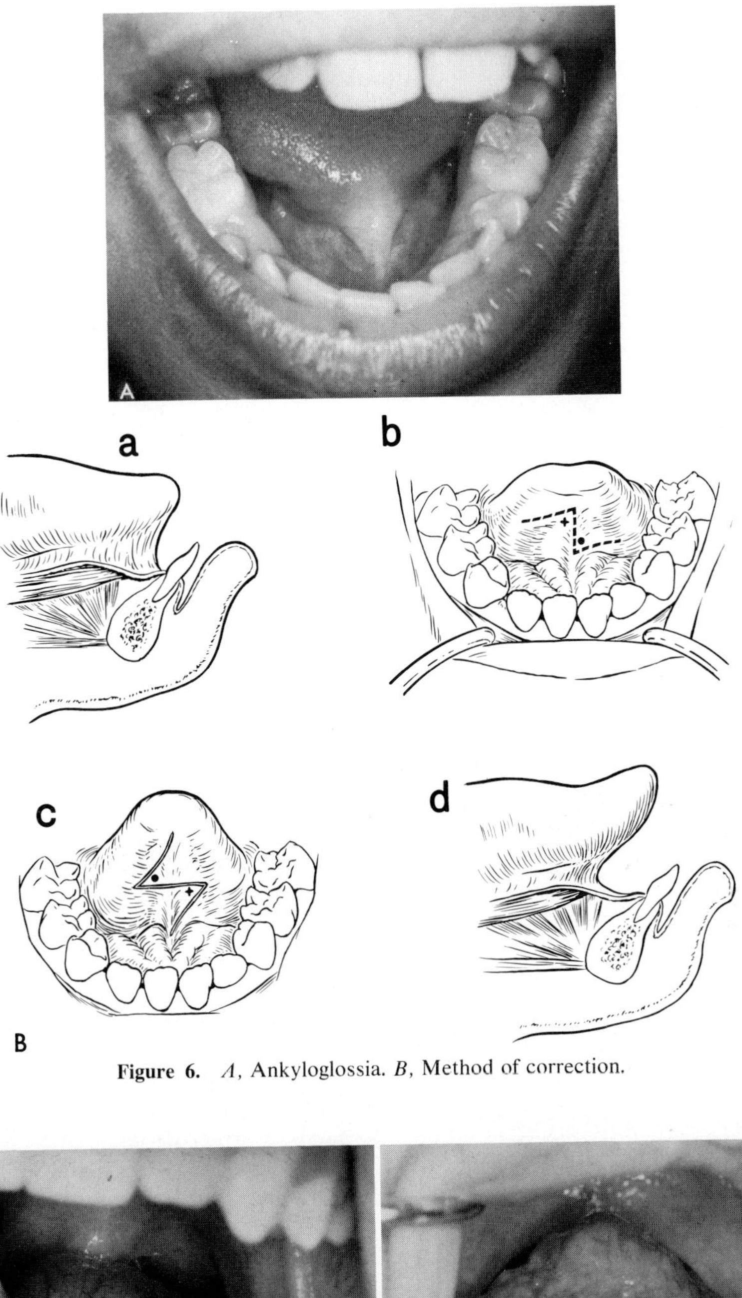

Figure 6. *A*, Ankyloglossia. *B*, Method of correction.

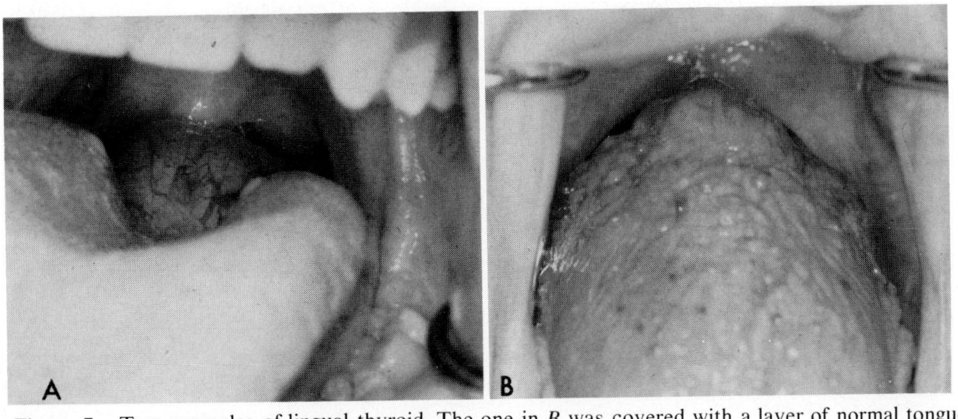

Figure 7. Two examples of lingual thyroid. The one in *B* was covered with a layer of normal tongue tissue.

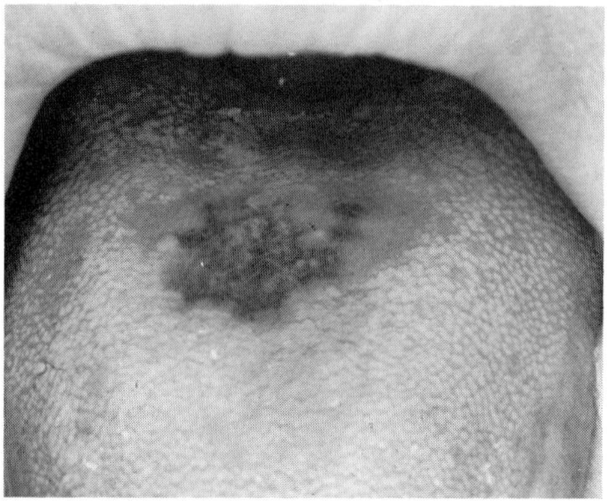

Figure 8. Median rhomboid "glossitis."

anteriorly in the midline, the dermoid cyst presents as a swelling on the undersurface of the tongue and often involves the floor of the mouth. It is commonly diagnosed in the second or third decade of life and may reach large proportions.

Epidermolysis Bullosa (Dystrophic Type). This rare condition is characterized by bullous and vesicular eruptions of the skin and mucous membranes and is manifested at or shortly after birth. The bullae usually heal by hypertrophic scars, leading to marked deformity of the oral cavity.

Palate

Clefts. Palatal clefts are described at the end of this chapter.

High Palatal Vault. This condition may be found in conjunction with micrognathia and glossoptosis (Robin's syndrome), and may present as a respiratory emergency of the newborn. Not infrequently, it may also be encountered in Turner's syndrome and in mongolism.

Hypoplasia of Velum. This is usually associated with submucous cleft palate.

Neuromuscular Agenesis. Both hypoplasia and neuromuscular agenesis may produce velopharyngeal incompetence. This may manifest itself very early in life by nasal regurgitation of food.

Lateral Fistulas. These fistulas are sometimes associated with congenital absence of the tonsils.

Cysts. These may be median or globulomaxillary, or they may involve the incisive canal.

Mucous Membranes and Connective Tissues

Defects include syphilitic stigmata, encephalofacial angiomatosis (Sturge-Weber syndrome), capillary or cavernous hemangioma, lymphangioma and hygroma.

CONGENITAL SYNDROMES OF THE MOUTH AND FACE

The number of syndromes involving stigmata of the mouth and the face is large, but many of them are quite rare. Only some of the commonest ones have been selected for brief description here. Most of these encompass lesions enumerated previously.

Mandibulofacial Dysostosis (Collins' Syndrome)

This condition involves mainly those structures that develop from the mandibular (first branchial) arch, groove and pouch. The facial appearance is characterized by downward sloping palpebral fissures, depressed malars, deformed auricles, retrognathia and unilateral or bilateral macrostomia. The palpebral fissures have an antimongoloid obliquity (downward lateral slope). In about 75 per cent of patients there is a coloboma in the outer third of the lower lid; about half of these have a deficiency of cilia medial to the coloboma. Iridial colobomata may also occur. Frequently, the lower orbital margins may also be defective laterally (Fig. 9).

The auricle is very often deformed, crumpled forward, or displaced forward and downward. Extra auricular tags and sinus tracts may occur anywhere between the tragus and the oral commis-

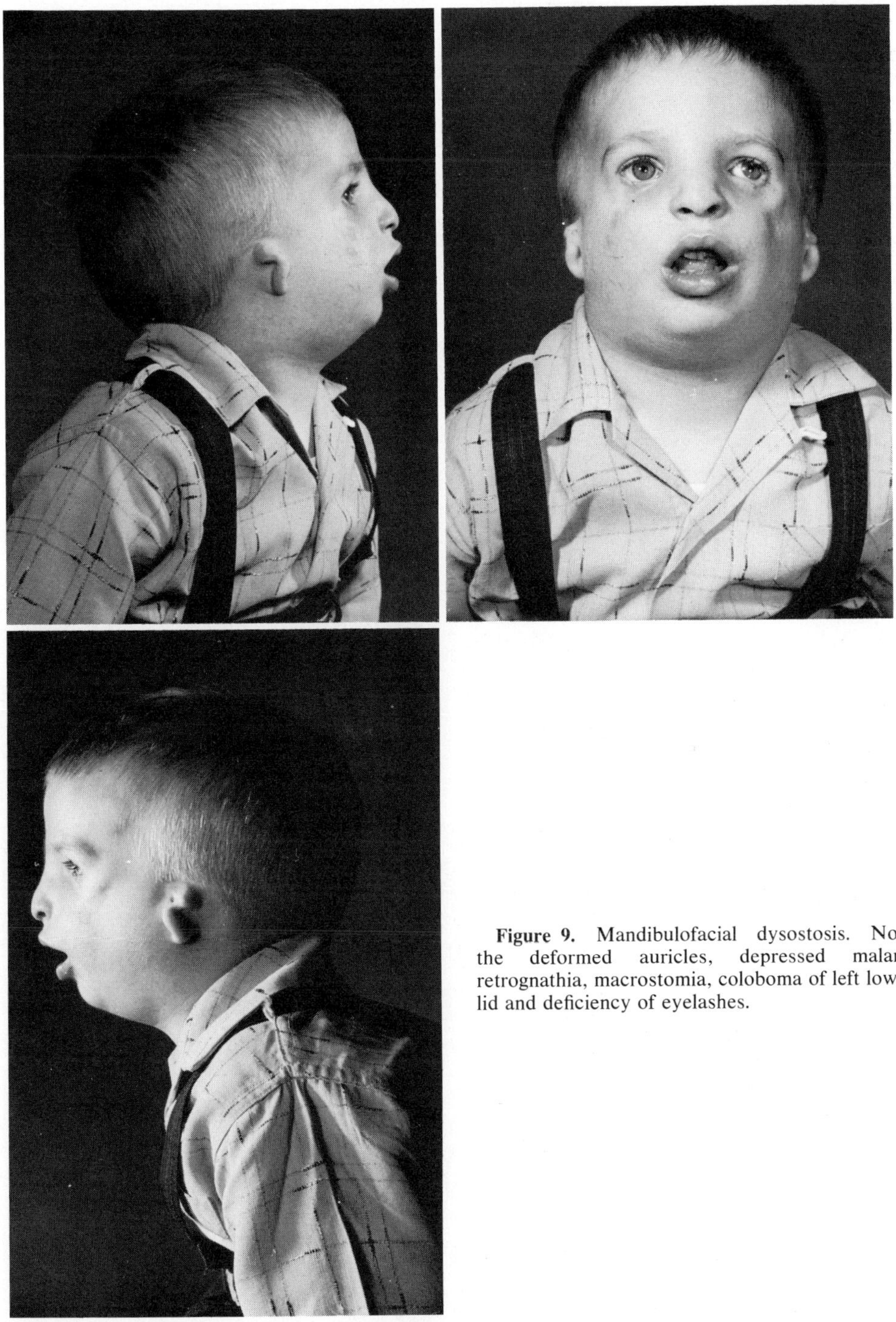

Figure 9. Mandibulofacial dysostosis. Note the deformed auricles, depressed malars, retrognathia, macrostomia, coloboma of left lower lid and deficiency of eyelashes.

sure. About one-third of patients have absence or marked stenosis of the external auditory canal and some tympanic and ossicular defect. There have been reports of nondevelopment of both the cochlear and vestibular labyrinths.

The nasofrontal angle is usually obliterated with a tendency toward a dorsal hump development at an early age. The nose may appear large because of the malar underdevelopment.

The mandible is almost always hypoplastic, with an obtuse angle and a deficient ramus. A marked antigonial angle is usually evident, giving the impression of concavity to the undersurface of the body. The palate is high or cleft in about 40 per cent of patients. Dental malocclusion is frequent.

Craniofacial Dysostosis (Crouzon's Syndrome)

This condition, characterized by exophthalmos and hypertelorism, produces a parrot-beaked nose, a short upper lip and a hypoplastic maxilla, resulting in an acute nasolabial angle. The maxillary dental arch is usually narrow and articulates within the mandibular teeth; an open-bite deformity may also be present. The palate is short and has a high arch. A number of cases present with palatal clefts.

Cleidocranial Dysostosis

In this condition the palate is extremely high-arched and may have a submucous or an actual posterior cleft. The maxilla is usually underdeveloped, giving the appearance of prognathism of the mandible. Nonunion of the mandibular symphysis has been reported.

Arachnodactyly (Marfan's Syndrome)

The face is usually long and thin, with prominent supraorbital ridges. The eyes may appear sunken, and frontal bossing is common. The auricles are often large, with abnormally thin helical rims. A high palatal vault is a very frequent finding.

Acrocephalosyndactyly (Apert's Syndrome)

In this condition, the middle third of the face appears underdeveloped, with a relative prognathism of the mandible

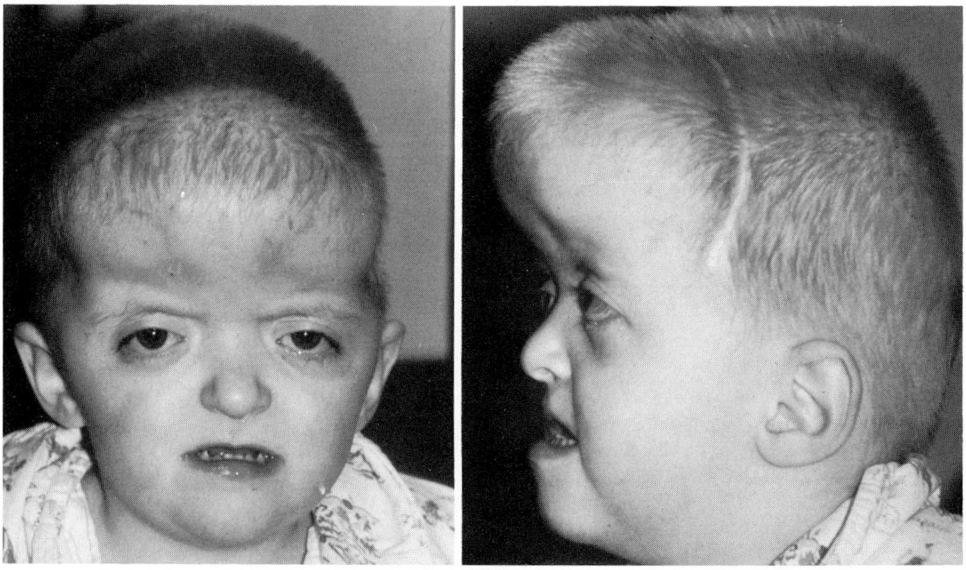

Figure 10. Apert's syndrome.

and depression of the lower forehead region. The nose is small. Hypertelorism, strabismus and proptosis are usually present. Frequently, there is a high-arched palate, and posterior clefts are found in at least 25 per cent of these subjects. The other common findings are oxycephaly and syndactyly (Fig. 10). There may be low intelligence, optic nerve damage, malformed auricles and deafness.

Congenital Facial Diplegia (Moebius' Syndrome)

In addition to the anomalies of the trunk and extremities, this complex entity consists of congenital facial paralysis, which is usually bilateral, and unilateral or bilateral loss of the ocular abductors. Frequently, other cranial nerves are involved, particularly the oculomotor, trigeminal and hypoglossal.

Although usually bilateral, the facial paralysis is frequently asymmetric and the lower face may be spared. Defects of the pinna have been reported. The angles of the mouth droop and drooling may be present. Atrophy, fasciculation and paralysis of the tongue, with resultant speech defects, are present in about a third of the patients.

Osteogenesis Imperfecta (Ekman's Syndrome)

Apart from the classic *fragilitas ossium* micromelia and poor healing of skin wounds with hypertrophic scars, this condition presents in the third decade of life with blue sclerotics, dentinogenesis imperfecta, and a form of otosclerosis in about half the patients.

Facial Hemihypertrophy (Curtius' or Steiner's Syndrome)

This condition, which may be noted shortly after birth, involves part or all of the face and may also be accompanied by enlargement of half of the body on the same side.

Mongolism (Down's Syndrome, Trisomy 21 Syndrome, G Trisomy)

The incidence of trisomy 21 is approximately one to two per 1000 births. The symptoms and signs are well known and have been adequately recorded in several reports. Since the clinical signs are rather numerous, reference should be made to detailed reviews.[3, 5]

The more familiar signs include short stature, brachycephaly, slanted and widespread eyes, epicanthus, strabismus, nystagmus, cataract, short nose, abnormal ear lobes, short neck, broad flat hands, clinodactyly and mental retardation. Poor development of the middle third of the facial skeleton produces a relative mandibular prognathism. The frontal and sphenoidal sinuses are underdeveloped or absent. Mouth breathing is often the rule, frequently with a large, fissured tongue thrust beyond the teeth. The lingual papillae are usually hypertrophied. The mandible is described as V-shaped, and the palate is often high-arched and narrow.

Genital Dwarfism (Turner's Syndrome)

This syndrome, consisting of short stature, gynecologic underdevelopment with primary amenorrhea, and cubitus valgus, is also characterized by pterygium colli and a low hairline at the back of the neck. It may also include coarctation of the aorta, mental retardation, deformed auricles and congenital deafness. The characteristic oral manifestations are a high palatal vault, micrognathia and downward displacement of the oral commissure due to the pull of the ptergium colli.

Gargoylism (Hurler's Syndrome)

The characteristic facies usually become apparent after one year of age. The head is large, with a prominent forehead and coarse features. Hypertelorism, heavy lids, a flat "pug" nose, a long upper lip, an open mouth with a prominent tongue, and a short broad neck characterize the facies. The lips are frequently thick. Upper respiratory infections are frequent, and chronic rhinitis is present from birth in many individuals, resulting in noisy mouth breathing.

Achondroplasia

This is characterized by a large head and broad skull, with frontal bossing and a prominent brow. The nose is small, with a saddle deformity of the dorsum. The maxilla is underdeveloped and the mandible appears relatively prognathic. Mild mental retardation is common.

Micrognathia, Glossoptosis and Cleft Palate (Robin's Syndrome)

The condition is accompanied either by a cleft of the secondary palate or by a highly arched palatal vault. The tongue appears large, since it cannot be contained within the small arch of the mandible. The relatively backward placement of the tongue tends to block the pharyngeal airway and may present as a neonatal emergency. A tracheotomy is not indicated. Securing the tongue in a forward position clears the airway, and the mandible usually assumes normal proportions within several months.

MAXILLOFACIAL CLEFTS

One of the most frequent of the serious congenital malformations, cleft lip or palate, or both, occurs approximately once in every 700 births. The incidence rises sharply when there is a familial history of a similar deformity. Oddly enough, cleft lip and palate is more common in males, but cleft palate by itself is more frequently found in females. Clefts are far more common on the left side – a factor unexplainable on the basis of our present knowledge of embryology.

EMBRYOLOGY. Knowledge of the relevant embryologic background aids in evaluation and understanding of the problem. In a normally developing fetus, the median nasal process fuses with the maxillary processes to form the upper lip, the premaxilla, and the corresponding segments of the alveolar process. The premaxilla and its alveolus form the primary palate (Fig. 11). The palatal processes fuse with each other – to form the secondary palate – as well as with the nasal septum and the premaxilla, between the eighth and tenth weeks. This fusion starts in the vicinity of the future incisive foramen, and from here it proceeds posteriorly and an-

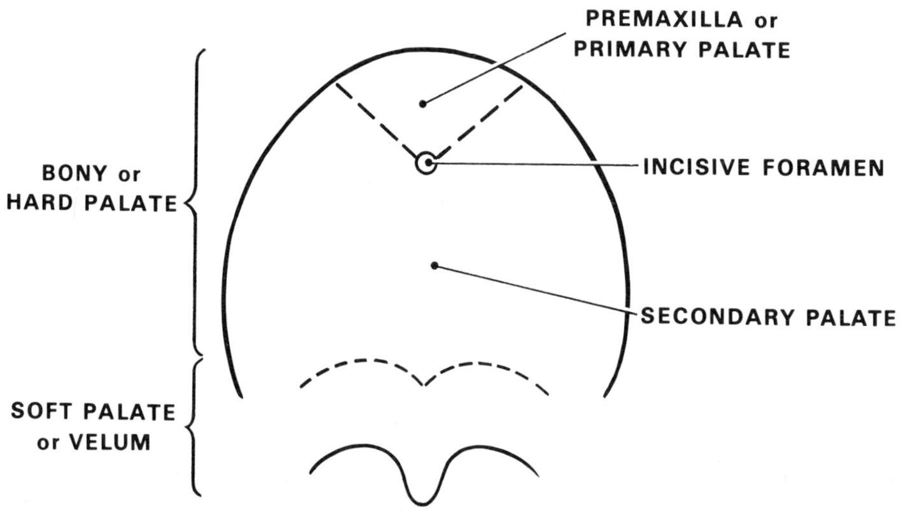

Figure 11. Components of the palate.

teriorly. In cleft cases, only a tenuous epithelial fusion is said to take place, but this breaks down because of the failure of ingrowth of mesodermal tissue. Cleft palate, therefore, results from a lack of cohesion of the palatal segments, and may be seen alone or in conjunction with clefts of the lip or alveolar process. Because embryonic fusion of the constituent segments is initiated at the incisive foramen, incomplete lip and palate clefts may be present only at the anterior or posterior edges of these structures—they do not appear as fistulas in the intervening areas.

Varieties of Clefts

Maxillofacial clefts have been classified in various ways. Figure 12 shows the classification and nomenclature used by the author. The illustrations are complementary to the following brief descriptions of types of clefts.

CLEFTS OF THE LIP. The simplest kind of cleft lip is that which does not have an underlying cleft of the premaxilla on the same side, although a notch may be present in the corresponding alveolar process. Such clefts may be partial or complete, unilateral or bilateral. Incomplete clefts of the lip may extend in varying degrees from the vermilion border to just short of the floor of the nasal vestibule (Fig. 13). Complete clefts extend into the floor of the naris, but these rarely occur without some degree of involvement of the underlying premaxilla. In a unilateral cleft involving only the lip and its corresponding alveolar process, the medial or premaxillary segment usually projects labially,

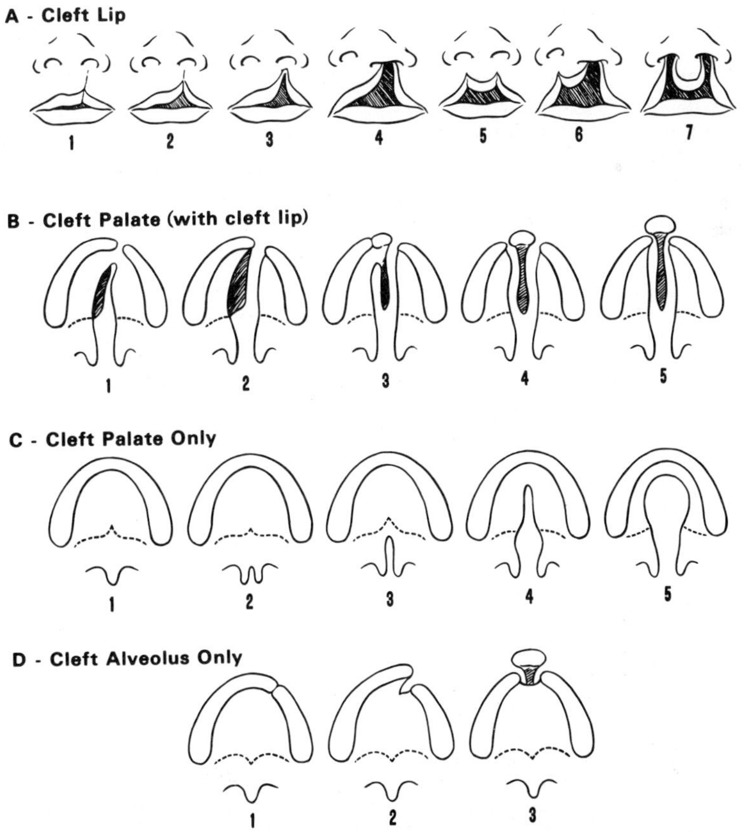

Figure 12. Classification of the cleft lip and palate.

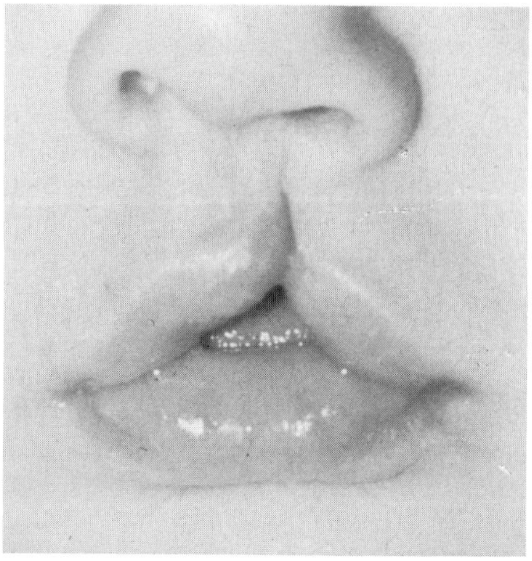

Figure 13. Partial cleft of the lip. Note the associated slight nasal deformity.

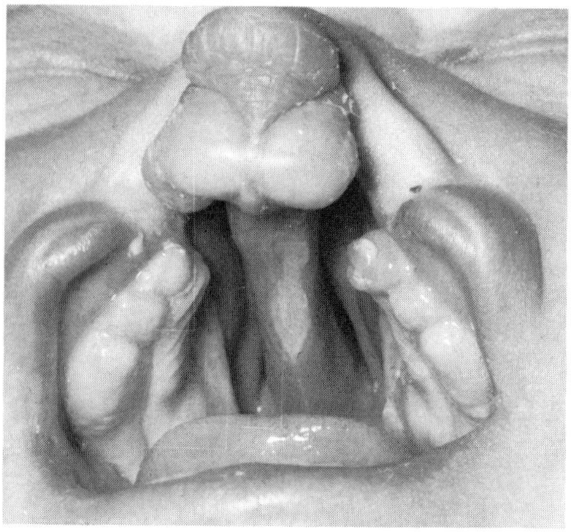

Figure 15. Complete bilateral cleft lip and palate.

apparently deflected in the direction of the muscle pull from the larger noncleft portion of the upper lip.

An overt nasal deformity accompanies most cleft lips, although this may not be readily apparent in some partial clefts, nor obvious to the inexperienced observer. Varying in degree with the severity of the cleft of the lip, the nasal defect usually consists of a depression in the lateral crus and possibly in the dome also, deflection of the tip toward the cleft, a shorter columellar border, a wider vestibular floor, and diminished size of the ala (Fig. 14).

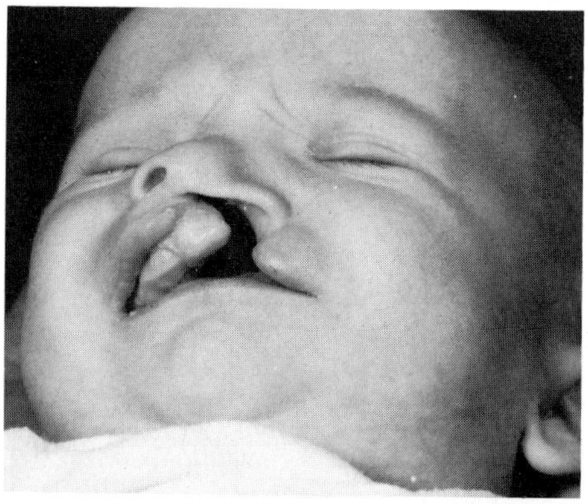

Figure 14. Complete unilateral cleft lip and palate. Note marked nasal deformity and rotation of premaxillary segment forward and upward.

When the lip is completely cleft on both sides, there usually is a complete bilateral cleft of the premaxilla also, and invariably one of the entire palate (Fig. 15). In such a case the premaxillary lip segment, or prolabium, is completely unrestrained by any attachment to either segment of the maxilla, and is attached to the tip of the nose by a very short or almost nonexistent columella. There is usually almost complete absence of any labial sulcus under the prolabium. Accompanying the bilateral cleft lip is a wide cartilaginous nasal vault, with flared alae that are stretched out across the maxillary cleft on each side.

COMPLETE UNILATERAL CLEFT PALATE AND LIP. Complete clefts of the palate are termed unilateral when the palatal process of the opposite side is fused with the nasal septum. In these cases the derangement in the palatal arch is characterized by the total lack of continuity of structure across the midline of the palate on the side of the cleft, and the premaxilla is separated from the alveolar process on the involved side. The vomer is characteristically horizontally inclined and is attached to the palatal process on the uncleft side, so that the oral cavity communicates only with the nasal chamber of the cleft side (Fig. 16 b). Very often, the free edge of the premaxillary segment protrudes into the cleft of

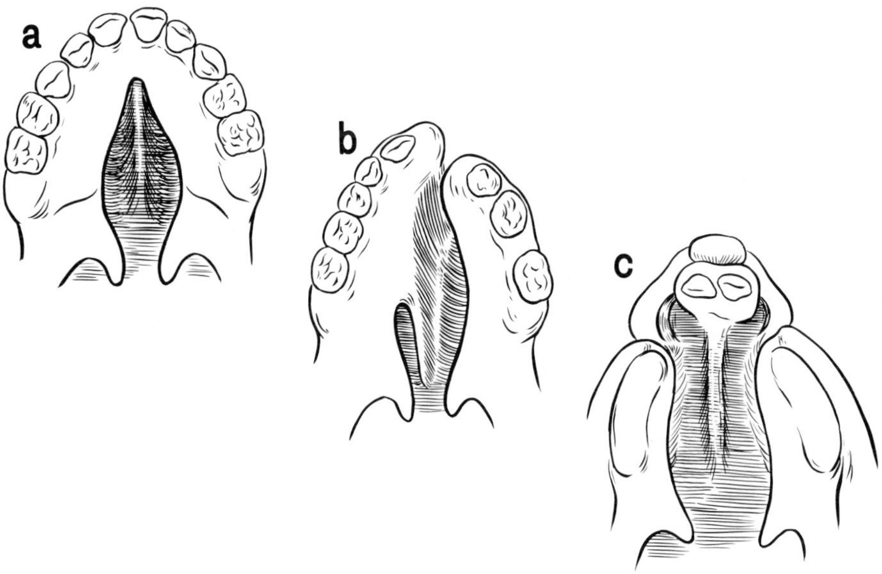

Figure 16. Common varieties of cleft palate. a, Cleft of secondary palate. b, Complete cleft of palate and alveolar process on the left. c, Complete bilateral cleft palate.

the lip and may also intrude into the void in the floor of the nasal vestibule (see Fig. 14). Occasionally, the premaxillary segment may appear to overlap the free edge of the alveolus of the maxillary segment, when the latter has rotated medially—a phenomenon that frequently follows repair of the lip.

Bilateral Cleft Palate and Lip. The frequency of bilateral clefts has been variously reported as being from 9.6 to 16 per cent of the entire maxillofacial cleft series. These infants present with the greatest deformity of all (see Fig. 15). The cleft through the secondary palate is in the midline and divides at the incisive foramen to separate the premaxilla from the rest of the palate. The small anterior segment of the palate thus remains suspended from the anterior portion of the nasal septum. Extending backward from the premaxilla, the inferior margin of the vomer is free and appears to be thickened, but it is vertical and in the midline (see Fig. 16 c). A bilateral cleft of the palate may be termed incomplete when the vomer is only partially attached to one of the palatine shelves.

The incidence of a protrusive premaxilla in bilateral cleft palate is high; not infrequently, the palatal segments appear small and retruded in relation to the premaxilla. There is often disproportion between the size of the premaxilla and the constituents of the secondary palate (see Fig. 15).

In some cases there may be adequate space between the anterior edges of the palate to accommodate the premaxilla, but in others the palatal segments may have collapsed immediately behind the primary palate, leaving no room for it in the alveolar arch.

Clefts of the Palate Only. Clefts that are limited to the secondary palate and that do not involve the alveolar process are a group by themselves, both genetically and morphologically. Their frequency is greater in females. It is this variety that exhibits a high incidence of mandibular micrognathia with glossoptosis—the so-called Robin syndrome.

Midline palatal clefts may vary in extent from a submucous cleft, through a bifid uvula, to a complete cleft of the secondary palate, as far forward as the region of the incisive foramen (Fig. 16 a).

Submucous Clefts. This refers to

a condition of midline mesodermal deficiency between the nasal and oral mucous membranes involving the velum and the posterior edge of the hard palate; the latter is manifested by varying degrees of notching where the posterior nasal spine would normally be present. Submucous palatal clefts invariably have accompanying deficiencies of the musculature of the soft palate, as may be evidenced by a short palatal velum. This condition frequently accompanies a bifid uvula. In fact, it has been my experience that every instance of a cleft of the soft palate has been associated with a submucous cleft of the hard palate of varying degree.

REFERENCES

1. Colby, R. A., Kerr, D. A., and Robinson, H. B. G.: *Color Atlas of Oral Pathology,* 2nd Ed. Philadelphia, J. B. Lippincott Co., 1961.
2. Gorlin, R. J., and Pindborg, J. J.: *Syndromes of the Head and Neck.* New York, McGraw-Hill Book Co., 1964.
3. Øster, J.: *Mongolism.* Copenhagen, Danish Science Press, Ltd., 1953, pp. 1–206.
4. Pindborg, J. J.: *Atlas of Diseases of the Oral Mucosa.* Philadelphia, W. B. Saunders Co., 1968.
5. Warner, E. N.: A survey of mongolism. *Canad. Med. Assoc. J.* 33:495, 1935.

Chapter Eighty-Nine

TUMORS

LEROY SMITH, M.D., and J. LATANE WARE, M.D.

Many lesions noted in the oral cavity are classified as tumors, since they present as a swelling of tissue. They may be neoplastic or non-neoplastic. We classify these lesions as (1) congenital, hereditary, and developmental tumors; (2) epithelial tumors; (3) benign connective tissue tumors; (4) malignant connective tissue tumors; (5) benign muscle and nervous tissue tumors; (6) malignant muscle and nervous tissue tumors; (7) odontogenic tumors; and (8) miscellaneous tumors.

CONGENITAL, HEREDITARY, AND DEVELOPMENTAL TUMORS

A number of tumors in this category are found in the mouth and associated structures. Some are associated with systemic pathology, but the majority represent a local condition.

Peutz-Jeghers Syndrome

Peutz-Jeghers syndrome is an unusual condition manifested by generalized intestinal polyposis associated with melanin pigmentation of the lips, oral mucosa, face, and sometimes the hands and feet. The pigmentation of the lips and mucosa may be present at birth. It looks like small brown speckles, less than 5 mm. in diameter. The intestinal polyps are generalized, have a low malignant potential, histologically appear to be hamartomas, and may cause abdominal pain and intestinal obstruction. The condition is inherited as a simple mendelian dominant characteristic without sex linkage. No treatment of the oral manifestations is required.

Fordyce Granules

These granules, which appear as small yellow spots, are most frequently found in a bilaterally symmetrical pattern on the buccal mucosa opposite the molar teeth. They are heterotopic sebaceous glands, which are presumed to have resulted from inclusion of ectoderm with skin potential in the oral cavity at the site of fusion of the maxillary and mandibular processes. It has been estimated that they are present in 80 per cent of the population, but they are usually not apparent until puberty. They are of no clinical significance and require no treatment.

Oral Epithelial Nevus (White Sponge Nevus; Familial White Folded Dysplasia of Mucous Membrane)

This uncommon condition is inherited as an autosomal dominant trait. It may be present at birth or appear later. It appears as thickened, folded, spongy mucosa with a white, opalescent hue and is located on the cheeks, palate, gingiva, floor of the mouth and tongue. Histologically, there is a generalized thickening of the epithelium with intracellular edema and an intact basal layer. The condition is benign with a good prognosis. No treatment is available.

Fibromatosis Gingivae

This is a rare malady. Most of the reported cases show autosomal dominant inheritance. Sporadic nonfamilial cases are seen. It usually makes its appearance when the permanent teeth are erupting, but a few cases have been reported in early infancy. In the majority of instances both arches are affected, although clinically the upper arch seems to be affected earlier. At the onset there is a slow, progressive thickening of the gingival structure, and as time passes, the teeth are partially covered. In some instances the entire palatal area may be involved. Examination reveals a smooth, rigid, hard, nontender mass involving the entire gingival structure. The mucous membrane appears to be normal or slightly hyperemic. As the deciduous teeth are shed, there is a delay in the eruption of the permanent teeth because of the enlargement of the gingiva. Microscopic examination shows a dense, fibrous network overlying the bone and covered with apparently normal epithelium. If no treatment is undertaken, the child has difficulty in eating, and general debilitation ensues. Surgical excision of the excessive amount of fibrous tissue is the treatment of choice, but recurrence may be expected.

Median Rhomboid "Glossitis"

This congenital anomaly of the tongue is an oval or rhomboid-shaped, slick red patch in the midline of the posterior portion of the tongue just anterior to the circumvallate papillae. Heavy coating of the papillae of the surrounding normal tongue mucosa makes this readily apparent; there are no papillae in the anomalous area, and such coating does not adhere to its surface. Actually, there is no infection, and therefore the term "glossitis" is a misnomer. This anomaly

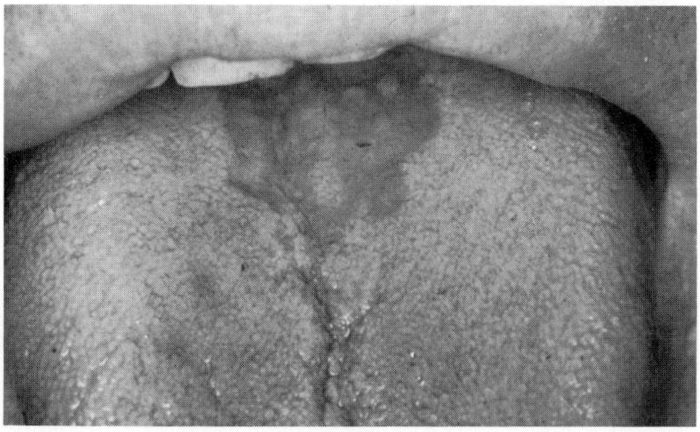

Figure 1. Median rhomboid glossitis. (Courtesy of Dr. Richard P. Elzay, Medical College of Virginia School of Dentistry.)

is due to failure of the tuberculum impar to retract before fusion of the lateral halves of the tongue. There are no symptoms, and no treatment is necessary (Fig. 1).

Thyroglossal Duct Cyst

Thyroglossal duct cysts usually arise in the anterior midline of the neck though they may present beneath the foramen cecum or in the floor of the mouth. Refer to Chapter 100.

Lingual Thyroid

This anomalous condition results from failure of a portion of the thyroid to descend from its normal embryologic point of origin in the foramen cecum. Only rarely does the remnant grow large enough to be of clinical significance, although follicles of thyroid tissue are not an uncommon finding at autopsy when the base of the tongue is examined. The condition is most commonly noted during puberty, adolescence or early maturity, but it has been recorded at birth. The lingual thyroid presents as a mass that has a smooth surface; it is deeply situated and is located near the base of the tongue in the vicinty of the foramen cecum. The presenting complaint is often dysphagia, dysphonia, hemorrhage or a feeling of fulness in the throat. Some patients with lingual thyroid have little or no normally located functional thyroid tissue. Microscopic examination reveals normal-appearing thyroid tissue or embryonal or fetal thyroid tissue. Surgical excision is the recommended treatment.

Oral Fissural Cysts

Five types of fissural cysts of bone, all similar in character, are found in the oral region. These cysts are true cysts. Their lining epithelium is derived from embryonic epithelium entrapped during fusion of bones at union lines. Surgical excision is the treatment of all fissural cysts. Adjacent teeth should not be extracted, since these cysts are not of odontogenic origin. These cysts are classified by location as: (1) median anterior maxillary cysts; (2) median palatal cysts; (3) globulomaxillary cysts; (4) nasoalveolar cysts; and (5) median mandibular cysts.

The median anterior maxillary cyst is found in the area of the incisive canal and is the most common of the fissural cysts. It may present as a mass in this area or as a draining fistula, or it may be noted on a routine dental radiograph. On microscopic examination it is lined by stratified squamous epithelium or pseudostratified ciliated columnar epithelium, or both.

The median palatal cyst is found in the midline of the hard palate. It presents as a visible mass clinically and as a radiolucent area on a palatal roentgenogram. Stratified squamous epithelium forms the lining.

The globulomaxillary cyst is found at the junction of the globular portion of the medial nasal process and the maxillary process. The cyst rarely presents clinical manifestations, but it is detected on oral roentgenograms. Columnar or squamous epithelium is seen on histologic examination.

The nasoalveolar cyst is a rare cyst and is not found within bone. It presents as a swelling in the mucolabial fold and the floor of the nose. This cyst arises at the junction of the globular process, the lateral nasal process and the maxillary process. On microscopic examination, squamous and columnar epithelium are present.

Median mandibular cyst is rare. It occurs, as its name indicates, in the midline of the mandible. It is usually clinically asymptomatic and is discovered on dental radiographs. Histologic examination shows stratified squamous epithelium.

Dermoid Cysts

The dermoid cyst is an oral developmental cyst that is derived principally from embryonic germinal epithelium. In some cases it also contains structures of the other germ layers. It is thus a form of

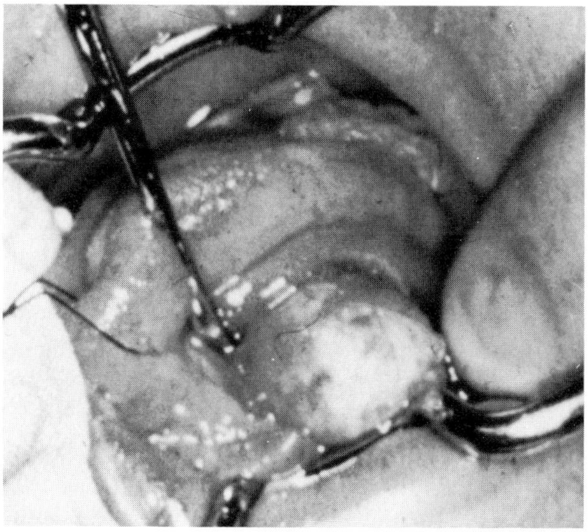

Figure 2. Dermoid cyst of the floor of the mouth.

cystic teratoma. The cyst is found in the floor of the mouth and the submaxillary and sublingual areas. It is presumed to be derived from entrapped epithelium during closure of the mandibular and hyoid arches. In the mouth, dermoids are seldom present at birth and are most common in early adulthood. The cyst may present as a bulge in the floor of the mouth, with elevation of the tongue, or as a bulge in the submental area. The histologic appearance is variable, depending on the complexity of the lesion. Surgical excision is curative (Fig. 2).

EPITHELIAL TUMORS

Benign and malignant epithelial tumors are found in the mouth. In children, malignant epithelial tumors are extremely rare, except possibly for the lympho-epithelioma found in the nasopharynx of adolescents and young adults. The two most common benign epithelial tumors are the papilloma and the pigmented nevus.

Papilloma

These are benign tumors arising from the epithelium of the mucous membrane of the oral cavity. They may be flat or pedunculated, but are usually small, wartlike projections. They may occur on any portion of the epithelium, but in children they are most frequently found around the mucous membrane of the lips and on the surface of the tongue. They may be either single or multiple. Irritation of a papilloma frequently causes bleeding and occasionally may result in infection. Although it has been asserted that these papillomas may be of viral origin, there is no evidence to show that they can be transmitted from one person to the other. They may disappear sponta-

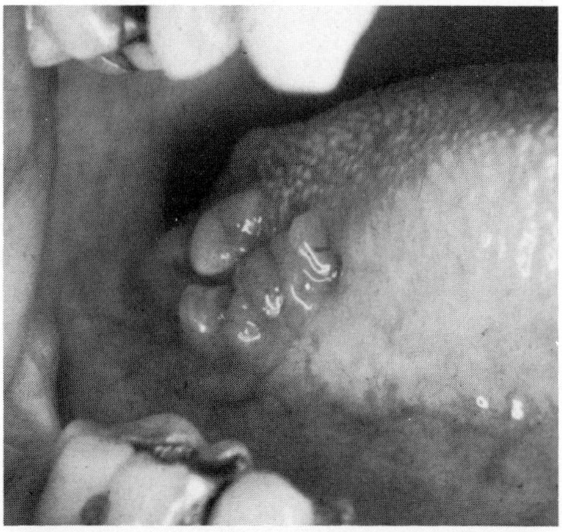

Figure 3. Papilloma of the tongue. (Courtesy of Dr. Charles Vincent, Medical College of Virginia School of Dentistry.)

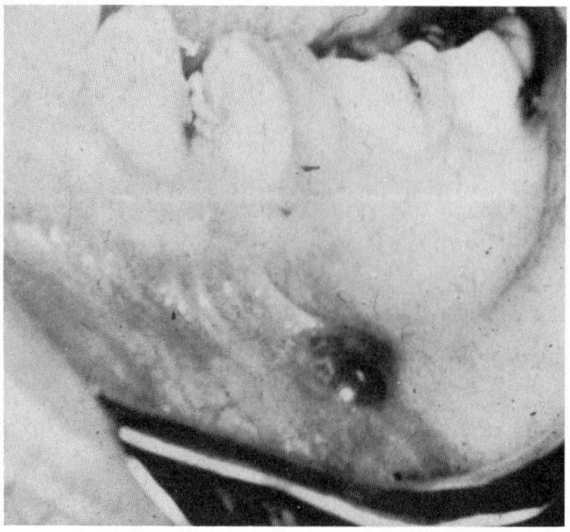

Figure 4. Nevus of the buccal sulcus. (Courtesy of Dr. Richard P. Elzay, Medical College of Virginia School of Dentistry.)

neously. Treatment consists of surgical excision or electrocoagulation, and in either procedure the pedicle at the mucous membrane level should be destroyed in order to prevent recurrence (Fig. 3).

Pigmented Nevus

This does not usually occur on the mucous membrane; however, when it does occur, the most frequent sites are the lips and the palate. The more common types are the intradermal and the junctional nevus, but occasionally amelanotic moles are found. The pigmented types are usually brownish red with a slick surface and usually are only slightly elevated above the mucous membrane surface. The percentage of malignancy in these tumors has not been established, but malignancy is rare, particularly before the advent of puberty. Treatment is by surgical excision (Fig. 4).

BENIGN CONNECTIVE TISSUE TUMORS

Tumors considered in this group arise from tissues of mesenchymal origin and are thus found in the soft tissues and bone.

Fibroma

This tumor of connective tissue is the most common benign soft tissue neoplasm arising in the mouth. The lesion may lie beneath the surface of the mucous membrane or present as a pedunculated, round, firm mass frequently with normal mucosal color. The tumor is essentially asymptomatic except for the presence of a slowly growing mass. In many instances, it is histologically indistinguishable from fibrous hyperplasia. Conservative surgical excision is usually curative (Fig. 5).

Juvenile Fibromatosis

This is a group of lesions characterized by massive proliferation of interstitial or subcutaneous fibrous tissue. The lesion may occur in any part of the body but is most commonly seen on the palms and soles and in the sternocleidomastoid muscle (congenital torticollis). Lesions in the neck may involve the mandible. Histologically, this benign lesion is very cellular, with many fibroblasts. The lesion is poorly demarcated and may be misinterpreted as sarcoma. Local excision is the preferred treatment. Though recurrence rates as high as 50 per cent have been found in the palms and soles, the recurrence rate in the neck is much lower.

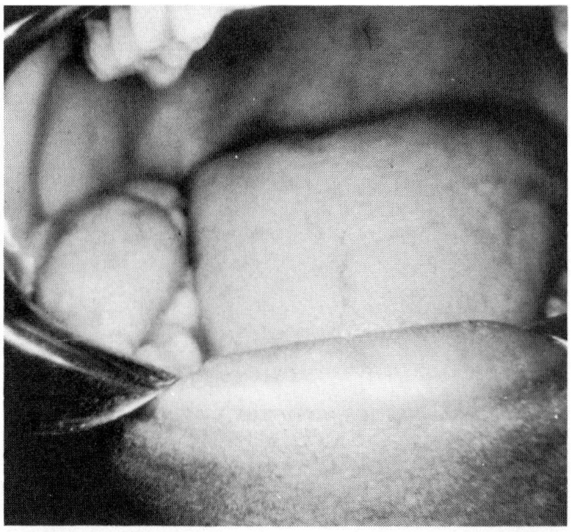

Figure 5. Fibroma of the buccal mucosa. (Courtesy of Dr. Richard P. Elzay, Medical College of Virginia School of Dentistry.)

Ossifying Fibroma of Bone

This central neoplasm is referred to by some authors as central fibro-osteoma and benign osteoblastoma. It probably is a distinct entity that is distinguishable from fibrous dysplasia of bone, which is not a neoplasm. Ossifying fibroma is one of the most common benign tumors of the bone in children and is most frequently seen in young adults, but it may occur at any age. This tumor produces a painless, slowly progressive swelling that may cause displacement of teeth. There is a predilection for the mandible, but either jaw may be involved. The bony cortical plate usually remains intact because of the slow growth. The radiographic picture is variable, depending on the stage of development. Early in its development the tumor is radiolucent; much later it is radiopaque. In the early lesion the microscopic appearance is that of interlacing collagen fibers interspersed by proliferating fibroblasts. The more mature lesion shows coalescing islands of ossification. Conservative excision is usually curative and recurrence is uncommon.

Giant Cell Epulis

This connective tissue tumor is also known as peripheral giant cell reparative granuloma. It is an unusual proliferative response of the tissues to injury rather than a true neoplasm. This lesion always occurs on the gingiva or alveolar process. It presents as a pedunculated or sessile lesion that is about 1 cm. in diameter and dark red in color, and it appears to arise from the periodontal membrane or mucoperiosteum. It may demonstrate rapid growth and show ulceration from irritation by teeth. The tumor is asymptomatic unless secondarily infected. It is more common in adults than children. Histologically, there is a nonencapsulated mass of connective tissue stroma with a large number of young connective tissue cells and multinucleated giant cells. Surgical excision that removes the base of the lesion also is the treatment of choice. Incomplete removal leads to a high recurrence rate. In recurrent cases the adjacent tooth may require removal (Fig. 6).

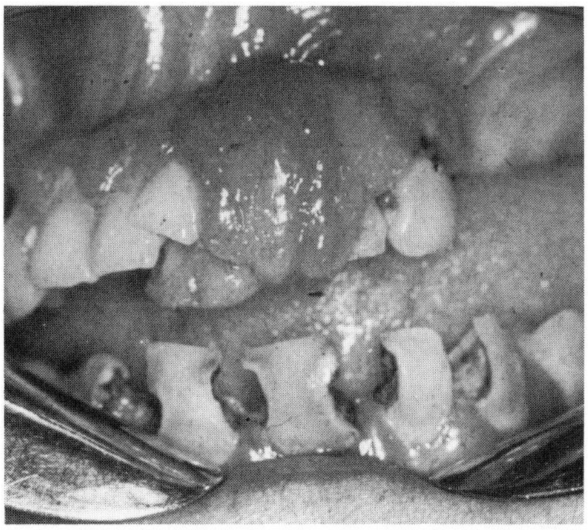

Figure 6. Giant cell epulis. (Courtesy of Dr. Charles Vincent, Medical College of Virginia School of Dentistry.)

Central Giant Cell Reparative Granuloma

There has been some dispute as to whether this lesion is a distinct entity. It occurs clinically in children and young adults and is more common in the mandible than the maxilla. The lesion may present with bulging of the jaw due to cortical plate expansion and with mild to moderate pain. Radiographically, there is a radiolucent area due to bone destruction. A loose connective tissue stroma with proliferating fibroblasts, small capillaries, multinucleated giant cells, and foci of new trabeculae of osteoid is seen on microscopic examination. Surgical excision or curettage is adequate treatment and the recurrence rate is low. Irradiation is contraindicated.

Aneurysmal Bone Cyst

This lesion, which is uncommon, is more frequently seen in children than in adults. There is frequently a history of trauma. Pain, tenderness, and swelling are common. On the radiograph, the bone is expanded and appears cystic with a honeycomb appearance. Microscopically, there is a fibrous connective tissue stroma with blood-filled spaces, numerous young fibroblasts and multinucleated giant cells. Surgical excision or curettage is the treatment of choice and recurrence may follow incomplete removal.

Lipoma

These tumors consist of fatty tissue proliferation and may originate anywhere that fat is found in the oral cavity. The most frequent sites are the cheeks and the lips. They are rare in children. The lesion is a slow-growing, rather firm, freely moveable mass beneath the mucous membrane and produces no symptoms. Treatment is surgical excision. Recurrence is rare. Multiple lipomas may occur under the mucous membrane of the cheeks (Fig. 7).

Hemangioma

Hemangiomas are usually congenital in nature and are characterized by a proliferation of blood vessels. Although the oral cavity is not as frequent a site of occurrence as the skin, hemangiomas may involve any of the oral tissues. The mucosa and submucosal tissues are most commonly involved. Central hemangiomas of the maxilla or mandible do occur and may be difficult to distinguish from other bone-destructive lesions. Carefully planned surgery is required to avoid exsanguinating hemorrhage when these central lesions are removed. The soft tissue lesions may present as flat or raised mucosal lesions that may be poorly circumscribed and are usually deep red or bluish in color. They vary in size from a small surface lesion to one that covers practically all of the oral cavity. In the oral cavity, most hemangiomas are either of the capillary type or the cavernous type.

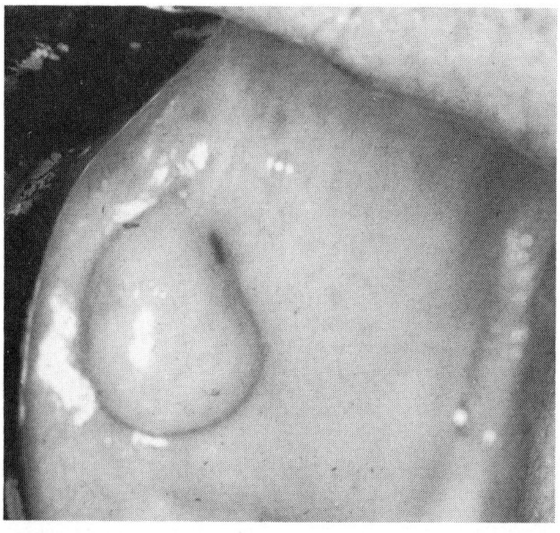

Figure 7. Lipoma of the cheek. (Courtesy of Dr. Richard P. Elzay, Medical College of Virginia School of Dentistry.)

Capillary hemangiomas are composed of many small capillaries lined by a single layer of endothelial cells and separated by a connective tissue stroma. They are found in the mucosa and submucosal tissue. The majority are present at birth and between 85 and 90 per cent make their appearance by the end of the first year of life. The tumor is slightly raised and intensely red or bluish red in color. On palpation it is soft and warm. If extension has occurred into the submembranous layers, a noticeable bulge of the underlying tumor can be demonstrated. The chief characteristic of the capillary angiomas is rapid growth. If untreated, they will often double in size within a period of four to six weeks. If traumatized, profuse bleeding may result. Although it is true that capillary hemangiomas will undergo spontaneous involution, one is never certain as to when or whether this will take place. Since the oral cavity is a self-limited space, excessive growth of the tumor may cause interference with feedings and the maintenance of an adequate airway (Fig. 8).

The destruction of capillary angiomas may be accomplished in several ways—surgical removal, irradiation, the local use of carbon dioxide snow and injection with sclerosing agents. If the lesion is superficial, the simplest treatment is the local application of carbon dioxide snow. If it is treated properly, little scarring results, and the procedure can be accomplished with little discomfort to the patient. Such treatment should be carried out every four to six weeks until the tumor has disappeared. Surgical excision

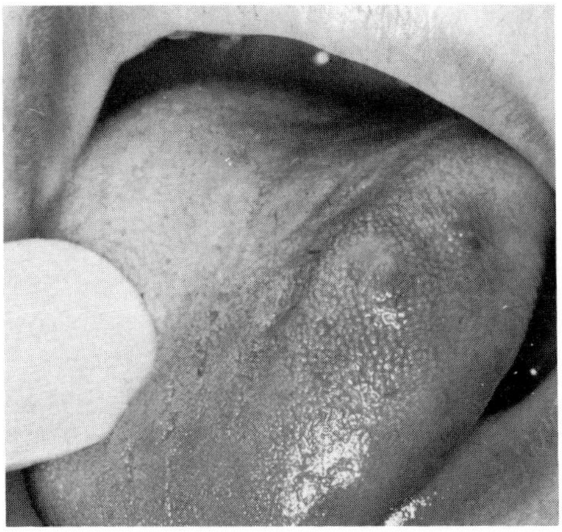

Figure 8. Hemangioma of mucosa and submucosa of tongue.

should be used when the tumor is small or when there is submucosal involvement. Small submucosal tumors may be treated by the injection of sclerosing agents. The solution most often used is sodium tetradecyl sulfate (Sotradecol). Irradiation is effective, but the danger of excessive radiation and of local slough makes this a less desirable method of treatment.

The cavernous hemangioma is composed of thin-walled, endothelial-lined, blood-filled sinusoidal spaces. They may extend into the surrounding tissue and involve muscle, bone, and the entire thickness of the tongue, cheek, or lip. Spontaneous regression is less likely than with capillary lesions. Untreated or unsuccessfully treated lesions may cause widespread destruction of the soft tissue and bone. Serious hemorrhage may result from intraoral trauma to the lesion. When possible, complete surgical excision of the lesion is the preferred treatment. Severe facial disfigurement should be avoided. The injection of sclerosing agents is effective in some cases. Other helpful measures are ligation of feeding arteries and the administration of cortisone derivatives to initiate involution. Recent studies using a cryoprobe hold hope for the future (Fig. 9).

Lymphangioma

This lesion is a benign tumor of lymphatic vessels and is far less common than hemangiomas. In the oral cavity, the common types are the simple lymphangioma and the cavernous lymphangioma. The majority are present at birth and nearly 90 per cent will be present by the end of the second year. The tongue is the most common oral site and the lips the second most common one. The tumor appears as a group of small, raised vesicles covering a portion of the surface of the mucosa. Some are grayish, some are translucent and others are hemorrhagic. The growth of the tumor is slow as compared with that of the hemangioma. Occasionally the submucosal layers are involved and, particularly when there is involvement of the tongue, may cause considerable enlarge-

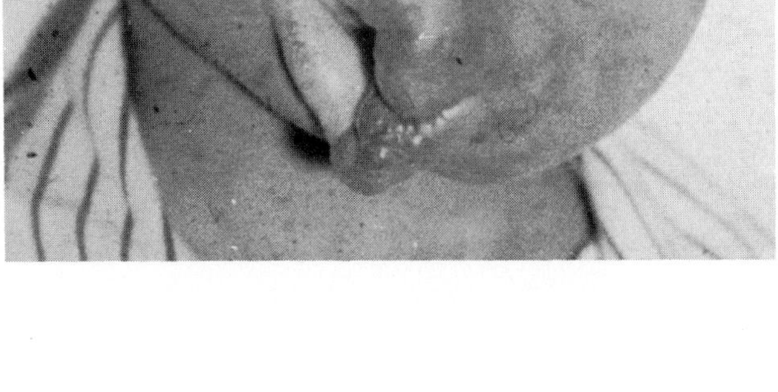

Figure 9. Cavernous angioma.

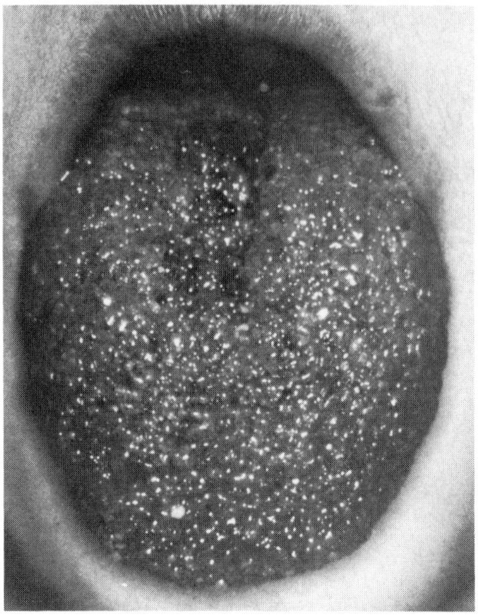

Figure 10. Lymphangioma of the tongue. (Courtesy of Dr. Richard P. Elzay, Medical College of Virginia School of Dentistry.)

ment (macroglossia). The cavernous lymphangiomas are more frequently found in the floor of the mouth and on the cheek. When present in the floor of the mouth, they may attain considerable size and affect the mobility of the tongue. Histologic examination shows a proliferation of lymphatic endothelial-lined spaces or numerous dilated lymphatics lined by endothelial cells and containing lymph. Surgical excision is the treatment of choice. Lymphangiomas are relatively radioresistant and insensitive to sclerosing agents. The incidence of recurrence is high. When there is extensive involvement of the superficial oral membranes and excisional surgery is not feasible, destruction of the tumor in stages by electrocoagulation may be adequate (Fig. 10).

Chondroma

Chondroma is a benign central tumor composed of mature cartilage. It is uncommon in the facial bones. In the maxilla it is usually found in the anterior portion near the midline; in the mandible it usually occurs in the body posterior to the cuspid tooth or in the coronoid or condylar processes. The lesion may occur at any age and is of importance because of its propensity to undergo malignant degeneration. There is bone destruction, and on the roentgenogram an irregular radiolucent lesion is seen. The histologic differentiation of the chondroma and the chondrosarcoma may be difficult. The chondroma shows a mass of hyaline cartilage with small cartilage cells that contain only single nuclei and show little variation in size, shape and staining. The tumor is radioresistant and should be treated by adequate, but not radical, surgical excision. The prognosis is good.

Osteoma

Although simple osteomas do occur in the maxilla, palate and mandible, they are not common. Clinically, this tumor presents as a bony prominence that is usually placed along the normal cortical edge or plate of the bone. It is asymptomatic and growth is slow. The radiograph reveals a well-defined, dense, bony lesion with no evidence of matrix. Microscopic examination reveals a well-circumscribed lesion of extremely dense compact bone or of coarse cancellous bone. Surgical excision is usually indicated and the lesion does not recur after complete removal (Fig. 11).

Exostoses

Torus palatinus and torus mandibularis are bony exostoses of unknown etiology. There appears to be a definite hereditary factor with a very high incidence (between 40 and 64 per cent) in children of parents with tori. The lesion is very common. Torus palatinus presents in the midline of the hard palate and may be flat, nodular, lobular or spindle-shaped. The overlying mucosa is normal unless traumatized. Torus mandibularis is found on the lingual surface of the mandible and varies greatly in size and shape. These lesions are composed of dense compact bone or a shell of compact bone with a center of cancellous bone. Since the lesion is benign and

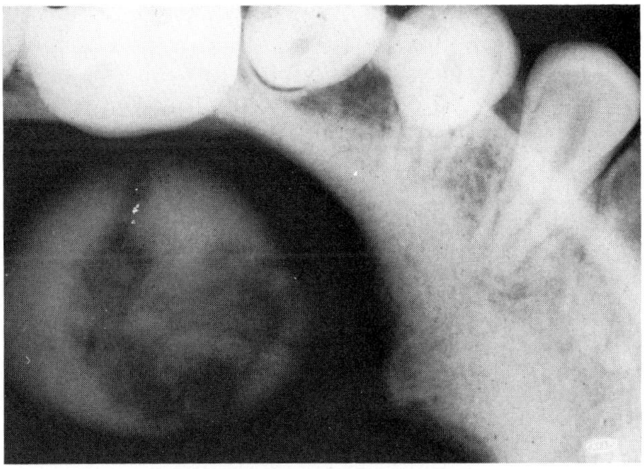

Figure 11. Osteoma of the mandible. (Courtesy of Dr. Richard P. Elzay, Medical College of Virginia School of Dentistry.)

never becomes malignant, treatment is indicated only when it causes difficulties in constructing and fitting dental prosthetic appliances. Surgical removal is curative.

Osteoid Osteoma

This is a benign tumor, possibly caused by trauma, which rarely occurs in the oral cavity. It is occasionally seen in children under the age of 10 years. Males are affected more often than females. The overlying mucosa is frequently tender and sometimes red. Severe pain out of proportion to the size of the lesion may be present. On x-ray examination there is a circular, dense area of bone with a translucent center. As growth continues, the surrounding sclerotic bone increases in size, and the center becomes larger. Calcification may arise

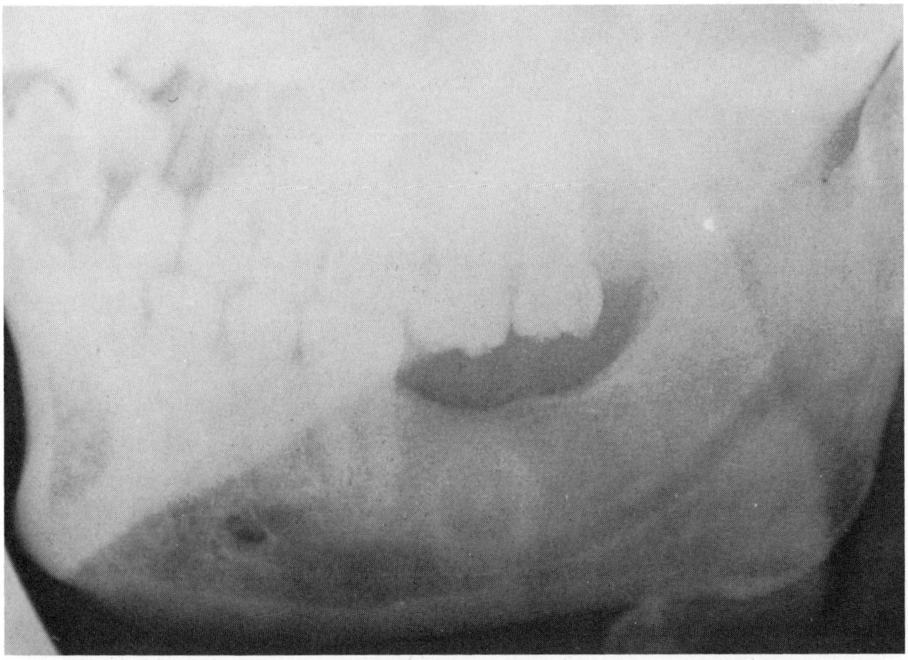

Figure 12. Osteoid osteoma of the mandible. (Courtesy of Dr. John I. Bowman, Jr.)

in the translucent area in tumors of long standing. Histologically, there is a central nidus of compact osteoid tissue with a varying degree of calcification and interspersed by a vascular connective tissue. The lesion should be treated by complete surgical excision and recurrence is uncommon (Fig. 12).

MALIGNANT CONNECTIVE TISSUE TUMORS

Sarcomas are relatively uncommon oral tumors. In general, sarcomas occur in younger patients than do malignant epithelial tumors. They have a tendency to metastasize through the bloodstream rather than the lymphatics.

Fibrosarcoma

Fibrosarcoma is one of the most common malignant tumors of connective tissue. Approximately 18 per cent of cases occur in the head and neck. This neoplasm may occur anywhere in the oral cavity. Although the rate of growth varies, it usually is fairly rapid in its invasion of the surrounding tissue. The tumor is a solid, smooth mass adjacent to the overlying mucous membrane and is so firmly attached to the surrounding tissues that the borders of the growth are difficult to establish. Ulceration of the mucous membrane is infrequent; but when it does occur, hemorrhage and secondary infection may follow. There are relatively few symptoms unless ulceration takes place. The tumor itself is not painful, and only after it has attained sufficient size to interfere with the function of the involved structures is there any complaint. The frequency of metastasis is not high; when metastasis occurs, it is usually late in the course of the disease. Histologically, there are proliferation of fibroblasts, formation of collagen and reticulin fibers, a variable degree of differentiation, spindle-shaped cells with elongated nuclei, and a variable number of mitotic figures.

Radical surgical excision is the preferred treatment. Radiation therapy is usually not effective. Survival and recurrence rates depend on the differentiation of the tumor. A recurrence rate of 75 per cent and a survival rate of 50 per cent may be expected with a poorly differentiated tumor. A 42 per cent recurrence rate and a 96 per cent survival rate have been reported with well-differentiated tumors for fibrosarcomas of all parts of the body (Fig. 13).

Hemangioendothelioma

This is a low-grade connective tissue neoplasm derived from endothelial cells. It may occur anywhere in the body, and primary lesions of the oral cavity, al-

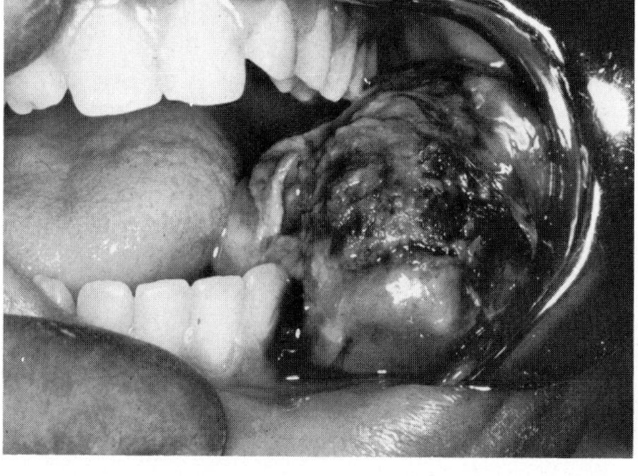

Figure 13. Fibrosarcoma of the buccal sulcus. (Courtesy of Dr. S. Elmer Bear, Medical College of Virginia School of Dentistry.)

though not common, have been reported in a variety of locations. The lesion may occur at any age. Those lesions present at birth or in early childhood (juvenile or infantile hemangioendothelioma) are a benign form of the malignant lesion and probably represent an immature stage in the development of the capillary hemangioma. This juvenile form can be expected to undergo transformation into the more common hemangioma. The malignant hemangioendothelioma resembles a capillary angioma and shows prominent capillaries extending along the surface of the mucous membrane with invasion of the submembranous tissues. The borders of the lesion are not circumscribed as they are in benign hemangiomas, and the rate of growth is much greater. When the lesion is adjacent to bone, early invasion is frequent. Metastasis is frequent especially in the recurrent lesions. Histological examination shows infiltration of surrounding tissues by the tumor, which is composed of masses of endothelial cells that are large, polyhedral or flattened, and have a round nucleus. Poorly defined capillary formation is present. Radical surgical excision is indicated. Radiation therapy has also been successful.

Hemangiopericytoma

This is an uncommon vascular neoplasm characterized by the proliferation of capillaries surrounded by masses of round or spindle-shaped cells. It occurs in many anatomic locations, including the mouth, and is seen at any age. The lesion usually presents as a firm, circumscribed, nodular tumor with rapid growth. Surgical excision is the preferred treatment, but 10 to 15 per cent of the tumors metastasize.

Ewing's Sarcoma

This is a rare malignant neoplasm, occurring as a primary bone tumor, but without osteoblastic properties. The majority of cases are seen in patients between 5 and 25 years of age. The jaw bones are involved in 13 per cent of cases. Pain and swelling are the presenting findings and the onset may be rapid. Roentgenographic examination shows an irregular, diffuse, radiolucent lesion that characteristically shows an onionskin appearance due to the formation of layers of new subperiosteal bone. Microscopic examination reveals a cellular neoplasm composed of solid sheets of small round cells with little cytoplasm, large round or ovoid nuclei, and frequent mitotic figures. The prognosis is poor and widespread metastases are common. The tumor is radiosensitive but rarely radiocurable. Radical surgery alone or with irradiation has produced poor results.

Chondrosarcoma

This lesion is the malignant counterpart of the chondroma. It is found in the maxilla and the mandible and is more common than the benign chondroma. Nevertheless, it is rare in children. This sarcoma may arise in a pre-existing benign chondroma or appear as a new lesion. Clinical differentiation of the benign and malignant lesion may be difficult. The tumor is invasive and destructive, and it metastasizes readily. Wide, radical excision offers the best chance of cure, but the tumor is difficult to control in the jaws. Radiation therapy is of little value.

Osteogenic Sarcoma

This is a rare neoplasm that may involve the bones of the face, particularly the mandible. It occurs in two forms, one an osteoblastic or sclerosing type and the other osteolytic. In the former there is an attempt at bone formation within the tumor, whereas in the latter there is no attempt at bone regeneration. Both tumors occur in young people. Occasionally there is a history of trauma before the onset of the tumor, but there is some question as to whether or not this is a factor in the causation. Pain and swelling producing facial asymmetry are early features of this tumor. Skin or mucosal ulceration is uncommon. Both types demonstrate bone destruction on a roentgenogram. In the osteoblastic form, irregular spicules of new bone may be seen radiating outward at the periphery of the lesion. This gives the characteristic sun-ray appearance. The osteolytic form has no characteristic roentgen appearance and so may cause difficulty in diagnosis.

The histologic appearance is variable. The osteoblastic lesion shows proliferation of both atypical osteoblasts and their less differentiated precursors. These neoplastic osteoblasts show variation in size, shape and nuclear staining. New tumor osteoid and bone formation are found in an irregular pattern. The osteolytic lesion shows proliferation of the spindle cell precursor of the osteoblast, prominent mitotic activity and bone destruction. Osteogenic sarcoma tends to metastasize by way of the bloodstream to the lungs and other bones.

Radiation therapy alone is of little value as a curative measure. Radical surgical resection is the treatment of choice. Survival rates of 20 to 30 per cent are reported.

Malignant Lymphoma

All varieties of the malignant lymphoma group of tumors are found in the head and neck. Both acute and chronic leukemias may present in a high percentage of cases with oral lesions such as gingivitis, gingival hyperplasia, hemorrhage, petechiae and mucosal ulceration. Hodgkin's disease frequently manifests itself in the neck, but oral manifestations are uncommon. Likewise, giant follicle lymphoma and reticulum cell sarcoma do not commonly appear in the mouth. The reticulum cell sarcoma does arise commonly in the tonsil and pharynx. Though multiple myeloma has frequently been reported in the jawbones, the lesion is rare in children. Solitary plasma cell myeloma (plasmacytoma) has been reported in all ages, but it is more common in the elderly. It may involve the jaw bones or the extramedullary form may present in the soft tissue of the oral cavity.

Lymphosarcoma

This tumor is common to all age groups and a relatively large number of cases occur in children. The majority of them occur in the male, the ratio being approximately two to one, and about one-fifth of all lymphosarcomas occur in the head and neck. In the oral cavity the most frequent sites are the tonsils, palate, gingiva, buccal mucosa and floor of the mouth. At the onset, the tumor appears to be a single mass beneath the mucous membrane, showing invasive characteristics by the fact that it is attached to the underlying structures early. It is not painful at first and the rate of growth is fairly rapid. In most instances, by the time the nodule is seen, there has already been evidence of lymph node metastasis. Pain does not occur until the tumor reaches considerable size. If invasion of the gingiva occurs, the teeth become loose and the gums bleed easily. Although ulceration does not occur until late, it will be seen eventually. These ulcers have irregular borders and become secondarily infected early, giving rise to a necrotic foul-smelling mass. At this time the tumor begins to grow above the level of the surrounding mucous membrane in a fungating pattern and is exceedingly friable, with hemorrhage from the growth resulting from the slightest trauma. The histologic appearance is variable. The prognosis is generally hopeless in children. Because the tumor is extremely radiosensitive, x-ray is the best method of palliative therapy.

Burkitt's Tumor

This lesion was first described in 1958 when it was found that this form of malignant lymphoma had a very high incidence in children living in British East Africa. The tumor originated in the jaw (usually the maxilla) in more than one-half of the cases, was found most commonly between the ages of 4 and 8 years, and was twice as frequent in males as in females. The lesions grow to tremendous size and invade and destroy surrounding structures, causing death in four to six months in untreated cases. Histologically, there are uniform primitive cells that appear to be lymphocyte precursors. They show no organization but are present in broad sheets. The tumor is very susceptible to chemotherapy and has demonstrated significant immunologic response; therefore, in treating those malignant tumors today, chemotherapy should be considered.

BENIGN MUSCLE AND NERVOUS TISSUE TUMORS

Benign muscle tumors of the mouth are uncommon. Leiomyomas are benign smooth muscle tumors and may arise from any anatomic site where smooth muscle is present. In the mouth they usually arise from blood vessel walls. The majority are found in the posterior tongue as slow-growing, painless lesions that are superficial and often pedunculated. They are treated by surgical excision. Rhabdomyoma is a benign tumor of striated muscle origin and is extremely rare in the mouth.

Traumatic neuromas are not neoplasms, but they may be seen in the oral structures following accidental or purposeful nerve sectioning. They usually present as small mucosal or submucosal nodules that may be quite tender on palpation. They should be excised.

Granular Cell Myoblastoma

This lesion is an uncommon tumor. Its origin is controversial, but it probably arises from connective tissue of nerves. The tongue is the most common site of occurrence. It presents as a single nodule within the substance of the tongue. Ulceration is uncommon. Microscopic study reveals a lesion made up of strands of large cells with granular eosinophilic cytoplasm. Surgical excision is curative.

Congenital Epulis of the Newborn

This lesion, which is present at birth, is considered by some to be a granular cell myoblastoma. The typical presentation is as a pedunculated mass of the maxillary gingiva. It is also found arising from the mandibular gingiva. It may be a few millimeters to several centimeters in diameter. It usually occurs in females. Histologic examination reveals an appearance very similar to that of granular cell myoblastoma. Surgical excision is the treatment of choice and recurrence is uncommon.

Neurofibroma

This is a benign tumor that arises from the nerve tissue. It may present as a solitary lesion or as one of many lesions in neurofibromatosis (von Recklinghausen's disease). Individual lesions may be pedunculated, smooth, superficial nodules or diffuse, deeply located lesions. Sarcomatous degeneration of the lesions is seen in about 15 per cent of patients with neurofibromatosis. Microscopically, the lesions are composed of delicate, intertwining connective tissue fibrils and occasional nerve fibers. Solitary lesions are treated by excision. In the diffuse form, it is feasible to excise only the lesions that are symptomatic or growing.

Neurilemmoma

This benign tumor arises from neurilemma. It is slow-growing and may occur at any age. The majority present as a painless circumscribed mass of varying size with no distinguishing features. Histologically, this is an encapsulated tumor containing small hyaline structures (Verocay bodies) and with palisading cells that have elongated nuclei (Antoni type A) or disorderly arranged cells and fibers with microcysts. The treatment is surgical excision. If complete removal would result in significant functional or cosmetic deformity, a partial excision is acceptable.

MALIGNANT MUSCLE AND NERVOUS TISSUE TUMOR

Malignant tumors of muscle or nervous tissue are rare in the oral cavity. Despite early radical treatment, the prognosis is very poor.

Rhabdomyosarcoma

This malignant tumor arises in striated muscle. In the head and neck, it is more common in children than in adults. A few cases are seen that arise in the mouth, but they mainly arise from the orbital, facial and cervical musculature as an embryonal type of rhabdomyosarcoma. In the mouth, the soft palate is the most common site, but lesions arising in the tonsil, the labial or buccal mucosa, the gingiva, the tongue and the floor of the mouth are seen. Cases are seen from early infancy through childhood. This tumor usually presents as a small, round, nontender nodule lying beneath the mucous membrane and fixed to the underlying muscle. Pain is not present initially unless there is sensory nerve involvement. Continuing growth may be relatively slow, but as the lesion enlarges, the color of the overlying mucous membrane will be slightly lighter than that of the surrounding nodules. Regional lymphadenopathy may present early or late. Blood stream metastases are also seen. The histologic appearance of the tumor is variable. In the embryonal type, the predominant cell is usually a spindle cell with very eosinophilic cytoplasm and glycogen vacuoles. The preferred treatment is wide surgical excision. This may be supplemented by postoperative irradiation. Irradiation as the sole modality has produced survivors. Chemotherapy may have a definite place in the treatment regimen. Survival rates of 20 to 30 per cent are reported.

Leiomyosarcoma

This malignant tumor of smooth muscle origin is extremely rare in the oral cavity. As with leiomyomas, they are thought to arise from smooth muscle in the walls of blood vessels when present in the mouth. They have been found in the tongue, floor of the mouth, and soft palate and usually present as a painless mass. Metastases are usually through the blood stream. Microscopic examination reveals plump and spindle-shaped cells arranged in interlacing bundles. Longitudinal myofibrils may be present. Radical surgical excision is indicated.

Alveolar Soft-Part Sarcoma

This rare malignant lesion occurs predominantly in young persons in their twenties and thirties. It is seen most commonly in an extremity, but lesions of the tongue and floor of the mouth have been reported. The origin and classification of this tumor are subject to debate. There are no distinguishing clinical features. A slow-growing, painless, well-circumscribed mass is the usual presenting picture. Metastasis by the blood stream or lymphatics may occur. The lung is a frequent site of spread. The treatment of choice is radical surgical excision. Radiation is of little value. The prognosis is variable, but in general it is poor.

Malignant Schwannoma

Malignant intraoral tumors of nerve tissue origin are very rare. Some of these lesions arise in previously benign lesions of neurofibromatosis and others appear spontaneously. The lesion occurs about the mandible more frequently than in the maxilla. The clinical picture may be one of a painless mass or there may be pain and paresthesias. When the mandible or maxilla is involved, there may be a radiolucent area on the roentgenogram. The histologic appearance closely resembles that of a fibrosarcoma, although palisading may be present. Wide surgical excision is the preferred treatment. Radiation therapy has been successful. Prognosis varies with the stage of the disease at which it is initially treated.

ODONTOGENIC TUMORS

Odontogenic tumors form a diverse group of lesions that reflects the complex development of the dental structures. These lesions are uncommon in children.

Odontogenic Cysts

Odontogenic cysts are not true neoplasms. They can be classified as follicular cysts (primordial cysts and dentigerous cysts), periodontal cysts (apical cysts and lateral cysts) and gingival cysts.

Primordial Cysts. This is the least common of dental cysts. It is found in place of a tooth and results from a malformation in the enamel organ before any calcified enamel forms. This cyst does not produce symptoms unless it becomes secondarily infected or produces looseness or sensitivity of adjacent teeth. On a roentgenogram the cyst presents as a round, well-demarcated, radiolucent lesion and is located where a tooth should be. There is a propensity for involvement of the third molar area. Surgical removal of the cyst with thorough curettage of the bone to remove any remnant of the lining is curative.

Dentigerous Cysts. This type of cyst is far more common than the primordial cyst. Dentigerous cysts are the result of a malformation of the enamel organ after a portion of enamel has formed. Usually only the crown of the tooth is present. The common locations of these cysts are the mandibular third molar area and the maxillary cuspid area. Symptoms are related to secondary infection, displacement of adjacent teeth, and occasionally facial asymmetry with bone expansion. A radiolucent area associated with an unerupted tooth crown is seen on a roentgenogram. The preferred treatment is surgical removal of the cyst and extraction of the malformed tooth.

Periodontal Cysts (Radicular Cysts). The apical periodontal cyst is the most common odontogenic cyst. These cysts form around the root of an erupted tooth and usually result from infection involving the pulp of the tooth. As growth progresses, the lesion may or may not cause pain, depending on the viability of the tooth. Inevitably the tooth becomes loose as the cyst increases in size. Clinical examination may reveal a bulge due to erosion of the cortex of the bone. Roentgenographically, the borders of the cyst are clear-cut and surround the root of the tooth. Extraction of the involved tooth and surgical removal of the cyst is the preferred treatment (Fig. 14).

The lateral periodontal cyst is rare. It appears to arise in the lateral periodontal membrane of an erupted tooth. This cyst is most often found in the mandibular cuspid-bicuspid area and may manifest itself as a lateral periodontal abscess. X-ray demonstrates a radiolucent area in apposition to the lateral surface of a tooth root. Surgical excision without extracting the associated tooth is the preferred treatment. Frequently, it is necessary to remove the tooth to excise the cyst.

Gingival Cysts. The gingival cyst arises from the dental lamina and is

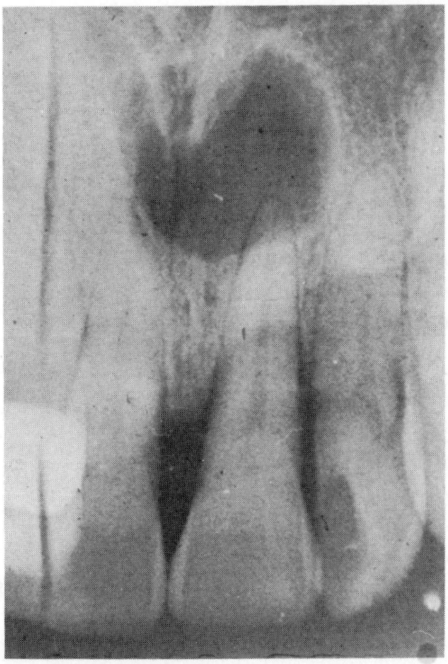

Figure 14. Apical cyst. (Courtesy of Dr. Charles Vincent, Medical College of Virginia School of Dentistry.)

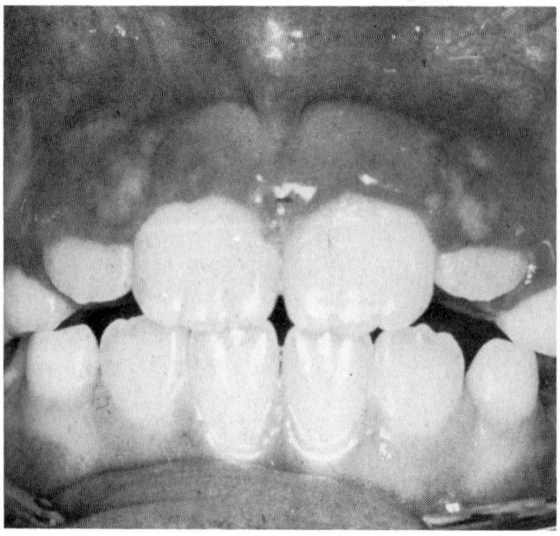

Figure 15. Gingival cysts.

found in any age group. The cyst is a lesion of the gingival soft tissue and presents as small, well-defined, painless nodule of the gum, covered with normal-appearing epithelium. In infants, the surface may appear blanched, and these cysts are referred to as Epstein's pearls or Bohn's nodules. In older children the treatment is surgical excision. In infants, however, these cysts usually undergo spontaneous degeneration, and then no treatment is required (Fig. 15).

Odontogenic Neoplasms

Although the following classification does not include several of the rare odontogenic neoplasms, it is useful. The three main types are ectodermal neoplasms (ameloblastoma or adamantinoma), mesodermal neoplasms (cementoma) and mixed tissue neoplasms (ameloblastic fibroma, odontoma, and ameloblastic odontoma).

Ameloblastoma. This tumor arises from enamel organ-type tissue and may occur at any age. It is a benign lesion but malignant degeneration has been reported. Half of the tumors occur between the ages of 20 and 40. There is a relatively even distribution between males and females, but there appears to be an increased incidence in blacks. The mandible is involved in 80 per cent of the cases and three-fourths of these are found in the molar-ramus area. In the maxilla, the molar area and floor of the nose are the most common sites.

Clinically, the tumor may appear as a cyst or as a solid tumor. Growth is insidious and there is usually no pain. As the tooth-occupying bone is involved, the teeth may become painful and loose. Ameloblastoma is a bone-destroying tumor; as the growth breaks through into the soft tissues surrounding the involved bone, the cortex is usually thinned out or, in advanced cases, completely eroded. Roentgen examination shows either a cystic tumor with multilocular areas throughout the involved bone and thinning of the cortex, or a solid tumor with the same picture except that the translucent appearance of the tumor on x-ray film is not as clear. Histologically, the typical ameloblastoma is composed of many small masses of tumor cells forming nests that are surrounded by a single layer of cuboidal or columnar cells that resemble ameloblasts.

Complete surgical removal is essential to prevent recurrence. When possible, complete excision of the tumor, leaving a rim of cortical bone intact for regeneration, is the preferred technique. Block excision of the lesion and adjacent bone with immediate bone graft is usually reserved for recurrent lesions. The tumor is radioresistant. The recurrence rate with surgical excision is approximately 10 to 15 per cent, but distant spread is uncommon (Fig. 16).

Adenoameloblastoma is an uncommon form of ameloblastoma that usually occurs before the age of 21 years and is more common in females than in males. The clinical and radiographic findings are similar to the simple ameloblastoma. Histologically, there is a formation of ductlike structures. The lesion has little or no tendency to recur and should be treated by conservative surgical excision.

Cementoma. This lesion is fairly common except in children. Its etiology is uncertain. Most commonly the lesion arises from the periodontal membrane around the apex of a mandibular incisor. Multiple lesions are common. The radiographic appearance is variable and may

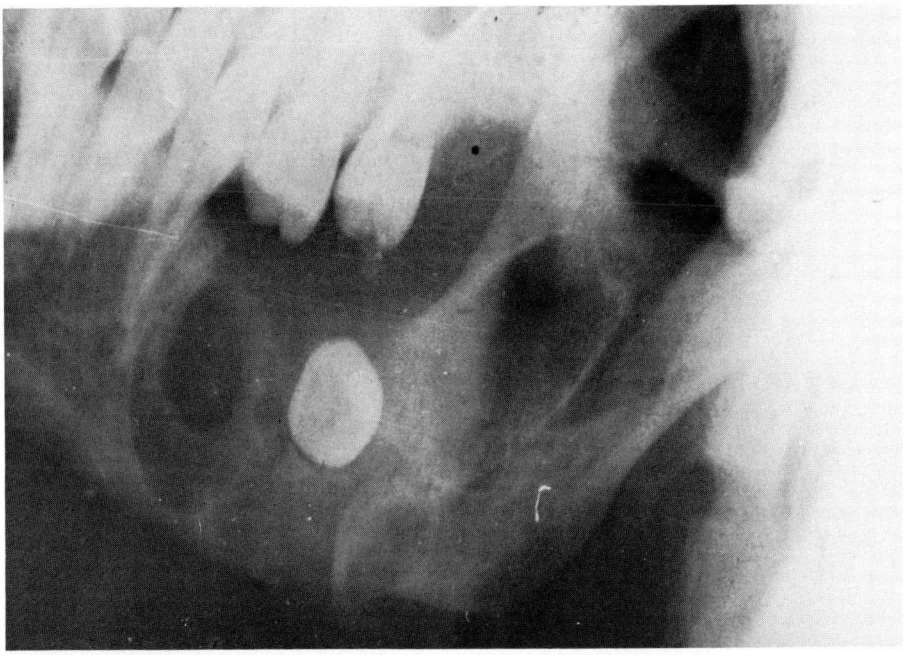

Figure 16. Ameloblastoma of the mandible. (Courtesy of Dr. Phillip Peters, Medical College of Virginia School of Dentistry.)

show osteolytic or calcified periapical lesions. No treatment is required for this harmless tumor.

Ameloblastic Fibroma. This uncommon tumor is a true mixed tumor characterized by the proliferation of both epithelial and mesenchymal tissue. The lesion occurs most commonly during the teenage years. Though somewhat slower growing than simple ameloblastoma, this lesion presents similar clinical and radiographic findings. Microscopic examination of the tumor reveals a variable pattern of scattered islands of epithelial cells closely resembling primitive odontogenic epithelium lying in a delicate, primitive connective tissue. Conservative excision is the preferred treatment and there is little recurrence.

The ameloblastic sarcoma is the malignant counterpart of the ameloblastic fibroma. The lesion is rare, tends to occur in children, grows rapidly, and has a poor prognosis even when radical excision is performed.

Odontoma. By definition, odontoma refers to any odontogenic tumor, but in common usage the term refers to a tumor in which the epithelial and mesenchymal cells exhibit complete differentiation and formation of enamel and dentin. Some refer to this lesion as a composite odontoma. This tumor may be found in any age group, even very young children, and shows no predilection for any location in the dental arch. It usually remains small. The radiograph is characteristic and shows an irregular mass of calcified material or a variable number of toothlike structures surrounded by a narrow radiolucent band and located between the roots of the teeth. Histologically the enamel matrix, dentin, pulp tissue and cementum are normal-appearing. Surgical removal should be curative.

Ameloblastic Odontoma. This rare tumor is a composite lesion formed by relatively undifferentiated neoplastic ameloblastic tissue and the highly differentiated tissue of an odontoma. The lesion occurs most commonly in children and is more frequent in the mandible than the maxilla. The slowly expanding lesion produces facial deformity, bone destruction, pain and delayed eruption of teeth. The radiographic appearance is similar to that of the odontoma. Histologically, there is a great variety of cells and tissue, with structures resembling tooth germs and sheets and cords of epithelial cells. The tendency to recur varies with the histologic subtype, but conservative surgical excision with close follow-up is probably the therapy of choice. A recurrence rate of 8 to 12 per cent is reported.

MISCELLANEOUS TUMORS

Under this heading we shall discuss several unrelated lesions that do not fall into any of the previous groups.

Retention Cysts

The mucocele (mucus retention cyst) is a relatively common oral lesion that is thought to be of traumatic origin. Trauma such as biting the lip or cheek may lead to severance and then closure of the duct of a mucous gland. A cystic lesion forms from retention of the gland secretions. This cyst most commonly presents as a cystic mass of the lower lip elevated above the overlying mucous membrane. The lesion less commonly is found on the tongue, palate, buccal mucosa or floor of the mouth. Some lesions regress and enlarge periodically or temporarily disappear after traumatic rupture with evacuation of the thick, mucinous contents. Histologically, the cyst is a circumscribed cavity in the submucosa that is usually lined by compressed fibrous connective tissue and fibroblasts. The lumen is filled by an eosinophilic coagulum. The proper treatment is surgical excision. Occasional recurrences requiring re-excision may be seen (Fig. 17).

The ranula is a retention cyst in either the submaxillary or sublingual ducts and, therefore, occurs only in the floor of the mouth. Clinically, it is characterized by a slow-growing mass on one side or the other of the lingual frenulum. As it bulges under the lining, it usually has a slightly bluish color. Except for its size, there are no particular symptoms. Treatment is by surgical marsupialization (Fig. 18).

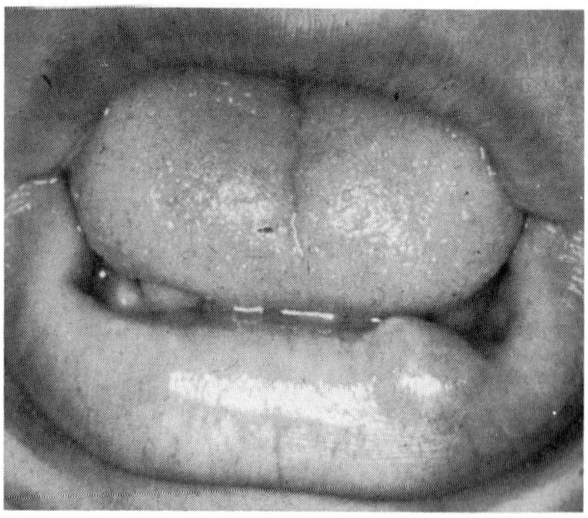

Figure 17. Mucocele of the lower lip.

Fibrous Dysplasia of Bone

Fibrous dysplasia of bone is a lesion of unknown etiology, uncertain pathogenesis and diverse histologic appearance. The disease is divided into monostotic and polyostotic forms. Two types of polyostotic fibrous dysplasia are described. If fibrous dysplasia involves a variable number of bones (while most of the skeleton is normal) and is associated with pigmented skin lesions, it is often referred to as Jaffe's type. A more severe form involving nearly all the bones of the skeleton and accompanied by pigmented skin lesions and endocrine disturbances is known as Albright's syndrome. Only the monostotic form will be discussed here.

Monostotic fibrous dysplasia is a benign bone lesion that is characterized by fibro-osseous connective tissue with varying degrees of osseous metaplasia replacing the normal substance of the interior of the bone. The etiology is unknown, but the lesion may represent a peculiar reparative reaction of bone to injury. Children are more often affected than adults and there is no sex predilection. A painless bulging of the jaw resulting from a swelling of the labial or buccal

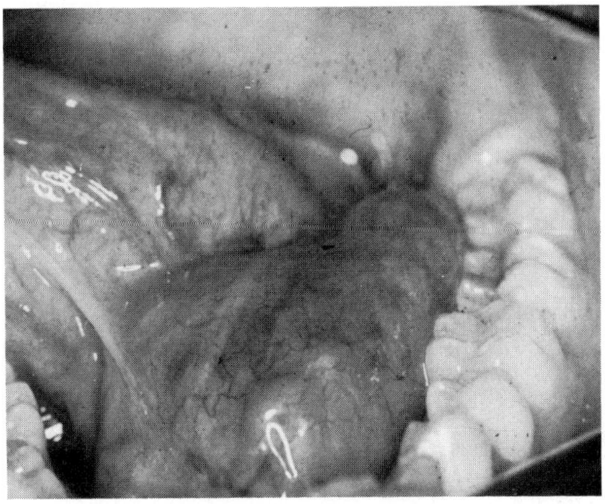

Figure 18. Ranula of the floor of the mouth. (Courtesy of Dr. S. Elmer Bear, Medical College of Virginia School of Dentistry.)

plate is the first clinical sign. Dental displacement and tenderness may develop. The mandible is affected more commonly than the maxilla. Radiographically, there is a radiolucent lesion that may show loculations or irregular foci of ossification. Thinning of the cortical plate (but without perforation) is seen. In the absence of a fracture, there is no evidence of periosteal reaction.

The lesion should be treated by surgical excision of the soft tissue mass. It will usually separate from the surrounding bone and there is little tendency to recur. If marked functional or cosmetic defects will result from complete resection, partial resection and curettage may be the treatment of choice. Progression of residual disease is seen in some patients after partial resection. Occasionally, the disease stabilizes at puberty and requires no treatment. Radiation is contraindicated because of the possibility of the late development of postradiation sarcoma.

Familial fibrous dysplasia of the jaws (cherubism) appears to be a related but distinct clinical entity. This hereditary disease is believed to be transmitted by an autosomal dominant gene with variable penetrance. This condition usually manifests itself at three or four years of age as a progressive, painless, symmetric swelling of the jaws that causes a fullness of the cheeks, firm protuberant intraoral masses and displaced teeth. Submaxillary lymphadenopathy is an early feature but tends to subside after 5 years of age. Roentgenograms reveal extensive bilateral bone destruction with cortical expansion and thinning. A multilocular appearance is common. Microscopic examination commonly shows numerous large multinucleated giant cells in a loose fibrillar stroma. Treatment is difficult because of the widespread involvement and rapid progression during early childhood. The best plan of treatment appears to be to observe tumor growth until it reaches a point of clinical or cosmetic intolerability and then proceed with curettement and recontouring. Repeated procedures may be necessary. The process has a tendency to become static after puberty.

Melanotic Progonoma (Melanotic Neuroectodermal Tumor of Infancy, Retinal Anlage Tumor, Melanoameloblastoma)

This unusual tumor of uncertain histogenesis is almost always found in infants 6 months of age or younger. It is probably of neural crest origin. The usual clinical picture is that of a rapidly growing, nonulcerated, darkly pigmented or deep red, firm anterior maxillary tumor, several centimeters in diameter in a small infant. Roentgenograms demonstrate bone destruction and displacement of teeth. Elevated levels of vanilmandelic acid have been found in the urine of some patients. Histologically there is a nonencapsulated, infiltrating tumor mass, with the tumor cells arranged in slitlike alveoli, lined by cuboidal cells that contain variable amounts of granules with melanin pigment. Conservative but complete surgical excision is indicated. The recurrence rate is low and recurrences should be treated by re-excision. There appears to be no tendency to metastasize.

REFERENCES

Archer, W. B.: Lymphangioma of the lips. *Oral Surg.,* 4:170, 1952.

Austin, L. T., Jr., Dahlin, D. C., and Royer, R. Q.: Giant-cell reparative granuloma and related conditions affecting the jawbones. *Oral Surg.,* 12:1285, 1959.

Bauer, W. H., and Bauer, J. D.: The so-called "congenital epulis." *Oral Surg.,* 6:1065, 1953.

Bernick, S.: Growths of the gingiva and palate. I. Chronic inflammatory lesions. II. Connective tissue tumors. III. Epithelial growths. *Oral Surg.,* 1:1029, 1098, 1948; 2:217, 1949.

Bhaskar, S. N.: Oral tumors in infancy and childhood. A survey of 293 cases. *J. Pediat.,* 63:195, 1963.

Bhaskar, S. N., and Akamine, R.: Congenital epulis (congenital granular cell fibroblastoma). *Oral Surg.,* 8:417, 1955.

Borcello, E. D., and Gorlin, R. J.: Melanotic neuroectodermal tumor of infancy—a neoplasm of neural crest origin. *Cancer,* 19:196, 1966.

Bruce, K. W., and McDonald, J. R.: Chondroma of the tongue. *Oral Surg.,* 7:1281, 1954.

Bruce, K. W., and Royer, R. Q.: Lipoma of the oral cavity. *Oral Surg.,* 7:930, 1954.

Burford, W. N.: Lymphosarcoma of the soft palate. *Amer. J. Orthodont. Oral Surg.,* 33:24, 1947.

Burkitt, D.: Sarcoma involving jaws in African children. *Brit. J. Surg.,* 46:318, 1958.

Campbell, J. A. H.: Congenital epulis. *J. Path. Bact.,* 70:233, 1955.

Christopherson, W. M., Foote, F. W., Jr., and Stewart, F. W.: Alveolar soft-part sarcomas. *Cancer,* 5:100, 1952.

Comerford, T. E., Jr., et al.: Nevus of the oral cavity. *Oral Surg.,* 17:148, 1964.

Cooke, B. E. D.: The giant-cell epulis: Histogenesis and natural history. *Brit. Dent. J.,* 93:13, 1952.

Coventry, M. B., and Dahlin, D. C.: Osteogenic sarcoma. *J. Bone Joint Surg.,* 39A:741, 1957.

Englart, R. D., and Leuin, I. S.: Diffuse osteofibromatosis: A symptom complex. *Oral Surg.,* 7:837, 1954.

Foss, E. L., Dockerty, M. B., and Good, C. A.: Osteoid osteoma of the mandible. *Cancer,* 8:592, 1955.

Freiberger, R. H., et al.: Osteoid osteoma: A report on 80 cases. *Amer. J. Roentg.,* 82:194, 1959.

Garn, S. M., and Hatch, C. E.: Hereditary general gingival hyperplasia. *J. Hered.,* 41:2, 1950.

Garrington, G. E., et al.: Osteosarcoma of the jaws. *Cancer,* 20:377, 1967.

Gorlin, R. J., and Goldman, H. M.: *Oral Pathology,* Vols. 1 and 2. St. Louis, C. V. Mosby, 1970.

Hamner, J. E., and Ketcham, A. S.: Cherubism: An analysis of treatment. *Cancer,* 23:1133, 1969.

Hamner, J. E., Scofield, H. H., and Cornyn, J.: Benign fibro-osseous jaw lesions of periodontal membrane origin. *Cancer,* 22:861, 1968.

Hiatt, W. H., and Orban, B.: Hyperkeratosis of the oral mucous membrane. *J. Periodont.,* 31: 96, 1960.

Hinds, E. C.: Noninflammatory bone disease. *J. Oral Surg.,* 28:27, 1970.

Hine, M. K.: Fibrous hyperplasia of gingiva. *J. Amer. Dent. Assoc.,* 44:681, 1952.

Hutter, R. V. P., et al.: Benign and malignant giant cell tumors of bone. A clinicopathological analysis of the natural history of the disease. *Cancer,* 15:653, 1962.

Johnson, A. E., Stenstrom, K. W., and Waldron, C. A.: Multiple lymphosarcoma (lymphoblastoma) of the oral and cervical regions. *J. Oral Surg.,* 4:159, 1946.

Kaufman, S. L., and Stout, A. P.: Congenital mesenchymal tumors. *Cancer,* 18:460, 1965.

Lighterman, I.: Hemangioendothelioma of the tongue; report of case. *J. Oral Surg.,* 10:163, 1952.

Litzow, T. J., and Lash, H.: Lymphangiomas of the tongue. *Proc. Staff Meet. Mayo Clin.,* 36:229, 1961.

Loring, M. F.: Hemangioma of the mandible. *Arch. Otolaryng.,* 85:92, 1967.

Maccomb, W. S., and Fletcher, G. H.: *Cancer of the Head and Neck.* Baltimore, Williams and Wilkins Company, 1967.

Meyer, G., Roswit, B., and Unger, S. M.: Hodgkin's disease of the oral cavity. *Amer. J. Roentg.,* 81:430, 1959.

Moore, O., and Grossi, C.: Embryonal rhabdomyosarcoma of the head and neck. *Cancer,* 12:69, 1959.

Pindborg, J. J.: Fibrous dysplasia or fibro-osteoma. *Acta Radiol.,* 36:196, 1951.

Pound, E., et al.: Fibrous dysplasia (ossifying fibroma) of the maxilla. *Ann. Surg.,* 161:406, 1965.

Ramsey, H. E., Strong, E. W., and Frazell, E. L.: Fibrous dysplasia of the craniofacial bones. *Amer. J. Surg.,* 116:542, 1968.

Rappaport, I., et al.: The significance of oral angiomas. *Oral Surg.,* 17:263, 1964.

Rise, E. N.: Dermoid cyst of the tongue and floor of the mouth. *Arch. Otolaryng.* 80:12, 1964.

Rush, B. F. J., Chambers, R. G., and Pavitch,

M. M.: Cancer of the head and neck in children. *Surgery,* 53:270, 1963.
Shafer, W. G., Hine, M. K., and Levy, B. M.: *A Textbook of Oral Pathology,* 2nd Ed. Philadelphia, W. B. Saunders Company, 1963.
Sharp, G. S., and Helsper, J. T.: Radiolucent spaces in the jaws. *Amer. J. Surg.,* 118:712, 1969.
Smith, J. F.: Fibrous dysplasia of the jaws. *Arch. Otolaryng.,* 81:592, 1965.
Stowens, D.: *Pediatric Pathology,* 2nd Ed. Baltimore, Williams and Wilkins Company, 1966.
Sutow, W. W., et al.: Prognosis in childhood rhabdomyosarcoma. *Cancer,* 25:1384, 1970.
Waldron, C. A.: Fibro-osseous lesions of the jaws. *J. Oral Surg.,* 28:58, 1970.
Waldron, C. A., and Shafer, W. G.: The central giant-cell reparative granuloma of the jaws. *Amer. J. Clin. Path.,* 45:437, 1966.
Walker, D. G.: Benign nonodontogenic tumors of the jaws. *J. Oral Surg.,* 28:39, 1970.
Ziegler, J. S., et al.: Treatment of Burkitt's tumor with cyclophosphamide. *Cancer,* 26:474, 1970.

Chapter Ninety

INFLAMMATORY CONDITIONS

LEROY SMITH, M.D., and J. LATANE WARE, M.D.

The majority of lesions of the mouth in childhood are inflammatory in origin. The lesions may involve one or more anatomic areas in the mouth and may be a manifestation of disturbances in growth and development, local infection, local physical or chemical irritation, allergic phenomena, systemic infection, metabolic disturbances or deficiencies, or processes of unknown etiology.

The congenital deformities of the oral and related facial structures are discussed in Chapter 89. For discussions of disturbances of development of the teeth and dental infections, the reader should refer to a text on dental medicine.

DISTURBANCES OF GROWTH AND DEVELOPMENT

In the newborn infant it is common to see "sucking pads" on the buccal mucosa and "sucking calluses" on the central portion of the lips. These lesions are usually present for only a few weeks. The alveolar ridges of the newborn are often capped by a thin, serrated, fringelike membrane. Small, firm, white epithelial pearls (Bohn's nodules) may be present on the gum margins but usually disappear spontaneously after a few months. Similar small nodules that disappear spontaneously may be present near the junction of the hard and soft palate (Epstein's pearls). Supernumerary or deciduous teeth, which are usually loosely attached and shed within a few days, may be present at birth (natal teeth) or may develop prior to the thirtieth day (neonatal teeth).

Several developmental lesions presenting as oral tumors were discussed in Chapter 89.

Ankyloglossia

The most common deformity of the tongue is ankyloglossia, or tongue-tie. In this condition there is a shortening of the lingual frenulum so that the tip of the tongue is tied to the floor of the mouth or to the posterior surface of the lower anterior alveolar arch. Movement of the tip of the tongue may be so restricted by the tongue-tie that speech is or will be impaired. In such instances surgical release

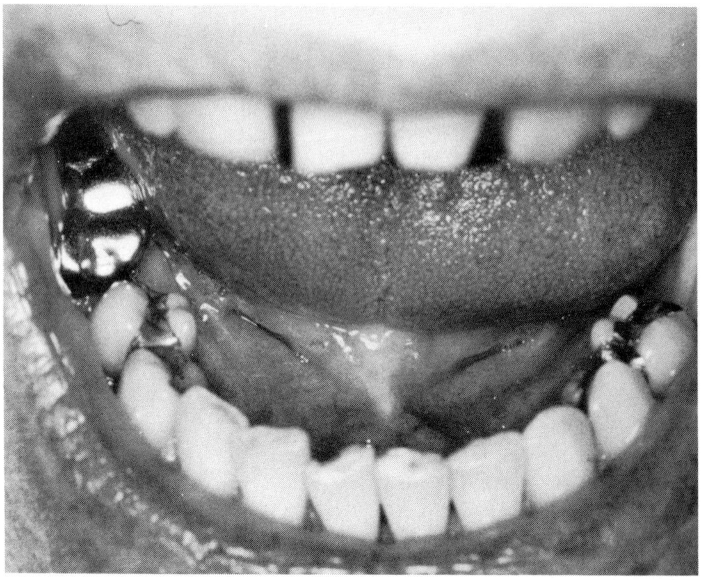

Figure 1. Ankyloglossia. (Courtesy of Dr. Richard P. Elzay, Medical College of Virginia School of Dentistry.)

of the tie will be necessary. Milder forms will usually not require treatment. Occasionally, complete ankyloglossia is present and will require extensive surgical release (Fig. 1).

Hypertrophied Maxillary Frenulum

This is an abnormal widening of the mucosa in the central portion of the upper lip where the maxillary labial frenulum normally occurs. The excessive width is frequently associated with a shortening of the frenulum. At its gingival termination there is a hypertrophied band of fibrous tissue that extends across the gingival arch; if the hypertrophy is extensive, there may be a resultant separation between the upper central incisor teeth when they erupt. The amount of separation depends upon the width of the arch and the size of the teeth. If nothing is done to correct such a marked hypertrophy of thick, fibrous tissue, the permanent teeth may be abnormally separated. If surgery is indicated, the operation should be performed before the time of eruption of the permanent teeth. Some pedodontists disagree with this approach, preferring to delay operation until the central incisors have erupted and the degree of separation can be visualized.

Epidermolysis Bullosa

This is an uncommon inherited dermatologic disorder characterized by the formation of bullae on the skin or mucous membrane. It may manifest itself at birth or during the early years of life. The oral lesions are most common in the dystrophic form. The bullae on the mucous membrane may follow minor trauma such as nursing and may be painful after rupture. No treatment is available.

LOCAL INFECTIONS

Noma (Gangrenous Stomatitis)

Noma is a relatively rare disease which occurs in debilitated children. It may be caused by fusospirochetal organisms, but other bacteria, such as streptococcus and staphylococcus, may be secondary invaders. The onset is sudden, and the lesion most often begins on the gingival border, but it may occur on the buccal mucosa or mucocutaneous

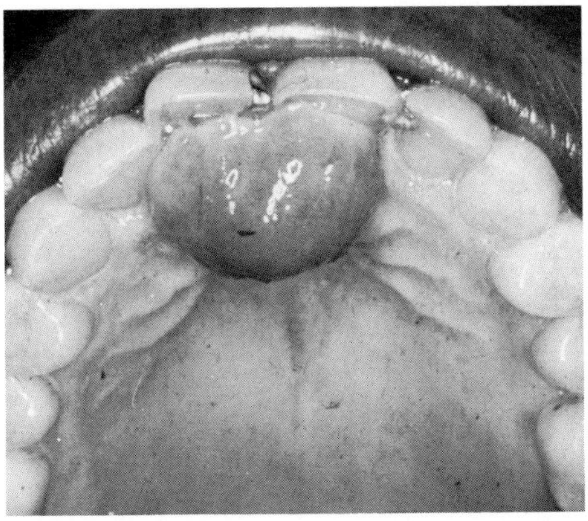

Figure 2. Pyogenic granuloma of the maxillary arch.

border. In the beginning there is a small ulcer. The tissues then become edematous, hard and grayish blue with a line of demarcation between the gangrenous process and the normal tissue. The gangrenous process continues to spread until the cheeks are perforated. It attacks both soft tissue and bone. Specific antibacterial therapy should be intensive and prolonged until all necrotic tissue has sloughed. Supportive therapy is a necessity, and plastic surgery will usually be indicated when there has been complete healing of the process.

Pyogenic Granuloma

The exact cause of this disease is not known; it has been suggested, however, that it may be traumatic irritation of the mucous membrane whereby bacteria, such as staphylococcus or streptococcus, may reach the deeper layers of the mucosa and then cause an overproduction of highly vascularized fibrous tissue. Any age group may be involved. The gingiva is the most common site, but the lesion may occur on the lips, tongue or buccal mucosa. Clinically, there is a smooth, slightly elevated, pedunculated or flat mass on the surface of the mucosa. As development ensues, the superficial layers desquamate, leaving a rather shallow, irregular, dirty gray membranous ulcer. Depending upon the degree of vascularity, irritation may or may not produce easy bleeding. The intact mucous membrane around the lesion becomes red or reddish purple. The granulomas develop rapidly for a short period and persist for long periods of time. They are rarely painful. The histologic picture is that of granulation tissue that is well localized and exuberant. Treatment consists in surgical excision and improvement of the oral hygiene (Figs. 2 and 3).

Herpes Simplex

It has been estimated that herpes virus hominis is present in approximately 90 per cent of the adult population. The virus is usually latent, but infection may become manifest in two forms: primary herpes simplex and recurrent or second-

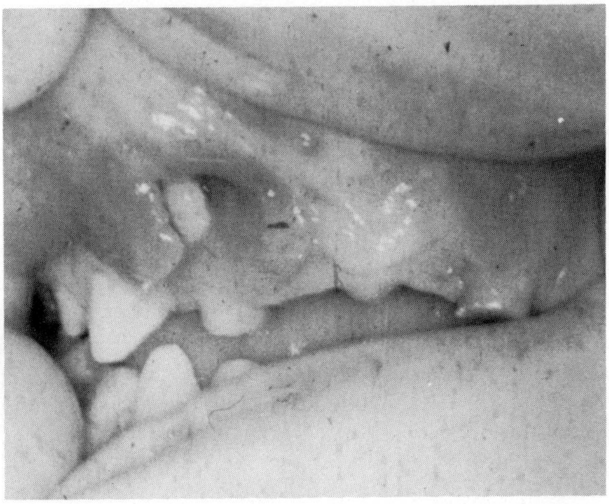

Figure 3. Ulcerating pyogenic granuloma.

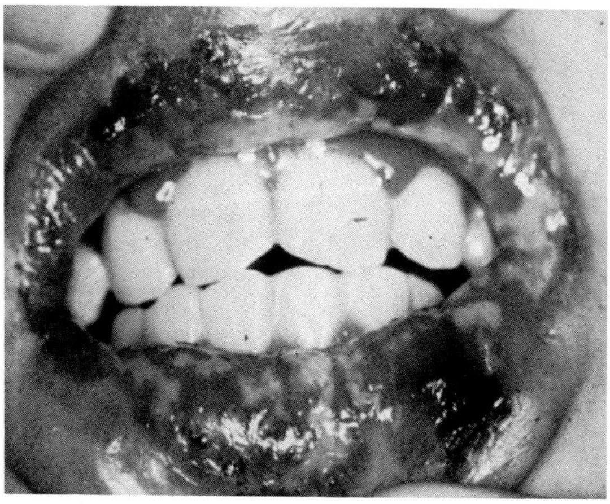

Figure 4. Herpes simplex. (Courtesy of Dr. Charles Vincent, Medical College of Virginia School of Dentistry.)

ary herpes simplex. In the former the first exposure of a susceptible host results in a subclinical infection without symptoms or in a general systemic reaction. Systemic infection usually occurs in a newborn infant or in a severely malnourished one. An infant with generalized disease may show fever or hypothermia, dyspnea, vomiting, jaundice, lethargy or convulsions. There may be hepatosplenomegaly, purpura and circulatory collapse. This severe form of the disease is usually fatal. Survivors may have chorioretinitis and mental retardation.

The more common course for primary herpetic stomatitis is less fulminating. In children (usually 1 to 6 years of age) there is fever, headache, cervical adenopathy and pain on swallowing. This is followed in several days by the development of inflammation and pain in the gingiva and other mucosal surfaces. Vesicles then appear but soon rupture to form shallow, painful ulcers covered by a gray membrane. Systemic symptoms subside in a few days and the oral lesions heal in one to two weeks (Fig. 4).

In the secondary (recurrent) form, the lesions are localized, and little or no systemic reaction occurs. These lesions are considered to be the result of the activation of latent virus by such stimuli as gastrointestinal disturbances, emotional upsets, febrile reactions, foods, changes in environment or menstruation. They occur only in persons who have already had a primary infection.

The vesicular lesions, which occur more often about the lips, may appear gradually over a period of several days. The vesicles rupture and shallow ulcers are left. In time, crusts cover the ulcerated areas and healing takes place. The course of the disease is usually seven to fourteen days.

When the vesicles appear on the buccal mucous membrane, they may simulate recurrent aphthous ulcers. Treatment is symptomatic.

Aphthous Stomatitis

Recurrent aphthous ulcer is a disease of unknown etiology that resembles herpes simplex in many respects but is probably not due to the herpes simplex virus. It appears that the tissue to be involved may be made susceptible by local trauma. In addition, psychologic stress, endocrine mechanisms, and hypersensitivity phenomena may be aggravating factors. Any of the oral mucosal surfaces may be affected by the painful, oral ulcerations that are usually less than one centimeter in diameter and covered by a grayish fibrinous exudate. Systemic manifestations are unusual, but they may be present. The ulcers heal in one to two

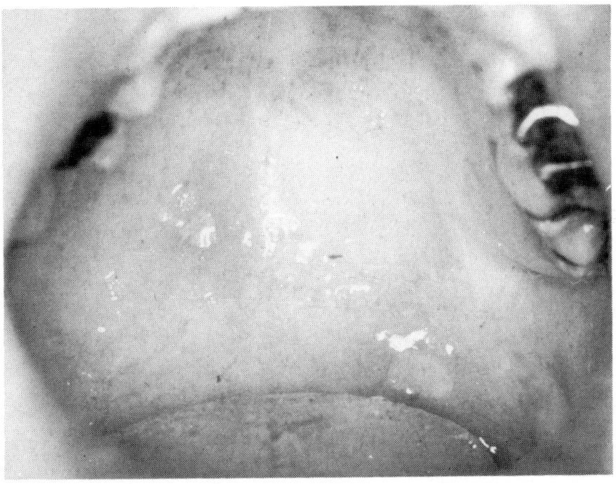

Figure 5. Recurrent aphthous ulcer.

weeks but recurrences are common. No specific treatment is available (Fig. 5).

Vincent's Infection (Trench Mouth, Acute Necrotizing Gingivitis)

This fusospirochetal disease primarily involves the free gingival margin, the gingival crest and the interdental papillae. Fusiform bacilli and an oral spirochete (*Borrelia vincenti*) coexist in a symbiotic relationship and are the causative organisms. Predisposing factors such as a decreased resistance to infection are important in the pathogenesis of this infection. Present opinion is that this is not a contagious disease. The disease is rare before 15 years of age and may be confused with primary herpetic gingivostomatitis. Severe pain and tenderness result from hyperemic, ulcerated friable gingiva. A fetid odor is present. Treatment consists of antibiotics, local oxygenating agents and local dental care.

Actinomycosis

The most common form of this fungus infection is cervicofacial actinomycosis. Five species of *Actinomyces* have been identified, but *Actinomyces israeli* is the cause of most human infection. This gram-positive organism, which has delicate mycelia, may be found in the oral cavity in the absence of clinical infection. Often there is a history of orofacial trauma or dental manipulation. The patient may present with a firm mass near the mandible associated with an abscess or draining sinus. Diagnosis is usually made by culture or biopsy, but one may find the diagnostic sulfur granules on smear. The organism is sensitive to penicillin.

Moniliasis

Moniliasis (thrush) is caused by the fungus *Candida* (*Monilia*) *albicans*. This fungus is a saprophyte in the normal oral cavity except in the newborn infant. The organism becomes pathogenic whenever there is sufficient impairment of tissue resistance; thus the disease is seen more often in weak, undernourished infants and children. Maternal vaginal moniliasis seems to be the main cause of infantile moniliasis, but cross-infection may result from poor nursery technique. Suppression of the normal flora of the oral cavity by long-term antibacterial therapy, especially with broad-spectrum antibiotics, may promote any fungal growth. Thrush develops on any membranous surface of the mouth and is characterized by soft, white, elevated plaques. These patches vary in size and frequently join to form large areas of involved membrane. A raw surface remains when the plaques are forcibly removed. The lesions are painless. Systemic symptoms are prominent only if

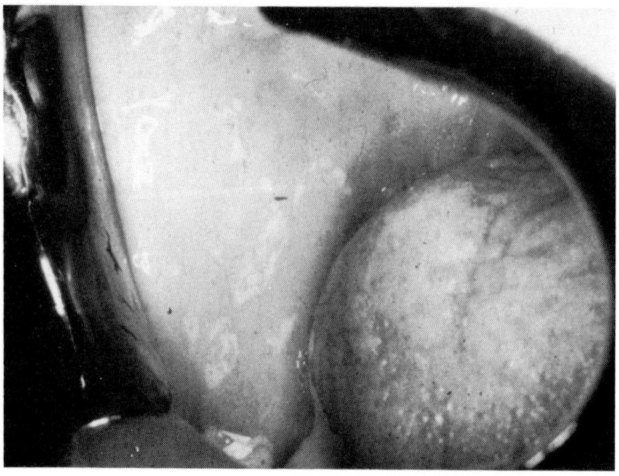

Figure 6. Moniliasis of the cheek. (Courtesy of Dr. Charles Vincent, Medical College of Virginia School of Dentistry.)

the infection spreads beyond the oral cavity. Pneumonitis and esophagogastritis may occur, but extensive spread of the infection usually occurs only in infants with an underlying debilitating condition (Fig. 6).

There is no completely effective therapeutic agent. Mycostatin given in a dosage of 200,000 units per milliliter and applied locally with a soft cotton swab three or four times daily (with the remaining portion swallowed by the infant), the local application of 1 per cent aqueous gentian violet, or the local application of 1:1000 aqueous solution of benzalkonium chloride (Zephiran) is usually effective. There may be recurrence with each of these therapeutic approaches.

Perleche

This is a lesion of varied etiology that may occur at any age and is manifested by a feeling of dryness and burning at the corners of the mouth. Local infection, local irritation and riboflavin deficiency may be etiologic factors. The lesions appear as fissures with a superficial crust lying in the corners of the mouth. Spontaneous remissions occur. Treatment depends on pinpointing the etiology.

Ludwig's Angina

Ludwig's angina is a severe cellulitis involving the submaxillary, sublingual and submental spaces. It is usually secondary to an infection of a mandibular molar but may result from a penetrating wound, mandibular osteomyelitis or other causes. Streptococci are found in most cases, either alone or with a mixture of organisms. Clinically, there is the rapid development of edema of the floor of the mouth, producing elevation of the tongue. This leads to difficulty in eating and swallowing and eventually makes breathing difficult. Edema of the glottis may result from progressive infection. Most cases respond favorably to large doses of antibiotics, especially penicillin, and rarely progress to the high mortality stage of disease seen in the pre-antibiotic drugs. The need for a tracheotomy must be considered and is still required in a few cases. Incision and drainage should be carried out when evidence of pus is present. This will usually be found between the mylohyoid and geniohyoid muscles or the geniohyoid and genioglossus muscles.

LOCAL PHYSICAL OR CHEMICAL IRRITATION

Dilantin Gingival Hyperplasia

Fibrous hyperplasia of the gingiva is seen as a side effect of anticonvulsant therapy with Dilantin. When good oral hygiene is maintained, this occurs in less

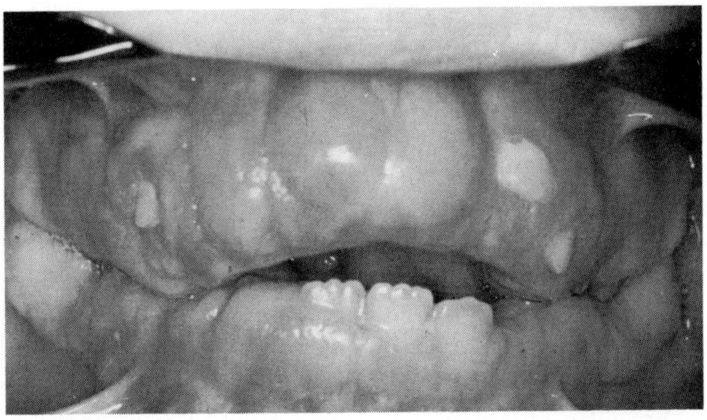

Figure 7. Dilantin gingival hyperplasia. (Courtesy of Dr. Charles Vincent, Medical College of Virginia School of Dentistry.)

than 10 per cent of cases. Usually the hyperplasia begins in the interdental papillae area as a painless enlargement of the gingiva some two or three months after treatment with the drug commences. The process continues and the gingival tissue becomes lobulated. Histologically, there are large bundles of collagen with fibroblasts and fibrocytes covered by a thick layer of stratified squamous epithelium with long, thin rete pegs. Therapy is directed toward improving dental hygiene if this is poor. When the lesion becomes esthetically or functionally objectionable, surgical excision is indicated. Recurrence is to be expected (Fig. 7).

Popsicle Panniculitis

This recently described benign condition is found in infants and presents as a deeply situated, movable, firm nodule in the cheek adjacent to the mouth. It apparently results from solidification of subcutaneous fat by ice (Popsicle). Induration diminishes over the period of a week and may be followed by transient light-brown hyperpigmentation of the overlying skin.

ALLERGIC PHENOMENA

Angioneurotic Edema

This disease may be either hereditary or nonhereditary. Psychologic factors and allergy to food may be precipitating causes. The edema is usually of rapid onset. It may be preceded by a feeling of itching and tenseness of the tissues; may involve any area, especially the lips, chin, eyelids and tongue; and usually lasts less than 36 hours. Treatment is directed toward eliminating any determined etiologic agent. Antihistamines are helpful in reducing the severity and duration of episodes.

Stomatitis Medicamentosa

This is the oral manifestation of a drug allergy and is less frequent than the cutaneous reaction. Although certain drugs may invoke reactions in a relatively high percentage of cases, practically every known drug is capable of producing an allergic phenomenon in sensitive patients. In the mouth there is usually diffuse erythema, vesicles, or ulceration. The gingiva, palate, lips and tongue are the most common oral sites. Antihistamines and cortisone derivatives may be used to treat the acute phase. The causative agent should be identified and eliminated.

SYSTEMIC INFECTIONS

In this section, only oral manifestations of the disease processes will be discussed. The reader should refer to a standard pediatric text for discussion of the systemic disease and treatment.

Scarlet Fever

This systemic disease is due to infection with beta hemolytic streptococcal organisms that elaborate an erythrogenic toxin. After an incubation of three to five days, the patient presents with pharyngitis, tonsillitis, headache, fever, chills and vomiting. Cervical adenopathy is present. The palatal mucosa is very red. The tongue initially appears to have a white coating, with the edematous, hyperemic fungiform papillae projecting above the surface (strawberry tongue). Later the coating is lost and the entire tongue is swollen and red (raspberry tongue). The red skin rash appears on about the third day and the duration of the illness is seven to ten days. Penicillin is the antibiotic of choice.

Diphtheria

Diphtheria is a rare disease today, but it must always be considered in any acute throat infection. See Chapter 98 for a discussion of diphtheria.

Syphilis

Acquired syphilis in children has become relatively rare since the advent of penicillin, but there are still cases that may demonstrate any one of the three intraoral manifestations. The primary stage is represented by a chancre that may occur on any part of the surface of the mucous membrane, but is more frequently present on the lip or tongue. This is a shallow, well-circumscribed, painless ulcer, often with a bright red base. If no treatment is instituted, the chancre usually disappears in two to three weeks.

The secondary or metastatic stage of the disease is represented by the so-called mucus patch. Whereas no part of the mucous membrane surface is exempt from these lesions, most of them are found on the lips or buccal mucosa. The lesion appears as a simple erosion of the mucous membrane surface covered by a silver-gray membrane and surrounded by a small area of inflammatory reaction. It is not painful. When the membrane is removed, the presence of the *Treponema pallidum* in the lesion can be demonstrated by dark-field examination. Other lesions of the secondary stage are condylomata (Fig. 8), which occur in the sulcus of both jaws and lips. These vary in size and are frequently detached by trauma, with resultant mild bleeding at the point of attachment to the mucous membrane. Fissures occur at the angles of the mouth, and there may or may not be maceration of the skin and mucous membrane. All lesions of this phase disappear spontaneously.

In late stages of syphilis, gummas may occur. These are found more frequently in the tongue and the tonsils. They are often confused with other tumors be-

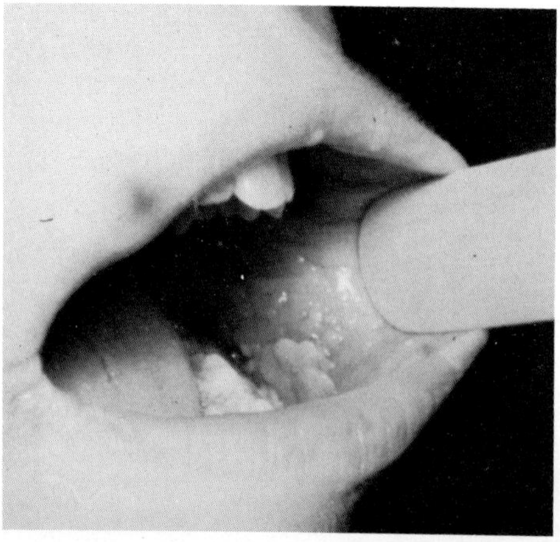

Figure 8. Condylomata of the left cheek.

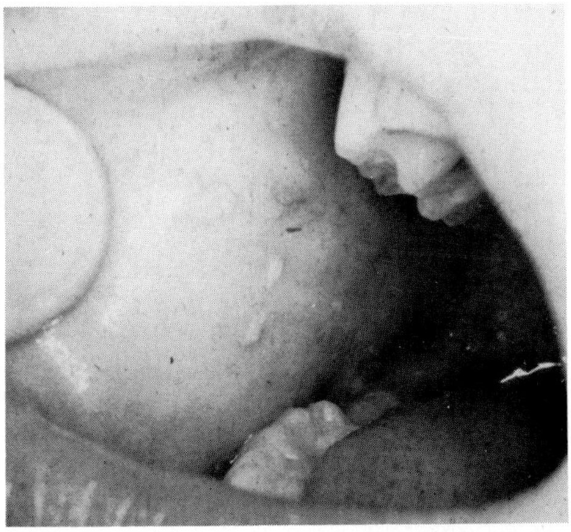

Figure 9. Koplik's spots. (Courtesy of Dr. Charles Vincent, Medical College of Virginia School of Dentistry.)

cause they are submembranous and adhere to the underlying tissue. On palpation there is little tenderness, and they increase in size fairly rapidly. Ulceration of the gumma may occur, giving rise to a necrotic ulcer that causes pain when the secondary infection occurs. A positive diagnosis of any one of the three stages is best made from serologic examinations and, when possible, from dark-field studies.

Measles (Rubeola)

In the prodromal phase of the disease there is a generalized swelling of the soft palate with a red mottling over the hard and soft palates. So-called Koplik's spots precede the appearance of that rash by one or two days. These Koplik's spots, the pathognomonic sign of measles, are bluish white or grayish white dots surrounded by an area of hyperemia. They are not elevated. The lesions tend to occur on the buccal mucous membrane opposite the lower molars, but they may occur anywhere on the buccal mucosa. They disappear rapidly (Fig. 9).

Chickenpox (Varicella)

The mucosa of the oral cavity is frequently involved in chickenpox. The pharyngeal wall is usually involved first, and later there may be involvement of much of the mucous membrane of the oral cavity. The lesion may first appear as small clear vesicles approximately 1 mm. in size. These rupture, and the resulting ulcerations are covered with a yellowish membrane. The mucous membrane between the lesions is intensely red, and the whole area becomes extremely painful. As the lesions spread over the entire oral cavity, the child usually refuses to eat or drink. These lesions gradually subside in seven to ten days. No local treatment is indicated.

METABOLIC DISTURBANCES OR DEFICIENCIES

In this section only the oral manifestations of the diseases discussed will be described.

Nonlipid Reticuloendothelioses

This group of diseases (eosinophilic granuloma, Letterer-Siwe disease, and Hand-Schuller-Christian disease) is of unknown etiology but appears to represent a disturbance of the reticuloendothelial system. The group is characterized by an inflammatory histiocytic proliferation. Eosinophilic granuloma occurs primarily in older children and young adults. It is found more commonly in males than in females, and it presents with local pain, swelling and tenderness in the jaw or soft tissues. Irregular radiolucent areas are seen on x-ray as a result of bone destruction. Curettage or radiation therapy is usually curative.

Letterer-Siwe disease is usually seen in infants and may present as a local or systemic disease. Nodular lesions occur in the jaws, with diffuse bone destruction. The prognosis is poor in this fulminating disease. No satisfactory therapy is available.

Hand-Schuller-Christian disease will occur most commonly in males prior to 10 years of age. Involvement of the viscera and skeletal system is seen. Facial asymmetry due to facial bone involvement is seen in association with exophthalmos and pituitary dysfunction. The radiograph reveals sharply outlined lesions with a sclerotic border. The prognosis is variable. Treatment is with curettage, irradiation, and corticosteroids.

Avitaminoses

The oral manifestations of vitamin A deficiency are primarily hyperplasia and keratinization of the gums. If this deficiency occurs to a serious degree before the sixth year, disturbance of tooth formation may occur.

The oral manifestations of vitamin B deficiency are usually those of the entire vitamin B complex. There is usually dryness, increased pain, and then burning of the lips. Fissures appear at the angles of the mouth, and the lining within the oral cavity becomes increasingly red and thickened. The tongue is somewhat swollen. Generally, the papillae are swollen and mushroom-shaped, but as the deficiency increases, the papillae take on an atrophic appearance. Swallowing becomes increasingly painful. Superficial ulcerations along the margins of the tongue may occur. They vary in size and have irregular borders. The gums bleed easily, and secondary gingivitis is a common finding.

Vitamin C deficiency is characterized by hypertrophy of the gums, which are soft and spongy and bluish red. These changes are most noticeable when the teeth have erupted. Slight pressure or irritation of the gums may cause bleeding. The teeth become loosened, and if the deficiency persists, actual loss of several or all of the teeth may occur.

Vitamin D deficiency may produce enamel hypoplasia in the infant. Retardation of the eruption of deciduous and permanent teeth is a manifestation of rickets.

There are no known oral manifestations of vitamin E deficiency. Vitamin K deficiency has no specific oral manifestation except possible increased bleeding following trauma, due to prothrombin deficiency.

LESIONS OF UNKNOWN ETIOLOGY

Cheilitis

Cheilitis glandularis is a lesion of the lower lip that presents as numerous small nodules caused by inflammatory obstruction of the small glands of the lip. This obstruction leads to dilatation and cystic formation in the glands.

Cheilitis granulomatosis is a chronic inflammatory condition of unknown etiology that may present in children or adults. There is painless, diffuse swelling of the lips, which are soft and frequently of normal color. Fissuring and vesicles are seen at the vermilion border in some cases. Histologically, there is similarity to sarcoidosis, with a chronic inflammatory cell infiltrate and focal granuloma formation with Langhans-type giant cells and epithelioid cells. No satisfactory treatment is known.

The triad of cheilitis granulomatosis, scrotal tongue, and facial paralysis is referred to as Melkerson-Rosenthal syndrome.

Fissured Tongue (Scrotal Tongue)

This malformation is manifested by numerous furrows on the dorsum of the tongue. The etiology of this condition is uncertain and it probably is not a developmental lesion. Clinically, there are usually no symptoms and no treatment is needed or available (Fig. 10).

Cleft of the Tongue

Median cleft of the tongue is a rare developmental anomaly in which there has been a fracture in union of the two halves of the tongue, resulting in a shallow or sometimes rather deep cleft in the midportion of the tongue. The cleft may

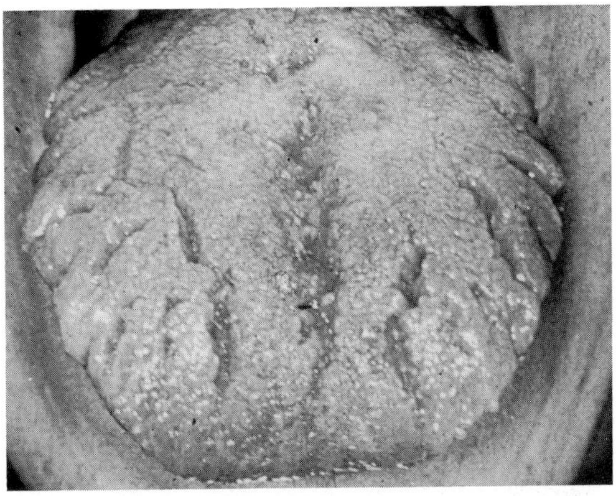

Figure 10. Fissures of the tongue (scrotal tongue).

be complete, but this is rare. The tip is usually not involved. Symptoms are few, but in some instances food may become lodged in the deep fissure, causing local irritation. In such an event, surgical removal of the fissure is advisable (Fig. 11).

Geographic Tongue

This lesion of unknown etiology is referred to by some authors as benign migratory glossitis. Though more common in adults, it is seen in young children. Clinically, there are areas of desquamation of the filiform papillae of the tongue in irregularly shaped patches. The central portion of the lesion is inflamed and the periphery lined by a thin white or yellow band. The patches of desquamation remain in one area for a variable period, heal, and then appear in another location. The total duration may be quite variable, lasting a few weeks or months, disappearing, and later reappearing. No definite treatment is available, and since the condition is benign, none is needed (Fig. 12).

Hairy Tongue

This unusual condition is of unknown etiology but may be a manifestation of hypersensitivity. In children it is most often seen in association with antibiotic therapy. In adults it is often seen in those who have received extensive head and neck irradiation and in heavy smokers. Thus, hairy tongue may be due to a change in the normal oral environment because of an alteration of the normal oral flora or a change in the composition and volume of saliva. There is a reactive hyperplasia of the filiform papillae and a

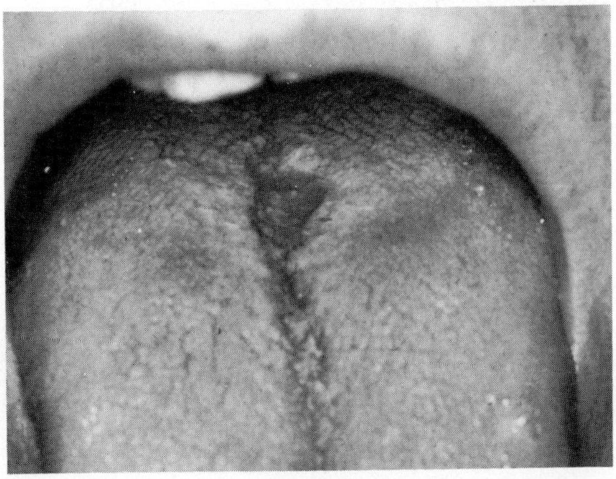

Figure 11. Median cleft of the tongue. (Courtesy of Dr. Richard P. Elzay, Medical College of Virginia School of Dentistry.)

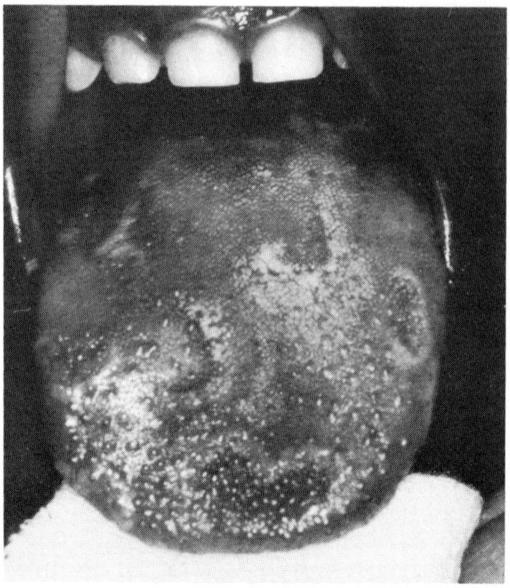

Figure 12. Geographic tongue. (Courtesy of Dr. Richard P. Elzay, Medical College of Virginia School of Dentistry.)

lack of normal desquamation. A thick, yellowish brown, matted layer of elongated papillae thus forms on the dorsum of the tongue. There is no specific treatment for this benign condition. Brushing the tongue with a toothbrush promotes desquamation.

Stevens-Johnson Syndrome

This disease complex of unknown etiology is related to erythema multiforme and is characterized by a cutaneous eruption, stomatitis, conjunctivitis and genital lesions. Mucosal vesicles form and then rupture, leaving ulcerations covered by a thick yellow exudate. Severe pain is a prominent symptom. No specific treatment is available for this self-limited disease. Antibiotics are indicated for secondary infections. Corticosteroids may reduce the acute inflammation and anesthetic lozenges may reduce discomfort.

REFERENCES

Barnett, H. L., and Einhorn, A. H.: *Pediatrics,* 14th Ed. New York, Appleton-Century-Crofts, 1968.

Bernick, S.: Growths of the gingiva and palate. I. Chronic inflammatory lesions. II. Connective tissue tumors. III. Epithelial growths. *Oral Surg.,* 1:1029, 1098, 1948; 2:217, 1949.

Brucker, M.: Studies on the incidence and cause of dental defects in children. III. Gingivitis. *J. Dent. Res.,* 22:309, 1943.

Brunner, H.: Eosinophilic granuloma of mouth, pharynx, and nasal passages. *Oral Surg.,* 4:623, 1951.

Burnett, G. W., and Scherp, H. W.: *Oral Microbiology and Infectious Disease,* 2nd Ed. Baltimore, Williams and Wilkins Company, 1962.

Cadham, F. T.: Vincent's disease: Infection due to fuso-spirillary invasion. *Canad. Med. Assoc. J.* 17:556, 1927.

Cahn, L. R., and Bartels, H. A.: Aphthae and herpetic gingivostomatitis. *Amer. J. Orthodont. Oral Surg.,* 28:140, 1942.

Calcaterra, T. C., and Strahan, R. W.: Stevens-Johnson syndrome: Oropharyngeal manifestations. *Arch. Otolaryng.,* 93:37, 1971.

Epstein, E. H., and Oren, M. E.: Popsicle panniculitis. *New Eng. J. Med.,* 282:966, 1970.

Glickman, I.: Acute vitamin C deficiency and periodontal disease. *J. Dent. Res.,* 27:201, 1948.

Gorlin, R. J., and Goldman, H. M.: *Oral Pathology,* Vols. 1 and 2. St. Louis, C. V. Mosby, 1970.

Hollander, L., and Goldman, B. A.: Syphilis of the oral mucosa. *Dent. Digest,* 40:135, 1934.

Kerr, D. A.: Stomatitis and gingivitis in the adolescent and preadolescent. *J. Amer. Dent. Assoc.,* 44:27, 1952.

Lichtenstein, L., and Jeffe, H. L.: Eosinophilic granuloma of bone. *Amer. J. Path.,* 16:595, 1940.

Shafer, W. G., Hine, M. K., and Levy, B. M.: *A Textbook of Oral Pathology,* 2nd Ed. Philadelphia, W. B. Saunders Company, 1963.

Ship, I. I., Ashe, W. K., and Scherp, H. W.: Recurrent "fever blister" and "canker sore." Test of herpes simplex and other viruses with mammalian cell cultures. *Arch. Oral Biol.,* 3:117, 1961.

Ship, I. I., Merritt, A. D., and Stanley, H. R.: Recurrent aphthous ulcers. *Amer. J. Med.,* 32:32, 1962.

Stammers, A. F.: Vincent's infections: Observations and conclusions regarding the aetiology and treatment of 1,017 civilian cases. *Brit. Dent. J.,* 76:147, 1947.

Stowens, D.: *Pediatric Pathology,* 2nd Ed. Baltimore, Williams and Wilkins, 1966.

Vaughan, V. C., and McKay, J.: *Textbook of Pediatrics,* 9th Ed. Philadelphia, W. B. Saunders, 1969.

Wollbach, S. B.: Pathologic changes resulting from vitamin deficiency. *J.A.M.A.,* 108:7, 1937.

Wollbach, S. B., and Bessey, O. A.: Tissue changes in vitamin deficiencies. *Physiol. Rev.,* 22:233, 1942.

Chapter Ninety-One

DISEASE OF THE SALIVARY GLANDS

FRANK D. LATHROP, M.D.

Disease of the salivary glands is not uncommon. Making the correct diagnosis and instituting the proper treatment often can be accomplished without difficulty. A careful history and clinical examination are all that are required to make a diagnosis in most instances. In others, the history and clinical examination may be suggestive but additional information about the nature of the pathologic process involving the glands must be obtained through the probing of the ducts, suitable roentgenograms, including sialography when indicated, and occasionally a representative biopsy. Assessment of the additional information obtained from such studies usually permits an exact diagnosis to be established.

DEVELOPMENTAL DISTURBANCES

Congenital abnormalities of the salivary glands are rare. Any conceivable malformation may occur, ranging from complete absence of the glands to failure of one or more to develop to full maturity, which could cause fistula formation, obliteration of salivary ducts or formation of cysts. Congenital tumors, such as hemangioma or lymphangioma, may occasionally involve a salivary gland and may almost entirely replace the glandular tissue. Branchiogenic cysts may be mistaken for either a congenital or an acquired cyst of a salivary gland; their true nature may not be discovered until surgical intervention has been accomplished. Aberrant salivary gland tissue is often found in the mouth and lips, and also may be situated in the lacrimal apparatus, eyelids, eyebrows and skin of the face and neck. It may undergo malignant degeneration.

The diagnosis of most of the developmental defects of the salivary glands is often self-evident. In some instances, however, when the diagnosis cannot be determined from the history and clinical and roentgen examinations, the diagnosis must depend upon exploratory operation when the symptoms justify such a procedure.

Surgery is often the best treatment for these lesions (except when the gland is absent). Radiation therapy, in my experience, has proved ineffective in controlling tumorous congenital lesions, even when the diagnosis has been established by biopsy. Similarly, sclerosing or electrocoagulation therapy of fistulas has more often than not proved fruitless, and has made subsequent surgical excision more difficult. Excision of every nodule of obscure origin situated beneath the mucous membrane of the mouth or lips is necessary if malignant degeneration of aberrant salivary gland tissue is to be minimized.

SECRETORY DISTURBANCES

The function of the salivary glands is to produce saliva. It has been calculated that the normal production of saliva during a 24-hour period in the human is about 1500 ml., of which about 69 per cent is contributed by the submaxillary glands. However, the quantity of saliva produced and its viscosity vary considerably during any given period of time, and are controlled by the secretory fibers to the glands from the sympathetic and parasympathetic nervous systems. The normal amount of salivary secretion is so constantly present in the mouth that we are likely to fail to appreciate its contributions to our comfort, our health and the ingestion of food. However, if any alteration occurs in the production of saliva or in our ability to swallow it normally, we immediately become aware of it.

Excessive salivation, or sialorrhea, is manifested by drooling of saliva from the corners of the mouth and by frequent swallowing. The same manifestations occur when an individual does not regularly swallow saliva that is secreted in normal amounts, as in patients who have painful lesions of the mouth or throat, paralysis of the tongue or pharyngeal constrictor muscles and stenosis or obstruction of the esophagus. True sialorrhea is encountered less frequently than these conditions and probably occurs as a result of reflex stimulation of the salivary glands.

Sialorrhea is normal in infants during teething and has been reported in the literature as occurring in diabetes and diseases of the stomach or pancreas. It commonly is a symptom of irritation of the tongue from jagged teeth, poorly fitting dentures or inflammation. Patients with organic disease of the central nervous system, such as motion sickness, tic douloureux, paralysis agitans, familial autonomic dysfunction and encephalitis lethargica, and patients with mental illness, such as schizophrenia, may exhibit troublesome sialorrhea. It is encountered also in advanced nutritional deficiencies, such as scurvy and pellagra, and often follows severe emotional stress.

Xerostomia, the antithesis of sialorrhea, is the term applied when salivary secretion is absent or markedly diminished in quantity. As a result, the mucous membrane of the mouth and tongue is relatively dry; the saliva is sticky in consistency when touched with a throat stick. Little secretion can be expressed from the principal salivary ducts and the secretion may be more viscid than normal. A common complaint of patients with pronounced xerostomia is difficulty in masticating and swallowing food.

Xerostomia is usually a temporary condition. Dryness of the mouth is a familiar complaint of public speakers and is purely nervous in origin, since it is present only while an address is delivered. Drugs such as belladonna, the opium derivatives and the antihistaminics, when administered therapeutically for disease, may cause a temporary decrease in salivary secretion. The dryness of the mouth, which is a frequent complaint of patients who have severe emotional disturbances, is usually a subjective symptom, but in some instances there may be an actual decrease in the secretion of saliva. Local inflammation or neoplastic disease of a salivary gland may produce an actual decrease in salivation, but rarely to the point that the patient is aware of it. Severe systemic infections or other diseases that cause either unrecognized or inadequately treated dehydration, such as those of the liver or kidneys, diabetes mellitus, diabetes insipidus, typhoid fever, cholera and systemic viral disease, often are accompanied by a decrease in the production of saliva and dryness of the mouth.

Xerostomia is most often a transitory symptom that disppears as soon as its cause is eliminated; however, when it follows radiation therapy for malignancy in the nasopharynx, the paranasal sinuses or the salivary glands, it may be more or less permanent. The xerostomia commonly associated with Mikulicz's disease and Sjögren's syndrome is permanent, and in the latter condition it may be the predominant symptom.

The treatment of sialorrhea and of xerostomia is primarily that of the underlying disease. Astringent mouth washes and the judicious use of small doses of atropine may be helpful in minimizing sialorrhea. The management of xerostomia when it is the predominating symptom of Sjögren's syndrome or follows extensive radiation therapy for malignancy of the head and neck is difficult. Under such circumstances, treatment is limited to improvement in the oral hygiene, the use of soothing mouth washes (such as those containing glycerin), supplementary vitamins and feedings to improve the nutritional status, and augmenting the fluid intake.

Similar therapy is also beneficial in cases of less severe xerostomia, when the salivary glands are still able to secrete a moderate amount of saliva. In such instances, mechanical and medical measures that normally increase salivary flow may be helpful. Chewing gum or sucking on sour-tasting hard candies is frequently of benefit in such cases. In addition, nicotinic acid in sufficient dosage to produce mild flushing or a sensation of warmth and pilocarpine in therapeutic doses to stimulate the salivary glands may produce a sufficient increase in salivary flow to permit relief.

CALCULI AND STRICTURES

Salivary calculi are not rare. Their most frequent location is the submaxillary gland or its duct, probably because of the nature of the secretion of this gland and the dependent location of its duct with relation to the duct orifice. A calculus located in the principal duct of a salivary gland produces symptoms characteristic of obstruction of the duct. The onset is usually associated with the ingestion of food and is ushered in by pain, followed by progressive enlargement and tenderness of the involved gland. These symptoms usually subside completely following the initial attack. As further attacks occur, the pain becomes less intense, the tenderness is constant and more pronounced and the gland remains swollen to some degree.

Secondary infection in some degree almost invariably occurs with recurrent obstruction, and purulent material can be expressed from the duct. On occasion, a calculus may be extruded spontaneously from the duct. When this occurs, relief from the acute symptoms of obstruction is obtained, but it may be followed by persistent enlargement of the gland and tenderness when eating as a result of the development of an inflammatory stricture at the site originally occupied by the calculus, which interferes with the normal flow of saliva from the gland.

Calculi within the substance of a salivary gland are likely to be larger than ductal stones and frequently are multiple. Although they may produce symptoms similar to those of duct calculi, the symptoms are usually less severe. They are more likely to be associated with chronic infection of the gland and the most prominent symptoms are those of inflammation of the gland rather than those caused by obstruction to the flow of saliva from the gland. Purulent material may be observed as flakes in clear secretion expressible from the duct or as intermittent clumps of cloudy, thickened secretion alternating with what appears to be normal saliva. When the infection is more severe, frank pus can be expressed from the duct. If the infectious process is allowed to proceed without interference or progresses in spite of therapy, the development of local abscesses and cellulitis is inevitable. Large calculi located in the deep portion of the submaxillary gland may, on occasion, erode through the adjacent muscles and mucous membrane of the floor of the mouth.

Calculi located in a duct, particularly when situated near the duct orifice, are usually palpable through the buccal mucosa. When they are situated in the substance of the gland, however, they cannot be palpated unless they are large or are incorporated in the buccal surface of the submaxillary gland. In most instances, the history is characteristic, and when coupled with a stone that can be palpated with the fingertip or a probe in the duct, the diagnosis is certain. When a stone cannot be palpated, roentgen examination, including an intra-oral occlusal film of the suspected gland and duct, often will demonstrate the calculus. Not all calculi are of sufficient density to be radiopaque, however, and when routine roentgen examination fails to demonstrate a suspected calculus, sialography will be successful in establishing the presence of a nonopaque calculus or of a stricture.

Calculi in the duct of the submaxillary or parotid gland can usually be removed intra-orally without difficulty if they are situated completely within the duct. Minute calculi may be expressed from the duct following dilatation of the duct with lacrimal dilators. When the stones are larger and cannot be removed by simple dilatation, a linear incision of the duct, guided by the largest lacrimal dilator that can be passed, will permit extraction of the stones.

This latter procedure also serves to rectify partial obstruction of a salivary duct secondary to stricture formation. When larger stones are situated in the submaxillary duct just after it leaves the gland or are in the substance of the gland but are palpable just beneath the mucous membrane of the floor of the mouth, removal through an intra-oral approach is possible, but it is more difficult and there is the possibility of injury of the lingual nerve and the spread of infection. If intra-oral removal of the calculus is attempted, one most be careful not to push the calculus further into the substance of the gland while attempting its removal. Passing a traction suture through the mucous membrane and substance of the gland posterior to the stone helps prevent this. When the suture has been placed, incision of the mucous membrane and gland substance directly over the surface of the calculus will frequently permit removal of the stone with forceps. If this procedure is unsuccessful, excision of the submaxillary gland and its contained calculus is indicated. If multiple calculi are present in the substance of the gland or if calculi reappear in the duct following previous removal, excision of the submaxillary gland is the treatment of choice. Calculi situated in the substance of the parotid gland are usually located near the beginning of Stensen's duct and are best removed through an external approach dirctly over the suspected location of the stone.

In every instance in which an acute infectious process is associated with calculus formation, the acute process should be controlled by antibiotics or other measures before surgery is instituted.

INFLAMMATION

Mumps (acute epidemic sialadenitis) is the prototype of inflammatory disease of the salivary glands. It is a communicable disease, usually occurring in epidemics, and is characterized by swelling, pain and tenderness of the parotid gland with associated fever. Mumps is caused by the mumps virus. Although it may affect persons of all ages, it occurs most frequently in patients between the ages of 5 and 15 years. The course of the disease is usually uneventful, but complications may occur. Orchitis rarely develops before the age of puberty, but in adults, during the course of an epidemic, the incidence may be quite high. Oophoritis rarely occurs. It is probable that some degree of pancreatitis occurs in nearly every case, since mumps is a systemic viral disease affecting many organs other than the parotid gland. Meningo-encephalitis may occur and affects patients of all ages. Deafness is occasionally a complication of mumps and is usually irreversible.

During epidemics the diagnosis of mumps is simple. Mumps occasionally involves the submaxillary glands, but when these glands alone are involved it is only during an epidemic that a diagnosis can be established at the time. The blood differential count usually exhibits a lymphocytosis, and this, together with complement fixation and skin tests, may be of help in establishing the diagnosis in the absence of an epidemic or in differentiating mumps from an acute sialadenitis of bacterial origin.

Bacterial inflammation of the salivary glands may be acute or chronic. The parotid gland is most commonly involved unless the suppurative process is secondary to a calculus, in which case the submaxillary glands are more frequently implicated because of the predilection of these glands for calculus formation. In my experience, acute parotitis has almost invariably been the sequel of dehydration in patients subjected to major abdominal operations or severe debilitating illness, in whom a lowered resistance to infection probably has contributed to the establishment of the infection.

The route bacteria follow to infect the gland has been considered to be either hematogenous or directly through the duct. It is my opinion that the latter route is the one most often implicated. When a patient is inadequately hydrated, it is quite conceivable that the gland, devoid of its protective flow of secretion, may become infected by retrograde extension of mouth flora through the duct, particularly in individuals with poor dental hygiene and septic oral cavities.

Usually only one of the parotid glands is involved by the inflammatory process, although, on occasion, both may be affected. The onset is sudden and is usually first noted by the patient as a tender swelling at the angle of the mandible. The swelling progressively enlarges and becomes painful. Fever is present and the skin overlying the gland becomes tense, reddened and shiny. Inspection of the mouth reveals the quantity of saliva to be less than normal, with the result that the tongue blade used for the examination tends to stick to the mucosa. The papilla of the duct is reddened and pouting. On palpation, the swollen gland is hot and exquisitely painful. When pressure is exerted from the back of the gland toward its duct, pus is expressed from its orifice.

The treatment of acute suppuration of the parotid gland consists of correcting dehydration if it exists and instituting adequate antibiotic therapy. Initially, the antibiotic is given intravenously or intramuscularly. If the results of the culture and sensitivity tests of the purulent secretion expressed from the parotid duct indicate that another antibiotic preparation might prove more effective, it is then changed. Whether the antibiotic is changed or not, it may be administered orally after these reports are received, if that is feasible. In addition, hot compresses are applied to the swollen gland and the patient is instructed in "milking" the gland. He is urged to do this several times a day. If the suppurative process appears to respond slowly or inadequately to this therapy, resolution may be hastened by dilating the parotid duct and irrigating the gland with a solution of the antibiotic. Roentgen therapy, in my experience, has been of little or no benefit in treating such cases.

On one occasion, the therapy described proved to be ineffective, and surgical intervention was necessary to effect a cure. Although a surgical procedure is rarely necessary, it can be accomplished without danger to the facial nerve. If surgery is indicated, it should be carried out without delay.

The surface of the parotid gland is easily exposed by reflecting the skin and subcutaneous tissue forward from an incision in the pretragal crease, beginning at the temporomandibular joint and extending inferiorly to terminate 2 or 3 cm. anterior to and below the angle of the mandible. Once the lateral surface of the gland has been exposed, numerous incisions are made in the substance of the gland, paralleling the course of the branches of the facial nerve. These incisions in the substance of the gland are then deepened and enlarged with blunt forceps to facilitate drainage. The wound is allowed to remain open and secondary closure is effected when the suppurative process has subsided.

Acute sialadenitis of the submaxillary gland is almost always secondary to obstruction of the duct by a calculus. If the stone is accessible and can easily be removed, the suppuration usually subsides rapidly. If phlegmon of the adjacent tissues is associated with the suppurative process of the submaxillary gland, however, medical treatment similar to that described for acute parotitis should be instituted and the more acute phase of the inflammatory process allowed to subside before any attempt is made to remove the stone surgically.

Chronic suppuration of the parotid gland occurs relatively infrequently. When present, it is exceedingly troublesome to the patient, and is characterized by acute exacerbations of the suppurative process alternating with periods of relative quiescence. Its etiology is unknown, but failure of the initial acute inflammatory process of the gland to subside completely or the presence of an inflammatory stricture of the parotid duct or its orifice is probably contributory. If the patient is seen during a quiescent stage, the gland may be only slightly enlarged and indurated with purulent secretion mixed with clear saliva expressible from the duct. When the patient is suffering from an acute exacerbation, however, it cannot be differentiated from an original acute parotitis except by the history of similar recurrent attacks.

Sialography always demonstrates some abnormality of the duct or the gland. A stricture of the orifice of the parotid duct is usually discovered only while dilating the duct in preparation for the instillation of radiopaque material for sialography. When properly carried out, sialography of a patient with chronic parotitis may demonstrate that the principal duct is stenosed or elongated, tortuous and dilated. In others, the parotid duct may appear normal and the smaller ducts are dilated and irregular in outline, with puddling of the radiopaque dye in the acini.

Treatment of chronic parotitis is difficult and often unsatisfactory. Even when an abnormality of the parotid duct, such as a stricture, can be eliminated, the suppurative process is usually so well established in the gland substance that, although the symptoms are improved, a cure is not obtained. Prolonged antibiotic therapy based upon culture and sensitivity tests frequently causes temporary abatement of the inflammatory process and occasionally results in a cure. Frequent "milking" of the gland and occasional irrigations of the duct to remove accumulated purulent secretions and enhance the salivary flow appear to be helpful in reducing the frequency of acute exacerbations of the infection. Ligation of the duct of the involved gland during a period in which the inflammatory process is relatively quiet has been reported to be beneficial. When all else fails, and the patient demands permanent relief from his symptoms, even though mild paresis of the facial nerve may ensue, total parotidectomy will effect a cure.

Chronic suppuration of the submaxillary gland is invariably the result of recurrent calculus formation or of extensive irreversible damage to the gland substance from a previous calculus. The treatment of choice is excision of the submaxillary gland.

NEOPLASMS

Neoplastic disease of the salivary glands is not common. It occurs less frequently in children than in adults. The majority of the neoplasms are situated in the parotid gland and are benign. Clinical differentiation between benign and malignant tumors of the salivary glands usually is not possible preoperatively, although the benignity or malignancy of the lesion may be suspect. Malignant tumors are usually more firm and have a greater tendency to be fixed to the adjacent tissues than do those that are benign. Pain occurs more frequently as a symptom of malignant disease, but cannot be relied upon for differential diagnosis, as it may be present when the tumor is benign. Facial paralysis is usually a preoperative indication of malignant disease, for it indicates that the neoplasm has infiltrated the facial nerve. However, this is true only if paralysis from prior surgery or Bell's palsy can be excluded.

Although the incidence of salivary gland neoplastic disease is less in children than in adults, the same variety of neoplasms is encountered in children as in adults. There are some differences. Neoplastic disease appears to grow more rapidly in children than in adults, even though the histologic appearance of the tumor is similar in both age groups. Hemangioendothelioma, which occurs frequently in children, apparently does not develop in adults, and undifferentiated carcinoma, which occurs most frequently in infants, seldom occurs in adults and probably is of a less malignant nature in the adult than in the child.[1] The mixed tumor, frequently encountered in adults, seldom occurs in children.

The mixed tumor is the commonest neoplasm affecting the salivary glands of adults. Although this tumor generally is considered to be benign, it exhibits a great propensity for recurrence. For this reason, it is important that every vestige of the tumor be removed at the time of its initial excision. The surgical management of mixed tumors is applicable to all benign tumors of the salivary glands, whether in an adult or a child. The involved gland should be widely exposed and the tumor, together with a wide margin of grossly normal salivary gland tissue surrounding it, should be excised. This is best effected by the performance of a superficial lobectomy when the tumor involves the parotid gland. However, it is not possible to remove all the surrounding normal salivary gland tissue when part of the capsule of the tumor contacts the facial nerve or when the tumor is very large. Wide excision is less likely to be followed by recurrent disease than any other method (with the possible exception of total parotidectomy).

Hemangioendothelioma is the most common benign tumor affecting the salivary glands in children. It most often appears during the first year of life; it apparently does not develop in adults. Management is identical to that described for mixed tumors in the adult. No other form of therapy, in my experience, appears to be as efficacious in eradicating neoplastic disease of the salivary glands as surgical excision.

Primary neoplastic disease involves the submaxillary gland much less frequently than the parotid gland. When a benign tumor of the submaxillary gland is present, whether in an adult or a child, its adequate removal is facilitated by complete excision of the gland.

Malignant tumors of the salivary glands do not occur as frequently as benign tumors. Malignant tumors are more difficult to manage successfully and are primarily of epithelial origin, although on rare occasions sarcomas may be encountered in these locations. Biopsy of a salivary gland tumor in order to establish diagnosis prior to definitive surgery is generally contraindicated, for the first surgical procedure employed should be instituted with the intention of eradicating the neoplasm. However, if at operation the benignity or malignancy of the lesion is questioned, biopsy is indicated.

When the findings at operation confirm the preoperative impression of malignant disease, or the frozen section unequivocally establishes the neoplasm as malignant, a more radical surgical procedure must be employed than that for benign tumors in an effort to effect a cure. The extent of this more radical procedure is influenced to a considerable degree by evidence of local invasion or lymphogenous spread as manifested by preoperative nonsurgical facial paralysis and cervical lymph node involvement. In general, these indicate the necessity for total excision of the gland, including resection of the facial nerve when the parotid gland is involved by malignant disease, and a radical neck dissection in continuity if the best opportunity for eradication of the disease is to be offered the patient. When the facial nerve has been sacrificed, it should be reconstructed, either as a part of the original operation or about a week later, in order that the patient may obtain relief from the facial palsy.

Unfortunately, there are instances in which it is impossible to excise all of the malignant disease because of involvement of adjacent structures that cannot be resected. This is particularly true when malignant disease invades the styloid group of muscles and the base of the skull. In addition, there are rare instances in which an encapsulated tumor that is removed was thought to be benign but is subsequently reported by the pathologist to be a malignant neoplasm. Under such circumstances, radiation therapy is indicated. My experience with two million volt radiation therapy suggests that it may be a valuable adjunct to the management of such lesions when most of the tumor has been excised.

MISCELLANEOUS CONDITIONS

There are a number of miscellaneous conditions that occur infrequently. These affect the parotid gland most often but may involve the submaxillary or sublingual glands on occasion. Nonsuppurative enlargement of the glands has been attributed to allergic factors, toxic reaction from drugs and associated with diabetes mellitus, the menopause, starvation and gout in adults. In addition, asymptomatic enlargement of one or more of the salivary glands may occur as a result of functional or familial hyperplasia or fatty replacement. Treatment of these conditions is unnecessary if enlargement by tumor can be excluded through biopsy. Enlargement of the salivary glands and ducts is seen on occasion in glass blowers and musicians who play wind instruments. Such cases require no treatment and are of interest only in that they occur as a result of an occupation. Occasionally, a lymphoma, branchial cyst, neurofibroma of the facial nerve or neurinoma arising from the nerves in the sublingual region will produce enlargement of a salivary gland. Their differentiation from specific disease of the gland can be established only by surgical intervention.

Mikulicz's disease is a rare condition that is characterized by symmetrical, progressive, painless enlargement of the parotid and lacrimal glands. The lacrimal glands are usually first involved, and for this reason patients with this disease are usually first seen by the ophthalmologist. The parotid glands may be enlarged without involvement of the lacrimal glands, and when this occurs the patient consults a surgeon or otolaryngologist. A positive diagnosis can be established only by biopsy. Treatment is usually required for cosmetic reasons only, and satisfactory reduction in the size of the parotid swellings can be obtained by total parotidectomy or x-ray therapy, the latter being the treatment of choice. The etiology of this condition is unknown, but there is evidence to suggest that it is a less highly developed variant of a larger symptom complex, known as Sjögren's syndrome. This syndrome usually affects menopausal women. It is characterized by the presence of keratoconjunctivitis, enlargement or atrophy of the parotid glands, dryness of the mucous membranes of the nose, mouth and throat and rheumatoid arthritis. Treatment is unsuccessful in reversing the pathologic changes present. Steroid therapy appears to be beneficial early in the course of the disease; nicotinic acid and pilocarpine in therapeutic doses, with an increased fluid intake when some salivary function remains, appear to be of benefit in relieving the dryness of the mouth that is a major complaint in more advanced stages of the disease. Uveoparotitis, or Heerfordt's disease, is a comparatively rare disorder characterized by firm, painless enlargement of the parotid glands with inflammation of both uveal tracts and a persistent low-grade fever. These symptoms are frequently accompanied by facial paralysis and irregular constitutional symptoms. The etiologic agent is unknown, but the condition is generally believed to be a manifestation of sarcoidosis. Treatment is largely confined to symptomatic relief. Cortisone may prove beneficial in some instances. Usually spontaneous recovery may be anticipated in the majority of instances, although visual impairment may persist.

In children, enlargement of the salivary glands may occur as a result of sialectasis, lymphoma, neurogenic tumors or cytomegalic inclusion disease, which is a widespread viral disease that produces symptoms infrequently. It appears to be largely harmless except when it occurs in infancy. Initially it was thought to be a disease of the salivary and lacrimal glands but now it is recognized as a generalized condition that produces a clinical picture resembling erythroblastosis or hepatitis in neonates.[2]

Sialectasis also occurs infrequently in childhood. The etiology is unknown, but it is thought that it may be congenital in origin, or may represent the end stage of chronic recurrent suppurative parotitis, or may be a late complication of mumps. The most common symptom is that of recurrent diffuse swelling of one parotid gland. Gland enlargement may slowly increase over many months or years. In an advanced stage of the disease, purulent secretion can be expressed from Stensen's duct.

The diagnosis of sialectasis can be accomplished only by sialography. Sialograms characteristically show ductal enlargement and sacculation within the regions of the intralobar ducts and acini. In this respect, the sialographic picture is similar to that observed in the sialogram of a patient with early Sjögren's syndrome.

Treatment consists of oral hygiene, hydration and "milking" the gland in order to evacuate stagnant secretion and to minimize the possibility of secondary infection. In an advanced stage, total parotidectomy with preservation of the facial nerve may become necessary.

CONCLUSIONS

The major salivary glands exhibit disease fairly often. In the majority of instances there is a disturbance in its development or function, calculus formation, imflammation or neoplastic process. Occasionally, the disease may be the result of tumors arising from nerves, blood vessels or lymphatics contained in the gland, or in rare instances it is a manifestation of an obscure condition of unknown etiology, such as Mikulicz's disease. Sjögren's syndrome or uveoparotid fever.

In general, the symptomatology and management of disease of the salivary glands is identical in children and adults. Significant differences do exist, however, in the incidence and behavior of neoplastic disease in children as compared to that in adults. Neoplasms appear to grow more rapidly in children than in adults. The most common benign tumor encountered in adults, the mixed tumor, is seldom observed in children, and hemangioendothelioma, the most common benign tumor of the salivary glands in children, is rarely, if ever, observed in the adult. In addition, undifferentiated carcinoma, the most common malignant tumor of the salivary glands in childhood, is encountered less frequently in adults and appears to be less malignant in the adult than in the child.

REFERENCES

Kauffman, S. L., and Stout, A. P.: Tumors of the major salivary glands in children. *Cancer,* 16: 1317, 1963.

Anderson, W. A. D.: *Pathology,* Vol. 2, 5th Ed., St. Louis, C. V. Mosby Co., 1966, chap. 25.

SECTION XV

THE PHARYNX

Chapter Ninety-Two

EMBRYOLOGY, APPLIED ANATOMY AND PHYSIOLOGY

CHARLES F. FERGUSON, M.D., F.A.C.S.

EMBRYOLOGY

The pharynx, like all other areas of the body, is not infrequently the site of congenital malformations due to errors of embryologic development. Many of these anomalies will be discussed also in other chapters. At one stage early in fetal life the nasal cavity is completely separate from the nasopharynx, and persistence of this separation into postnatal life results in *congenital choanal atresia* (see Chapter 86). Early in embryonic life, a dorsal outpocketing of the primitive oral cavity (stomadeum) joins an evagination from the floor of the brain to form the pituitary gland (Rathke's pouch). The *craniopharyngeal canal* (see Chapter 99) may persist as a communicating tract, and from this area tumors or cysts may arise (Fig. 1). Likewise, the path of the primitive notochord opening just below the pharyngeal tonsil may leave a depression *(Thornwaldt's bursa)* that may later become a source of infection or the location of a cyst.

Malformation of the branchial arches with their intervening clefts and pouches may result in a *cervical cyst* or a *branchiogenic sinus tract* that still retains its communication with the tonsillar fossa (see Chapter 100). In the midline of the neck a sinus tract may persist as a patent *thyroglossal duct,* and its related cyst is often misdiagnosed as an abscess, lymph node or dermoid, unless the process of embryologic development is recalled (see Chapter 100). Around the second or third week of embryonic life, four (or possibly five) parallel clefts or grooves develop on each side of the neck, separated by solid branchial arches, each with its own blood and nerve supply. These clefts are matched internally by outpocketings of the foregut, forming pouches that do not extend completely through to the corresponding cleft, but are separated by a thin mem-

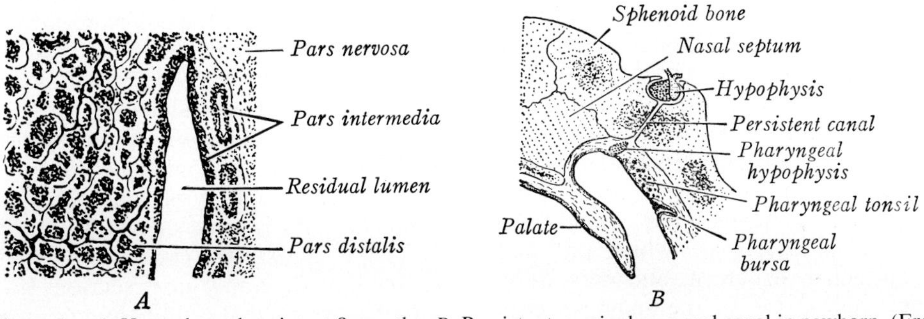

Figure 1. *A,* Hypophyseal region at 8 months. *B,* Persistent craniopharyngeal canal in newborn. (From Arey, L. B.: *Developmental Anatomy,* 7th Ed., W. B. Saunders, 1965.)

brane. The first pouch and dorsal portion of the second give rise to the eustachian tube, the tympanic cavity and its related structures, and the mastoid cells. The first cleft is the precursor of the external auditory meatus. The ventral portion of the second pouch forms part of the tonsillar fossa, and the first branchial arch gives rise to the maxillary and mandibular processes, the anterior portion of the tongue, various muscles, glands and arteries.

The second arch produces part of the auricle, stapes, a portion of the tongue and various muscles. The third external cleft forms the pyriform sinus, the inferior thyroid and the thymus glands. The fourth pouch forms the superior parathyroid and thymus glands and portions of the upper esophagus. The third arch produces most of the hyoid bone, the posterior portion of the tongue, and other vascular and muscular structures.

The fourth arch gives rise to the upper portion of the thyroid cartilage, the cricothyroid and some pharyngeal muscles, as well as the arch of the aorta on the left and the subclavian artery on the right. The fifth and sixth arches produce the lower portion of the thyroid cartilage, the cricoid cartilage, the pulmonary artery, and the recurrent laryngeal branch of the vagus nerve.

The great majority of congenital fistulas in the neck arise from the second branchial cleft or pouch, as the tract usually runs up to the base of the tonsil or along the posterior pillar. It is said that as many as 95 per cent of these branchial anomalies are produced by the second pouch and groove, therefore lying between the internal and external carotid arteries. However, some of these fistulous tracts are situated anterior to the carotids and pass upward to the supratonsillar fossa or the posterior pillar.

THE PALATINE TONSILS. These develop in the primitive tonsillar fossae, which are the regions of the second pharyngeal pouches. The tonsil originates from ectoderm, which produces its epithelial structure, and mesoderm, which gives rise to the mass of mesenchyme beneath the epithelial layer. During the third fetal month, solid ingrowths of epithelium burrow into this mesenchyme, and then these solid epithelial cords branch out and later establish crypts by resolution of the interior cells. Lymphocytes which originate from mesoderm start to infiltrate these crypts during the fourth month. This lymphocytic proliferation and infiltration is associated with further development of the crypts, and these processes continue until the time of birth.

THE NASOPHARYNGEAL TONSIL. This tonsil, called the adenoid, develops from entoderm lining the nasopharynx and longitudinal ridges of mesenchyme. It appears around the sixth month. Lymphocytic infiltration and proliferation similarly occur in this tissue at a very rapid rate, and continue for about six months after birth. A second spurt of growth occurs around 2 years of age. From then on, general physiologic enlargement progresses until 4 to 6 years of age, after which the lymphoid tissues remain relatively the same until the onset of puberty.

THE LINGUAL TONSIL. This originates on the pharyngeal surface of the tongue between the second and third branchial arches. It consists of lymphoid tissue surrounded by mucous glands, but crypts are not prominent and are not branched.

APPLIED ANATOMY

The pharynx is a common passageway from the nasal and oral cavities to the larynx and to the esophagus. It conducts air into and out of the lower respiratory tract, and also transports food, fluid and saliva into the upper digestive system. Traditionally, it is divided into three component parts, all of which are in direct continuity: the nasopharynx, the oropharynx (mesopharynx) and the hypopharynx (laryngopharynx) (Fig. 2).

THE NASOPHARYNX. The nasopharynx is the uppermost section. It is a small air space that is quite immobile and

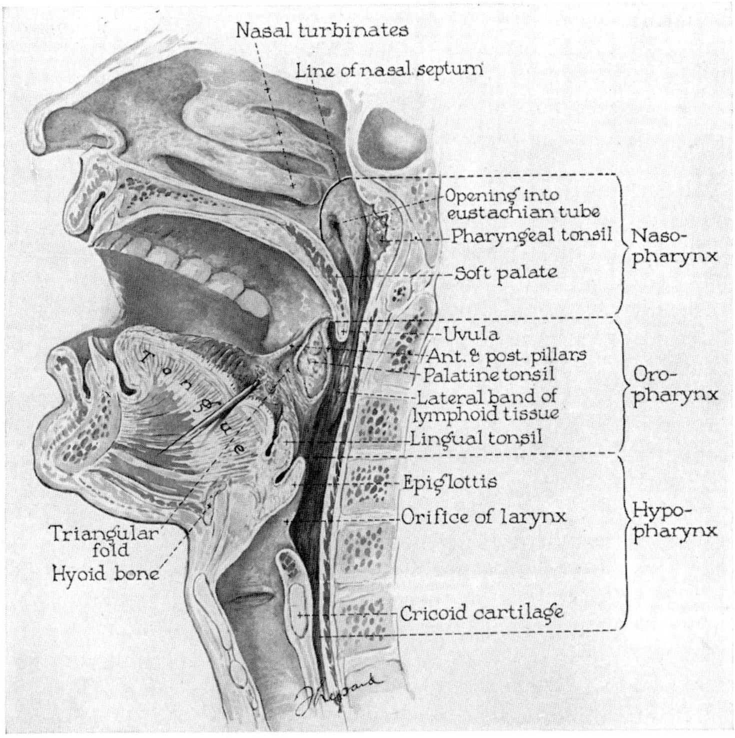

Figure 2. Sagittal section of the pharynx, showing its three subdivisions. (From Jackson, C., and Jackson, C. L.: *Diseases of the Nose, Throat and Ear,* 2nd Ed., W. B. Saunders, 1959.)

rigid, except for the soft palate, which comprises its inferior floor. The soft palate is a muscular organ that can completely close off the nasopharynx from the oropharynx. The nasopharynx extends from its vault at the basal process of the occipital bone, just beneath the sphenoid sinus, downward to the free edge of the soft palate, opening anteriorly into the nasal cavities through the two posterior choanae, and communicating laterally into the tympanic cavities through the two eustachian tubes. Below, it opens into and is continuous with the oropharynx.

The nasopharynx contains the pharyngeal tonsil (or adenoids). This large mass of lymphoid tissue is more prominent in infancy and childhood than at any other time, as it undergoes involution around puberty. The pharyngeal tonsil is located in the vault of the nasopharynx and on the upper part of the posterior nasopharyngeal wall. It also extends laterally into the fossa of Rosenmueller, and even over the openings of the eustachian tubes, thereby predisposing to recurrent attacks of otitis media and hearing impairment in the young patient. It overlies the superior pharyngeal constrictor muscle, but is not separated from it by a true capsule. This mass of tissue is composed of lymphoid structures with many longitudinal fissures or cryptlike depressions, lined by ciliated columnar epithelium (which probably removes debris, desquamated cells and infectious agents).

On each lateral wall of the nasopharynx is located the pharyngeal opening of the eustachian tube. The cartilaginous portion of this auditory tube, covered with mucous membrane, is located lateral and superior to the tubal orifice. It is easily visualized and may be palpated during surgery. Behind and above the cartilaginous torus of the tube is situated the pharyngeal recess (fossa of Rosenmueller). Bands of lymphoid tissue also extend downward on the lateral walls of the nasopharynx into the oropharynx. The midline adenoid mass extends down to a horizontal muscular constriction just behind and above the uvula (Passavant's ridge), which is important in the surgery of the nasopharynx.

THE OROPHARYNX. The oropharynx, or mesopharynx, extends from the soft palate to the hyoid bone or upper surface of the epiglottis, directly communicating above with the nasopharynx, anteriorly with the buccal cavity and inferiorly with the hypopharynx. It contains the palatine tonsils, which are located laterally in the fauces between the anterior and posterior pillars which separate the oropharynx from the oral cavity. The palatine tonsil is a large mass of lymphoid tissue with deep crypts branching into its depths. There are 10 to 20 of these crypts, lined with stratified squamous epithelium that constantly desquamates, carrying along with it white blood cells and food debris. Surrounding the crypts are follicles that, in the very young patient, show very prominent germinal centers.

The tonsillar fossa is bounded anteriorly by the glossopalatine muscle, which forms the anterior pillar, posteriorly by the pharyngopalatine muscle, which forms the posterior pillar (a larger, earlier developed and more important structure) and laterally by the superior constrictor muscle of the pharynx. Extending from the lower pole of the tonsil to the tongue between the two pillars is the lymphoid tissue of the triangular plica (extracapsular). The tonsil is always regarded as an encapsulated structure, yet anatomically there is no true "capsule," but merely a reflection of the buccopharyngeal fascia at its upper portion, separating the tonsil from the aponeurosis of the superior constrictor, but not actually enclosing the tonsil. It produces a helpful plane of cleavage for the extirpation of the tonsil.

The glossopalatine and pharyngopalatine muscles are important in contraction of the palate and elevation of the pharynx and larynx during swallowing and speaking. The tensor veli palatinus tightens the anterior part of the soft palate and opens the eustachian tube during the act of swallowing. The levator veli palatinus causes narrowing of the pharynx, and also widens the orifices of the auditory tubes. Surrounding the pharynx posteriorly are the three constrictor muscles of the pharynx (the superior, the middle, and the inferior), which overlap from below upward. The stylopharyngeus muscle elevates the larynx on swallowing and widens the pharynx, and the pharyngopalatine muscle also elevates the inferior portions of these structures during swallowing. Internally, the pharynx is lined by stratified squamous epithelium that is not ciliated, as is the mucosa of the nasopharynx.

THE HYPOPHARYNX. The hypopharynx, or laryngopharynx, is a continuation of the oropharynx downward, extending from the upper surface of the epiglottis to the lower border of the cricoid cartilage at the level of the sixth cervical vertebra. It merges directly into the esophagus posteriorly at the cricopharyngeus muscle, and also connects directly with the larynx anteriorly. At the base of the tongue are two pockets known as the valleculae, located between the median and lateral glosso-epiglottic ligaments. Along the posterior portion of the tongue is the lingual tonsil, with very shallow, nonbranching crypts. These are lined with stratified squamous epithelium, as are the crypts of the palatine tonsils. The lateral bands of lymphoid tissue continue downward posterior to the pharyngopalatine muscles, and the posterior pharyngeal and hypopharyngeal walls are studded with solitary lymphoid follicles.

The *blood supply* to the palatine tonsils and surrounding areas of the pharynx comes from the external carotid artery through the lingual artery (dorsalis linguae) and the ascending pharyngeal artery, the external maxillary artery (through the ascending palatine and tonsillar arteries) and the internal maxillary artery through the descending palatine artery.

Sensation to this area is supplied through the glossopharyngeal (ninth cranial) nerve. The motor nerve to the pharynx is the vagus (or tenth nerve), but the tensor veli palatinus is supplied by the mandibular branch of the trigeminal (or fifth nerve).

The *lymphatic drainage* of the pharynx is extensive. The nasopharynx drains mostly into the deep posterior cervical nodes behind the sternocleidomastoid muscle, and in infants it drains also into the temporary retropharyngeal nodes of Henle in the potential retropharyngeal space between the posterior pharyngeal wall and the prevertebral fascia. This is an area of loose areolar tissue, which contains several lymph nodes in infancy and early childhood, that disappear after the age of three. The lymphatics of the anterior pharynx and tonsillar areas drain into the anterior cervical nodes in front of the sternocleidomastoid muscles. There are probably no afferent vessels to the tonsils.

Lateral to the retropharyngeal space and immediately adjacent to it, separated only by thin membrane, is the pharyngomaxillary fossa. This is bounded medially by the superior constrictor muscle, and laterally by the internal pterygoid muscle, the ascending ramus of the mandible and the parotid gland. It contains the great vessels of the neck and the vagus nerve. This space may become infected by extension from the tonsils or pharynx, and this is a serious complication.

Surrounding the entrance to the upper air and food passages is a complete circle of lymphoid structures designated as *Waldeyer's ring*. This includes the pharyngeal tonsil (adenoids) superiorly, the two palatine tonsils laterally and the lingual tonsil inferiorly. Together these structures, along with the many solitary lymphoid nodules on the posterior pharyngeal wall and the lateral bands of lymphoid tissue, form this important ring so strategically located. All the lymphoid tissue composing Waldeyer's ring undergoes considerable hypertrophy during early childhood, a period when exposure to infection is frequent and immune processes are developing. This hypertrophy reaches a peak at 4 to 6 years of age, and later on, unless chronic infection is present, the structures undergo involution and decrease greatly in size. In fact, in most instances, after adolescence the adenoid for all practical purposes has disappeared as a troublesome entity.

PHYSIOLOGY

The functions of the pharynx may be considered four-fold: respiration, deglutition, conduction of mucus from upper nasal passages, and assistance in speech articulation and voice resonance.

RESPIRATION. The pharynx conducts air into the lower respiratory tract during inspiration, and out from the lung and trachea on expiration. The tongue, when approximated against the palate, completely separates the mouth from the pharynx, thereby occluding the oral airway. Respiration, however, is adequate as long as the nose and nasopharynx are clear. If a person is relaxed, as during sleep, and his mouth falls open, the air column may vibrate the relaxed palate and produce stertorous respirations (snoring). If the nasal passageways are obstructed, as by a large mass of adenoid tissue or tumor, or even by an upper respiratory infection, this oral and pharyngeal airway alone is perfectly adequate for respiration. Mouth breathing, as noted in the discussion of choanal atresia, is not innate, but is an acquired function that has to be learned and developed.

DEGLUTITION. Food, fluid, saliva and secretions are conducted from the oral cavity into the digestive tract through the lumen of the pharynx by muscular contraction of its mobile walls. Food is masticated in the mouth and mixed with saliva by the process of chewing, which turns the food into a soft, moist bolus. (The infant obtains nourishment merely by sucking, which is a normal instinctive process.) The food bolus, after being formed in the mouth, is then voluntarily brought to the base of the tongue and forced past the pillars of the soft palate by upward pressure of the tongue against the hard palate, and by compression of the cheeks, which narrows the oral cavity.

Contraction of the myelohyoid muscle along with the pharyngeal constrictors raises the tongue, hyoid bone and thyroid cartilage. The pillars (glossopalatine and pharyngopalatine muscles) contract to close the nasopharynx, and force the bolus downward into the oropharynx. (Contraction of the tensor veli palatinus opens the eustachian tube at this point and produces intermittent aeration of the middle ear cavity). The sphincteric inlet of the larynx (aryepiglottic folds, ventricular bands and vocal cords) closes as the epiglottis is raised in order to protect the airway from foreign material.

Contraction of the superior and middle constrictors of the pharynx, the pharyngopalatine and salpingopharyngeal muscles, narrows the nasopharynx and forces the bolus downward along its path. As the tongue, thyroid cartilage and larynx involuntarily rise, the epiglottis projects into the hypopharynx and allows food to go laterally through the pyriform sinuses. These sinuses now open as the larynx is elevated, since the esophagus is attached to the cricoid cartilage. The cricopharyngeus involuntarily relaxes on stimulation of the bolus. As a vacuum develops in the upper esophagus, food is sucked downward, so at first it requires no peristaltic propulsion.

Contraction of the striated muscle in the upper third of the esophagus continues to force food downward until it is picked up by the peristaltic waves of the smooth muscle layers of the middle and lower thirds of the esophagus. Longitudinal contraction of the esophageal muscles also propels the bolus along its path until the diaphragmatic "sphincter" opens and lets it into the stomach. Fluid merely falls downward by gravity and requires no peristaltic activity.

CONDUCTION OF MUCUS. Mucus is formed in the nasal passageways, the nasal sinuses and the nasopharynx, and is carried along by ciliary action into the pharynx, as the cilia beat downward toward the oropharynx. Once in the pharynx, it is swallowed like other liquids.

SPEECH ARTICULATION AND VOICE RESONANCE. For proper speech, complete velopalatal closure is necessary. This demands adequate functioning of the palatal muscles, as well as a soft palate that is sufficiently long and mobile enough to approximate the posterior pharyngeal wall. In a patient who has a submucous cleft of the palate, or who has had a congenital cleft of the palate repaired, the adenoid mass is of great importance in adding bulk to this region and assisting in the closure by approximating the short palate to its pad. The integrity of Passavant's ridge in contributing to this closure is also most important.

REFERENCES

Arey, L. B.: *Developmental Anatomy,* 7th Ed. Philadelphia, W. B. Saunders Co., 1965.

Boies, L. R., Hilger, J. A., and Priest, R. E.: *Fundamentals of Otolaryngology,* 4th Ed. Philadelphia, W. B. Saunders Co., 1964.

Coates, G. M., and Schenck, H. P.: *Otolaryngology.* New York, Harper & Row, 1956.

Gross, R. E.: *The Surgery of Infancy and Childhood.* Philadelphia, W. B. Saunders Co., 1963.

Jackson, C., and Jackson, C. L.: *Diseases of the Nose, Throat and Ear,* 2nd Ed. Philadelphia, W. B. Saunders Co., 1959.

Proctor, B., and Proctor, C.: Congenital lesions of the head and neck. *Otolaryng. Clin. N. Amer.,* 3:221, 1970.

Van Alyea, O. E.: *The Embryology of the Ear, Nose and Throat.* Chicago, American Academy of Ophthalmology and Otolaryngology Publications, 1949.

Chapter Ninety-Three

METHODS OF EXAMINATION

CHARLES F. FERGUSON, M.D., F.A.C.S.

Examination of the Pharynx

Examination of the pharynx is relatively simple as compared with the investigation of other otolaryngologic areas. A thorough and systematic inspection is always indicated, and the physician should not be satisfied merely with a fleeting glimpse of the tonsils. The mucous membranes of the mouth and pharynx should always be examined for color (pallor, inflammation, cyanosis or jaundice), exudate, enanthemata, ulceration or perhaps a gross local lesion. Note should be taken of the appearance of the tongue and gums and of the physical condition and alignment of the teeth. The orifices of the salivary ducts should also be inspected, noting any edema, pouting or inflammation, as well as the possibility of milking out any abnormal secretion from the gland. The tonsils are then examined as to size, degree and extent of inflammation or ulceration, dilatation of vessels of the pillars, and the type of exudate or debris in the crypts. Cheesy material can easily be expressed with slight pressure on the tonsil or pillar by a tongue depressor without causing undue discomfort or anxiety to the patient. If the patient has undergone a tonsillectomy, the condition of the fossae and pillars should be noted, especially if there are any infected tonsillar remnants. If indicated, bacteriologic cultures may be obtained at the same time, especially to confirm the presence or absence of the group A beta hemolytic streptococcus.

The movements of the palate should not be neglected, as this evaluation may give a clue as to the presence of a submucous cleft, so frequently missed even on an otherwise detailed examination. Tonsillectomy and adenoidectomy in the presence of such an undiagnosed malformation may be disastrous for future speech, yet, unfortunately, this diagnosis is frequently not made until ill-advised surgery has already been performed. The palate with a submucous cleft is short, and the uvula also short, wide, stiff, and occasionally bifid. The palate and uvula do not reach the posterior pharyngeal wall, indicating too deep a nasopharynx. Movements of the palate are stiff and somewhat limited. There may be a faint white line resembling a midline scar running the length of the palate, with or without some depression or apparent thinning. Occasionally a perforation may be noted. A V-shaped midline defect of the *hard* palate may also exist, and this defect is palpable or may even be visible as the velum retracts during phonation. The condition of the lingual tonsil and lateral bands of lymphoid tissue, the solitary follicles on the posterior pharyngeal wall, and any localized swelling in this area should be carefully noted. The character and amount of any postnasal discharge should also be evaluated, and possibly a bacteriologic culture should be taken.

For adequate examination of any otolaryngological area, bright illumination is a prime necessity. Facility in the proper use of a head-mirror should be developed early in one's medical career, since this simple instrument gives excellent axial illumination of otherwise darkened recesses. The light source preferably should come from a "bullseye" bulb, which intensifies the beam. This instrument leaves the examiner's hands free to manipulate the tongue depressor with one hand and a suction tube, probe or throat swab with the other. Sometimes the use of the extra hand merely to steady the patient's head is of great value. An electric headlight (such as the "Goodlite") serves the same purpose.

A word about the use of the tongue depressor is in order. Probably more pediatric patients have a real phobia about "the stick" than any other commonly employed diagnostic instrument, yet this is usually the only equipment needed for a satisfactory examination of the oropharynx. Many children, unfortunately, have been unfavorably conditioned to apprehension and fear, precipitated by previous improper and indelicate use of this commonest of all examining aids. The child should *not* be asked to protrude his tongue (unfortunately, this is often the first direction the examiner gives him!), because this procedure instantly stiffens and thickens the tongue, necessitating more pressure on the dorsum by the stick to obtain a proper view. This extra pressure merely elicits discomfort as well as the gag reflex and often vomiting. The tongue should be left relaxed in its normal position on the floor of the mouth, and the patient asked merely to breathe rapidly and pant ("like a dog on a hot day"). Only later is he asked to say "ah," to bring out better the physiological movements of the palate. The anterior portion of the tongue is not at all sensitive, but if the stick is applied too far back over the dorsum, the gag reflex is inevitably initiated. The tongue should not be pushed backward into the hypopharynx, but merely depressed firmly to the floor of the mouth. Extreme gentleness and true consideration for the natural anxieties of a child who has previously been frightened will pay great dividends in obtaining his confidence. Giving the child a few tongue depressors to practice with at home is a valuable investment that pays good dividends in the future.

Examination of the Hypopharynx

The hypopharynx is easily seen with a properly placed throat stick or, better yet, by a right-angled metal tongue depressor, if the patient breathes deeply. Many times the lingual tonsil and epiglottis are easily visible, as well as the lateral bands of lymphoid tissue and the solitary follicles of the posterior pharyngeal wall. Any abnormal swelling should also be noted in this region. All of these deeper structures, of course, are seen better with the laryngeal mirror. The mirror should have been previously warmed, preferably by dipping it in a glass of warm water (less frightening than heated in an alcohol flame), or rubbed with pHisoHex, which prevents fogging.

Examination of the Nasopharynx

Examination of the nasopharynx is somewhat more difficult than the visualization of the oropharynx. With a little patience, however, and a relatively cooperative child, there is no problem in obtaining good evaluation of the nasopharynx at any age. In the past, digital palpation of the nasopharynx was more commonly employed, but this at best is an uncomfortable procedure for anyone, and occasionally frightening to even the most cooperative or placid child. At the same time, the examiner obtains little specific information, except regarding the size of the adenoid mass. The use of a small nasopharyngeal mirror (Fig. 1) may not be feasible in the very young, but in the older child this is a most valuable instrument. The child should be in a sitting position facing a beam of bright light from the head-mirror. A small nasopharyngeal mirror is then inserted along the stick or metal tongue depressor close to the posterior pharyngeal wall below the uvula, and rotated in various directions between the thumb and forefinger to obtain a composite view of the entire nasopharynx. The tongue should not be touched, for that will initiate the gag reflex.

The electric nasopharyngoscope (Fig. 2) is one of our most valuable instruments for the examination of this area, and ordinarily may be used without difficulty at any age, even in infants. If the child is allowed to handle the in-

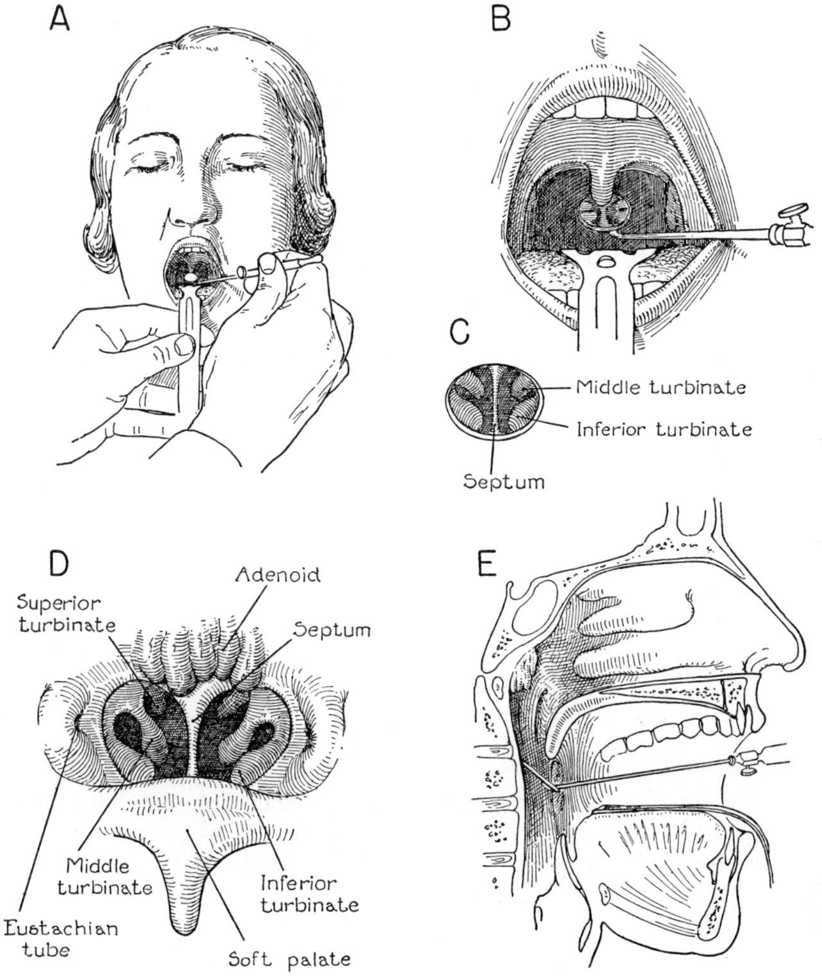

Figure 1. Mirror examination of the nasopharynx. (From Richards, L. G.: *Otolaryngology in General Practice,* Macmillan, 1939.)

strument before its insertion into the nasopharynx, its use is properly explained, and he is allowed to look through it himself and visualize his own fingernail, his apprehension is greatly reduced. In the older child, this instrument is employed while he sits upright in the chair, but the infant is best examined, properly restrained, in a supine position. One side of the nose is first sprayed with a single squirt of a local anesthetic, such as 0.5 per cent xylocaine solution. In a minute or two a small cotton-tipped applicator moistened with the anesthetic solution is gently guided along the floor of the nose into the nasopharynx, avoiding the posterior wall. The small telescopic instrument may then be similarly inserted along the floor of the nose, care being taken not to touch the turbinates or the posterior wall.

One advantage of the nasopharyngoscope is that excellent, direct visualization of the orifices of the eustachian tubes may be obtained, as well as the extent of any adenoid tissue. A careful evaluation of the fossae of Rosenmueller can be made, and the presence of any obstructing lymphoid tissue noted, as well as infection or adhesions about the tubal

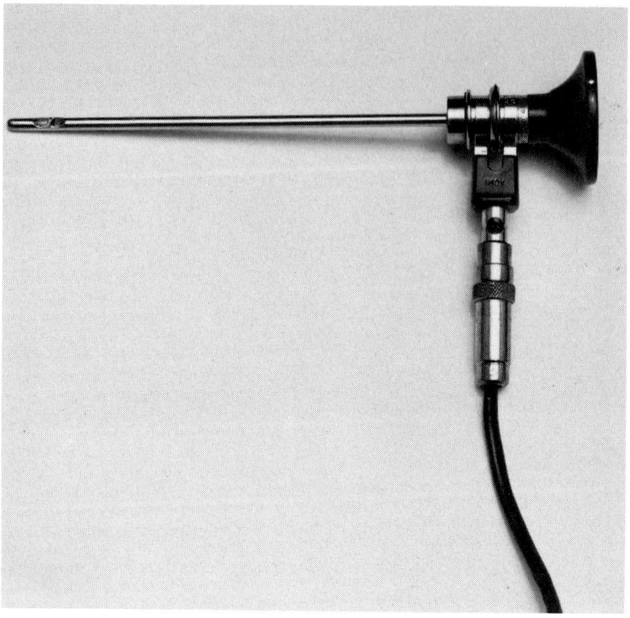

Figure 2. The electric nasopharyngoscope.

orifices. The nasopharyngoscope is then rotated 180° to visualize the opposite eustachian orifice and pharyngeal recess. If indicated, the opening may be easily catheterized under direct vision. The posterior choanae and the posterior portion of the septum are noted, as well as any exudate, inflammation, choanal polyp or tumor. On rare occasions a nasopharyngeal bursa or cyst may be discovered. If the patient is under anesthesia, such as at the time of surgery, a Love palatal retractor or the larger Yankauer speculum will assist in direct inspection of the nasopharynx. On occasion, a lateral roentgenogram of the nasopharynx taken by a technique to visualize soft tissues is of great assistance if direct nasopharyngoscopy is not possible. The film should always be taken during inspiration and with the head extended (see Chapter 64). Care in the interpretation of such films must be used, as abnormal masses, posterior-wall fullness or other shadows are often erroneously diagnosed, especially if the head is flexed or if the films are taken during expiration, when a phantom "mass" may appear. Cineradiography is helpful not only in discovering local pathology or obstruction, but also in studying and recording palatal movements and the degree of nasopharyngeal closure.

Examination of the Neck

Examination of the pharynx and nasopharynx has not been completed until the neck is carefully inspected and palpated externally for the presence of sinus tracts, abnormal masses or enlarged lymph nodes. In general, the nasopharynx drains through the lymphatic vessels into the chain of nodes posterior to the sternocleidomastoid muscle, and in infants it drains also into the retropharyngeal nodes just behind or below the uvula. The palatine tonsils and the surrounding structures drain into the anterior groups of cervical nodes, especially the "tonsillar node" at the angle of the jaw. Chronic enlargement of these lymphatic structures is of clinical significance.

Chapter Ninety-Four

THE TONSIL AND ADENOID PROBLEM

WILLIAM A. HOWARD, M.D.

The palatine and pharyngeal tonsils are part of a mass of lymphoid tissue encircling the nasal and oral pharynx known as Waldeyer's ring. Acute infections and conditions involving these tissues have been described elsewhere. In this chapter, interest is centered on the possibility of chronic and persistent tonsil and adenoid involvement and the desirability or necessity of surgical removal of these structures as a method of treatment.

Pathogenesis

The lymphoid tissue of Waldeyer's ring undergoes physiologic hypertrophy and hyperplasia, usually greatest between two and five years of age, in response to infections in this general area. Whether or not this lymphoid tissue is a constituent of the bursal system of immunity, such hyperplasia is associated with an increase in lymphocytes in these tissues and with increased immunologic activity of the host in response to specific infections. These infections of the tonsils and adenoids are most prevalent during these early years, and as increasing resistance to infection develops, the frequency and severity of respiratory infections diminish rapidly, usually with a corresponding decrease in the size of the lymphoid mass. Under the stress of acute infection, tonsils and adenoids may undergo rapid enlargement, but as infection subsides, they generally return to their former state. One should not judge the tonsil by viewing it only under the stress of acute infection.

Clinical Manifestations

Chronic infection in the tonsils and adenoids may be associated with a variety of clinical manifestations. There may be recurrent bouts of acute infection manifested by a sore throat or a more or less continuous low-grade involvement, with or without fever. Some degree of cervical adenitis is often present, and there may be a history of recurring middle ear infections, with or without some degree of hearing loss. Mouth breathing may occur as a result of adenoid enlargement, and a heavy, fetid breath may be noted in the morning. Though less common than formerly, peritonsillar and retropharyngeal abscesses may develop adjacent to the chronically infected tonsil or adenoid.

A variety of other symptoms have been ascribed to diseased tonsils and adenoids, including fatigue, loss of appetite, failure to gain weight, so-called growing pains, difficulty in swallowing, chronic cough, frequent upper respiratory tract infections, postnasal drip, "clearing of the throat" and many others.

Physical findings generally relate to the size of the tonsils, which may be large or small, and of the adenoids, which are usually enlarged. The chronically infected tonsil cannot be diagnosed by a single, simple inspection, and usually a careful chronologic history is essential for a proper evaluation of the nature and degree of infection present. Additional findings will include varying degrees of cervical adenitis, nasal obstruction, occasional hearing loss, and not infrequently a collection of serous fluid behind the tympanic membrane, the so-called serous otitis media. When nasal obstruction has been present for a considerable period of time, there may be a thoracic deformity, usually a simple funnel chest of varying depth, involving the lower portion of the sternum, the xiphoid and the neighboring rib cartilages. Some depression also may be noted at the level of attachment of the diaphragm. Malocclusion of varying degree, associated with enlarged adenoids and nasal obstruction, may help in producing what is termed the adenoid facies.

Many of these signs and symptoms can be produced by other causes, the most common of which is allergic involvement of the upper respiratory tract. It should be emphasized again that a careful history is most important in making a decision about the removal of tonsils and adenoids.

Indications for Adenotonsillectomy

Based upon an abundance of available evidence, a few salient facts may be noted.

Although a more conservative attitude has developed toward adenotonsillectomy, the operation is still extremely common, and probably is performed much too frequently.

The wide variation in the reported incidence of adenotonsillectomy in different groups rated according to age, geographic location, socioeconomic status, medical insurance and educational levels is such that one cannot escape the conclusion that the operation must at times be performed for reasons other than those purely medical.

Indications for operation vary greatly, emphasizing the lack of understanding of the basic function of this lymphoid tissue and the consequences of its early removal.

It is extremely difficult to assess the results of adenotonsillectomy because of the wide variety of indications for its performance and the lack of long-term follow-up by those who perform the operation, and because it is usually done at an age when gradual but spontaneous improvement in response to exposure to infection is to be expected.

Adenotonsillectomy is not without danger, 200 to 300 deaths being reported each year from this elective procedure.

Tonsillectomized persons are neither more nor less susceptible to streptococcal infections, nor is the clinical course of streptococcal disease modified. There is also no effect on the development of rheumatic fever or rheumatic valvular heart disease. Streptococcal infections are less readily recognized in tonsillectomized children, who may thereby escape adequate treatment.

The degree of antibody response in the nasopharynx to orally administered polio vaccine appears to be significantly higher when the vaccine is administered to children with intact tonsils. Also, pre-existing levels of local antibody may fall sharply after tonsillectomy, and may persist at these levels for several months. These observations may provide an explanation for the observed epidemiologic relationship between tonsillectomy and bulbar and paralytic poliomyelitis, and would suggest that the recently tonsillectomized child may still be more susceptible to natural infection with poliovirus.

With due consideration of the foregoing discussion, it is possible to give a brief résumé of the various situations that have been considered indications for adenotonsillectomy.

PERITONSILLAR ABSCESS. Once this complication has been diagnosed, there is fairly general agreement that a second attack should not be risked, and that adenotonsillectomy should be done as soon as feasible.

RECURRENT TONSILLITIS. Recurrent acute tonsillar infections, with fever, cervical adenitis and possibly otitis media, may constitute a sound indication for operation, especially if there is persistent evidence of chronic involvement between acute attacks. There exists the possibility, however, that such attacks represent new infections with differing etiologic agents, and that they constitute an immunologic experience that might occur regardless of the presence or absence of the tonsils. In spite of its failure to modify streptococcal disease, operative removal should be considered when tonsillitis is due to proven recurrent streptococcal infections.

RECURRENT "COLDS." Recurrent upper respiratory tract infections resembling the common cold generally are not controlled by adenotonsillectomy, and operation is not recommended.

RECURRENT OTITIS MEDIA. If ear infections are frequent, and there is any evidence of *hearing loss* adenoidectomy alone should be considered the operation of choice. Removal of the tonsils should not be done at the same time unless there are specific indications.

HYPERTROPHIED TONSILS. Tonsillar enlargement alone, especially under the age of 5 to 6 years, is seldom if ever sufficient indication for operation. An exception to this may be when tonsils are so large as to affect swallowing and breathing, as suggested by the increasing number of reports of cor pulmonale resulting from tonsillar hypertrophy and airway obstruction.

ADENOID ENLARGEMENT. If adenoid enlargement is sufficient to cause noisy mouth-breathing, snoring, and persistent low-grade nasal congestion and discharge, removal of the adenoids is considered proper, provided one can be assured that the symptoms are not produced by allergic involvement in the same area.

CERVICAL ADENITIS. Chronic infection in the cervical lymph nodes, with frequent acute flare-ups, are fundamentally an indication of persistent infection in the pharyngeal area. Depending on the appearance of the tonsils and the degree of infection present, cervical adenitis may then constitute a valid indication for tonsillectomy.

In considering the indications for adenotonsillectomy, it becomes apparent that there will be many instances in which removal of the adenoids may be the only surgical procedure indicated, and that results may be more satisfactory and much less disturbing if tonsillectomy is avoided. Also, in making a decision about operation, the possibility of an allergic cause of the signs and symptoms must be considered. Nasal obstruction, frequent upper respiratory tract involvement resembling "colds," serous otitis media, enlargement of tonsils and adenoids and diminished hearing may all appear on the basis of nasal allergy. Adenotonsillectomy may be indicated in the allergic child as well, but the indications for operation should be *at least* as stringent as those for the nonallergic child, if not more so. It is the consensus among pediatric allergists that adenotonsillectomy should not be undertaken in the allergic child until there has been a period of definitive treatment of the underlying allergy, and adequate treatment of any accompanying infection. After three to six months of such treatment, the indications for operation may have lessened a great deal or even may have disappeared entirely. Removal of tonsils and adenoids in a child with untreated nasal allergy may be followed by the development of bronchial allergic symptoms.

Complications

Complications from adenotonsillectomy are relatively infrequent, with the exception of postoperative hemorrhage. Blood loss occasionally may be sufficient to warrant replacement by transfusion. Pneumonia, lung abscess, atelectasis and septicemia have occurred. As indicated earlier, death may occur, usually as a result of cardiac arrest, hemorrhage or infection. The psychologic reaction to the trauma of hospitalization and operation should not be overlooked.

Results from Adenotonsillectomy

Although the incidence of epidemic respiratory infections is not altered by the removal of the tonsils and adenoids, there may be a decrease in the number and severity of throat infections and in the amount of fever that accompanies them. Obstructive symptoms may be relieved, especially by adenoidectomy, but relief from recurrent otitis media is variable. There is generally a gradual disappearance of cervical adenopathy, and bouts of acute adenitis are decreased or absent. There may be gain in weight and apparent benefit to general health and appetite, but multiple factors may be involved in this general improvement. It is unwise to promise too much as a result of adenotonsillectomy.

REFERENCES

Bakwin, H.: The tonsil-adenoidectomy enigma. *J. Pediat., 52*:339, 1958.

Canby, J. P.: Acquired fibrinogenemia. An unusual cause of post-tonsillectomy and adenoidectomy hemorrhage. *J.A.M.A., 183*:282, 1963.

Chamovitz, R., Rammelkamp, C. H., Jr., Wannamaker, L. W., and Denny, W. F., Jr.: The effect of tonsillectomy on the incidence of streptococcal disease and its complications. *Pediatrics, 26*:355, 1960.

Chobot, R.: Infectious aspects of asthma in children. In Prigal, S.: *Fundamentals of Modern Allergy*. New York, McGraw-Hill Book Company, Inc., 1960.

Clein, N.: Influence of tonsillectomy and adenoidectomy on children, with special reference to the allergic implications. *Ann. Allergy, 10*:568, 1952.

Gellis, S. L.: Personal communication to the author.

Howard, W. A.: Childhood complications of respiratory allergies. *Clin. Proc. Child. Hosp., D.C., 8*:210, 1952.

Idem: Diagnosis and treatment of nasal obstruction in children. *Postgrad. Med., 21*:136, 1957.

Lelong, M.: Asthma et amygdalectomie. *Lille Med., 9*:77, 1964.

Ogra, P. L.: Effect of tonsillectomy and adenoidectomy on nasopharyngeal antibody response to poliovirus. *New Eng. J. Med., 284*:59, 1971.

Ravenholt, R. T.: Poliomyelitic paralysis and tonsillectomy reconsidered. *Am. J. Dis. Child., 103*:658, 1962.

Reid, J. N., and Donaldson, J. A.: The indications for tonsillectomy and adenoidectomy. *Otolaryng. Clin. N. Amer., 3*:339, 1970.

Sherman, W. B., and Kessler, W. R.: *Allergy in Pediatric Practice*. St. Louis, C. V. Mosby Company, 1957.

Sobel, G.: Adenotonsillectomy in the allergic child. In Prigal, S.: *Fundamentals of Modern Allergy*. New York, McGraw-Hill Book Company, Inc., 1960.

Chapter Ninety-Five

TONSIL AND ADENOID SURGERY

CHARLES F. FERGUSON, M.D., F.A.C.S.

Tonsillectomy and adenoidectomy are still the most frequently performed surgical operations throughout the world. Often they are regarded as merely "minor" procedures, and this attitude results in unnecessarily high mortality. When these operations are performed by an adequately trained surgeon, in a well-equipped and competently staffed hospital, with proper indications and precautions, the results are most gratifying, and both morbidity and mortality should be at a minimum. It must always be remembered, however, that the operation is carried out in a very vascular field, located in the all-important airway, and this vital air passage must be kept perfectly clear at all times. Hemostasis must always be careful and complete, not only throughout the operative procedure, but during the recovery period as well.

In a textbook of this scope it is obviously impossible to describe all the various surgical techniques employed.

Today there is more standardization as to anesthesia, position of the patient, surgical equipment and technical maneuvers than in former days. The procedure now used more generally at The Children's Hospital Medical Center in Boston will be described in some detail.

A well-taken complete medical history is the most important factor in proper evaluation of the indications for the operation. This history should include a very careful consideration of any bleeding problem, both in the patient and in the family. Epistaxis, bleeding from the gums, hemoptysis, hematemesis, hematuria, easy bruising or other abnormal bleeding symptoms should be investigated carefully, as well as any family history of bleeding tendencies, transfusions or unusual hemorrhagic complications during or after surgical procedures. In such cases special coagulation studies should be carried out preoperatively under the direction of the Hematology Department, in addition to routine complete blood counts and blood smears. Specific allergies should always be looked for in both patient and family, including eczema, urticaria, asthma, hayfever and drug reactions. The history of persistent colic or chronic diarrhea in infancy is always suggestive of an allergic background.

A complete physical examination should be done well in advance of hospitalization in order to determine whether any special investigations are in order before surgery is performed. After admission of the patient to the hospital, the preoperative examination should include the taking of temperature, pulse, respirations and blood pressure, as well as inspection for evidence of present infection or contagion. Blood and urine studies should also be performed. The anesthesiologist should confer with the patient, and preferably also with the family, during the afternoon or evening of admission, and develop much needed rapport and confidence. Preoperative medication consists of pentobarbitol according to age, weight and general physical condition, given one hour beforehand, followed by proper doses of morphine and atropine one-half hour preoperatively. (The patient should have received nothing by mouth for at least eight hours.)

The most common general anesthetic agent used today is halothane, preferably given by endotracheal intubation. This gives the anesthesiologist the best control of the patient, and assures a clear airway throughout the operative procedure. Ether has stood the test of time as having the widest margin of safety of any generally used anesthetic agent, especially in the hand of the less experienced anesthetist. It is, however, used very little at the present time, mainly because of hazards with possible legal complications due to its flammability.

The operation today is usually done with the patient lying supine on the operating table, which is tipped somewhat in Trendelenburg position (25 to 30 degrees). The true "Rose" position (with marked hyperextension of the head) makes removal of the adenoid tissue very difficult, since the cervical spine is arched too far anteriorly. The potentially dangerous sitting position, which is most "unphysiologic" for a patient under general anesthesia, has now been nearly abandoned. With the patient in slight Trendelenburg position, the surgeon sitting at ease at the head of the table has excellent exposure of the brightly-illuminated oral cavity, and is in a good position to aspirate secretions and blood as necessary.

The sterile tray of instruments (Fig. 1) is placed in front of the surgeon over the chest of the patient. The patient's mouth is kept open by a Brown-Davis mouth gag, the Ring tongue blade* of which has a V-shaped groove to hold the endotracheal tube firmly in place, but well out of the way of the surgeon. The proper-sized tongue blade should be selected, depending on the diameters of the oral cavity, in order to give complete ex-

---

*Ring Instrument Company, Salt Lake City, Utah.

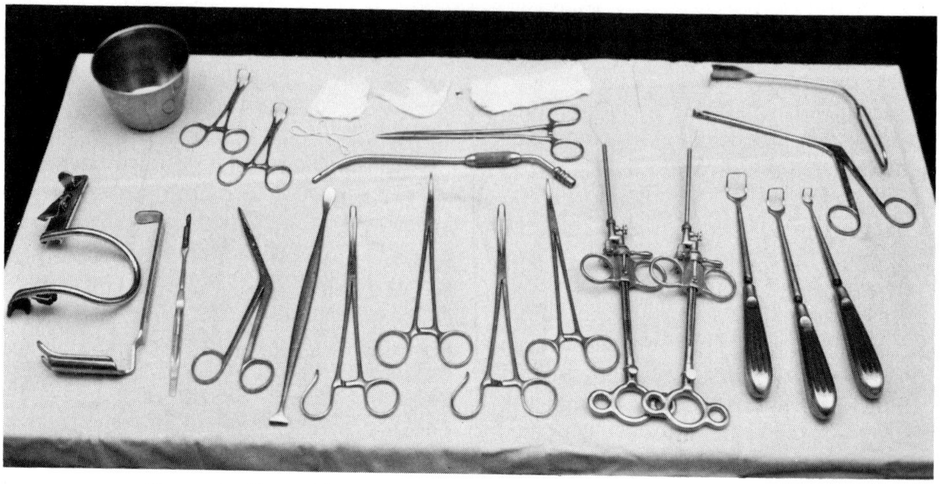

Figure 1. Tray of instruments for tonsillectomy and adenoidectomy.

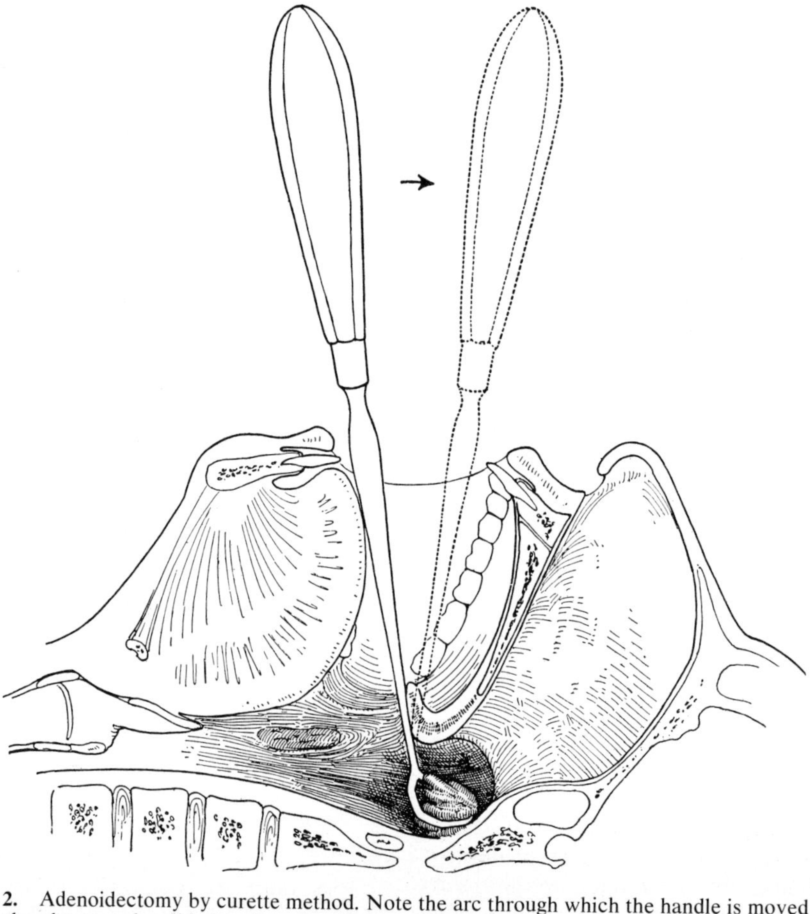

Figure 2. Adenoidectomy by curette method. Note the arc through which the handle is moved to avoid injury to the pharyngeal wall below the adenoid mass. (From Richards, L. G.: *Otolaryngology in General Practice,* Macmillan, 1939.)

posure of both tonsils without impinging on them. Great care should be used in the insertion of the gag, noting or even removing any loose teeth, and at the same time protecting the lips from being pinched.

If adenoidectomy is performed prior to tonsillectomy, the greater vascular area of the nasopharynx should ordinarily be perfectly dry at the end of the operative procedure. A Barnhill or Beckman curette is inserted behind the soft palate and passed upward in the midline as far as the posterior edge of the nasal septum, but the septum should not be scraped (Fig. 2). The sides of the curette are curved to prevent engaging the thin, horizontal cutting blade too deeply. By firm pressure on this blade the adenoid mass is engaged, and by a sweeping motion following the anatomic curve of the nasopharynx, using firm steady pressure, this lymphoid structure is completely removed. Care must be taken to lighten pressure on the curette as the inferior edge of the adenoid is reached, in order not to injure Passavant's ridge.

Adenoid curettes must always be very sharp so that the tissue mass will be cleanly removed and no tags left behind. Incomplete removal of the adenoid mass is the most common cause of primary postoperative hemorrhage. If the curette is not sharp, the mucosa at Passavant's ridge may be stripped all the way down into the oropharynx.

After the central mass of adenoid has been removed, another similar application of the curette is usually necessary, first to one side of the midline and then to the other, taking care not to injure the tori of the auditory tubes. The cutting blade must always be applied squarely to the posterior wall, for if it is turned laterally it will cut into the torus. Small curettes can easily be passed posterior to the torus without injury, if the blade is always kept flat against the posterior wall.

Small tags or solitary lymphoid follicles may be cleanly removed under direct vision by a flat, triangular ring-punch as the soft palate is retracted for careful visual inspection of the nasopharynx with a mirror or Yankauer speculum. Bleeding may be controlled by electrocoagulation of individual vessels or temporary tamponade by gauze sponges, always used with the attached strings hanging out of the mouth. (These strings are good insurance against dangerously abandoning a foreign body in the nasopharynx.) The LaForce box-adenotome may be used in place of the curettes, but in our experience a cleaner removal of all of the lymphoid tissue can be accomplished with the curettes with less danger of damage to the tori.

Following adenoidectomy, the tonsils are removed by scissors dissection, followed by the application of a snare. A right-angled tenaculum firmly and squarely grasps the tonsillar mass, care being taken not to catch either pillar in its blades. The tonsil is then momentarily retracted into the middle of the pharynx, keeping in mind the edge of the now stretched anterior pillar. A small, very superficial vertical incision is made in this area, where the pillar would ordinarily fold back on itself, going only through the mucosa and exposing, but not injuring, the tonsillar capsule. One sharp straight cut with a right-angled blunt scissors carries this very superficial incision inferiorly all the way to the tongue along the pillar edge.

The scissors are then reversed and the incision carried upward around the upper pole of the tonsil, and then, with the blades closed, the incision is taken a bit deeper down to expose the upper portion of the posterior pillar. (A curved tonsil knife may be used for this maneuver in place of the scissors.) The tonsil is then pushed laterally and deeper into its bed, and this scissors incision continued just inside the edge of the posterior pillar downward all the way to the junction of the posterior pillar with the lateral pharyngeal wall (Fig. 3). The tonsil is then peeled away from the fossa by blunt dissection with a dissector or the nearly closed scissors, using small sponges in the fossa and constant suctioning for hemostasis until the tonsil is entirely free from all attachment, except at its lowermost pole. This blunt dissection should now be carried below the lower margin of the tonsil and should

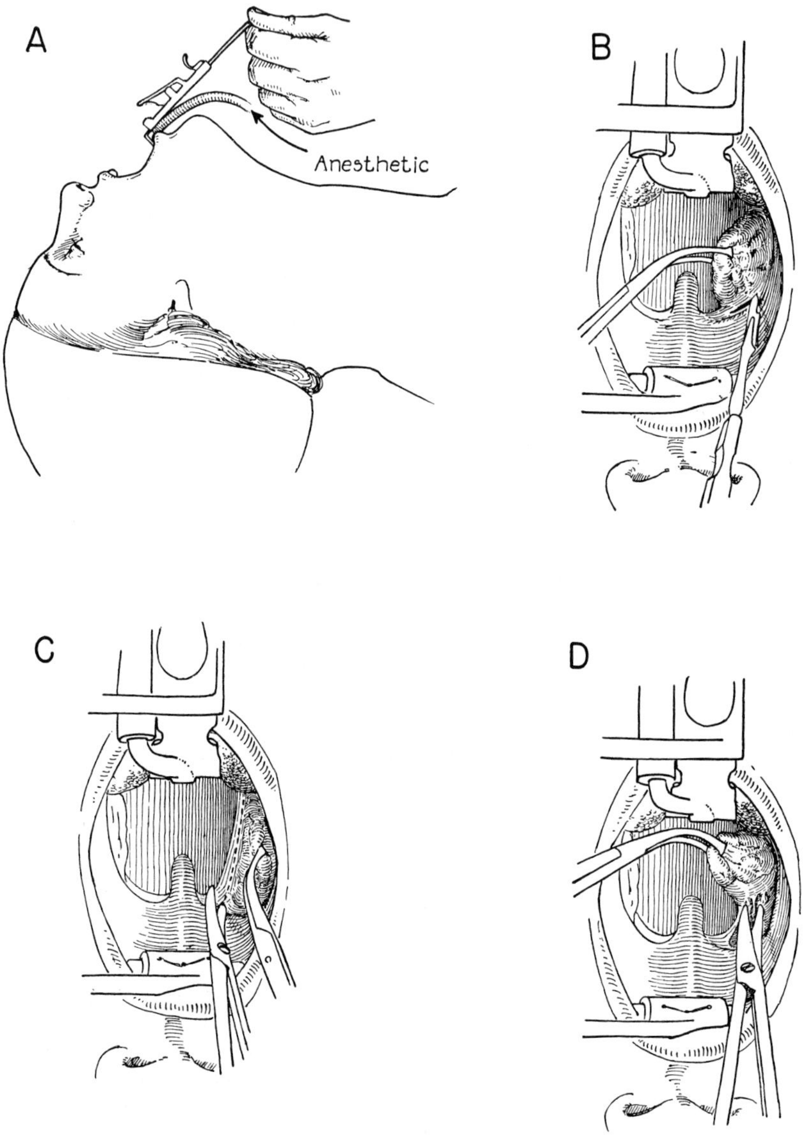

Figure 3. Tonsillectomy. *A,* Gag and endotracheal tube in place, supported by anesthesiologist (drapes omitted). *B,* Incision of anterior pillar carried down to tongue. *C,* Continuing incision of posterior pillar around superior pole. *D,* Dissection of tonsil from bed. (From Richards, L. G.: *Otolaryngology in General Practice,* Macmillan, 1939.)

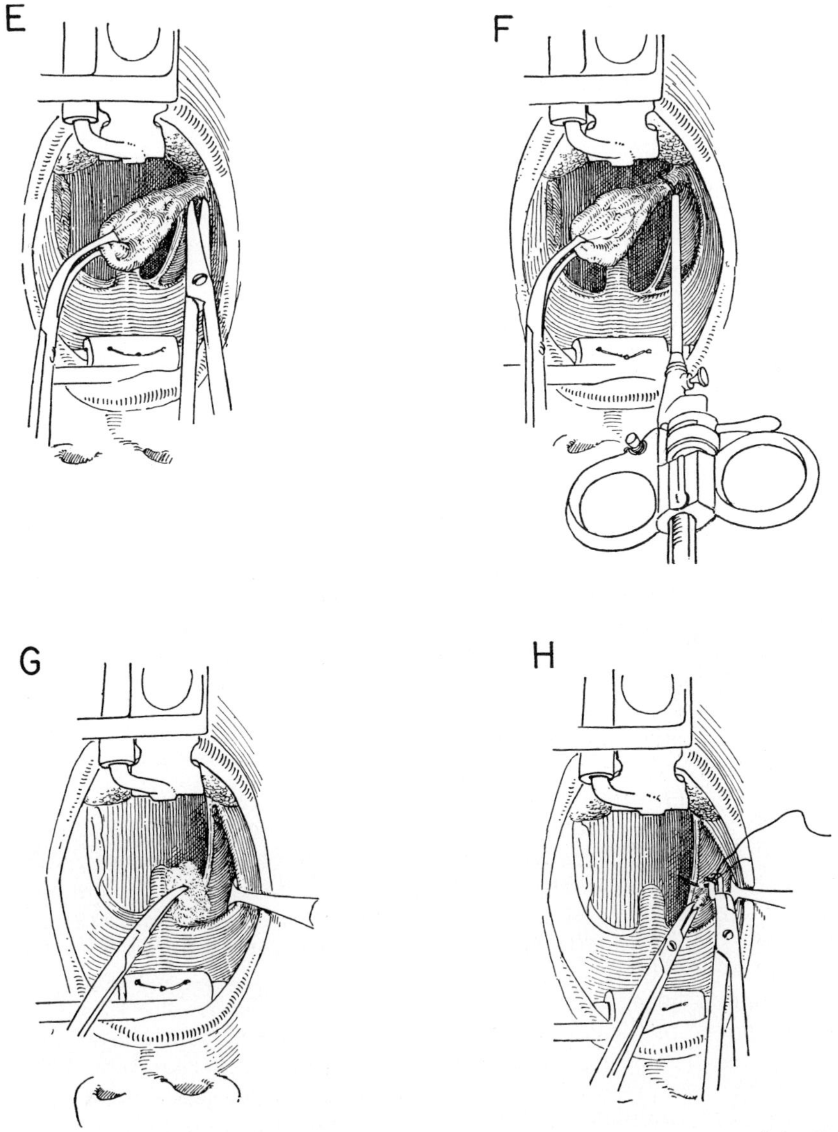

Figure 3. *Continued.* *E,* Dissection completed to pedicle. *F,* Application of snare to pedicle. *G,* Inspection of fossa and application of sponge for hemostasis. *H,* Ligation of bleeder with "figure 8" catgut stitch. (From Richards, L. G.: *Otolaryngology in General Practice,* Macmillan, 1939.)

include the thinner layer of lymphoid tissue of the triangular plica. Otherwise, a later "recurrence" of the tonsil may be charged to the surgeon. A snare passed over the tenaculum will cut the pedicle flush with the tongue and include the plical tissue. This maneuver should leave no lymphoid tissue at the base if the wire loop is pushed down as far as possible at the same time that the tenaculum grasping the tonsil is pulled upward as firmly as possible.

In the dissection of the tonsil from its bed, connective tissue and vessels should always be cut close to the tonsil in order not to injure the aponeurosis of the constrictor muscle as it is being pulled out into the throat. As much mucosa as possible should be left along the edges of the pillars, and the primary incisions along the anterior and posterior pillars should always be 1 to 2 mm. from the actual edge.

Arterial bleeders usually retract and occlude by contraction of their muscle fibers, but venous bleeders may be more troublesome and oozing may persist or recur later on. If temporary sponging and pressure does not produce adequate hemostasis, each bleeder should be grasped with a fine-tipped hemostat, and either ligated or, better still, sutured with a figure-8 stitch around the vessel, using 000 plain catgut on a small-curved malleable needle. Such a needle will not break, and if the catgut is swaged onto the needle, there is no danger of its becoming unthreaded and lost. The postnasal sponges should now be removed and counted, as one of the strings may have been clipped during the procedure, leaving the sponge in the nasopharynx. The patient should not be extubated or returned to the recovery room until hemostasis has been complete in all areas for at least a few minutes, during which the mouth gag has been relaxed to take away tension from the pillars, which may have been obliterating possible bleeding.

Postoperative Care

The two most important factors in the postoperative management of the tonsillectomy and adenoidectomy patient are constant maintenance of a clear, dry airway and persistent checking for bleeding. By keeping the jaws forward and the tongue away from the roof of the mouth, the airway will remain patent. (An artificial airway should be in place until the patient has recovered.) He should lie on his side with his anterior chest at a 45-degree angle with the bed, possibly with a sandbag or folded blanket supporting the chest, with the jaws and tongue falling forward and the mouth open. In this position even slight bleeding can be quickly observed. Suctioning of excessive secretion is always essential to the maintenance of a clear airway. Pulse and blood pressure should be checked very frequently (possibly at 15-minute intervals), but these efforts should never detract from constant observation of the airway as well as the mouth and nose for bleeding. Any bleeding should always be detected and controlled long before a significant rise in pulse and certainly before a fall in blood pressure. After recovery, proper doses of Demerol may be used as a sedative and analgesic, and if vomiting occurs, a 25 mgm. thorazine suppository will usually control it satisfactorily.

Postoperative Bleeding

If bleeding occurs, it will usually be within the first 24 hours postoperatively (primary bleeding) or not until the fifth to ninth days (secondary bleeding). Primary bleeding should be extremely rare if adequate precautions have been taken during surgery. Secondary bleeding, which is usually due to low-grade infection causing premature separation of the fibrinous eschar, should occur in less than 1 per cent of cases. The use of prophylactic antibiotics for a week postoperatively should prevent secondary bleeding.

In either primary or secondary bleeding, the adenoid area is more commonly involved than the tonsillar fossae. In any case, the clot must first be carefully removed by suction through each nostril or by extraction through the mouth. If this does not stop the bleeding promptly, a postnasal pack is inserted if the bleed-

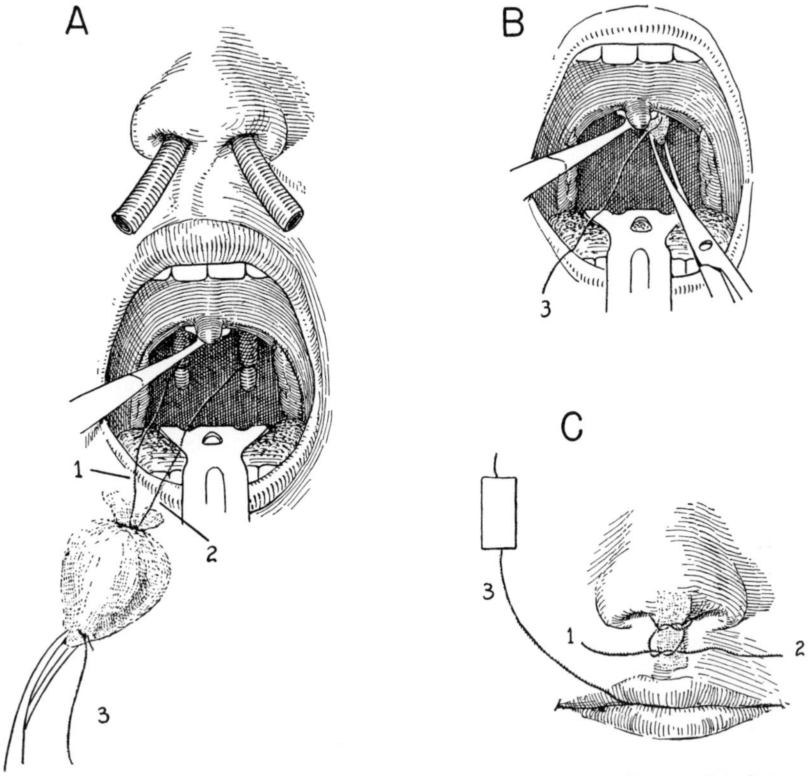

Figure 4. Postnasal pack for adenoid bleeding. *A,* Pack-strings attached to nasal catheters. *B,* Pack pulled firmly up into place behind palate. *C,* Two strings tied about columella (1 and 2) and attached to cheek (3) for later removal of pack. (From Richards, L. G.: *Otolaryngology in General Practice,* Macmillan, 1939.)

ing is all from the nasopharynx. This is a three-stringed gauze sponge rolled into a firm pack. It should be just large enough to fill the nasopharynx snugly. A soft rubber catheter is passed through each nostril until both tips are seen in the pharynx. These tips are then grasped with forceps and pulled just outside the mouth while two of the strings are quickly attached, one to each catheter tip. By pulling on the nasal ends of both catheters, the pack is raised up into the nasopharynx and tightly secured by tying the two strings over a small sponge at the nasal columella (Fig. 4). The uvula should not be caught by the pack or troublesome edema will result. The third string is tied to a piece of adhesive attached to the cheek and will assist in removal of the pack a few hours later.

With the postnasal pack tightly occluding the nasopharynx, there is always the danger of potential airway obstruction unless the tongue and jaws are constantly in proper position. This danger can be completely eliminated by the insertion of a flexible endotracheal tube along the floor of the nose with its tip just visible below the uvula, but extending beyond the pack. The external end of the tube may be cut off close to the nares and the intranasal tube fixed by tape to the upper lip. This procedure may be a life-saver if the patient should change his position when temporarily unattended.

A tonsil bleeder may stop when the clot is removed and a sponge moistened with xylocaine and epinephrine is held firmly against the fossa for a few minutes. A definite bleeding point may be sealed with a silver nitrate stick or a chromic acid bead. If this procedure is not successful, the bleeder may be snapped and tied with 000 plain catgut, as during the original operative procedure.

Chapter Ninety-Six

PHARYNGEAL INFECTIONS

HENRY G. CRAMBLETT, M.D.,
and
CHARLES F. FERGUSON, M.D., F.A.C.S.

PHARYNGITIS AND TONSILLITIS

Although pharyngitis frequently heralds the onset of a biphasic illness in which the principal manifestation is aseptic meningitis, gastroenteritis or exanthem, this chapter will deal only with those infections in which the primary sites of infection are the pharynx and tonsillar areas.

Etiology

The principal bacterial cause of pharyngitis is group A *Streptococcus pyogenes* (Table 1). In the nonimmunized person, *Corynebacterium diphtheriae* causes sporadic cases of disease. In the debilitated patient or the patient with underlying disease, such as leukemia or cystic fibrosis of the pancreas, *Staphylococcus aureus* or *Diplococcus pneumoniae* may occasionally be recovered in pure culture from patients with a pseudomembranous type of tonsillitis. In the otherwise healthy child, these organisms are unlikely causes of primary pharyngitis.

Many viruses have been associated with pharyngitis, including adenoviruses, influenza viruses, Coxsackie viruses and parainfluenza viruses. Other viruses in which the proof of etiologic association is not conclusive include respiratory syncytial virus, rhinoviruses and reoviruses. Pharyngitis may occur early in the course of infectious mononucleosis, a disease that has been recently established as having a viral etiology.

Manifestations

From the clinical standpoint, in order to assess possible causation, it is helpful to divide pharyngitis into severe, moderate and mild categories, depending upon the presence of certain physical findings.

SEVERE PHARYNGITIS. Severe pharyngitis includes the unequivocal findings of fever, exudate, and erythema of the pharynx, or fever and erythema of the pharynx associated with a scarlatinal rash. Most studies indicate that about 90 per cent of the patients with severe pharyngitis who are older than 3 years have this disease as the result of infection by group A beta hemolytic strep-

TABLE 1. ETIOLOGIC CLASSIFICATION OF ACUTE TONSILLITIS AND PHARYNGITIS

Bacterial	Viral
Group A beta hemolytic streptococci	Adenoviruses
Corynebacterium diphtheriae	Coxsackie viruses
Staphylococcus aureus and *Diplococcus pneumoniae* (rare)	Infectious mononucleosis
	Influenza viruses
	Parainfluenza viruses
	Reoviruses (?)
	Respiratory syncytial virus (?)
	Rhinoviruses (?)

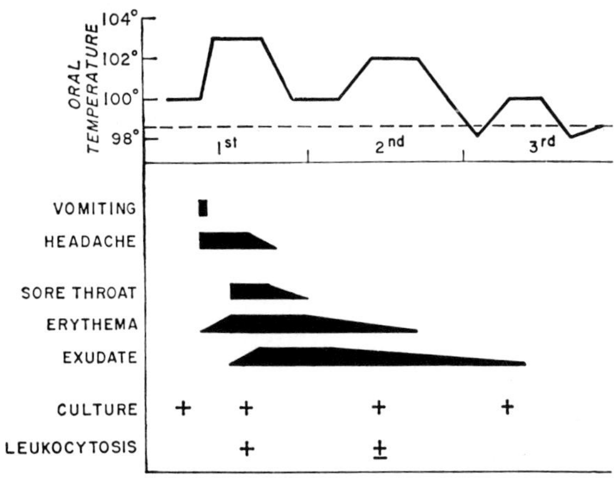

Figure 1. Typical clinical pattern of streptococcal pharyngitis in school-age children. (From Moffet, H. L., Cramblett, H. G., and Smith, A.: Group A streptococcal infections in a children's home. II. Clinical and epidemiologic patterns of illness. *Pediatrics, 33*:11, 1964.)

tococci. It is usual for the exudate to appear after the onset of erythema or the actual complaint of sore throat (Fig. 1). Early in the course of streptococcal pharyngitis, the younger patient may complain of headache accompanied by vomiting before the obvious signs of severe pharyngitis are present. Therefore, the likelihood of the presence of the aforementioned signs depends upon how early in the illness the patient is seen. The peripheral white blood cell count is usually elevated during the first two days of illness. Other physical findings suggestive of a streptococcal etiology include edema and petechiae of the soft palate and uvula and tender, enlarged tonsillar lymph nodes.

MODERATE PHARYNGITIS. In moderate pharyngitis there are two of the three characteristics of fever, erythema and exudate. From the etiologic standpoint, approximately 50 per cent of the patients with moderate pharyngitis have this disease as a result of infection with group A beta hemolytic streptococci, and in the other 50 per cent the disease is caused by a virus. Factors favoring a viral origin of moderate pharyngitis include a normal white blood cell count, absence of regional lymphadenopathy, and the presence of hoarseness and rhinitis. Hoarseness rarely if ever occurs in streptococcal infections. Moreover, in viral pharyngitis (with the exception of infectious mononucleosis) there is usually little or no edema of the soft palate.

MILD PHARYNGITIS. Mild pharyngitis is defined as the subjective complaint of sore throat or evidence of mild pharyngeal erythema on physical examination, without fever or exudate. Such patients commonly have minor complaints of cough or rhinorrhea. From the etiologic standpoint, at least 85 to 90 per cent of the cases of mild pharyngitis is due to a virus. There is nothing clinically distinguishable between mild pharyngitis due to one virus from that due to another, except in herpangina caused by Coxsackie A viruses; in this disease vesicular or ulcerated lesions may be present in the pharynx.

Table 2 lists the diagnoses in school-age children from whose throat cultures 10 colonies or more of group A beta hemolytic streptococci were recovered. It should be stressed that in younger children there may be an undifferentiated febrile illness due to streptococcal infections in which there are no signs or symptoms of pharyngitis. In the study from which the data in Table 2 were derived, it was concluded that the carrier rate of streptococci in the children studied was approximately 10 per cent. Hence, those diseases from which 10 per cent or less of the positive cultures were obtained probably have no etiologic importance.

Diagnosis

Since the only significant bacteriologic cause of pharyngitis is group A *Strep-*

TABLE 2. DIAGNOSES ASSOCIATED WITH RECOVERY OF MORE THAN 10 COLONIES OF GROUP A BETA HEMOLYTIC STREPTOCOCCI

Clinical Diagnosis	Children (no.)	Positive Cultures (no.)	Positive Cultures (%)
Pharyngitis, severe	99	87	88
Pharyngitis, moderate	83	44	53
Undifferentiated febrile illness	46	13	23
Acute otitis media	33	5	15
Pharyngitis, mild	65	8	12
Headache only	30	3	10
Vomiting without fever	88	9	10
Vomiting with fever	34	3	9
Nausea	24	2	8
Bronchitis or pneumonia	27	2	7
Febrile rhinitis	16	1	6
Other*	51*	3	6
Other*	51*	3	6
Diarrhea	23	1	4
Cough only or rhinitis	73	2	3
	692	182	

*Other: otitis externa, 16; laryngitis, 11; conjunctivitis, 10; asthma, 5; sinusitis, 3; urinary tract infections, 3; herpes simplex, 2; arthralgia, 1.

tococcus pyogenes, a precise diagnosis may be made by culture of the pharynx. A dry swab may be rubbed over the tonsillar and pharyngeal areas and then plated on 5 per cent sheep blood agar. Although immediate plating of the specimen is optimum, it has been shown that swabs taken in this manner may be kept in a tightly stoppered container overnight in the refrigerator or at room temperature and plated the following morning. The characteristic beta hemolytic streptococcal colonies can be recognized with a little practice. In order to assure that the beta hemolytic streptococcus is indeed group A, the organism may be subcultured onto a plate containing a bacitracin disk. At least 95 per cent of group A beta hemolytic streptococci are sensitive to bacitracin, whereas other beta hemolytic streptococci are usually resistant.

Prognosis

It has been demonstrated that patients with streptococcal pharyngitis need not be treated immediately in order to prevent the complication of rheumatic fever. As a matter of fact, if therapy is instituted within six days after the onset of symptoms of streptococcal pharyngitis, there will be ample time to prevent this complication in most patients. Under any circumstance, the efficacy of antibiotic therapy in preventing post-streptococcal nephritis is much less. Figure 1 presents a diagrammatic representation of the typical clinical pattern of streptococcal pharyngitis in school-age children. Many patients improve rapidly and are well within 24 hours without specific antibiotic therapy.

Treatment

If cultures are not obtained for the purpose of therapy, all patients with severe pharyngitis should be considered to have streptococcal infection. As indicated, of those with moderate pharyngitis, approximately one-half will have disease caused by streptococci, and in the other one-half, disease will be the result of virus infection. It is usually impossible to differentiate between these two groups, and unless throat cultures or leukocyte counts are available to aid in differentiation, they should probably all be treated as if they are caused by the streptococcus. Those patients with mild pharyngitis who do not have throat cultures should be considered to have virus infection and not be subjected to treatment.

For those patients who are not allergic to penicillin, this antibiotic is the agent of choice for the treatment of streptococcal pharyngitis. One of the two following regimens may be chosen for the treatment of streptococcal pharyngitis: (1) oral administration of penicillin, 400,000 units (250 mg.) three times daily for 10 days, or (2) intramuscular injection of benzathine penicillin, 600,000 units for children under 6 years of age, 900,000 units between 6 and 9 years, and 1.2 million units over 9 years of age.

In order to achieve a rapid level of penicillin in the blood and therefore more rapid clinical improvement, administration of three doses of an oral penicillin such as phenoxymethyl penicillin in the amount of 200,000 units each may be given to those patients receiving benzathine penicillin. Of the two regimens, the one utilizing benzathine penicillin is preferable. The only disadvantage is that an injection must be given, which is sometimes painful. With the oral regimen the child improves rapidly, and there is a tendency for the parent to disregard the instructions to administer the 10 days of therapy necessary to completely eradicate streptococci and to prevent recurrence of the streptococcal infection.

If the patient is allergic to penicillin, erythromycin may be given. Erythromycin estolate given in doses of 10 to 20 mg. per kilogram per day for 10 days has been shown to produce results comparable to those achieved with a 10-day course of phenoxymethyl penicillin.

DIPHTHERIA

Diphtheria today is a rare disease, but it must always be considered in any acute or subacute throat infection, especially when a membrane is present. In recent years, however, more than sporadic cases are being encountered. Proper and prompt treatment of this infection early in its course is imperative in order to prevent serious complications, such as postdiphtheritic paralysis or myocarditis. The history of a negative Schick test is not always reliable, since "permanent" immunity may have run out. If the patient then comes in contact with a particularly virulent organism, he may contract the disease. Diphtheria has a short incubation period of only two to five days.

The presenting symptom is sore throat, ordinarily not as severe as in scarlet fever or other streptococcal infections. Fever usually is low-grade and rarely goes above 101 degrees, although the pulse rate may be proportionately much more rapid. This low-grade temperature elevation and soreness of the throat persist for several days, along with increasing swelling of the anterior cervical nodes. Associated symptoms are headache, nausea with occasional vomiting, increasing toxemia, general malaise and (very rarely) chills.

Examination of the throat shows a very characteristic coalescent, dirty-gray membrane over the tonsils, extending also over the pillars, or even onto the soft palate. At first this soft white coating may resemble ordinary cryptic exudate, but within a day or two it forms a tough, dirty membrane. When this membrane is traumatized with a culture swab, it bleeds and leaves an oozing raw base. It is a firm, fibrinous structure and will rapidly reform over the bleeding surface if removed. This membrane has a characteristic musty odor, and older practitioners could make a diagnosis merely by "sniffing" the patient. Ulcerations are not common and sloughing to any great extent is never encountered.

Direct cultures should always be obtained for routine studies and also for incubation on a Klebs-Loeffler medium, and smears should immediately be stained and examined for the specific organism. If at first diphtheroids are reported, further investigation must always be carried out, using various sugar media to determine whether the organism is actually *C. diphtheriae*. This should always be accompanied by a virulence test performed by injection into a guinea pig.

Meanwhile, as the diagnosis is being made in the laboratory, the patient should be completely isolated because of the contagiousness of this disease. If there is any clinical suspicion, or certainly if the smears are questionable, the patient should be promptly treated with specific diphtheria antitoxin to neutralize any circulating toxin already produced by this particular organism. Otherwise, late complications of a serious nature may ensue before the correct diagnosis has become definite. It is unfortunate that penicillin, the commonest antibiotic used in throat infections today, may be fairly effective in relieving symptoms and eradicating the organisms, thereby ruining a later culture and the chance of proper diagnosis. However, penicillin is totally ineffective against the circulating diphtheria *toxin.* If diphtheria antitoxin is used, penicillin is not necessary, but may be employed to prevent secondary infection. Twenty thousand to thirty thousand units of diphtheria antitoxin are usually given intramuscularly after a skin test is done for possible allergy. The patient must always be observed for need for possible tracheotomy until the membrane has been removed or coughed out. In 15 to 20 per cent of cases, temporary postdiphtheritic paralysis of the soft palate or muscles of the larynx, eye, diaphragm or extremities may ensue, or the more serious complication of diphtheritic myocarditis may develop. This could be a fatal complication.

SCARLET FEVER

Scarlet fever (scarlatina) is a disease due to group A beta hemolytic streptococcus infection in which an erythrogenic toxin is elaborated. The exotoxin liberated by the particular strain of this organism produces a characteristic punctiform scarlet blush more evident in the skin folds, but still generalized over the entire body. It is a diffuse erythematous rash, appearing ordinarily in 24 to 48 hours of the onset of an acute sore throat. Circumoral pallor is ordinarily noted, swallowing is difficult because of the inflammation, and there is toxemia, high fever, headache, vomiting and occasionally chills. However, depending on the degree of immunity of the patient to the streptococcus, these symptoms may be lessened. An incubation period of two to five days is usual.

Examination discloses a diffuse punctate rash over the palate, and the tonsils and pharynx show an acute inflammatory reaction. There may be whitish exudate in the crypts of the tonsils, and the tongue shows enlarged, red papillae, producing the characteristic "strawberry tongue." The anterior cervical lymph nodes, especially at the angle of the jaw, are enlarged and tender. Direct throat cultures and smears are positive for the group A beta hemolytic streptococcus, unless the patient has been treated with proper antibiotics immediately preceding the taking of the culture. The Dick test (an intradermal injection of dilute scarlet fever streptococcus toxin) will give a positive skin reaction, but is seldom used today, as most antibiotics are so effective for treatment.

Penicillin in full doses (as described for streptococcal infections without scarlet fever) is specific for the disease, and the clinical response is usually rapid and complete. On occasion, however, the patient may become a streptococcus carrier in spite of prolonged and adequate antibiotic therapy and tonsillectomy may then be indicated. Before the advent of antibiotics, scarlet fever resulted in many serious complications, such as glomerulonephritis, otitis media and severe destructive mastoiditis. These complications today are very rare if treatment is prompt and thorough.

VINCENT'S ANGINA

Sometimes a differential diagnosis of the sore throat of acute tonsillitis, agranulocytosis, herpetic infection or Vincent's angina is difficult to make on inspection alone, since all of these conditions may produce ulcerations or membranes. Poor oral hygiene, neglected teeth in older patients, and general lowered resistance to infection are contributing factors. In Vincent's angina, a dirty, grayish yellow membrane covers the tonsils or fossae and on occasion even the palate, and the underlying tissues show a bleeding tendency when the false membrane is removed. Removal, however, is much easier than when dealing with a diphtheritic membrane, since it is not so adherent. In Vincent's angina there are usually deep, sharply punched out ulcerations with a surrounding band of inflammation and edema, and there is considerable sloughing.

Presenting symptoms are sore throat, dysphagia, excessive salivation, cervical glandular enlargement and a characteristic odor to the breath. The submaxillary nodes are particularly involved. The ulcerative lesions are seen on the mucous membrane of the pharynx, as well as of the tonsils, and often on the gingival and buccal membranes, producing gingivitis and stomatitis as well. Fever is usually low-grade, but in a patient who is particularly toxic it may be high, and it is accompanied by associated headaches.

Cultures show a combination of a fusiform bacillus and a characteristic long, thin spirochete. There are many differences of opinion as to whether these organisms (which are sometimes found in the normal mouth) are the causative agents of this disease. When they are found in symbiosis, however, the diagnosis is most probable. It has also been suggested that Vincent's angina may be due to an anaerobic streptococcus.

Penicillin for a week or 10 days is usually effective, as are the tetracyclines and other broad-spectrum antibiotics. Oxidizing agents, such as hydrogen peroxide, diluted 1 to 1, and used as a gargle, or sodium perborate applied locally as a moist paste several times a day gives a good result. Formerly, 10 per cent silver nitrate, 10 per cent copper sulfate and Salvarsan in glycerine were favorites for local therapy. The disease is self-limited, but highly contagious, and deserves adequate precautions as well as proper treatment.

FUNGUS INFECTIONS

In the very young child, fungus infections of the mouth and pharynx are frequent. Some of these infections follow delivery if the mother has had a recent vaginitis due to the Candida organisms. If this infection in the mother is noted before delivery, it should be treated vigorously to prevent its being passed on to the baby at birth. Poor hygiene in the newborn, along with improper sterilization of nipples or bottles, may lead to rapid spread of this infection throughout the nursery. Fortunately, today most of the supplies are prepackaged, so sterility is more certain. In older children, orally administered antibiotics may disturb the normal flora of the mouth and allow the ever-present fungi to overgrow. Thrush, due to *Candida albicans,* is manifested by small, white, curdlike patches or plaques adherent to the gums, buccal mucosa, tongue, lips or pharynx. Moniliasis may involve the entire respiratory tract, and often the gastrointestinal tract becomes infected. Improvement here is slow, and long courses of therapy are necessary to relieve these troublesome symptoms.

Treatment consists of elimination of the oral antibiotics if they are the cause, and the local use of 1 per cent aqueous gentian violet is a time-honored remedy. However, this is a messy type of therapy and is not as effective as mycostatin used by dropping 1 ml. of an aqueous suspension (containing 100,000 units per ml.) into the mouth four or five times a day for 10 days, and continuing for three or four days after the lesions have disappeared. Rather than using drops, the mycostatin solution may be applied locally by swabs. Recurrences, however, are frequent, and long-continued therapy may be necessary.

REFERENCES

Moffet, H. L., Cramblett, H. G., and Black, J. P.: Group A streptococcal infections in a children's home. 1. Evaluation of practical bacteriologic methods. *Pediatrics, 33*:5, 1964.

Moffet, H. L., Cramblett, H. G., and Smith, A.: Group A streptococcal infections in a children's home. 2. Clinical and epidemiologic patterns of illness. *Pediatrics, 33*:11, 1964.

Chapter Ninety-Seven

PHARYNGEAL ABSCESSES

CHARLES F. FERGUSON, M.D., F.A.C.S.

RETROPHARYNGEAL ABSCESS

The common throat abscess in infancy and very early childhood is the acute retropharyngeal abscess. This condition is very rare after 2 to 3 years of age, but even in this age group it is now much less common than in former years. Early in life the potential retropharyngeal spaces (of Gilette) on either side of the midline of the posterior pharyngeal and nasopharyngeal wall, lying between the posterior wall and the aponeurosis of the cervical prevertebral fascia (C_2 and C_3), contain several lymph nodes ("glands of Henle"). These nodes are present at birth, but tend to disappear usually by 2 or 3 years of age. Lymphatic drainage from the posterior nasal passages, the nasopharynx and the eustachian tube areas is received by these nodes. They are located just lateral to the midline, because the prevertebral fascia and posterior pharyngeal wall are adherent down the midline of the pharynx. Following an upper respiratory infection or acute pharyngitis, especially the type resulting from the group A beta hemolytic streptococcus, these nodes may become infected and enlarged. If this infection is not controlled, the nodes very often break down, rupture and extrude pus into the loose areolar tissues of the retropharyngeal spaces. Occasionally, an acute retropharyngeal abscess may result from trauma, such as an accidental perforation of the posterior pharyngeal wall, or from an embedded foreign body.

Symptoms are high fever, rapid pulse, and stridor on both inspiration and expiration. There is also considerable dyspnea from airway obstruction, as well as dysphagia and even refusal to swallow. Considerable toxemia is ordinarily present, and the infant is extremely irritable and restless from pain and obstruction. He lies with his head hyperextended (sometimes in true opisthotonus) in order to obtain a better airway, especially if the abscess is down near the larynx. There is no trismus in a retropharyngeal abscess, which is a characteristic finding in the true peritonsillar abscess. Respirations are labored, rattling and gurgling, as excessive mucus keeps accumulating in the mouth and pharynx. Severe respiratory obstruction may occur, especially if the abscess is located in the hypopharyngeal region. Rupture may result in aspiration of pus, with flooding of the tracheobronchial tree, serious pulmonary infection or asphyxia.

An abscess in the nasopharynx with considerable obstruction may be manifested by a marked bulging of the soft palate. The round, firm, red bulging mass on the posterior wall, just slightly lateral to the midline, is usually easily visualized simply with a tongue depressor, since the mouth can be easily opened. In the early stages of cellulitis, however, before suppuration has occurred, the diagnosis may be obscure. Digital palpation of any throat abscess in order to determine fluctuation may be fraught with danger, unless the patient is examined in Trendelenburg position and with suction readily available in case of rupture. A lateral roentgenogram may be helpful in diagnosis, but this should always be taken during inspiration with the head extended, since films in expiration may give an erroneous impression of the thickness of the posterior pharyngeal wall ("phantom masses") (Fig. 1).

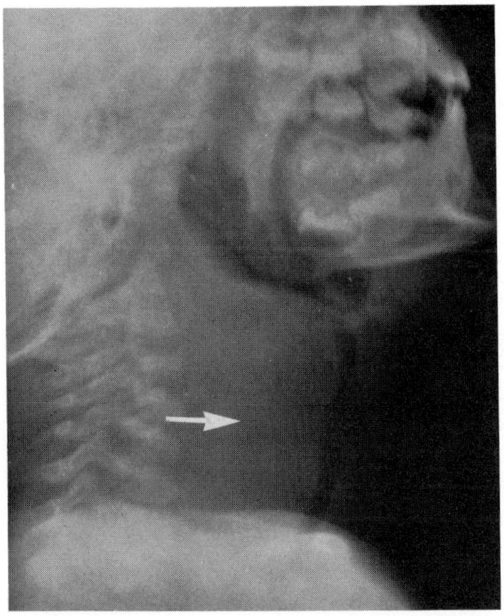

Figure 1. X-ray of retropharyngeal abscess. (Courtesy of Dr. John Kirkpatrick.)

Treatment of retropharyngeal cellulitis or adenitis consists of adequate antibiotic therapy, preferably with parenteral penicillin or ampicillin in high doses. In most instances today this therapy alone is effective. Local treatments, such as the use of gargles or throat irrigations, are not necessary or even practical in infants. If or when fluctuation occurs, however, surgical drainage is indicated. Anesthesia is ordinarily not advisable or necessary, and simple incision and drainage of the abscess can easily be performed with the baby wrapped in a blanket. Formerly it was recommended that a quick incision be made with the infant in a sitting position, immediately inverting him for drainage. A preferable method is to start with him in extreme Trendelenburg position and with strong suction in hand. A vertical incision is made over the most fluctuant area, and then quickly spread deeper with a hemostat, constantly aspirating the pus and other secretions (Fig. 2). Care must be taken not to make too deep an initial incision. Since no drains are used, another spreading of the incision may be indicated in a day or two if the fullness does not completely subside. If general anesthesia is employed, an endotracheal tube should always be carefully introduced beforehand, but this procedure in itself may be dangerous.

If inadequately treated, infection may

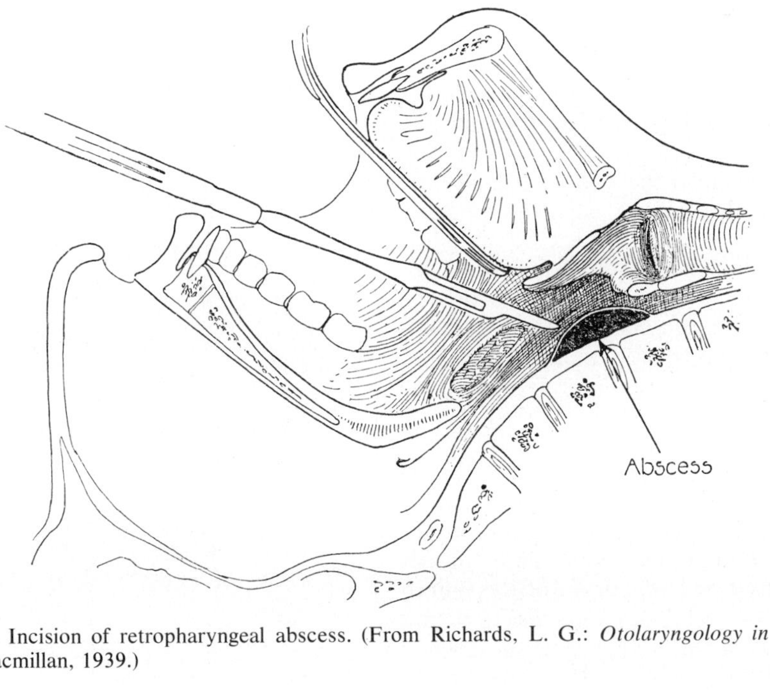

Figure 2. Incision of retropharyngeal abscess. (From Richards, L. G.: *Otolaryngology in General Practice*, Macmillan, 1939.)

extend laterally into the pharyngomaxillary space by rupture of a thin dividing membrane, or even descend down around the esophagus into the posterior mediastinum. External rupture has also occurred behind the sternocleidomastoid muscle at the angle of the jaw. Serious recurring hemorrhage has on rare occasions also been reported.

A retropharyngeal swelling in an older child today suggests foreign body or trauma. In former years, tuberculosis of the cervical spine always had to be considered, as did tuberculous adenitis of the upper deep cervical chain which was even more common. This was before the days of pasteurization of milk, when bovine tuberculosis was an ever-present problem.

PERITONSILLAR ABSCESS

The true peritonsillar abscess ("Quinsy sore throat"), which is the commonest abscess of adults, is rare in children under 10 to 12 years of age. It is almost nonexistent in infants. In this condition, pus localizes in the supratonsillar region in the loose areolar tissue between the tonsil and the muscle wall. It is actually an abscess located in the soft palate itself. It may follow acute tonsillitis (especially that due to the group A beta hemolytic streptococcus) or may extend from behind an infected, adherent tonsil remnant if the patient has already had a tonsillectomy.

After the original attack of tonsillitis seems to have improved, especially if antibiotic therapy is inadequate in dosage or given over too short a period, a sudden rise in temperature and pulse occurs, along with severe unilateral pain in the throat. This pain frequently radiates to the ipsilateral ear. Because of the proximity of the pterygoid muscles, severe trismus develops and the patient cannot open his mouth sufficiently for a proper examination. Excessive saliva drools constantly from the corner of the mouth in these miserable, anxious and toxic patients. Dyspnea is apparent, the speech is very thick and muffled, and the breath is foul. Externally in the neck there are enlarged tender nodes and the neck itself is stiff; the head is usually held toward the affected side (torticollis). If the mouth can be opened even a little, it will be seen that the pharynx is very asymmetrical, with a very edematous uvula displaced almost to the opposite tonsil by a bright red bulging of the supratonsillar area of the palate, almost obscuring the tonsil itself. (Fig. 3). If fluctuation is present, a tiny yellow area may be seen over the most bulging portion. This abscess may rupture into the throat, or laterally through the superior constrictor muscle into the parapharyngeal space, and then downward into the medias-

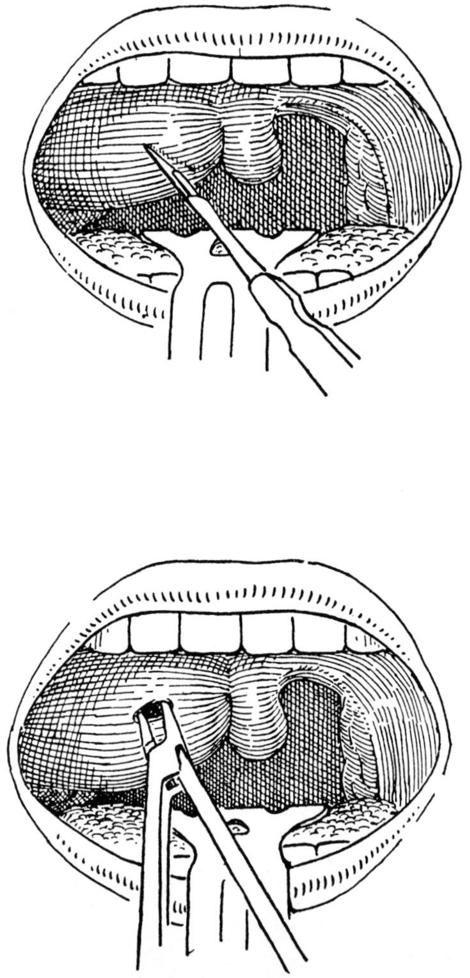

Figure 3. Peritonsillar abscess, incised. (From Richards, L. G.: *Otolaryngology in General Practice*, Macmillan, 1939.)

tinum through a continuing pathway that Mosher used to term the "Lincoln Highway of the neck."

Treatment consists of the parenteral use of large doses of penicillin or ampicillin, warm throat irrigations if possible, hot compresses to the neck, and analgesics for pain and apprehension, followed by surgical incision and drainage of the abscess if and when it becomes fluctuant. This is best performed under local anesthesia or possibly endotracheal general anesthesia. In children, however, a suspected peritonsillar abscess usually is found to be a lateral pharyngeal abscess.

LATERAL PHARYNGEAL ABSCESS

Lateral pharyngeal abscess is the common throat abscess of childhood, much as the retropharyngeal abscess is the common abscess of infancy. As the name implies, the localization is deep in the lateral pharyngeal wall, posterior to the fossa and pillars, although the entire tonsil, soft palate and uvula may be considerably displaced medially, and the pharynx presents an asymmetrical appearance somewhat similar to that of peritonsillar abscess. The tonsil and supratonsillar region, however, are not involved in the swelling, and trismus from spasm of the pterygoid muscles is absent, so the mouth is easily opened. It is the entire pharyngeal wall that is displaced medially, and the swelling is localized *behind* the posterior pillar rather than in the palate. There is usually considerable acute cervical adenitis as well.

Since most abscesses of the throat are caused by the group A beta hemolytic streptococcus, the drug of choice is penicillin G or ampicillin, unless individual sensitivity contraindicates its use. The drug should be given parenterally at first and continued in full doses for at least 10 days. Frequently warm saline irrigations to localize the infection and hot compresses externally to the involved side of the neck are comforting in older children, but not generally tolerated by youngsters. Aspirin or Tylenol will help to alleviate the discomfort and fever. A culture should be taken and sensitivity tests are also performed. If a resistant *Staphylococcus aureus* is the causative organism, methicillin or sodium oxacillin should be prescribed instead of penicillin. As in the retropharyngeal abscess, most of the time satisfactory resolution will occur, but occasionally, if there has been inadequate or tardy treatment, incision and drainage will be necessary. If general anesthesia is used, the abscess should be evacuated with the patient in the Trendelenburg position, and under endotracheal intubation. Adequate suction should always be available, along with an anterior commissure laryngoscope (already lighted) for possible aspiration of the trachea.

PARAPHARYNGEAL ABSCESS

It is fortunate that this is a relatively rare abscess, because the mortality is high. It follows extension of infection from the more superficial areas of the throat through the lateral pharyngeal wall and superior constrictor muscle into the parapharyngeal space, and frequently downward into the posterior mediastinum. The patient is very toxic, has a high fever and may even be in shock. Significant signs of airway obstruction are present. Harlowe stated that there were 25 deaths in 125 cases of such abscesses—a very high mortality. Incision of the abscess is usually carried out externally in the neck behind the sternocleidomastoid muscle, and a drain can be inserted here. Massive doses of penicillin or ampicillin should be employed, unless sensitivity tests decree otherwise, and continued for some time after the abscess has healed in order to prevent a troublesome recurrence, which is not infrequent.

REFERENCE

Harlowe, H. D.: Complications following tonsillectomy. *Laryngoscope, 58*:861, 1948.

Chapter Ninety-Eight

PHARYNGEAL MANIFESTATIONS OF SYSTEMIC DISEASE

CHARLES F. FERGUSON, M.D., F.A.C.S.

AGRANULOCYTOSIS

This disease is relatively rare in infants and children, but today it is being seen more commonly as increasingly potent drugs are being used. A sore throat with visible exudate, membrane formation or ulceration and high fever may not indicate an acute infectious process, but rather lead to suspicion of a generalized systemic disease.

The first manifestation of agranulocytosis is often a sore throat suggesting acute pharyngitis or tonsillitis. Unless a blood examination is performed, the correct diagnosis will be missed. The mouth, tongue, pharynx and tonsils may show a grayish-white or yellowish exudate, similar to that of Vincent's or another exudative throat infection. Later on, this area may become necrotic, mucosal hemorrhages are frequent, and glandular enlargement is common. Severe deep pain as well as pain on swallowing occurs and dysphagia is a presenting symptom. The patient is usually very toxic and prostrated, even though the fever may be only slight. In fulminating cases, however, fever may be very high and unresponsive to antibiotics, and severe chills may occur. In contrast to the lesions in Vincent's infection, there is rarely a surrounding red, inflammatory reaction, although ulceration may be extensive and the mucosal areas may be diffusely involved. The pathologic mechanism here is more a sloughing of tissues rather than inflammation.

This serious disease is due to depression of the granulocytic series of white blood cells, manifested in the peripheral blood and bone marrow as well, with a granulocytic leukopenia of 2000 cells or less. Although the nucleated cells and myeloid elements in the bone marrow are depressed, the red cell precursors and megakaryocytes are usually normal. This signifies a toxic bone marrow depression, frequently following sensitization to certain drugs, especially those with a benzine ring, such as aminopyrine, some of the sulfanilamides, chloramphenicol, penicillamine, and occasionally some of the antihistamines.

After discontinuation of any offending drug, large doses of antibiotics are usually effective in preventing secondary infection, which is the serious complication. This allows the myeloid tissue to regenerate. In some patients transfusions are indicated. The course may be shortened and symptoms minimized by the use of adrenocortical hormones or even splenectomy. Pentnucleotide, liver extract, vitamins and extract of bone marrow have all been used with very questionable benefit. Removal of the underlying causative agent is the most important part of treatment, along with antibiotic and adrenocorticoid therapy.

ACUTE INFECTIOUS MONONUCLEOSIS

This is an acute systemic infectious disease, presumably due to a herpetic type of virus. It is usually first manifested by pharyngeal symptoms, and occurs for the most part in young adults as "glandular fever." It is recognized not infrequently in children, and has been seen as early as the first year of life, once confirmed by laboratory studies at 6 months of age. It is relatively contagious and may spread rapidly through schools or other institutions. The virus probably enters through the nasopharynx. Fever, usually to 103° or 104°, is common, and headache, general malaise, and muscular aches are marked as the sore throat develops into an acute tonsillitis or pharyngitis. Fever may persist for a week or 10 days, or even longer, before the diagnosis is suspected. Occasionally, chills are encountered, and excessive perspiration is common.

Small patches of superficial exudate may be noted. Occasionally, even membrane formation with superficial ulceration is found, but there is no underlying bleeding surface, as in diphtheria. Early in the course of the disease, the cervical glands become enlarged or tender, especially in the posterior chains, and this is followed by a generalized lymphadenopathy, including enlargement of the liver and spleen. The spleen may even rupture. Jaundice may develop on rare occasions, and this ordinarily indicates hepatitis. There may be an abnormal Bromsulphalein retention. A generalized purpuric type of rash may be noted. The lymphoid structures of the throat are markedly enlarged, including sometimes tremendous swelling of the adenoid tissue, completely closing off the nasopharynx.

Blood studies by the fourth or fifth day should show a high white blood cell count, with a preponderance of large atypical lymphocytes and monocytes in the peripheral blood (up to 70 per cent). The abnormal large lymphocytes are characteristic of the disease and may persist for 10 days; they comprise up to 20 per cent of the circulating lymphocytes. On rare occasions there may be a leukopenia as well as an anemia. Early in the disease, the relatively simple spot test is positive. By the second or third week, the Paul-Bunnell heterophile agglutination test becomes positive (1 to 30 or more), and may remain positive for weeks, then returning to a normal level (1 to 14 or less) in 8 to 10 weeks. In 1965, Hoff and Bauer developed a simpler test that uses heat-inactivated serum from patients. In mononucleosis, the serum agglutinates horse red cells treated with formalin. Sedimentation rate is elevated and the SGOT may also be elevated.

The disease usually persists for several weeks and recovery is slow, although serious complications are rare. Relapses, however, are frequent. Supportive and systemic treatment only is indicated, and antibiotic therapy should be reserved for the rare bacterial complications, such as a streptococcal throat infection. Throat irrigations are helpful and the ice collar diminishes discomfort. Corticosteroids may shorten the period of indisposition, but routine use of these drugs in this otherwise self-limited disease is open to question. Complications, however, may include hemolytic anemia, thrombocytopenic purpura, and on rare occasions, myocarditis or orchitis in the older patient.

ACUTE LEUKEMIA

Examination of the pharynx may give the first clue to this serious systemic blood disease. The acute pharyngeal symptoms are often confused with the sore throat, fever and cervical adenitis of an ordinary bacterial infection, but ulcerations of the tonsils or pillars may quickly become apparent. The oral and gingival mucous membranes may show similar ulcerations not unlike those seen in agranulocytosis. There is a foul odor to the breath, nosebleeds are common, and persistent bleeding from any mucosal surface may occur. The mucosa is very pale. The cervical lymph nodes are swollen, and the spleen and liver are unusually enlarged. Blood smears and white blood cell counts will usually provide the diagnosis, but bone marrow puncture is always indicated. This disease should be suspected when an apparently ordinary acute throat infection fails to respond properly to treatment. The white blood cell count is usually very high, except in aleukemic stages. The peripheral blood smear shows typical myeloblasts, lymphoblasts or monoblasts, depending upon the type of leukemia, and there is inevitably an associated anemia and thrombocytopenic purpura.

At present, various chemotherapeutic agents consistently establish and prolong periods of remission, but so far the disease has always been fatal. Steroids have also been used, but the folic acid antagonist, Methotrexate (amethopterin), or the purine antagonist, 6-mercaptopurine (Purinethol), is much more effective in prolonging these periods of remission. Methotrexate is less toxic but has a wider margin of safety than the original aminopterin.

REFERENCES

Hoff, G., and Bauer, S.: A new rapid slide test for infectious mononucleosis. *J.A.M.A., 194*:351, 1965.

Selawry, O. S., et al.: New treatment schedule with improved survival in childhood leukemia. *J.A.M.A., 194*:75, 1965.

Smith, C. H.: *Blood Diseases of Infancy and Childhood.* St. Louis, C. V. Mosby Co., 1966.

SECTION XVI

HEAD AND NECK MASSES

Chapter Ninety-Nine

THE BRANCHIAL ARCHES–NORMAL DEVELOPMENT AND ABNORMALITIES

BURTON F. JAFFE, M.D.

NORMAL DEVELOPMENT

The branchial arch structures contribute greatly to the development of the head and neck region (Fig. 1). The human embryo has four well-developed arches and a fifth arch that is poorly defined. Arey calls this poorly defined arch number 5,[1] but Patten[2] calls it number 6 and Langman[3] states that number 5 does not develop. This confusion abounds in the literature. The arches appear as masses along the lateral side of the embryo in the lower head and

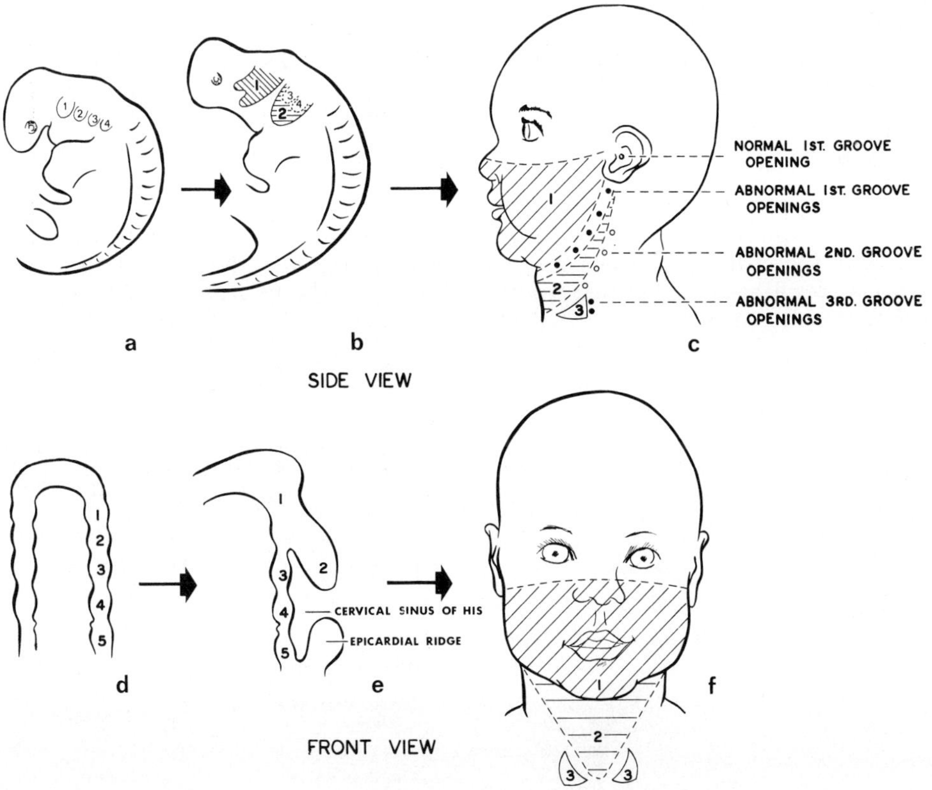

Figure 1. Normal and abnormal branchial arch development.

neck regions. The arches are separated externally by four grooves, also known as pharyngeal clefts. Inside the pharynx and opposite all four grooves is a pharyngeal pouch, but the fourth pouch is bilobed and therefore is referred to as the fourth and fifth pouches.

Our attention should be focused on the second branchial arch, because it grows more than the other arches and its migration is responsible for the production of many congenital anomalies associated with the branchial arches. The second arch is located at the side of the neck, and as it grows inferiorly it overlaps the third and fourth arches (Fig. 1 a and b), creating a space called the sinus of His (Fig. 1 e). Then it migrates anteriorly toward the midline of the neck and fuses with the opposite second arch (Fig. 1 f). In a sense, the second arch usurps almost the entire external covering of the neck from all other arches. Anteriorly, the second arch fusion is related to the formation of the midline thyroglossal duct cyst and midline dermoid cyst. Laterally, the second arch creates the cervical sinus of His, which gives rise to branchial cleft sinuses, fistulae and cysts.

Ectoderm

The ectoderm over the arches becomes the skin of the lower face (arch 1) and the skin of the neck (arch 2), except for a small area of the lower neck (arch 3) (Fig. 1 c and d). *The ectoderm over the grooves* plays a smaller role in the mature fetus. Groove one becomes the external auditory canal and the epithelium of the tympanic membrane. The ectoderm of groove two, groove three, and groove four are normally obliterated as the ectoderm of arch two compresses the underlying arches.

Endoderm

The endoderm lining the branchial arches becomes the mucosa of the nasopharynx, oropharynx and hypopharynx (Fig. 2). *The endodermal lining of the pharyngeal pouches* develops into structures of the pharynx (Fig. 2) and into specific adult organs (Fig. 3).

Abnormal Groove-Pouch Development

In the developing human embryo, the grooves and pouches never communicate. Arch 2 grows inferiorly over the third and fourth arches, fuses with the epicardial ridge in the lower part of the neck, creates the cervical sinus of His, and obliterates the second, third and fourth grooves. Should this cervical sinus fail to obliterate, four types of anomalies can develop (Fig. 4). A *fistula* develops when no obliteration occurs and saliva can leak from the pharynx to the skin of the neck. An *external sinus* or *internal sinus* results from partial failure of obliteration of the sinus of His. A *cyst* develops when the epithelial lining of the cervical sinus of His fails to obliterate.

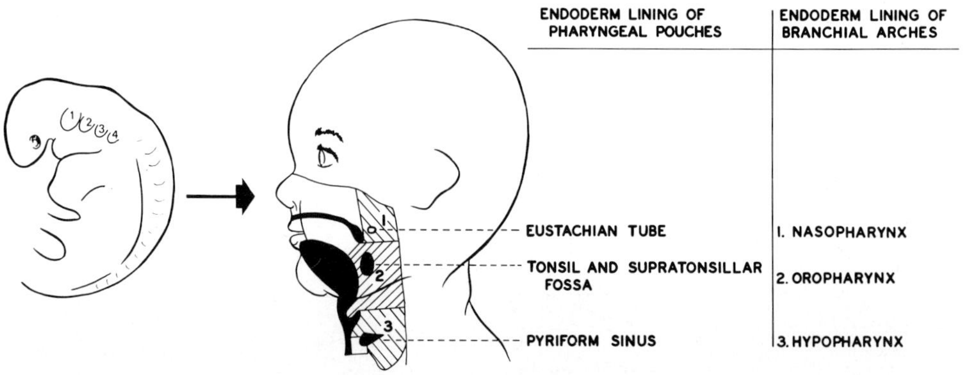

Figure 2. Endodermal derivations from the pharyngeal pouches and the branchial arches.

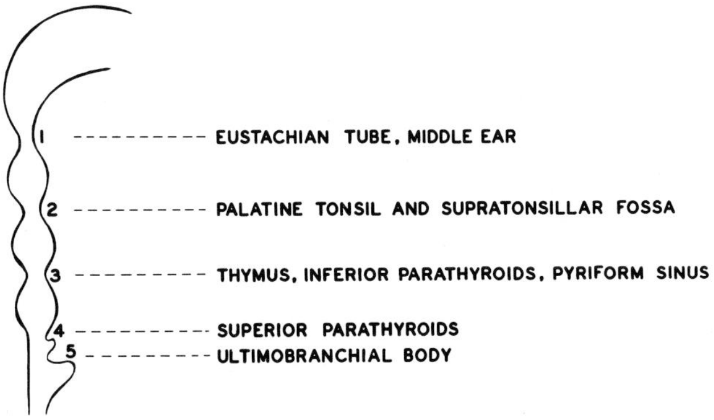

Figure 3. Endodermal derivatives from the pharyngeal pouches.

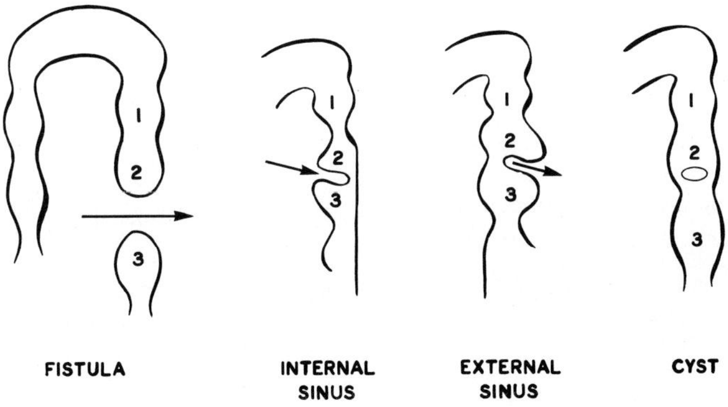

Figure 4. Abnormal branchial pouch–groove anomalies.

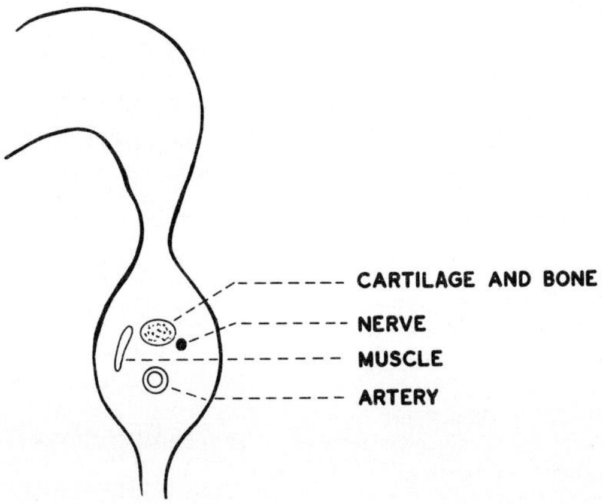

Figure 5. The basic components of the branchial arches.

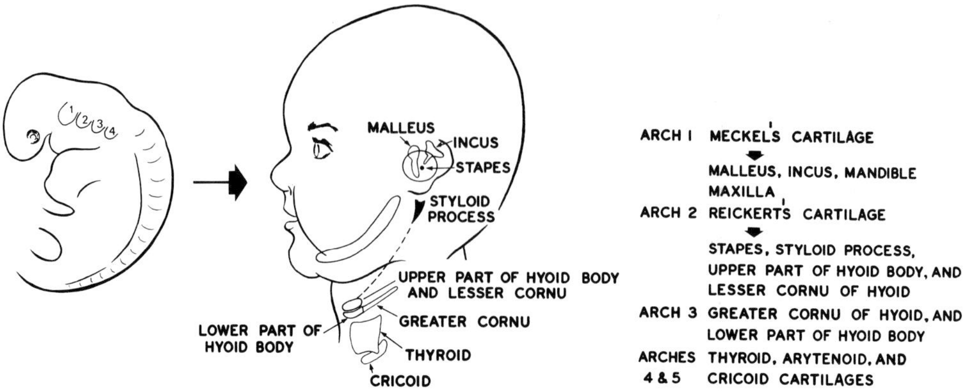

Figure 6. Structures derived from the branchial arches.

Branchial Arch Mass

Each branchial arch is composed of four structures: one set of cartilages and bones, one set of muscles, one cranial nerve and one aortic arch (Fig. 5).

Arch 1 divides into two cartilaginous processes (a smaller maxillary process and a larger mandibular process) and is quite prominent, since it contributes to the skeletal structure of the lower face. The other arches develop into much smaller structures (Fig. 6).

The muscles of each arch are listed in Table 1. Once again, arch 2 becomes of major importance. The muscles of facial expression develop from arch 2, and they must migrate from the neck along with the facial nerve to the face. In so doing, the facial nerve is pulled superior to the first branchial groove, and when a first branchial fistula develops, it will have a relationship to the facial nerve, lying medial or lateral to the facial nerve.

There is a cranial nerve associated with each branchial arch. These nerves are outgrowths from the brain and innervate the muscles derived from each arch (Fig. 7).

The single artery of each arch is called an aortic arch. There are a dorsal and a ventral component to each aortic arch, and all except a very few will disappear (Fig. 8).

TABLE 1. MUSCLES DERIVED FROM BRANCHIAL ARCHES

Arch	Muscles
Arch 1	Muscles of mastication (temporalis, masseter, pterygoids) Tensor veli palatini Tensor tympani Anterior belly of digastric
Arch 2	Posterior belly of digastric Muscles of facial expression Stapedius
Arch 3	Superior pharyngeal constrictor
Arch 4	Inferior pharyngeal constrictor Intrinsic laryngeal muscles

BRANCHIAL ARCH ANOMALIES

First Branchial Arch Anomalies

In conjunction with the frontonasal process, arch 1 anomalies will give rise to cleft lip and cleft palate (see Chapter 88). Arch 1 anomalies may also give rise to an abnormal pinna (see Chapter 67) or to a malformed malleus and incus, producing congenital conductive deafness. (see Chapter 69).

First Branchial Groove Anomalies

Anomalies of this groove are not common. Clinically, they present below the

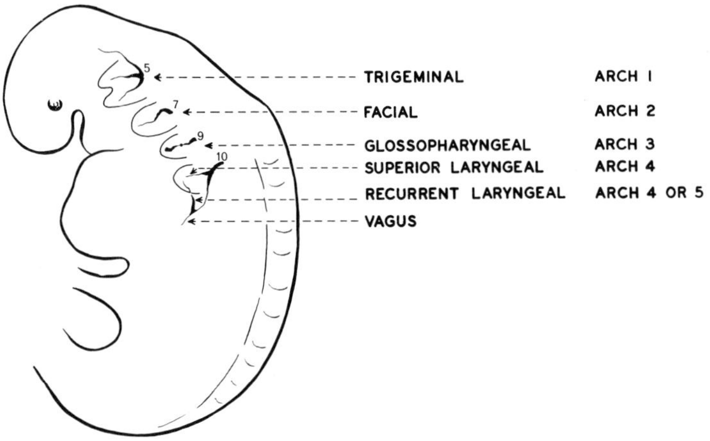

Figure 7. Cranial nerves associated with each branchial arch.

pinna, near the angle of the mandible, or along the lower border of the mandible into the submaxillary triangle. Anomalies present in three different ways. *An external sinus* may present as a pinpoint opening in the skin. The medial extension is variable, but it typically approaches the cartilage of the external auditory canal. Rarely, it may extend into the ear canal and be associated with drainage from the ear, or extend slightly posterior to the pinna and present as a cyst behind the pinna. (Note: The preauricular sinus is not a branchial arch derivative, but is derived from a malformation of the hillocks forming the pinna. The excision is relatively simple, since it extends from the helix to the periosteum of the temporal bone, and does not involve the facial nerve or parotid gland.) *A skin lesion,* like a birthmark, may be the only external evidence of a sinus tract. When activated by infection, however, the birthmark may convert to a draining sinus, revealing the true nature of this lesion. Treatment consists of antibiotics and heat during the acute stage. *A cyst* can develop below the pinna or in the submaxillary triangle. These usually become prominent during acute infections and are often confused with cervical adenitis or a suppurative node. Excision and drainage will only lead to a recurrence, since the cyst wall persists.

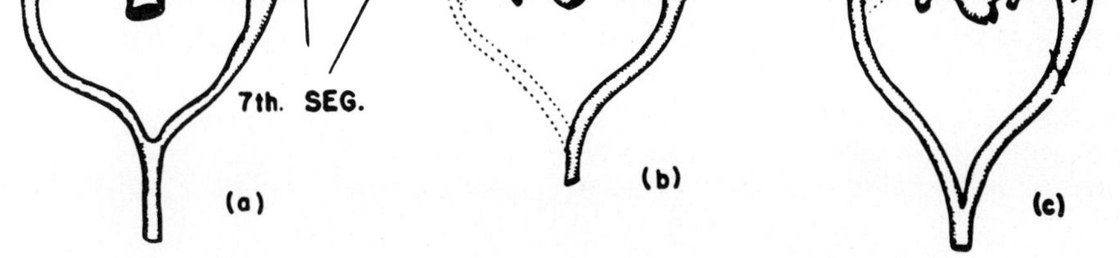

Figure 8. Development of the vasculature from the branchial arches.

Recurrent infection with or without drainage should alert one to a branchial cleft cyst.

OPERATIVE REMOVAL OF THE FIRST BRANCHIAL GROOVE EXTERNAL SINUS. The first groove sinus tract should be totally excised. An elliptical transverse incision is made around the sinus opening and along the lower border of the mandible, with an extension anterior to the pinna, ending at the top of the tragal cartilage. The tract can be identified by placing a small probe into it (Fig. 9) or by injecting diluted methylene blue through a polyethylene catheter into the tract. An anterior skin flap is elevated, exposing the parotid gland.

Wide exposure is often needed in cases with extensive fibrosis from prior infections, in order to facilitate exposure of the facial nerve. The surgeon must be prepared to dissect the facial nerve trunk and its bifurcation if intense fibrosis is present or if the tumor mass lies medial to the facial nerve. In more difficult cases with a deep-lying tract or cyst, resection of the tail of the parotid or even greater resection of portions of the parotid gland are necessary to allow for visualization. In these cases, the sinus tract is dissected up to the facial nerve, pushed under the facial nerve, and grasped from the superior aspect, as a pull-through technique. The tract is divided at the cartilaginous external ear canal, and the opening into the canal is sutured. A temporary weakness of the ramus mandibularis branch may occur as well as a total facial paralysis. A wound infection will occur if the lesion is excised during an inflammatory episode.

Pathologic examination reveals a tube lined with stratified squamous epithelium, hair follicles, sweat glands and sebaceous glands. Hyaline cartilage surrounds the tract, indicating a contribution from the surrounding branchial arches. Acute or chronic inflammatory infiltrates are also seen.

OPERATIVE REMOVAL OF FIRST BRANCHIAL CYSTS. A transverse incision with dissection of the cyst is performed, but one should look for a medial extension of the tract, which would take a course similar to that of the external sinus tract just described.

First Pharyngeal Pouch Anomalies

Anomalies of the eustachian tube have not been reported, although one would expect them to occur, especially in cleft palate patients.

Second Branchial Arch Anomalies

Of great interest to the otolaryngologist are the second branchial arch anomalies, such as the malformations of the stapes (see Chapter 69) and the mal-

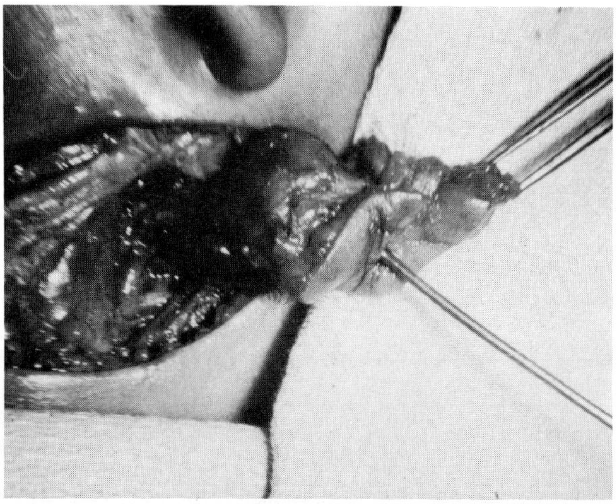

Figure 9. Surgical removal of a first branchial sinus tract.

formations of the pinna and external auditory canal leading to microtia and aural atresia (see Chapter 67).

DERMOID CYSTS. These develop when the second branchial arch fuses in the midline anteriorly, and traps epithelium in the midline below the surface of the skin. The cyst develops in this subcutaneous plane superficial to the geniohyoid and mylohyoid muscles comprising the floor of the mouth. A transverse incision is made over the cyst and then, using sharp and blunt dissection, the cyst is freed from the underlying tissues. All bleeding should be controlled so that no drain is needed. Dead space is avoided by appropriate suturing in layers.

THYROGLOSSAL DUCT CYSTS. As the second branchial arch grows and fuses in the midline of the neck, it develops into the hyoid bone and surrounds the descending tract of the thyroid gland, as it descends from the foramen cecum of the tongue. A thyroglossal duct or cyst may develop, which will be described in detail in Chapter 100.

Second Branchial Groove Anomalies

These are the most common of the branchial anomalies. Clinically, they present at the anterior border of the sternocleidomastoid muscle from the level of the hyoid bone to the lateral border of the thyroid cartilage. Anomalies present in three different ways. An *external sinus* appears as a nondraining dimple in the newborn. Early removal is not mandatory, since infection is uncommon in the external sinus. A *fistula* will extend from the neck to the supratonsillar fossa. This fistula creates a problem for the mother because saliva drips from the neck orifice, constantly soaking the baby's nightgown. Excision relieves this annoying problem and should be considered from age six months on. A *cyst* present since birth has a clinical onset at 13 years of age on the average. I have seen one occur first at the age of 34. The late clinical onset cannot be explained easily if one assumes that they were there since birth as a persistent cervical sinus of His. Therefore, a current alternate theory states that branchial cysts arise from cystic formation of epithelial inclusions lying within lymphoid tissue. The cysts often present during upper respiratory infections as the cyst wall participates in the inflammatory reaction. A soft cystic mass develops, but I have sometimes found the mass to be surprisingly hard, probably due to tension from the increased fluid. Transillumination of the cyst will not occur when the fluid content is cloudy. There is no reason to delay excision except when infection is present.

OPERATIVE REMOVAL OF SECOND BRANCHIAL GROOVE EXTERNAL SINUS OR FISTULA. A transverse elliptical incision is made around the external opening. The skin incision is carried through the subcutaneous tissue, the platysma muscle and the fascia. The tract can be identified by placing a small probe into it, or by injecting diluted methylene blue through a polyethylene catheter into the tract. A hemostat placed on the opening of the tract can be used to tent up the tissue to follow the tract as far medially as it extends. Knowledge of the embryologic development of the second branchial cleft fistula will allow one to understand the complex route for the dissection between the internal and external carotid artery, lying lateral to the hypoglossal and glossopharyngeal nerve, and passing beneath the styloglossal muscle to the supratonsillar fossa (Fig. 10). Failure to remove the entire fistulous tract will once again result in recurrent neck infections. The opening into the supratonsillar fossa is closed with a chromic suture.

OPERATIVE REMOVAL OF SECOND BRANCHIAL CLEFT CYSTS. This begins with a transverse incision over the cyst and dissection through the platysma to the cyst. Using blunt and sharp dissection, the tissues are freed from the cyst wall. I find it easier to open the cyst wall, place hemostats on the sac (much as in a hernia repair), and then pull on the cyst to identify an ascending tract of taut tissue if it is present. In approximately 20 per cent of cases a fistulous tract can be identified ascending between the internal and external carotid arteries, lying lateral to the hypoglossal and glossopharyngeal nerve and passing beneath the styloglossal muscle to the supratonsillar fossa (Fig. 10). The operation is simplified when there is no fistulous tract; however, failure to find an existing fistulous tract will result in recurrent lateral neck infections.

Second and Third Pharyngeal Pouch Anomalies

Failure of development of the second and third pharyngeal pouches was suspected in a case of thymic hypoplasia with hypothyroidism. Clinically, no tonsils were visualized in the infant.[4]

Third, Fourth, Fifth Branchial Arch Anomalies

Malformations of these arches will give abnormalities of the larynx, which will be discussed in Chapter 103.

Third Branchial Groove Anomalies

Third branchial groove anomalies are rare and may present as a tiny opening with a blind sac, a fistulous tract, or a cyst—all located on the anterior border of the sternocleidomastoid in the lower one-third of the neck. The symptoms and signs are exactly like those in second branchial groove anomalies. An understanding of the embryology will allow the surgeon to appreciate the tortuous course that the fistulous tract follows from the lower one-third of the neck to the upper one-third of the neck and then back down to the middle third of the neck, where it enters into the pyriform sinus, just lateral to the larynx (Fig. 11).

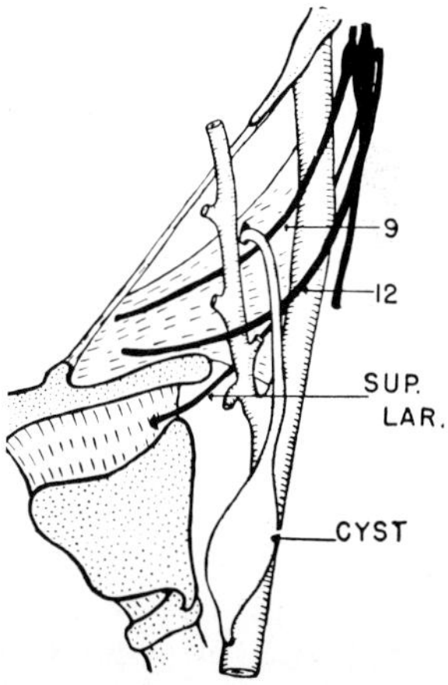

Figure 10. The course of the tract associated with the second branchial cleft cyst.

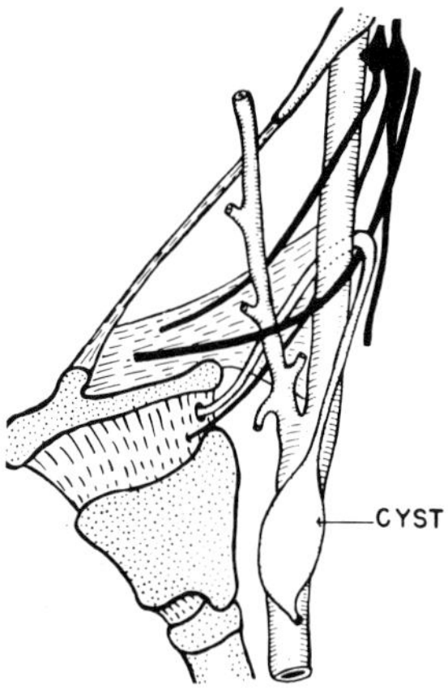

Figure 11. The course of the tract associated with the third branchial cleft cyst.

Third and Fourth Pharyngeal Pouch Anomalies

Failure of development of the third and fourth pharyngeal pouches leads to absence of the thymus and parathyroid glands (DiGeorge's syndrome).[5] Cellular immunity is abnormal; humoral antibody synthesis and serum immunoglobulins are normal. Convulsions with hypocalcemia in the neonatal period, chronic rhinitis, diarrhea and moniliasis may occur. A right aortic arch and an anomalous subclavian artery may also be present.

REFERENCES

1. Arey, L. B.: *Developmental Anatomy; a Textbook and Laboratory Manual of Embryology*, 7th Ed. Philadelphia, W. B. Saunders Co., 1965.

2. Patten, B. M.: *Human Embryology,* 3rd Ed. New York, McGraw-Hill, 1968.
3. Langman, J.: *Medical Embryology: Human Development—Normal and Abnormal,* 2nd Ed. Baltimore, Williams & Wilkins, 1969.
4. Hong, R., Gatt, R., Rathbun, J. C., and Good, R. A.: Thymic hypoplasia and thyroid dysfunction. *New Eng. J. Med.,* 282:470, 1971.
5. DiGeorge, A. M.: Discussion in *J. Pediatrics,* 67:907, 1965.

Chapter One Hundred

NECK MASSES AND MALIGNANT TUMORS OF THE HEAD AND NECK*

BURTON F. JAFFE, M.D.

NECK MASSES

A lump in the neck is a common, challenging diagnostic problem. A careful history is the single most important diagnostic aid. The physical examination is also important, since size, position, hardness, tenderness, and mobility of the neck mass are guides to a proper diagnosis.

In many cases, removal of the mass is performed for definitive diagnosis of treatable infections, for suspicion of a tumor, for cosmetic correction, or for a definite therapy for a recurrent painful lesion.

CONGENITAL TUMORS

Thyroglossal Duct Cyst

Thyroglossal duct cysts are very common in children, second in occurrence only to cervical adenitis.

An understanding of the embryology will not only make the surgeon's operation more complete, but will relieve the need for multiple procedures. The thyroid gland develops from the area of the foramen cecum at the base of the tongue and descends as an epithelial tract into the neck by the sixth week of life. Typically, the epithelial tract obliterates and disappears; if it persists, a thyroglossal duct remains. Any pinching off of the duct leaves a closed segment that can fill up with secretory fluid or pus. The second branchial arch (also known as the hyoid arch) grows anteriorly and fuses, completely surrounding the epithelial tract and trapping the thyroglossal duct if it persists. On occasion, the tract lies anterior or posterior to the hyoid bone. External fistulas are not developmental, since the thyroglossal duct does not communicate with the skin. It is only after spontaneous drainage or operative incision of an abscess that an external thyroglossal duct sinus or fistula develops.

Of all thyroglossal duct cysts, about 50 per cent present before 10 years of age and 65 per cent present under 20

*The technical assistance of Sandra Stolt is greatly appreciated.

years of age.[1] A thyroglossal duct cyst may even be present at birth. The sex frequency is equal. The distribution by ages is shown in Table 1.

The typical history in 80 per cent of the patients consists of an asymptomatic mass that, because of its exposed site, becomes a cosmetic problem for the patient and his family. Fear of a tumor sometimes grips the parents and they seek surgical advice. About 10 per cent will present as an infected cyst, appearing either as a tender, inflamed mass or as a fluctuant abscess following an upper respiratory infection. The history may include treatment with an antibiotic and successful resolution of the mass. However, recurrent infections may then ensue, and the mass will alternately swell and decrease in size. About 10 per cent appear as draining sinuses. These sinuses do not develop embryologically, as mentioned before, but follow an incision and drainage of the infected abscess, or occasionally follow spontaneous rupture of the abscess. A mucoid or purulent discharge from the sinus may occur. In infants, dysphagia and even death have been reported due to a large cystic mass.[1]

Thyroglossal Duct Cyst Location

Classically, the thyroglossal duct cyst appears as a cystic mass in the midline of the neck just below the hyoid bone, although frequently this is not its location. Ward[2] reported the following locations of fifty-three midline and nineteen lateral cysts (Table 2).

TABLE 1. DISTRIBUTION OF THYROGLOSSAL DUCT CYSTS BY AGE

Age	Number
0–10	448
11–20	138
21–30	103
31–40	119
41–50	61
51–60	37
61–70	2
71–90	4

TABLE 2. LOCATION OF THYROGLOSSAL DUCT CYSTS IN SEVENTY-TWO PATIENTS

Lingual	0	Transhyoid	2
Submental	2	Infrahyoid	45
Suprahyoid	18	Suprasternal	5

LINGUAL LOCATION. These occur in the base of the tongue at the foramen cecum. Differentiation from ectopic thyroid is confirmed by the absence of I^{131} uptake on a thyroid scan.

SUBMENTAL AND SUPRAHYOID LOCATION. This is a relatively common site for the thyroglossal duct cyst. Differentiation from a dermoid cyst is clinical. Protrusion of the tongue will elevate the thyroglossal duct cyst, which is attached to the tongue, but will not elevate the dermoid cyst, which is in the subcutaneous tissue.

INFRAHYOID LOCATION. These occur between the hyoid bone and the bottom of the thyroid cartilage. The cyst may be "pushed" laterally by the sloping thyroid cartilage.

SUPRASTERNAL LOCATION. These cysts are often confused with thyroid tissue. A thyroid scan will aid in differentiation.

LATERAL LOCATION. This location occurs uncommonly, and the link to the hyoid bone is not apparent preoperatively. The anatomic extent of a lateral thyroglossal duct cyst was carefully identified by a meticulous dissection in one patient.[3] A 2-year-old presented with a mass at the anterior border of the right sternocleidomastoid muscle at the hyoid level. At operation, a median extension of the primary mass passed posterior to the omohyoid and sternohyoid muscles. After dividing these muscles, a smaller contiguous cyst was found with a fibrous band coursing inferiorly to the pyramidal lobe of the thyroid and superiorly to the hyoid bone.

Differential Diagnosis

ECTOPIC THYROID GLAND. This may simulate a thyroglossal duct cyst.[4]

A 2-year-old girl was evaluated for a nodule below the hyoid bone, which was excised with the suspected diagnosis of a thyroglossal duct cyst. Pathologic diagnosis was "thyroid adenoma." Within two months after surgery, the mild constipation that had been present preoperatively became so severe that Hirschsprung's disease was suspected. Over the next 10 months, her growth nearly ceased and the bone age was only 1 year at a chronological age of 3 years. At age 5 years, the serum cholesterol value was 514 mg. per cent, BEI was 0.5 μg. per cent, and the PBI was 4.3 μg. per cent. Hypothyroidism was diagnosed and treatment was begun with desiccated thyroid, which definitely reversed the diseased state. In three other cases, a similar pattern also revealed that the ectopic thyroid gland functions significantly well under the age of 1 to 2 years with symptoms of only mild hypothyroidism (constipation, hoarse voice, delayed dentition, anemia and growth retardation), but within two months of surgery full-blown signs of hypothyroidism had developed in all four cases. A preoperative thyroid scan would have made the diagnosis. Should thyroid removal be performed, no great harm is done, since these ectopic thyroid glands function poorly and lifetime thyroid hormone would have been needed anyway. However, when the pathological report shows thyroid adenoma or colloid goiter, immediate thyroid substitution should be started to avoid severe postoperative hypothyroidism.

The differential diagnosis also includes a pyramidal lobe of the thyroid, midline thyroid adenomas, lipoma, papillary or follicular adenocarcinoma of the thyroid, squamous cell carcinoma, Hashimoto's thyroiditis, lymphosarcoma, and Boeck's sarcoid.[1, 5]

Operative Procedure

The cyst should be removed as soon as it is detected to prevent recurrent infections, to achieve better cosmetic appearance and to establish a histologic diagnosis. Prior to 1920, recurrences were common because the dissection took the central part of the hyoid bone but then proceeded to isolate the epithelial tract from the hyoid bone to the base of the tongue. Inadvertent tears of this delicate tract left enough duct tissue in the base of the tongue and suprahyoid area to regenerate and form recurrent cysts, or mucoid draining sinuses. In 1920, Sistrunk[6] advocated a block dissection involving not only the central portion of the hyoid bone but also a block of tissue from the hyoid bone to the base of the tongue, without actually dissecting the duct. Interestingly, Sade pointed out only recently that eleven out of twenty patients had three or more ducts going from the hyoid bone to the foramen cecum.[7] This again emphasized the need for a block dissection from the hyoid bone to the base of the tongue.

The operative procedure is begun with a transverse incision in the skin crease below the cyst and beyond the lateral margin of the cyst. The dissection is continued through the subcutaneous tissue and the platysma muscle and the upper flap is elevated. Dissection of tissue 1 cm. around the thyroglossal duct cyst and usually including the tissue between both sternohyoid muscles is advocated. The cyst and the surrounding tissue are then elevated to the hyoid body and 2 cm. of the midportion is removed with Mayo scissors. It is important not to go laterally at the level of the hyoid bone, since the hypoglossal nerve curves in close to the greater cornu. At this time, the assistant dons a second operative glove and pushes intraorally on the base of the tongue so that the base of the tongue is easily within the field of the surgeon. Using a Bovie with combined cutting and coagulation currents (or using a scalpel), a 1 to 2 cm. wide block of tissue at the base of the tongue is removed, including part of the geniohyoid and the genioglossus muscles. If the tongue mucosa is open, it should be closed with a figure-eight or purse-string chromic suture. Perfect hemostasis is needed; the surgeon can use suture ties or coagulation. Then he sews the base of the tongue and closes each layer separately. No drains are needed if the field is dry.

Pathology

The histology of the excised lesion is varied. In the series shown in Table 3, adjacent tissue involvement included 34 per cent with thyroid tissue, 17 per cent with lymphoid, and 6 per cent with hematomas, foreign body giant cells and salivary tissue. The adjacent thyroid tissue varied from a few scattered follicles to large islands and was located around the ducts, around the cyst or in the center of the hyoid bone.

Mucous glands, sometimes impressive in number, have been found along the tract from the cyst to the base of the tongue in twelve out of twenty specimens serially sectioned, and mucus was demonstrated in the lumen in eighteen out of twenty specimens using the PAS stain, alcian blue and colloidal iron. This explains the mucus content of the cyst as well as the postoperative mucoid cyst or mucoid sinus that develops if the ducts are not completely excised.

Results

In most patients the incision heals well. There is no dysphagia or alteration of the speech pattern, as might be expected from removal of tissue at the base of the tongue and removal of the body of the hyoid bone. Cystic recurrence, however, is the major postoperative problem, and that occurs in less than 10 per cent of patients after the Sistrunk procedure. Redissection is more difficult and a wider block dissection must be performed to include unseen multiple or more laterally placed thyroglossal ducts. Complications may be cellulitis, wound abscesses and hematomas. Uncommon complications include osteomyelitis of the hyoid bone, hypoglossal nerve palsy and croup secondary to transient epiglottic edema.

TABLE 3. HISTOLOGY OF THE LINING OF THE THYROGLOSSAL DUCT CYSTS[2]

	Number	Per Cent
Pseudostratified ciliated columnar respiratory epithelium	74	61
Stratified squamous cell epithelium	47	38
Transitional epithelium	8	7
Cuboidal epithelium	8	7
Other	18	15
Granulation tissue	14	
Abscess formation	4	

Branchial Cleft Cyst

This congenital lesion does not typically appear until adolescence. It often presents as an inflammatory mass. It is discussed in Chapter 99.

Cystic Hygroma

About 50 per cent of cystic hygromas are present at birth and 90 per cent appear before the end of the second year of life. On rare occasions, a huge congenital cystic hygroma can cause dystocia during delivery. Most cystic hygromas appear in the posterior triangle of the neck, although extensions into the mediastinum or up into the floor of the mouth do occur. The mass is fluctuant and transilluminates easily.

Cystic hygromas are believed to develop embryologically from a large lymphatic space in the neck of the embryo, called the jugular lymph sac, which fails to communicate with the internal jugular vein or the thoracic duct. This sequestered lymphatic tissue accumulates fluid and increases in size either by absorbing interstitial fluid or by secreting the fluid itself (although secretory cells have not been described on the histological examination). As the cystic hygroma fluid content increases, it seems to weave and insinuate itself into fascial planes around muscles, into the carotid sheath, circumferentially around the esophagus, pharynx or trachea, and then, with gravity aiding it, into the mediastinum. The fluid is usually clear and slightly yellow, identical to lymph. Blood-stained fluid is not surprising, since capillaries and even cavernous venous spaces are often intimately associated with the cystic hygroma and mild trauma easily creates a hemorrhage.

The cystic hygroma, although admittedly a cosmetic problem, is even more significantly related to acute fatal airway obstruction if a hemorrhage occurs into the cyst, or if the cystic hygroma swells after becoming infected secondary to an upper respiratory infection.

In one study, spontaneous regression occurred in seven out of forty-four patients (15 per cent).[8] However, it is unwise to postpone surgery, since most cystic hygromas persist, and acute crises can be superimposed on an otherwise stable cystic hygroma.

Special preparations for surgery should include having blood ready for transfusion, using transparent plastic drapes for the face to allow observation in order to detect facial nerve twitching, having a facial nerve stimulator, and being ready to perform a tracheotomy if needed during or after the operation. Surgical excision in *acute cases* with airway obstruction is limited to partial excision and a tracheotomy. However, surgical excision in *elective cases* should be as complete as possible, with removal of all pseudopods in order to reduce the recurrence rate. The tumor may infiltrate the brachial plexus, cervical muscles and cranial nerves, and it is reasonable to leave as small an amount of tumor as possible, yet sparing these vital structures. Opened, partially removed cysts usually stop leaking lymph after an initial postoperative lymph accumulation. Since this tumor is not malignant and since total excision is virtually impossible, a grossly mutilating procedure is not justifiable. Submucous cysts of the pharynx and larynx should be removed if possible. Cystic hygromas extending into the mediastinum can often be removed from the neck without a thoracotomy.

Subcutaneous suction catheters and postoperative antibiotics are needed. Complications include wound infections, ramus mandibularis paresis, Horner's syndrome, hoarseness secondary to recurrent laryngeal nerve paralysis, and strictures secondary to entering the esophagus with later fibrosis. Recurrent cystic hygromas develop in 15 per cent of the patients when gross incomplete excision has been performed, but these recurrences are usually small in size.

Dermoid Cyst

This uncommon cyst may be present in infancy. It typically appears in the midline in the submental area. It contains skin, the skin appendages, hair and desquamated epithelium appearing as a cheesy white material. Surgical removal is discussed under second branchial arch anomalies (see Chapter 99).

Sebaceous Cyst

This cyst may occur on a congenital basis. Like the dermoid cyst, this contains a cheesy material and sebaceous glands. However, unlike the dermoid cyst, the sebaceous cyst has no hair and no skin appendages in the wall. These occur principally in or around the pinna. The cyst may become inflamed, and surgical removal at a later time is indicated.

Epidermoid Cyst

This cyst is identical to the sebaceous cyst, except that no contiguous sebaceous glands can be found—only a stratified squamous epithelial lining and cheesy debris.

INFLAMMATORY MASSES

Viral Infections

These upper respiratory tract infections in children are very frequently associated with multiple adenopathy in both the anterior and posterior triangles of the neck. The nodes are frequently tender and move around like marbles under the skin. It is surprising at times to see these nodes persist for weeks, months or even years. Most important is the fact that no growth of the nodes occurs after the viral infection ceases.

INFECTIOUS MONONUCLEOSIS. This is an outstanding example of a viral infection with huge nodes in the neck that resolve completely with time. There are many atypical lymphocytes in the peripheral blood, increased heterophil antibody titers, and occasionally hepatomegaly and splenomegaly. Treatment with local heat and analgesics will comfort the child. Suppuration may occur in the nodes.

Bacterial Infections

Cervical adenopathy frequently accompanies bacterial infections of the head and neck. Common sites of infection are the tonsils, pharynx, ear and scalp. Treatment is usually for a gram-positive agent unless a specific culture and sensitivity report indicate otherwise.

An interesting study was performed to determine which agents caused large neck nodes. Dajani et al. studied thirty-four consecutive cases of cervical lymphadenitis in patients under 15 years of age, without antibiotics, and with a node at least 3 cm. by 3 cm.[9] A needle aspiration was obtained from each node and bacteriological, TB, and atypical TB studies were performed. No viral studies were done. The distribution from node aspirations is shown in Table 4.

TABLE 4. BACTERIOLOGIC RESULTS FOLLOWING ASPIRATION OF LARGE CERVICAL LYMPH NODES IN CHILDREN

	Number of Cases	Percentage
Group A beta-hemolytic streptococcus	15	44
Staph. aureus	4	12
Group A beta-hemolytic streptococcus and *Staph. aureus*	1	3
Mycobacteria tuberculosis	1	3
Scotochromogenic mycobacterium	1	3
Cultures negative	12	35

When nose and throat cultures as well as antistreptolysin-O titers were totaled, 25 (74 per cent) were possibly due to Group A streptococci. In this series, fluctuance or pus was present in five of sixteen patients with a streptococcal infection and in four of five with a staphylococcal infection (a total of nine of twenty-one, or 43 per cent).

Atypical Mycobacteria Tuberculosis

Four groups of atypical mycobacteria have been described by Runyon.

Group I or Photochromogens. These produce yellow to orange or brick red pigment when exposed to light and are known as the "yellow bacilli." They occur in neck nodes and in the lung. Two bacteria have been classified as *M. kansasii* and *M. luciflavum.*

Group II or the Scotochromogens. These are yellow-orange from the onset of growth in the dark and are known as the "orange bacilli." They occur in neck nodes.

Group III or the Nonchromogens. These have weak or no pigmentation and are known as the "Battey bacilli." They occur in neck nodes and in the lung.

Group IV or Rapid Growers. These grow out in forty-eight hours at room temperature from small inocula.

Neck node involvement with atypical mycobacteria is far more common in children than involvement with typical mycobacteria tuberculosis. The disease is localized to one side of the neck and the nodes are usually separate and discrete. This contrasts with typical mycobacteria, which give conglomerate masses of lymph nodes. Associated with the neck mass is a chronic draining sinus with or without granulation tissue at the orifice. Usually the nodes involved include the jugulodigastric, submandibular and submental nodes, but a few cases have originated in the parotid gland region.[10]

Skin testing with antigen from the atypical strains will reveal a positive reaction, whereas the standard PPD reveals a negative or up to 5 mm. reaction. A chest x-ray is normal and contact with other people with tuberculosis is absent.

The role of surgery is varied. If diagnosis is in doubt, excisional biopsy is needed. When a fluctuant node occurs, aspiration should be performed for culture and sensitivity. If the node fails to respond to treatment, it should be excised. Careful dissection is needed to avoid the ramus mandibularis nerve, which is adjacent to the nodes in the submaxillary and jugulodigastric areas. Transient cranial nerve paralyses may occur. A child with an atypical mycobacterial infection is not contagious, and a tonsillectomy is not indicated. Histology reveals a caseating epithelioid granuloma. Treatment with antituberculous drugs for a year or two is indicated.

Mycobacterium Tuberculosis

Neck node involvement with a tubercle infection is part of a generalized disease that follows the primary lung infection. Mycobacterium tuberculosis is less common in children than the atypical strains. The nodes are in the posterior triangle and are matted together. Evidence of pulmonary lesions will be present, along with a positive PPD skin test and even a positive gastric washing. A history of close contact with a patient with TB is usually obvious, and this contrasts with a negative history found in the atypical strains. A neck node biopsy may be needed if there is any doubt about diagnosis. A fluctuant node should be aspirated, especially when pressure necrosis of the skin is imminent. Treatment with antituberculous drugs for one or two years is indicated. If the nodes fail to resolve after therapy, surgical removal is indicated.

Syphilis

Single or multiple tender neck masses may be the presenting symptom of this disease in adolescents. A positive history of contact may be denied and the primary intraoral chancre may not be found. Serologic testing will confirm the diagnosis. Appropriate antibiotic therapy causes the neck mass to begin to resolve in one to two weeks.[11]

Cat Scratch Fever

A child with this disease presents with an enlarged, usually tender node in the neck or the preauricular or submandibular area.[12] Approximately one-third of the patients have multiple nodes and one in every eleven has a suppurative node. A positive history of a contact with a cat is necessary, although a scratch or bite is not necessary. A primary lesion occurs at the inoculation site as a 2 to 5 mm. red papule about seven to twelve days after contact. This primary lesion does not itch (unlike insect bites) and it persists for one week to three months. Occasionally, a linear pattern of papules is seen, as if left by a scratch. A skin test (Hanger and Rose test) is almost always positive if done at least one week after the onset of adenitis. Expectant treatment without antibiotics is recommended. Surgery is indicated when a suppurative node exists and aspiration is needed; when a node with a draining sinus exists, and the node and tract should be excised; or when a malignancy is suspected and tissue diagnosis is needed.

Actinomycosis

A draining sinus is characteristically found, although an underlying mass may or may not be present. This sinus is usually in the submaxillary area of the neck.

Other Granulomas

Histoplasmosis and other fungi may rarely present as a neck mass. Sarcoidosis rarely occurs in children, but it can present as a neck mass.

METABOLIC

The thyroid gland may be involved in children in a variety of ways. This will be a brief review.

Diffuse Enlargement

HYPERTHYROIDISM, OR GRAVES' DISEASE. Symptoms of hyperthyroidism include eye, neuromuscular, cardiac and gastrointestinal complaints. In children, hyperthyroidism is treated with propylthiouracil and subtotal thyroidectomy.

COLLOID GOITER IN ADOLESCENTS. This is a soft mass that is clinically euthyroid.

HASHIMOTO'S DISEASE. This is thought to be secondary to a congenital defect of iodothyronines in some cases, yet it is uncommon in children. With increasing damage to the gland, hypothyroidism occurs.

Multinodular Masses

MULTINODULAR COLLOID GOITER. The diffuse colloid goiter converts to a multinodular form at about age 20. Approximately 4 to 17 per cent of these are malignant and can be suspected if one hard nodule, a dominant hard nodule unresponsive to therapy, a delphinian node, or a cold nodule on scan exists. If tumor is suspect, a subtotal thyroidectomy should be performed.

Solitary Nodule

When a single nodule is palpated, surgery is indicated. However, on histological examination, 50 per cent are multinodular goiters, 40 per cent are benign adenomas and 10 per cent are carcinomas. Of the carcinomas, about 50 per cent are papillary adenocarcinoma, with a good prognosis after total thyroidectomy and suppression thyroid hormone therapy. About 25 per cent are follicular adenocarcinoma, with a poor prognosis, and about 25 per cent are undifferentiated carcinomas, with the worst prognosis.

Ectopic Thyroid Tissue

Laterally placed masses in the neck may be ectopic thyroid tissue, and after the histologic report a primary tumor is suspected in the normally positioned thyroid. Midline masses in the subhyoid area appear like the thyroglossal duct cyst. Removal may be inadvertent, and early thyroid hormone therapy is mandatory. Table 5 shows the interrelationship between the previously mentioned thyroid masses.

TABLE 5. THYROID MASSES PRESENTING IN THE NECK

Diffuse Goiter	Multinodular	Solitary Nodule
Hyperthyroidism		Multinodular goiter (50%)
Colloid goiter —age 20→	Multinodular colloid goiter	Benign adenoma (40%)
	↘ 4–17% ↘	
Hashimoto's disease →	10% →	Carcinoma (10%)
		Papillary adenocarcinoma
		Follicular adenocarcinoma
		Undifferentiated
		Small cell
		Giant cell
		Hurtle
		Anaplastic

VASCULAR

Hemangioma

These may occur in any head and neck area in subcutaneous tissues. They may be associated with intraoral, intrapharyngeal or intralaryngeal hemangiomas. One variety occurs in the parotid area. They may be seen at birth, but generally they disappear by 2 years of age. Surgery is indicated only if bleeding occurs or if a large cosmetic problem exists. The role of cryosurgery is being investigated for these masses in order to reduce the scarring that follows operative removal.

Carotid Body Tumors

Most carotid body tumors occur in adults and it is difficult to establish the incidence in children. One large series reported 7 out of 38 (18 per cent) under age 21.[13] All patients with carotid body tumors have a symptom besides the mass, as outlined in Table 6.

Physical examination reveals a mass that moves from side to side but not up and down. A bruit can be heard. Characteristic arteriograms establish the diagnosis by the densely vascularized tumor at the carotid bulb level. The blood supply is frequently by the ascending pharyngeal artery. Bilateral tumors occur in 10 per cent of patients and malignant tumors occur in about 10 per cent of patients.

Surgical excision is advocated in children, since increasing growth with age would lead to huge tumors with symptoms of vascular compression, such as syncope, airway obstruction, or dysphagia. Usually, the dissection can progress under the adventitial layer of the carotid artery. If arterial resection is needed, an internal shunt is used while a saphenous vein replacement is sutured in place.

Venous Ectasia

This unusual lesion feels like a soft bag of worms. It increases in size while the patient is lying down or coughing. It decreases in size when the patient is sitting up. Surgical excision is indicated if it is a cosmetic problem.

TRAUMA

Hematoma

Inadvertent injury to the neck can tear a small vein, which produces a hematoma in the neck. The mass is moderately soft, and gradual resolution will occur after a few days or a week.

Aneurysm and Arteriovenous Fistula

Following stab wound or penetrating injury of the neck, an expanding lesion of the neck occurs, associated with a bruit. An arteriogram confirms the diagnosis and surgical ligation of the fistula is indicated.

TUMOR

Benign tumors may occur including fibromas, lipomas and neuromas. The

TABLE 6. SYMPTOMS OF CHILDREN WITH CAROTID BODY TUMORS[13]

Age	Symptoms	Age	Symptoms
9	mass and pain	19	syncope
12	mass, pain, syncope	20	mass, pain, syncope
14	mass, dysphagia	20	syncope
19	syncope		

diagnosis is a histologic one made from the excised tissue. Malignant tumors will be discussed in detail immediately. Suffice it to say here that in the neck one may see primary tumors as in thyroid, salivary, or carotid body tumors; secondary tumors as in rhabdomyosarcomas metastatic from other head and neck primary sites; or "systemic" tumors as in lymphosarcoma or Hodgkin's disease.

MALIGNANT TUMORS OF THE HEAD AND NECK

The otorhinolaryngologist who deals with tumors in children must have a much different fund of information than the otorhinolaryngologist managing tumors in adults. In children the common head and neck malignancies are lymphoid tumors (Hodgkin's disease or lymphosarcoma) and sarcomas (rhabdomyosarcoma and fibrosarcoma); the tumor-cell type in adults is predominantly squamous cell carconoma. Interestingly, certain tumors are found almost exclusively in children, i.e., the embryonal rhabdomyosarcoma and the neuroblastoma. Even a newborn may have a malignant tumor. The intrauterine or immunologic factors which are so deviant as to allow this to occur are unknown.

Malignant head and neck tumors in children are not rare. A number of reports with large series of patients can be found, although many institutions have not reported their experience. Unfortunately for these children, the tumors present with symptoms that are common in children and belie the serious nature of these lesions. An earache may precede an obvious rhabdomyosarcoma of the ear, and nasal obstruction may be the earliest symptom of a rhabdomyosarcoma of the nasopharynx. These symptoms are frequently overlooked until a metastatic node is identified. The fact that the infant cannot express his complaints compounds the delay in diagnosis and therapy.

The workup for children with malignant tumors differs from the workup in adults. The malignant tumors of the lymphoid system require lymphangiography, laparotomy and bone marrow aspirations in order to stage the clinical spread of the disease. Sarcomas spread by bloodstream and occasionally by the lymphatics; therefore, metastasis is sought frequently by performing a bone marrow aspiration as well as by taking laminograms of the lung.

Surgical excision in the infant is sometimes met with resistance by both parents and physicians, yet for many tumors surgery is clearly the best treatment. Performing wide resection for some tumors may pose psychological and cosmetic issues that must be discussed openly with the parents. It is surprising how very well some children adjust functionally and psychologically following these operations. Resection of certain organs may also pose unusual questions, such as: How will a 3-year-old child learn to speak if a laryngectomy is performed?

Radiation therapy is commonly used in pediatric tumors, and a long life post-therapy may present new problems, such as a late-occurring radiation-induced tumor.

Chemotherapy is much more important in dealing with children, and both the chemotherapeutic agents and their capacity to cause remission or cure should be known to the surgeon.

All our tumor patients are seen at the Children's Cancer Research Foundation (The Jimmy Fund), and chemotherapy is recommended and carried out under the expert guidance of their staff. Daily attention is paid to the blood count.

The word "cure" and the phrase "five-year cure" are used throughout this chapter. One must recognize that "control" or "five-year control" is actually more realistic, since late recurrences may and do occur.

This chapter will deal with malignant tumors but will not include brain, orbital or odontogenic tumors. However, all other tumors which occur primarily in the head and neck area will be discussed. On occasion, metastatic head and neck tumors will be included if they commonly present first in the head and neck region. The frequency of each tumor is listed in Table 7.

MALIGNANT NEOPLASMS OF THE LYMPHOID TISSUE

Malignant neoplasms of the lymphoid tissue are the most common solid tumors found in the head and neck area in children. The tumors included in this section are malignant lymphomas (lymphosarcoma, reticular cell sarcoma, and follicular lymphoma), Hodgkin's disease, and Burkitt's lymphoma. The presenting sign may be *nodal*, such as a mass in the neck, or *extranodal*, such as in Waldeyer's ring, the maxillary sinus or the parotid gland.

Malignant lymphoma is more common in children than Hodgkin's disease. However, since Hodgkin's disease presents about 80 per cent of the time with a neck mass and lymphomas present only about 40 per cent of the time with a neck mass, the occurrence of a neck mass is about equal in both groups.

The criteria for clinical staging were adopted at the Symposium in Rye, New York in 1965 and were revised in 1970 (Table 8). Stages I through IV are divided into Group A (no systemic symptoms) and Group B (systemic symptoms, such as fever, night sweats and pruritus). Pruritus, however, is rare in children, and if it occurs, it is only in adolescents. The concept of staging is well established for Hodgkin's disease and is less important for lymphosarcoma. An evaluation of subdiaphragmatic lymph nodes is made by bilateral lower leg lymphangiograms, but because false-positive and false-negative lymphangiograms have been found, a laparotomy with splenectomy, liver biopsy and retroperitoneal node biopsies are needed for proper staging.[14]

Malignant Lymphomas

Malignant lymphomas in the head and neck area can occur in all age groups; about 6 per cent occur in children.[15] In children, the head and neck sites account

TABLE 7. MALIGNANT HEAD AND NECK TUMORS*

Tumor	Number of Patients
Malignant neoplasms of the lymphoid tissue	97
Hodgkin's disease (46)	
Lymphosarcoma (43)	
Reticulum cell sarcoma (7)	
Burkitt's lymphoma (1)	
Rhabdomyosarcoma	20
Fibrosarcoma or neurofibrosarcoma	11
Thyroid malignancies	9
Neuroblastomas of the head and neck	9
Squamous cell carcinoma	7
Melanoma	4
Ewing's sarcoma (endothelial myeloma)	3
Malignant histiocytoma	2
Osteogenic sarcoma and chondrogenic sarcoma	2
Malignant hemangiopericytoma	2
Malignant hemangioendothelioma	2
Parotid malignancies	2
Malignant Schwann cell tumors	2
Malignant teratomas	1
Miscellaneous tumors	5
	178

*From the Children's Hospital Medical Center, Boston, Massachusetts from January 1, 1960 to December 31, 1969.

TABLE 8. CLINICAL STAGING FOR HODGKIN'S DISEASE AND MALIGNANT LYMPHOMAS

	Stage	Example
Stage I	Involvement of a single lymph node region (I) or of a single extralymphatic organ or site (I–E)	One side of neck
Stage II_n	Involvement of two or more lymphoid regions, but limited to one side of the diaphragm (the subscript $_n$ indicates the number of regions involved) or solitary involvement of an extralymphatic organ or site and of one or more lymph node regions on the same side of the diaphragm (II–E)	Both sides of neck or left preauricular node and right side of neck
Stage III	Involvement of lymph node regions on both sides of the diaphragm (III) which may also be accompanied by involvement of the spleen (III–S) or by solitary involvement of an extralymphatic organ or site (III–E) or both (III–SE)	Neck nodes and abdominal nodes
Stage IV	Multiple or disseminated foci of involvement of one or more extralymphatic organs or tissues, with or without associated lymph node involvement	Neck nodes, abdominal nodes and lung parenchyma

for 40 per cent of the malignant lymphomas and about twice as many males as females are affected.

The malignant lymphomas are classified as shown in Table 9. The lymphocytic lymphosarcoma is the most common type of malignant lymphoma in the head and neck area in children. In our series, thirty-one lymphosarcomas presented in neck nodes, and twelve were in extranodal sites. Reticulum cell sarcoma is approximately one-sixth as common. In our series, two presented with neck nodes alone; in five children the neck nodes were shown to be part of a systemic involvement. The follicular form is

TABLE 9. HISTOLOGIC CLASSIFICATION OF MALIGNANT LYMPHOMAS

Predominating Component Cell(s)	Rappaport Classification	"Old Classification"
Primitive reticular cell	Malignant lymphoma, reticulum cell type, undifferentiated*	Large cell lymphosarcoma; reticulum cell sarcoma
Histiocyte	Malignant lymphoma, reticulum cell type, histiocytic*	
	(Malignant lymphoma Hodgkin's type)*	
Histiocyte and lymphocyte	Malignant lymphoma, mixed cell type (histiocytic-lymphocytic)	Large cell lymphosarcoma; lymphoblastic lymphosarcoma
Lymphocytic cells Poorly differentiated lymphocyte	Malignant lymphoma, lymphocytic type, poorly differentiated*	
Differentiated lymphocyte	Malignant lymphoma, lymphocytic type, well-differentiated*	Small cell lymphosarcoma; lymphocytic lymphosarcoma
*Malignant lymphomas with follicular pattern have been integrated into this classification and are designated by adding follicular to the cytologically appropriate term		(Giant) follicular lymphoma

quite rare and therefore will not be discussed in detail; the prognosis has been so good in children that one wonders if it represents an overdiagnosis for a benign extraordinary hyperplasia of a lymph node.

Lymphosarcoma and Reticulum Cell Sarcoma

These tumors will be discussed together because they arise in the same sites (although their clinical courses may differ).

NECK NODES. About 40 per cent of patients with lymphosarcoma or reticulum cell sarcoma present with a neck node as an initial symptom. At first, the node is rubbery and firm, painless and discrete. Later, large conglomerates of nodes occur. Lymphosarcoma neck nodes are unilateral in 75 per cent (involving the upper cervical and submaxillary nodes in 90 per cent of these cases and the supraclavicular nodes in 10 per cent.)[16] Bilateral neck nodes were present in 25 per cent. In reticulum cell sarcoma, by contrast, the neck nodes are unilateral in 94 per cent (involving the upper cervical and submaxillary nodes in only 56 per cent of cases and the supraclavicular nodes in 44 per cent). Bilateral nodes occurred in only 6 per cent.

EXTRANODAL (HEAD AND NECK). The solitary primary lymphosarcoma is especially common in the head and occurred in 110 patients (8.7 per cent) of Rosenberg's series of all ages.[15] A 52 per cent five-year survival rate in fifty patients has been reported.[17] This compares favorably to the five-year survival rate of 28 per cent for all lymphosarcoma patients.

Tonsils. The tonsil is the most common primary extranodal site, occurring in ninety-seven patients (7.7 per cent) of the Rosenberg series.[15] The tonsils were large, and often the tumor appeared to be a peritonsillar abscess. Ulceration of the tonsil does not occur. Tonsillectomy may have been performed for diagnosis. This treatment alone has produced a 50 per cent cure in cases in which no neck nodes were present.

Nasopharynx. This primary site occurs in 5.4 per cent of all patients. Local spread to adjacent structures occurs, and when that happens the five-year survival rate drops to 30 per cent.

Parotid and Submaxillary Glands. Lymph nodes occurring in these glands rarely develop a malignant lymphoma. A unilateral, rapidly growing, rubbery mass suggests the lymphoma. Needle biopsy, open biopsy or a superficial parotidectomy may be performed for diagnosis. A parotidectomy has achieved a cure for this solitary tumor.[18] Radiation therapy may also be used.

Maxilla and Maxillary Sinus. The maxilla and maxillary sinus will be considered together, since the precise site of origin is difficult to ascertain. Lymphosarcoma attacks the maxilla more often than any other bone in the head and neck area; the mandible is the second most commonly involved facial bone. Radiation therapy produces a 25 per cent cure rate. If the sinus becomes seriously infected, drainage via a Caldwell-Luc operation may be needed for relief of pain.

Tongue. The lingual tonsils in the base of the tongue may give rise to a malignant lymphoma. What appears to be a primary head and neck extranodal malignant lymphoma may really be part of a widespread malignant lymphoma; this is especially true with presentation in the thyroid gland, the orbit and the skin. In our experience at Children's Hospital Medical Center, 1960–1970, three had extranodal sites at lymphosarcoma in the tonsils, two in the skin of the scalp, one in the skin of the forehead, one in the nasopharynx, one in the cheek, one in the suboccipout, and one in the temporal area. No solitary extranodal sites for reticulum cell sarcoma were recorded.

Hodgkin's Disease

Hodgkin's disease in the head and neck area can occur in all age groups; 10 to 15 per cent occur in children. About

80 per cent of children with Hodgkin's disease present with nodes in the head and neck site. The five-year survival is 54 per cent, which is better than the adult five-year survival of 15 to 38 per cent.

The disease progresses through successive flare-ups and regressions. A bad prognosis occurs when liver, lung or bone marrow is involved, but a solitary bone lesion is not necessarily a bad sign. Terminal infections are common, since the immunologic status deteriorates.

The histologic classification listed in Table 10 was conceived by Lukes and Butler.[19] The old classification listed on the right was of no help in prognosis, since most of Hodgkin's disease fell into the granuloma type. The cellular types are related to the prognosis, the worst prognosis being at the bottom of the list. Progression from one cell type to another may occur down the list, but progression up the list with better diagnosis does not seem to occur. The Reed-Sternberg cell, an abnormal reticulum cell, is essential for the diagnosis of Hodgkin's disease.

NECK NODES. About 80 per cent of children with Hodgkin's disease present with a neck node as an initial symptom. Unilateral nodes are present in 82 per cent (involving the upper cervical and submaxillary nodes in 51 per cent, the supraclavicular nodes in 25 per cent and preauricular nodes in 6 per cent.)[16] Bilateral nodes occurred in 18 per cent. When the lower third of the neck is involved, mediastinal adenopathy is frequently present. Excisional biopsy establishes the diagnosis, and then the extent of the involvement is established by using the staging previously described. Slaughter[20] reported a 50 per cent five-year cure rate following radical neck dissection for localized unilateral neck lesions. Radiation therapy, however, is currently the treatment of choice because it also treats the contiguous node areas; this will allow a greater number of children to live. In our series, forty-one children presented with a neck node.

EXTRANODAL (HEAD AND NECK). These extranodal sites are less common in Hodgkin's disease than in lymphosarcoma or reticulum cell sarcoma. A large report in adults lists eleven solitary extranodal sites (tonsils, four; main stem bronchus, one; trachea, one; nasal septum, one; palate, one; base of tongue, one; and submaxillary salivary gland, one).[21] A slightly erythematous tumor was found in ten patients, and a tender ulcer with raised edges was seen in the nasal septum in the eleventh patient. In our series, two were in the nasopharynx and one was in the thyroid gland.

Radiation Therapy

Radiation therapy is the principal modality for stage I or stage II lymphomas or Hodgkin's disease. Radiation therapy for Hodgkin's disease is remarkable, since only 3400 to 4000 rads will make the tumor disappear, and this sensitivity is almost unique to this tumor. Kaplan[22] has emphasized that the spread of Hodgkin's disease is generally orderly and involves contiguous areas rather than spreading capriciously. Radiation therapy in Hodgkin's disease is directed to-

TABLE 10. HISTOLOGIC CLASSIFICATION OF HODGKIN'S DISEASE

New Name (Lukes and Butler)	Old Name (Jackson and Parker)
Lymphocytic predominance (22%)	Paragranuloma (7%)
Nodular sclerosis (12%)	
Mixed cellularity (54%)	Granuloma (90%)
Lymphocytic depletion (12%)	Sarcoma (3%)

ward involved nodes and also to one contiguous uninvolved area of nodes. This concept has provided cures in a much higher percentage of patients than would otherwise be possible.

Chemotherapy

Chemotherapy is used to prolong survival in stages IIIb and IV. For Hodgkin's disease, the MOPP program of nitrogen mustard, vincristine (Oncovin), prednisone and procarbazine (Natulan) is used. If the patient fails on the MOPP program, BCNU [1,3-bis(2-chloroethyl)-1-nitrosourea] may be used. Chemotherapy for lymphomas often uses cyclical vincristine, Cytoxan and prednisone. Other forms of treatment include trials with methotrexate, Velban or MOPP.

Surgery

Biopsy of a neck mass must be performed with a high regard for the pathologist's difficulties in diagnosing these tumors. Confusion exists not only between tumor and inflammation but also between tumor cell types. Sometimes only a minute focus of Hodgkin's disease exists in a node. Therefore, a needle biopsy or incisional biopsy would probably be nondiagnostic. Removal of the largest node is most likely to be diagnostic. However, removal of multiple nodes is even better since a node with only reactive hyperplasia will frequently be found next to a node with tumor. Gentle handling of the specimen is mandatory since the capsular details, such as focal obliteration of subcapsular sinuses, provide the pathologist with much information. Even cutting the node in half and placing it in formalin will help to preserve the minutest details.

Surgery for cure is limited to stage I neck nodes or extranodal sites in the head and neck for lymphosarcomas or reticulum cell sarcoma. However, in stage I Hodgkin's disease, radiation therapy has replaced the radical neck dissection for localized disease of the neck, since contiguous nodes are frequently present.

Surgery for palliation may become necessary. Bailey[21] lists four instances in which removal or excision is necessary: bulging tumors of the tonsil or base of tongue interfering with swallowing; nasal and tracheobronchial tumors obstructing the airway; large cervical nodes compressing the trachea or esophagus; and sinus tumors which are grossly infected and pose the threat of intracranial infection.

Cryosurgery for palliation seems reasonable for accessible lesions in the preceding cases.

Burkitt's Lymphoma

This tumor is now considered a malignant lymphoma of an undifferentiated type.[23] Much has been learned since 1958 when Burkitt described the endemic African childhood jaw tumor that progressed to a generalized fatal aleukemic disease.[24] A "starry sky" pattern due to histiocytes containing phagocytized material is seen. The maxilla is involved twice as often as the mandible, and the first site in the maxilla is usually located posteriorly. Growth upward to the orbit with proptosis and anterior erosion into the cheek are typical. Although the jaw tumor is the first clinical sign of the disease, it is often a late manifestation of tumor which involves the retroperitoneum and viscera. Uncommon sites of involvement are the peripheral lymph nodes, Waldeyer's ring, the mediastinum and the spleen. A cloudy maxillary sinus may be present.

Burkitt's tumor is now recognized in the U.S. and in other parts of the world. Jaw involvement is less common in the U.S. (15 per cent) than in Africa (50 per cent). On the other hand, involvement of Waldeyer's ring is reported in the U.S. but is rare in Africa. Chemotherapy alone or in combination with surgical removal of large masses may be successful as treatment in a small percentage of patients. Cytoxan given for two to four days will cause remarkable regression in the tumor, but it often recurs in a few months.

RHABDOMYOSARCOMA

Rhabdomyosarcomas (RMS) are the second largest group of solid tumors in the head and neck area. RMS occur at all ages, but the embryonal form occurs primarily in the pediatric group. Even congenital RMS can occur.[25]

The embryonal rhabdomyosarcomas have a predilection for the head and neck area as well as the genitourinary region in children. Alveolar rhabdomyosarcomas are most often found in the head and neck area or the extremities of children and young adults. Pleomorphic rhabdomyosarcomas are rare in children, but when present, they chiefly involve the extremities and similar sites of involvement found in adults. The tissue of origin for the majority of RMS is probably from totipotential mesenchyme rather than from adult or mature skeletal muscle. Cross-striations, if found, are the hallmark of the diagnosis and PTAH staining (phosphotungstic acid-hematoxylin) reveals these cross-striations. The demonstration of cross-striations, however, is not considered essential for diagnosis. The presenting signs and symptoms of RMS depend on the locale of the primary site, and this will be discussed subsequently. There is a wide spectrum of growth rates so that a slowly growing tumor may present with just local signs and symptoms and a rapidly growing tumor may present with widespread complaints, including anorexia and weight loss. Table 11 shows our experience during the past ten years.

Nasopharynx

The nasopharynx is a common site for RMS in children. Symptoms are divided into the following four groups: local symptoms, neck nodes, cranial nerve paralysis and systemic symptoms.

Local symptoms occur first but are often overlooked. The botryoid tumor expands in the relatively small nasopharynx, quickly occluding the eustachian tube (giving a silent serous otitis media) and occluding the posterior choana (giving epistaxis or a nasal speech sound and a nasal discharge similar to that with a common cold or large adenoids). These early symptoms, so common in many infants, are easily overlooked. Indeed, one patient had a two-year history of local symptoms before the tumor spread to the neck, and only then did it become recognized. In an infant or young child, digital palpation of the nasopharynx can be performed. Three tongue blades are placed sideways between the teeth to keep the mouth open while the finger is inserted. The examining index finger can pass behind the soft palate and feel a bulging mass (Figs. 1 and 2). In an older child the nasopharynx can be examined by indirect nasopharyngoscopy using a nasopharyngeal mirror.

Neck nodes occur in the upper third of the neck, first unilaterally and then bilaterally. Typically, it is at this stage that a tumor is suspected and the biopsies are obtained. Unfortunately, the primary site is undetected at this time and will be sought only after pathological diagnosis is made.

Cranial nerve paralysis occurs by direct tumor spread or by metastasis.

TABLE 11. RHABDOMYOSARCOMA OF THE HEAD AND NECK*

Location	Number	Location	Number
Nasopharynx	6	Tongue	2
Ear and mastoid	4	Orbit	2
Soft tissues of face	3	Maxilla	1
Mastoid area (2)		Nose	1
Temporal area (1)		Peritonsillar	1

*From the Children's Hospital Medical Center between 1960 and 1970.

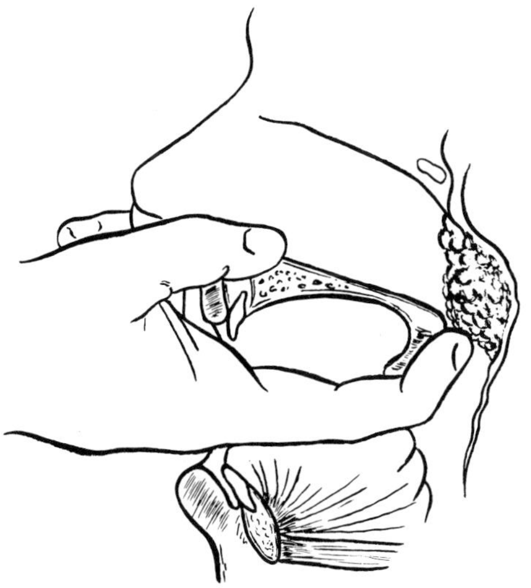

Figure 1. Detection of a mass in the nasopharynx by digital palpation.

Cranial nerves V to VII are involved by direct intracranial spread, with involvement of nerve VI, most commonly giving a "lazy eye." Cranial nerves IX to XII are involved by large high neck nodes compressing the nerve trunks between the tumor mass, the vertebral bodies and the base of the skull near the jugular foramen.

Systemic symptoms occur as the tumor metastasizes to the hilum, to the lungs or widely throughout the body. The role of surgery is limited to a nasopharyngeal examination under general anesthesia using a soft palate retractor and a biopsy using a forceps. A bone marrow study at this time should be done to rule out metastasis. A neck dissection may be indicated if the primary tumor is controlled by radiation therapy but the neck nodes persist.

Radiation therapy to the nasopharynx and upper neck and chemotherapy are the treatments of choice. In our study, almost all children received actinomycin D and vincristine as well as radiation therapy. Methotrexate is also useful. Promising results have been reported with the combined use of vincristine, actinomycin D, and Cytoxan (VAC).

A gloomy prognosis for these patients can be seen in Table 12, in which some larger series of cases have been reported. There are no five-year survivals out of

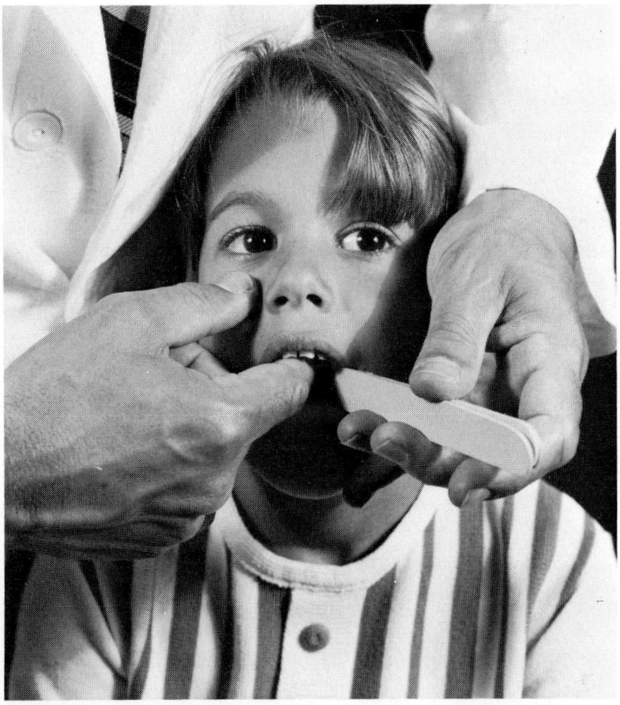

Figure 2. Digital palpation of the nasopharynx in a child.

TABLE 12. SURVIVAL IN RHABDOMYOSARCOMA OF THE NASOPHARYNX

Source	Total Number	Number Alive at Five Years	Number of Years Reviewed
Mayo Clinic[27]	11	0	16
M. D. Anderson Hospital[28]	8	0	16
Children's Hospital Medical Center, Boston (Current Report)	6	0*	10
University of Michigan Medical Center[29]	2	0	10
Emory[30]	2	0	10

*Two alive at less than five years.

the twenty-nine patients in these five series. However, a single five-year survival was reported by Edland[26] in 1968 using 6750 rads of radiation therapy and actinomycin D—a total of 3.0 mg. over twelve days (75 μg./kg. total).

Middle Ear and Mastoid

Rhabdomyosarcoma in the middle ear and mastoid is an uncommon, uniformly lethal neoplasm that occurs almost exclusively in children. By 1969, thirty-seven well-documented examples had been recorded in the literature.[31] In these patients, the earliest symptom was an earache; twenty patients complained of an aural discharge, often bloody; sixteen patients manifested a "polyp" in the ear canal or a mass near the ear. In five patients the cervical lymph node metastases were the initial presenting symptoms. Rapid progression developed in fifteen children, as evidenced by an initial presentation with a cranial nerve palsy (primarily nerve VII).

Neck masses below the pinna may represent direct extension by erosion through the floor of the external auditory canal, middle ear or mastoid. If a tumor of the petrous portion of the temporal bone erodes inferiorly, it presents lateral to the pharynx as a contiguous parapharyngeal mass. In some cases this parapharyngeal mass bulges into the nasopharynx; in other cases it bulges into the oropharynx and pushes the tonsil medially or bulges into the soft palate.

Until recently RMS of the middle ear and mastoid bone have been uniformly fatal. Conte and Sagerman reported a three-and-a-half-year cure following radical mastoidectomy and radiation therapy.[32]

In our series, four patients with middle ear RMS have been seen during the past ten years. Patient #1 has been free of tumor for two years following combined radiation therapy and chemotherapy (vincristine and actinomycin D). Patient #2 had a recurrence after radiation therapy and chemotherapy and subsequently had a total temporal bone resection; thirteen months after operation there is no evidence of tumor. Patient #3 died after radiation therapy, chemotherapy and a temporal bone resection. Patient #4 died after combined radiation and chemotherapy.

Surgery is important in the management of this tumor. *Biopsy* of a polypoid lesion in the ear canal may reveal RMS. A *mastoidectomy* performed in some patients with chronic suppurative otitis media may unexpectedly reveal tumor when the surgeon suspects typical "granulation tissue." *Temporal bone resection* may be indicated after radiation therapy and chemotherapy fail. Laminograms of the temporal bone will reveal areas of erosion; if erosion is more medial than the petrous tip (as in erosion of the posterior sella turcica), a resection would not be indicated. A retrograde eustachian tubogram will detect the presence of tumor growing down into the eustachian tube. An internal carotid arteriogram will reveal the extent of the tumor in the carotid canal at the base of the skull. A retrograde jugular venogram will detect any tumor erosion inferiorly into the jugular bulb or sigmoid sinus structures.

Soft Tissue of the Face

These primaries occur as painless, rapidly expanding hard masses. The rapid growth will eventually produce pain by invading nerves or eroding bone. Our experience in the ten years was limited to two in the parotid area and one in the temporal area. The role of surgery is limited to the total excision of localized masses and is generally followed by radiation therapy or chemotherapy. Occasionally, five-year cures have been documented after superficial or total parotidectomies as well as after excisions at other sites.

Intraoral

RMS may present as a violet-red exophytic mass of the tongue, palate, tonsil or peritonsillar areas. Surgical excision of a localized lesion followed by radiation therapy and chemotherapy is the treatment of choice. In our series, in the past ten years there have been two tongue RMS treated, and both are alive five and ten years post-therapy. One patient with peritonsillar RMS died after partial excision, radiation therapy and chemotherapy.

Larynx

These primaries are extremely rare. Fortunately, however, when they do occur, hoarseness is an early symptom and often results in early examination and early diagnosis. Therefore, occasional cures have been mentioned in the literature. One five-year cure followed total laryngectomy.[28] However, a real enigma is the problem of voice rehabilitation in children. A seven-and-a-half-year cure following radiation therapy for a laryngeal and subglottic tumor was also reported.[27] Certainly radiation therapy is the preferred means of treatment, but if recurrence occurs, a total laryngectomy would be indicated.

Orbit

This is the most common site for head and neck RMS.[33] However, in our series, only two patients were seen with this tumor. This bias represents the known referral pattern to the Massachusetts Eye and Ear Infirmary for orbital tumors. Five-year cures have been reported following combined orbital exenteration, radiation therapy and chemotherapy.

Soft Tissues of the Neck

Primary tumors in the neck have occurred, but none were present in our series. A complete examination of the ear, nose and throat, x-rays of the sinuses and mastoid, and biopsies of the nasopharynx are needed to rule out an occult primary site.

Recent developments in the treatment of RMS justify aggressive combined therapy with surgery, radiation therapy and chemotherapy.

FIBROSARCOMA AND NEUROFIBROSARCOMA

Fibrosarcoma in the head and neck area can occur in all age groups, and 25 per cent occur in children.[33] In children, the head and neck site accounts for 25 per cent of all fibrosarcomas.[35] Congenital fibrosarcoma can occur; one appeared as a mass on the cheek of a newborn.[38]

Fibrosarcomas are composed of two histologic types: the differentiated fibrosarcoma (fibromatosis), which grows locally and invades other tissues but can be cured; and the undifferentiated fibrosarcoma, which metastasizes and is difficult to cure.

In a large series of head and neck fibrosarcomas in patients of all ages, the following distribution occurred: face, eighteen; neck, fourteen; maxilla and mandible, six; nose and sinuses, five;

scalp, five; oral mucosa, four; and larynx, two.[34]

In our series, eleven children with fibrosarcomas and neurofibrosarcomas of the head and neck were seen. In three the mandible was affected, the cheek was affected in three, the neck in two, the pharynx in one, the nose in one, and the forehead in one. All were fibrosarcomas except two in the cheek and one in the neck which were neurofibrosarcomas.

Surgical excision is the treatment of choice, since the tumors are not curable by radiation therapy or chemotherapy. For *mandibular lesions,* a mandibulectomy with reconstruction is indicated. A neck dissection is not routinely performed because neck metastases are rare. For *primary neck lesions,* a radical neck dissection is performed to obtain a satisfactory surgical margin around the tumor, but not to remove other tumor-containing nodes, since metastases are rare. For a *maxillary sinus or maxillary bone lesion,* a subtotal or total maxillectomy is performed, depending on the site, growth and histologic characteristics of the tumor. In general, the more undifferentiated the tumor, the greater the need for a radical excision.

In the head and neck area, a five-year cure rate of 79 per cent for the differentiated fibrosarcomas contrasts with the 33 per cent rate for the undifferentiated fibrosarcomas. Fortunately, the differentiated variety is three to four times as common as the undifferentiated type. One should not be deceived, however, by the benign appearance of the differentiated fibrosarcomas, since they are the direct cause of death in 20 per cent of the cases, by local recurrence and invasion. Even late recurrences after fifteen years of an apparent "cure" have been reported.[37]

THYROID MALIGNANCIES

This is a relatively common type of head and neck tumor in children. Although usually twice as many females as males are affected, in our series there were five females and four males.

The occurrence of thyroid malignancies following radiation therapy is well known. Even very low dose radiation therapy in the range of 200 rads can be followed in one or two decades by a thryoid malignancy.

The age and tumor type are listed in Table 13. There were two medullary carcinomas, six mixed papillary and follicular adenocarcinomas, and one pure papillary adenocarcinoma.

At operation, a search for enlarged nodes along the jugular chain should be made for frozen section report. If negative, a total thyroidectomy is advocated followed by thyroid replacement. If positive nodes are found, a total thyroidectomy and a neck dissection should be performed, although this is controversial. If a neck dissection is decided upon, a "conservative" neck dissection can be performed, leaving the internal jugular vein, the spinal accessory nerve and the sternocleidomastoid muscle.

TABLE 13.

Age	Male or Female	Type
14 months	M	Medullary
7 years	F	Mixed papillary and follicular
9 years	F	Mixed papillary and follicular
10 years	F	Mixed papillary and follicular
11 years	M	Mixed papillary and follicular with neck nodes
11 years	F	Mixed papillary and follicular with neck nodes
13 years	M	Papillary
14 years	F	Mixed papillary and follicular
17 years	M	Medullary

NEUROBLASTOMA

Neuroblastoma is one of the most common solid tumors in children; yet, it is relatively uncommon in the head and neck region (excluding intracranially). The neuroblastoma is derived from the primitive sympathetic neuroblast of neural crest origin, presenting in the adrenals, the ganglia of the spinal nerves, or in sympathetic ganglia which are present in the neck and thoracic, retroperitoneal or pelvic areas. Histologic variations range from differentiated to undifferentiated cell types. Under 1 year of age, a head and neck *primary neuroblastoma* was found in 7 per cent (6 of 82) in our hospital between 1948 and 1971. Five were in cervical and one in a nasopharyngeal primary site. *Secondary neuroblastoma* representing metastases to the head and neck area occurred in 6 per cent of Gross' series (twelve to neck nodes and one to the nasal cavity)[38] reviewed from 1920 to 1957 in our hospital. In our series from 1960 to 1970 there were nine primary and twenty metastatic neuroblastomas to the head and neck.

The fascinating picture of this tumor results from many unusual characteristics. (1) Neuroblastoma in situ has been found in 1 in 200 routine infant autopsies but never in infants over the age of 3 months.[39] An overt neuroblastoma occurs in 1 in 10,000 children, and thus, for each clinical case, about forty-nine neuroblastomas in newborns spontaneously disappear. (2) Neuroblastoma is an embryonal tumor and may be diagnosed at birth. Ten per cent of neuroblastomas are congenital and 50 per cent of all congenital tumors are neuroblastomas. (3) Multicentric tumors occur, adding confusion to diagnosis, therapy and prognosis, since differentiation from metastases is difficult. (4) Hemorrhage, either spontaneous or traumatic, is frequently due to the vascular nature of the tumor. Proptosis with orbital and periorbital ecchymosis is a characteristic sign of a neuroblastoma metastasis. (5) They cause increased urinary excretion of catecholamines, 3-methoxy-4-hydroxymandelic acid (VMA), and cystathionine. After successful therapy catecholamine, VMA and cystathionine, if elevated, may return to normal. Recurrence of tumor may be accompanied by recurrent high levels of metabolites. (6) An immune reaction to neuroblastoma has been demonstrated by Hellstrom by analyzing the patient's lymphocytes and plasma. (7) Early pulmonary metastases, common in Wilms's tumor, are uncommon with neuroblastoma.

Prognosis is variable, but certain factors are harbingers of a better prognosis. (1) A well-differentiated tumor has a better prognosis. (2) Infants under 1 year of age survive more commonly. Under 1 year of age 62 per cent survive, but over 1 year of age only 16 per cent survive. (3) Patients with tumors in extra-abdominal sites, such as the neck and mediastinum, have a better rate of survival than those with abdominal tumors, probably because of earlier diagnosis and earlier therapy. (4) Neuroblastomas have the highest rate of spontaneous regression of any type of malignancy. Disappearance of the tumor cells may occur. (5) Maturation to a benign ganglioneuroma may also occur. (6) Liver metastasis, although not the sign of a good prognosis, is not a fatal sign if seen under 1 year of age. (7) Even widespread metastases on occasion can be successfully treated with vincristine and Cytoxan. If breakthrough occurs, nitrogen mustard is useful. (8) Localized tumors can be treated successfully by surgical resection and with radiation therapy when total surgical resection is impossible.

Primary Neuroblastoma of the Neck

Primary masses may occur at any level of the neck from the submaxillary triangle to the supraclavicular area. Even when the neck mass is considered primary, a search for mediastinal or abdominal neuroblastoma should be undertaken. The neck mass is usually progressively enlarging, firm and painless, although pressure on nerve routes can produce pain. An x-ray may reveal a mottled calcification. Early neurologic signs are present with primary tumors of the neck, since the ganglia of nerves are the origin of this tumor. This is in contrast to the cervical metastases from neuroblastomas; these typically do not produce early neurologic signs because they spread instead to the lymph nodes. For example, an early Horner's syndrome occurs when the point of origin is a cervical sympathetic ganglion. High mediastinal masses may also present with a Horner's syndrome. Various neurologic symptoms occur when the primary site is the ganglion of cranial nerve IX, X, XI or XII. Origin from the ganglion nodosum of the vagus nerve has been reported in detail,[40] and recurrent laryngeal nerve paralysis will produce an abnormal cry, hoarseness or difficulty in breathing. Dysphagia may result from a parapharyngeal space tumor, i.e., a large deep neck mass bulging against the pharyngeal constrictor muscle and present simultaneously in the pharynx and the neck.[41]

Diagnosis is made by open biopsy. Partially differentiated neuroblastomas, called ganglioneuromas, are found in 75 per cent of the neuroblastoma neck masses and treatment by wide surgical excision provides a fair prognosis. Undifferentiated neuroblastomas, called sympathicoblastomas occur in 25 per cent of the neuroblastoma neck masses. They are highly malignant, and the prognosis is poor, even following wide surgical excision, because of widespread metastasis. However, a radical neck dissection is still recommended to achieve some cures.[42] When the undifferentiated tumor infiltrates the vertebrae and brachial plexus only a subtotal removal should be performed, followed by radiation and chemotherapy. Conley stressed the need to preserve all cranial nerves when performing wide surgical excision.[40] In his case, surgery produced transitory injury to the cranial nerves X, XI and XII and loss of pharyngeal sensation, leading to aspiration and pneumonitis. A feeding gastrostomy was necessary to overcome the swallowing difficulty, and a tracheotomy was needed to provide bronchial care.

Secondary Neuroblastoma of the Neck

A mass in the left supraclavicular area, Virchow's node, in an infant or child should alert the physician to the possibility of a variety of tumors. Neuroblastomas should be considered, and in these cases a bone marrow, urine for VMA and cystathionine, and a skeletal metastatic series should be done.

Primary Neuroblastoma of the Head

In our series, covering ten years, there were nine primary and twenty metastatic neuroblastomas of the head and neck. The nine primary tumors affected the neck (three), the nasopharynx (two), the maxillary sinus (one), the nose (one), the scalp (one), and the lip (one).

One of the primary tumors was present in the neck at birth. Of the twenty metastatic tumors of the head and neck, twelve involved the neck nodes. Also, one benign ganglioneuroma was found in the pterygoid fossa.

NOSE. The olfactory esthesioneuroblastoma is a specialized neuroblastoma. The origin is the neuroepithelial cells of the olfactory placode or the vestigial organ of Jacobson or the sphenopalatine ganglion, but this is less likely. Clinically, it presents as an intranasal mass, such as a polyp, and is associated with epistaxis and sinusitis. As it enlarges, the tumor erodes the maxilla, causing the cheek to swell, and later enters the orbit, producing proptosis and diplopia. Finally, it spreads intracranially to the frontal lobe, producing increased intracranial pressure, intracranial infections or stroke.[43] Metastasis to neck nodes occurs in 30 per cent of the patients and pulmonary metastasis may also occur. The olfactory esthesioneuroblastoma is the most sensitive of all neuroblastomas to radiation therapy, and this modality remains the primary treatment of choice. Chemotherapy should also be considered. On occasion, surgical excision is also performed.

NASOPHARYNX. The nasopharynx is stated as being the most common site of primary extracranial neuroblastoma, yet it is still very rare. Neither Gross[38] nor Fortner[42] reported any primary nasopharyngeal neuroblastomas.

ORBIT, MAXILLARY SINUS, LIP, MANDIBLE, PALATE AND MASTOID. Only isolated case reports mention these sites.

Secondary Neuroblastoma of the Head

MANDIBLE. This is the most common site for metastasis in the head (excluding the CNS), and the angle of the mandible is the most involved portion. A hard mass bulges from the jaw either lingually or labially, loosening the teeth. Typically, this metastasis is found in a child between 2 and 8 years of age, and it forebodes a grim future, since death almost always occurs within months.

MAXILLA, NOSE AND CHEEK. Only isolated case reports mention these sites.

SQUAMOUS CELL CARCINOMA

In the head and neck area of children, only 4 per cent of the tumors are squamous cell carcinoma (SCC). This contrasts vividly with adults, in whom 80 per cent or more of head and neck tumors are SCC. The predominance of sarcomas in children is unexplained unless there is a developmental or immunologic etiology in children.

Squamous cell carcinoma may occur in the nasopharynx, skin, larynx and maxilla. It may also develop in the wake of xeroderma pigmentosa, a congenital sensitivity to sunlight affecting the skin. In our series, three patients had nasopharynx primaries [ages 14 (two) and 16 (one)], and neck nodes were present in all three. Radiation therapy and chemotherapy are the modalities of choice for nasopharynx SCC. Bliomycin is the chemotherapeutic agent preferred at the present time. Surgical excision of persistent neck masses is indicated if they fail to respond to radiation therapy and if the primary site is controlled. Two children, aged 10 months and 14 years, had SCC in neck nodes with occult primary sites. Another child, 8 years old, had an undifferentiated carcinoma of the maxillary sinus. One child had an anaplastic carcinoma of the larynx.

MELANOMA

Only 2 per cent of all melanomas occur in children in the head and neck area.[44] Of all pediatric melanomas, 60 per cent are in the head and neck area[45] (compared to 20 per cent in the head and neck area in adults).[46] Sites of origin may be in the skin or in mucous membranes. A melanoma may arise from the junctional element of a *pre-existing nevus*. A melanoma may also arise *de novo* from a melanocyte. Although melanomas may be amelanotic (appearing as a benign lesion or as an enlarging, raised and ulcerated lesion) or melanotic, all four of our patients in the series exhibited the pigmented variety.

Melanomas spread by local, nodal and distant metastasis even after many years of an apparent cure. There are two special varieties of spread. One is *satellitosis*—multiple melanotic nodules of tumor in dermis and epidermis signifying local recurrences, and associated with a 10 per cent cure rate. The other type is *melanomatosis*—widespread dissemination of single cells or clumps of tumor cells into bloodstream organs; this is fatal. Biopsy for a small lesion consists of a local excision with a 3- to 4-mm. margin. A frozen or permanent section is obtained, and if it is positive for melanoma, a larger excision is necessary. In large lesions it is not practical to do an excisional biopsy, so an incisional biopsy is obtained from the most suspicious area.

Scalp melanomas also occur. A 5- to 6-cm. margin with a primary skin graft and a composite neck dissection are indicated. If the tumor is anteriorly placed on the scalp, a superficial parotidectomy should be done, but if preauricular metastases are present, a total parotidectomy is needed. If the melanoma is posteriorly placed on the scalp, the dissection includes the suboccipital nodes. *Face* melanomas have a low rate of metastases and are treated by local resection with only a 1-cm. margin, and then direct closure, skin grafts or local flaps are needed. *Neck* melanomas require a wide local resection with a neck dissection. *Ear* melanomas may be superficial, requiring only a partial pinnectomy, or invasive, requiring total pinnectomy, parotidectomy and a neck dissection. If the top of the pinna or the conchal cartilage is involved, a total pinnectomy is required. If only the lower part of the pinna is involved, the upper part of the pinna may be saved to support sunglasses or eyeglasses. Mucous membrane lesions can be treated with electrodesiccation, but there is little chance of a cure.

Radiation therapy and chemotherapy have little to offer. The role of immunologic therapy is being investigated.

In our series there were two tumors on the scalp, one on the ear and one on the neck.

EWING'S SARCOMA (ENDOTHELIAL MYELOMA)

About 50 per cent of Ewing's sarcoma occur in children, and the majority of these are over 10 years old. About 5 per cent occur in the head and neck area.[47] This is a malignant tumor of bone that is thought to arise from the primitive mesenchymal framework of bone. Recent evidence suggests that it may be a myelogenous neoplasm similar to a plasma cell myeloma, and this would account for its clinical pattern of multicentricity, involving many bones at one time.[48] In a majority of cases, a positive PAS stain is present in Ewing's sarcoma and negative in reticulum cell sarcoma, neuroblastoma, and undifferentiated osteosarcoma. Clinically, fever, pain, and swelling make it appear to be an inflammatory lesion, and x-rays reveal a lytic bone lesion.

Head and neck sites of involvement are skull, cervical vertebrae, and facial bones (especially the mandible and maxilla). In our series, one primary tumor involved the scalp, one was metastatic to the mandible, and one arose as a neck mass. Radiation therapy is the treatment of choice. Wide surgical excision, such as a radical maxillectomy, on occasion has established a cure. Chemotherapy includes Cytoxan, vincristine, and actinomycin D. Less than 10 per cent survive more than five years.

HISTIOCYTOMA

This tumor occurs in children and approximately 45 per cent are in the head and neck area.[49] Kauffman and Stout, in following their patients, found that although these are usually benign tumors, approximately 20 per cent had a malignant course.[49] This is a solid tumor of histiocytes and fibrous tissue involving the skin, subcutaneous tissue, muscles and lung. It not only histologically looks like reticulum cell sarcoma, but may behave like it. Pseudonyms are reticulohistiocytomas and reticulohistiocytic granulomas.

Kauffman reported five scalp (four benign and one malignant) and two lip (both benign) histiocytomas. In our series, two children were diagnosed with histiocytomas. One, aged 9 months, had a tumor of the eyelid; the other, aged 14 months, had tumor behind the ear. Local recurrence as well as erosion into the underlying bone or metastasis to the neck nodes or lung may occur. Therefore, surgery should be performed not merely to "shell out" the tumor but also to excise a wide margin of tissue around the histiocytoma. Radiation therapy and chemotherapy have also been used.

MALIGNANT HEMANGIOPERICYTOMA

About 10 per cent of hemangiopericytomas occur in children.[50] Of all pediatric hemangiopericytomas 30 per cent occur in the head and neck area.[51] Stout and Murray described this entity in 1942.[52] These tumors are usually benign but about 20 per cent are malignant. They may even be present at birth. Clinically, the tumor presents as a slow-growing, painless mass.

The hemangiopericytoma is a vascular tumor in which the tumor cells are derived from the pericytes of Zimmerman, which lie outside the capillary walls and which fill in the intercapillary spaces. Reticulin stain surrounds each dense proliferation of capillaries and the reticulin stain surrounds each pericyte.

Head and neck sites of origin include the nose and paranasal sinuses (present with nasal obstruction and epistaxis), oral cavity (slow-growing reddish mass), orbit, neck, skull and scalp, pinna and in isolated cases the larynx and nasopharynx. In our series, one patient, aged 11 months, had a tumor of the neck, which was treated with wide excision. A 13-month-old patient had a tumor of the soft palate with neck nodes. It underwent widespread dissemination, and death resulted.

As stated by Farr,[53] "The clinical course cannot be gauged by the histologic appearance or the relatively benign title of hemangiopericytoma. It is a malignant tumor, not in a five year but in a ten year concept, with ability to recur locally, and metastasize to regional nodes, and via the blood stream to lungs, bone, brain, and liver." Of eleven patients reported by him, two were dead at five years and seven more were dead at 10 years (the tenth was alive with the disease and the eleventh is free of tumor after a maxillectomy). Surgically, it is important to include a wide margin around these tumors, since the tumor is poorly encapsulated, infiltrates local structures, and often recurs locally. Radiation therapy may be useful in large lesions. Cryosurgery is being considered as a mode of treatment.

OSTEOGENIC SARCOMA AND CHONDROGENIC SARCOMA (MALIGNANT CHONDROID TUMORS)

These tumors occur in the jaws or in the skull and are very rare in children. A comparison of these two types of tumor shows the following: *Osteogenic sarcoma* is the more common. Radical excision is necessary, and 35 per cent have a five-year survival. *Chondrogenic sarcoma* is less common, and only 15 per cent have a five-year survival. Treatment is radical excision and radiation therapy.

In our series, there was a 19-year-old patient with a chondrosarcoma of the mandible, a 5-year-old male with a primary osteogenic sarcoma of the skull, and a 17-year-old with osteogenic sarcoma metastatic to the scalp (three years earlier he had undergone a hemipelvectomy for osteogenic sarcoma of the ischium).

Tumors of the mandible offer a better survival than tumors of the maxilla because an earlier diagnosis can be made and a better margin of the resection is possible. Antral lesions are fatal, although maxillary alveolar lesions are somewhat less morbid because of the surgeon's ability to obtain a margin around the tumor.

Each case must be considered separately. The philosophy of treatment may be compared to the treatment of osteogenic sarcoma of the extremities. In some institutions, immediate surgery is performed. In other institutions initial radiation therapy is given, followed by a waiting period (e.g., six months). If no pulmonary metastases have occurred during this waiting period, surgery is performed.

MALIGNANT HEMANGIOENDOTHELIOMA (ANGIOSARCOMA)

Of all hemangioendotheliomas (HET), approximately 15 per cent occur in children, and of these about 30 per cent are in the head and neck area.[54] Congenital HET may occur in the newborn. Benign and malignant HET (angiosarcoma) occurs. Well-differentiated angiosarcomas have a better prognosis than poorly differentiated tumors. Infants and children usually have the benign type; adults usually develop the malignant variety.

Stout described the tumor in 1943.[55]

The benign HET does not demonstrate the prominent capillary anastomoses, and the capillaries are more separated. The reticulin stain impregnates the capillary wall. The tumor cells are located intravascularly and within the reticulin sheath. No reticulin stain appears around individual cells as it does with pericytes of the hemangiopericytomas. The malignant HET has pronounced anastomosing capillaries lined by neoplastic endothelial cells (endothelioblasts) and papillary infoldings into the lumina. The malignant HET may have histologic features suggestive of Kaposi's sarcoma.[56]

Head and neck sites of origin include the scalp (slowly enlarging submucosal or purple-blue mass), neck nodes (painless growth), mouth (purplish mass) or, rarely, the antrum, thyroid, inner canthus of the eye, or developing in portwine stains. Local growth horizontally in the dermis produces the advancing violaceous discoloration of the skin. It is one of the few sarcomas that metastasize to regional nodes.

In our series there were seven benign and two malignant tumors. Of the benign group, there were two in the parotid gland, one in the neck, one on the scalp, one over the eyebrow, and two in unlisted sites. One malignant HET in a 10-year-old boy involved the right cheek with erosion into the floor of the orbit, and the second, in a 10-year-old girl, involved the temporal area.

Treatment consists of wide surgical excision. In the less malignant variety a cure is usually obtained. In the malignant variety, five-year cures have only occasionally been reported. If the tumor cannot be excised, radiation therapy may be effective. When metastases to neck nodes or lungs occur chemotherapy with actinomycin D or vincristine has been employed.

PAROTID AND SUBMAXILLARY GLAND MALIGNANCIES

About 10 per cent of all parotid tumors in children are malignant,[57] and these may even be present in the newborn. Clinically, they are rapidly growing and sometimes painful, and they may produce a facial nerve paralysis. If malignancy is suspected, an open biopsy is indicated. A positive report dictates a radical parotidectomy, since five-year cures have been observed.[57] The most common malignancies in the literature have been mucoepidermoid carcinoma; next in frequency are undifferentiated carcinoma, undifferentiated sarcoma, adenocarcinoma, adenocystic carcinoma and malignant mixed tumors.

Welch reported thirty years of experience at Children's Hospital Medical Center. In that time he found eight children with malignant parotid tumors and two with malignant submaxillary gland tumors. They were distributed as follows: adenocarcinoma, three; mesenchymal sarcoma, two; adenocystic carcinoma, one; neurofibrosarcoma, one; duct cell carcinoma, one; mixed maligant, one; and carcinoma (no type listed), one.

During the past ten years, one child was seen with a malignant duct cell parotid tumor. She had a radical parotidectomy and was free of tumor after five years. Another child had a mesenchymal sarcoma of the parotid gland.

MALIGNANT SCHWANN CELL TUMORS

This rare tumor develops about half of the time in patients with von Recklinghausen's disease; the other half of the time it occurs without associated neurofibromatosis. Multiple sites may develop as breakdown occurs in the multiple neurofibromas. In our series there was a 3-year-old male and a 10-year-old female, each with malignant Schwann cell tumor of the neck. Radical surgical excision was performed and one survived, but one died.

MALIGNANT TERATOMAS

These tumors are composed of three or more tissues (trigerminal) in an ectopic site and may resemble a fetus.[58] Neural tissue is present in 70 per cent of the cases. Other tissues found have been muscle, bone, cartilage, fat, respiratory epithelium and squamous epithelium. A "dermoid" is a benign cystic teratoma and should not be confused with a "dermoid cyst," which is composed of only one germinal layer and is not a teratoma. Benign teratomas are more common than malignant teratomas.

Neck teratomas are the most common variety. They occur at birth and are rare over 1 year of age. They may be asymptomatic or they may present with either compression of the trachea, producing dyspnea, stridor and cyanosis or pressure on the esophagus, producing dysphagia. On physical examination, the neck teratoma is a large, semi-cystic or solid mass in the anterior triangle of the neck. X-rays may reveal calcifications. Local excision is a treatment of choice for benign teratomas.[59] Malignant neck teratomas are exceedingly rare, and a radical excision is indicated. *Nasopharyngeal teratomas* are associated with deformities of the skull. Local excision, if possible, is the treatment of choice. *Tonsil teratomas* have all been benign and local excision is the only form of therapy needed.[60] *Orbital teratomas* rarely occur.

MISCELLANEOUS TUMORS

Beyond the more common categories of tumors discussed already, certain very rare and unusual or nonspecific tumors have been grouped together.

An *undifferentiated tumor* of the trachea was found in a child 11 years old. Two unspecified *mesenchymal tumors* of the nasopharynx were identified. One *undifferentiated sarcoma* of the retrotonsillar area has been recorded, and *basal cell carcinoma* of the forehead has also been reported.

NONMALIGNANT, BUT POTENTIALLY FATAL, TUMORS

This section will be limited to two lesions which are not considered malignant tumors but which can be fatal.

ANGIOFIBROMAS OF THE NASOPHARYNX

The angiofibroma of the nasopharynx is a tumor of adolescent males. However, it has occurred under the age of 10, and 16 per cent occur over the age of 20 (even up to 79 years of age!). This lesion rarely, if ever, affects a female.

The original tumor site is the roof of the nasopharynx. There is a spectrum of tumor sizes; the tumor may remain small or grow extensively, destroying the bony walls of the sinuses, orbit and skull. The spread of growth is depicted in Table 14.

TABLE 14. ANATOMIC PATHWAYS BY WHICH THE JUVENILE ANGIOFIBROMA SPREADS

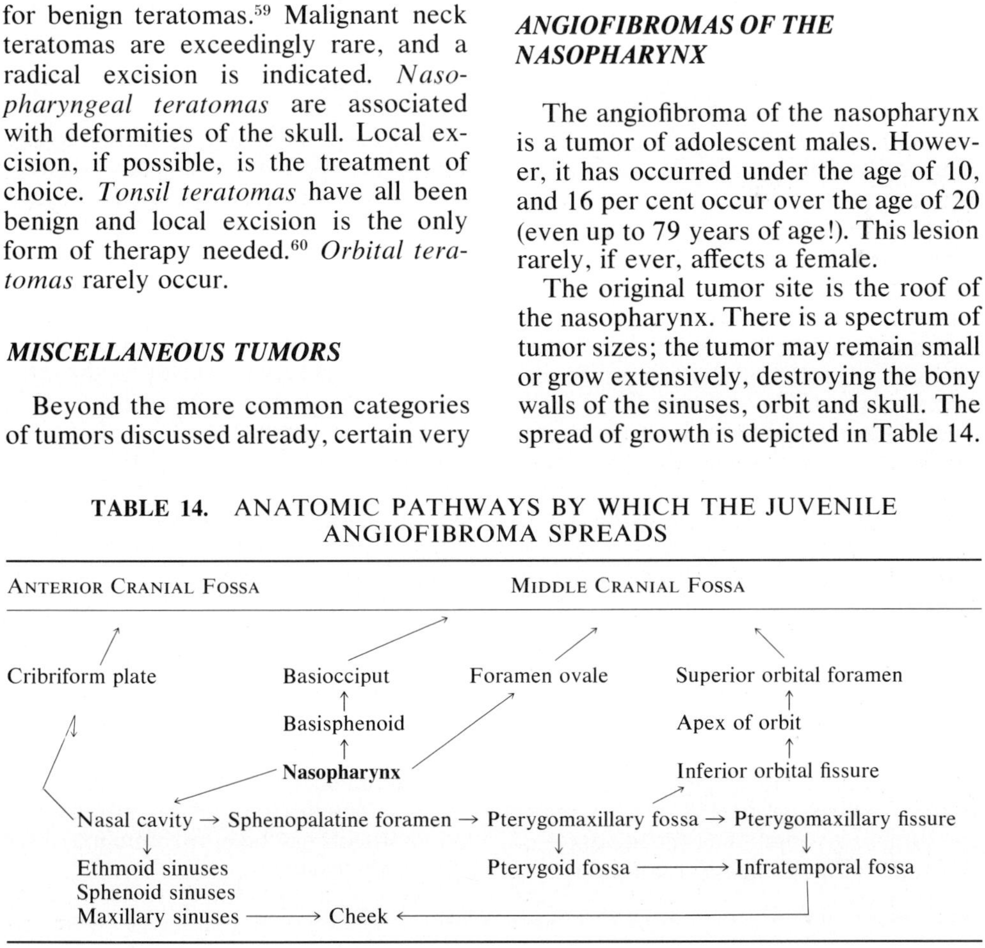

Symptoms depend on the extent of the lesion and will be discussed in detail later. The morbidity from the tumor can be severe.

The tumor consists of thin-walled vessels in a fibrous stroma. Electron microscopy demonstrates that the vessel is lined by a single layer of endothelial cells and dark staining perithelial cells. There is no elastic tissue in the walls of the tumor vessels.

Hormonal dependency was postulated long ago, since the tumor characteristically occurs in the adolescent male. Hormonal therapy preoperatively has proved beneficial in some cases by decreasing the vascular channels, thereby decreasing the bleeding during surgery. Hormonal therapy has occasionally helped in cases of recurrent tumor or intracranial extension by slowing tumor growth or causing tumor regression. Different hormones can be tried. Estradiol, 0.3 mg. daily; stilbestrol, 5 mg. three times a day; and testosterone, 200 mg. every two weeks, have been advocated to ameliorate the symptoms of extensive tumor growth. If tumor recurs after stopping drugs, the hormones may be restarted.[61]

Surgery should be performed only after four-vessel arteriography has been performed and x-rays of skull and sinuses with laminography and polytomography have been taken in order to assess the extent of the tumor. Severe hemorrhage during operation demands that 10 units of blood be available before starting the operation. Two intravenous lines with large bore needles are necessary so that simultaneous infusion can be given. When large tumors are to be excised, a preliminary tracheotomy is needed to prevent aspiration and to maintain a good airway. Controlled hypotension using Arfonad assists in reducing blood loss. Cryosurgical tips have been designed for these tumors, and although cryosurgery is an aid in removal of the tumors, massive bleeding still occurs, unfortunately. It is important for the surgeon to appreciate the life cycle of the tumor. Spontaneous remission may occur; therefore, one should not perform radical surgery that might compromise the optic nerves or the patient's life. Postoperative recurrences frequently occur, but the recurrence rate has been drastically reduced by using good exposure and by exploring all the sinuses and the pterygomaxillary fossa. Small foci of residual tumor may never grow and may become asymptomatic. If the tumor should recur (as it will in 30 per cent of the patients), it will most often recur in the first year. A two-year free period after operation is enough to consider the patient cured.

Radiation therapy is not advocated for this lesion. Post-therapy sarcomas as well as dry mucosal surfaces are undesirable.

The multiple clinical aspects of the nasopharyngeal angiofibroma can be described according to several anatomic sites.

Nasopharynx

The earliest nasopharyngeal angiofibroma is asymptomatic. Then it grows, and severe recurrent epistaxis occurs. Later, the tumor abuts against the posterior choanae, producing unilateral or bilateral nasal obstruction, a nasal voice ("adenoid speech"), mouth breathing and a nasal discharge. Lateral extension in the nasopharynx occludes the eustachian tube orifice, producing a mild hearing loss secondary to an atelectatic middle ear or to serous otitis media. Physical examination by indirect nasopharyngoscopy reveals a pink to reddish bulging mass in one or both sides. A view of the eustachian tube orifice is precluded by the tumor. The mass may also be seen by anterior rhinoscopy. A soft tissue lateral of the nasopharynx will reveal the tumor mass.

Excisional biopsy is indicated if local extension is ruled out by clinical signs and radiographic studies. Removal similar to adenoidectomy or via a transpalatal approach has been recommended for this early lesion.

Conley submits that some tumor masses progress beyond the local nasopharyngeal stage, are undetected clinically, and then regress spontaneously after the age of 20. This dynamic growth and resolution could therefore go unrecognized and untreated.

Local Extension

NASAL CAVITY. Extension into the nasal cavity is easily seen by anterior rhinoscopy. However, the tumor may adhere to the turbinates or septum and not remain free within the nasal airway. The symptoms are nasal obstruction, denasalized speech, mouth breathing, nasal discharge and epistaxis. A unilateral or bilateral rhinotomy incision is used with medial and lateral osteotomies to carefully inspect the interior of the nose. Resection of the tumor, the septum or the turbinates is performed as needed. The nasopharyngeal mass is visualized and removed.

PARANASAL SINUSES. An expanding angiofibroma of the ethmoid sinuses may widen the bridge of the nose and also may produce headaches. X-rays may show a cloudy sinus, even if the sinus is free of tumor. The clouding is due to obstruction of the sinus ostium with secondary infection and a thickened membranous lining. Polytomography may reveal minor degrees of bony erosion. A conservative surgical philosophy is to examine each sinus to obtain biopsies. A lateral rhinotomy incision is followed by ligation of the anterior ethmoidal artery, an external ethmoidectomy and a sphenoidectomy. A Caldwell-Luc approach to the maxillary sinus via the canine fossa is also needed.

PTERYGOMAXILLARY FOSSA. Extension into the pterygomaxillary fossa is common and is not accompanied by localized symptoms. One must therefore rely on laminograms to reveal a soft tissue mass in the pterygomaxillary fossa or to reveal an anterior bowing of the posterior wall of the maxillary sinus. The pterygomaxillary fossa should be examined operatively in all cases via a canine fossa-transantral approach with removal of the posterior wall of the maxillary sinus.[62] If tumor is identified, a Weber-Ferguson incision is made so that a lateral cheek approach can allow the surgeon to remove the pterygoid plates and pterygoid muscles.[63] An alternate operation is to split the mandible in the midline and then approach laterally to the retromaxillary area.

Extension Beyond Pterygomaxillary Fossa

INFRATEMPORAL FOSSA. Tumor extension laterally from the pterygomaxillary fossa via the pterygomaxillary fissure to the infratemporal fossa is evidenced by cheek or temple swelling.[64] Arteriography, either four-vessel or by selective external and internal carotid injections, will demonstrate the size, location and blood supply of the tumor. Enlargement of feeding vessels occurs, as in an enlarged internal maxillary artery. Successful management consists of blunt finger dissection following a lateral cheek approach with a Weber-Ferguson incision.

PTERYGOID FOSSA. Tumor extension posteriorly from the pterygomaxillary space destroys the pterygoid plates and fills up the pterygoid fossa (located posterior to and between the internal and external pterygoid plates). Following a Weber-Ferguson retromaxillary approach, sharp and blunt dissection is needed to remove tumor.

INFERIOR ORBITAL FISSURE AND APEX OF ORBIT. Extension superiorly from the pterygomaxillary space places the tumor at the inferior orbital fissure and apex of the orbit. Clinically, eye pain, exophthalmos and hypesthesia over the cheek occur. Orbital x-rays and laminograms reveal widening of the infraorbital fissure and orbital wall thinning. Angiography will show an enlarged ophthalmic artery and possibly an anastomotic supply from internal and external carotid systems. The tumor may be shelled out of this area via a Weber-Ferguson retromaxillary approach.

Base of Skull and Intracranial Extensions

Basi-occiput and Basi-sphenoid Erosion. Headache and V_2 anesthesia occur secondary to compression at the foramen ovale. Radiographically, the foramen may be enlarged and bony erosion may be seen in the base of the skull underlying the middle cranial fossa. Operative excision is not possible. Hormonal therapy, radiation and watchful waiting are advocated.

Anterior Cranial Fossa Extension. This extension occurs via the ethmoid sinuses or the cribriform plate. It may be asymptomatic or accompanied by intracranial symptoms and signs. Hormonal therapy, surgery (combined intra- and extracranial procedures in association with a neurosurgeon) and radiation therapy have been advocated.

Superior Orbital Fissure Syndrome. Extension from the apex of the orbit to the superior orbital fissure occurs, followed by extensions into the middle cranial fossa. Passing through the superior orbital fissure are cranial nerves III, IV, V and VI, the sympathetic nerves and the ophthalmic vein. Diplopia first occurs with pain around the eye and forehead. Lastly, ophthalmoplegia is noted. On examination, papilledema is detected along with the multiple cranial nerve palsies. The accessible tumor is extirpated, leaving the tumor in the superior orbital fissure untouched. Hormonal therapy can be used postoperatively.

Conclusion

The anatomic spread of a nasopharyngeal angiofibroma is complex and closely involves the anatomy of the pterygomaxillary fossa. The surgeon must study this area in anatomy texts or by cadaver dissections.

The key to cure in this disease is a precise preoperative assessment of the anatomic region involved so that the operative field will allow the surgeon to remove all or almost all of the tumor. Multiple surgical approaches may be necessary to excise the tumor. Each approach has its application.

Nature may assist if tiny islands of tumor are left behind, but one should not depend on spontaneous regressions of residual tumor, since postoperative recurrences are known to occur so typically.

HISTIOCYTOSIS X

Most cases of histiocytosis X occur in children, yet it is still a very rare disease. This group of non-neoplastic, inflammatory diseases is characterized by a proliferative disorder of histiocytes affecting one or more organ systems. When it is localized to bone, it is called eosinophilic granuloma; when it is widespread and chronic, it is called Hand-Schuller-Christian disease; and when it is acute, widespread and fatal it is called Letterer-Siwe disease. Conversion from a localized to a systemic form does occur.[65]

Eosinophilic Granuloma (Localized Histiocytosis)

Localized eosinophilic granuloma of bone is the most common variety of histiocytosis X. The lesion can involve any bone, beginning in the bone marrow and gradually eroding the cortex. Histology reveals an admixture of histiocytes and eosinophils.

In the head and neck area the temporal bone is classically involved, and a mastoid mass presents as a moderately tender, slightly erythematous lesion.[66] X-rays reveal a lytic lesion of the mastoid and sometimes the petrous pyramid. A biopsy confirms the diagnosis and radiation therapy of 600 R. is effective treatment. If localized to the mastoid bone, curetting or mastoidectomy may be curative. Other head and neck sites include the mandible and the orbit. The patient must be observed frequently, since multiple new sites may develop with a conversion from a localized to a systemic histiocytosis.

Hand-Schuller-Christian Disease (Chronic Disseminated Histiocytosis)

This is the most common variety of generalized histiocytosis X. The diagnosis is made when more than one system is involved and multiple lytic bone histiocytic lesions exist. Only 10 per cent of patients present classically with the triad of skull lesions, exophthalmos and diabetes insipidus. Usually a lifelong chronic disease exists, but a few patients have been cured and a few patients have died.

In the head and neck area, the temporal bone is the most common site. It was the site in six of sixteen (37 per cent) patients with Hand-Schuller-Christian disease.[67] Frequently, it affects both mastoids either synchronously or metachronously. The main symptoms are a draining ear or a mass behind the ear. Physical examination reveals polypoid tissue in the external auditory canal eroding from the mastoid. Facial nerve paralysis occurs uncommonly. Treatment with radiation therapy (600 R.) is curative and even cranial nerve VII function may recover. When middle ear fluid is present a tympanotomy tube improves hearing. Large cervical nodes may occur, and they respond to radiation therapy. Later, involvement of the alveolar ridge of the mandible or maxilla may occur with loosening of teeth, soreness and ulceration of the gingiva. The paranasal sinuses may also be involved. Diabetes insipidus and exophthalmos are usually late and uncommon problems.

Letterer-Siwe Disease (Acute Disseminated Histiocytosis)

This is the least common type of generalized histiocytosis X. Onset is in infancy and may occur as early as two months of age. Drainage from the external auditory canal is an early symptom and is quickly followed by multiple symptoms and signs. Examination reveals external otitis with or without granulation tissue or otitis media. Marked cervical node enlargement may mimic a lymphoma.[68] A seborrheic rash, hepatomegaly, splenomegaly and anemia are found. Radiation therapy to localized lesions can be given. However, when widespread systems are present as multiple bone, skin, lung and visceral involvement, systemic chemotherapy as with vincristine, Velban, nitrogen mustard, prednisone or methotrexate should be given. Death usually occurs in one to three years.

REFERENCES

1. Sammarco, G. J., and McKenna, J.: Thyroglossal duct cysts in the elderly. *Geriatrics,* 25:98, 1970.
2. Ward, P. H., Strahan, R. W., Acquarelli, M., and Harris, P. F.: The many faces of cysts of the thyroglossal duct. *Trans. Amer. Acad. Ophth. Otol.,* 74:310, 1970.
3. Thompson, C. A., and Smith, J. W.: Thyroglossal duct cyst presenting laterally. *J.A.M.A.,* 201:565, 1967.
4. Strickland, A. L., Macfie, J. A., VanWyk, J. J., and French, F. S.: Ectopic thyroid glands simulating thyroglossal duct cysts. *J.A.M.A.,* 208:307, 1969.
5. Snedecor, P. A., and Groshong, L. E.: Carcinoma of the thyroglossal duct. *Surgery,* 58:969, 1965.
6. Sistrunk, W. E.: Technique of removal of cysts and sinuses of the thyroglossal duct. *Surg. Gynec. Obstet.,* 46:109, 1928.
7. Sade, J., and Rosen, G.: Thyroglossal cysts and tracts: A histological and histochemical study. *Ann. Otol. Rhinol. Laryng.,* 77:139, 1968.
8. Broomhead, I. W.: Cystic hygroma of the neck. *Brit. J. Plast. Surg.,* 17:225, 1964.
9. Dajani, A. S., Garcia, R. E., and Wolinsky, E.: Etiology of cervical lymphadenitis in children. *New Eng. J. Med.,* 268:1329, 1963.
10. Olson, N. R.: Atypical mycobacterial infections of the neck. *Laryngoscope,* 77:1376, 1967.
11. Yarington, C. T., and Jensen, O. C.: Syphilis as a differential diagnosis of neck masses. *Arch. Otol.,* 86:219, 1967.
12. Carithers, H. A., Carithers, C. M., and Edward, R. O.: Cat-scratch disease. *J.A.M.A.,* 207:312, 1969.
13. Chambers, R. G., and Mahoney, W. D.: Carotid body tumors. *Amer. J. Surg.,* 116: 554, 1968.
14. Lowenbraun, S., Ramsey, H., Sutherland, J., and Serpick, A. A.: Diagnostic laparotomy and splenectomy for staging Hodgkin's disease. *Ann. Int. Med.,* 72:655, 1970.
15. Rosenberg, S. A., Diamond, B. D., Jaslowitz, B., and Craver, L. F.: Lymphosarcoma: A review of 1269 cases. *Medicine,* 40:31, 1961.
16. McNelis, F. L., and Pai, V. T.: Malignant lymphoma of head and neck. *Laryngoscope,* 79:1076, 1969.
17. Catlin, D.: Lymphosarcoma of the head and neck. *Amer. J. Roentg.,* 59:354, 1948.

18. Lipton, A., and Lee, B. J.: Prognosis of stage I lymphosarcoma and reticulum cell sarcoma. *New Eng. J. Med.,* 284:230, 1971.
19. Lukes, R. J., Butler, J. J., and Hicks, E. B.: Natural history of Hodgkin's disease as related to its pathological picture. *Cancer,* 19:317, 1966.
20. Slaughter, D. P.: Surgical management of Hodgkin's disease. *Ann. Surg.,* 148:705, 1958.
21. Bailey, B. J., and Brindley, P. C.: Manifestations of malignant lymphomas in the head and neck. *Trans. Amer. Acad. Ophth. Otolaryng.,* 74:283, 1970.
22. Kaplan, H. S.: Clinical evaluation and radiotherapeutic management of Hodgkin's disease and the malignant lymphomas. *New Eng. J. Med.,* 278:892, 1968.
23. Histopathological definition of Burkitt's tumor. Memoranda. *Bull. World Health Org.,* 40:601, 1969.
24. Burkitt, D.: A sarcoma involving the jaws in African children. *Brit. J. Surg.,* 46:218, 1958.
25. Kauffman, S. L., and Stout, A. P.: Congenital mesenchymal tumors. *Cancer,* 18:460, 1965.
26. Edland, R. W.: Embryonal rhabdomyosarcoma. Five year survival of a patient treated by radiation and chemotherapy. *Amer. J. Roentg.,* 99:400, 1967.
27. Mahour, G. H., Soule, E. H., Mills, S. D., and Lynn, H. B.: Rhabdomyosarcoma in infants and children: A clinicopathologic study of 75 cases. *J. Ped. Surg.,* 2:402, 1967.
28. MacComb, W. S., and Fletcher, G. H.: *Cancer of the Head and Neck.* Baltimore, Williams & Wilkins Co., 1967.
29. Jaffe, B. F.: Personal review.
30. Nelson, A. J., III: Embryonal rhabdomyosarcoma. Report of twenty-four cases and study of the effectiveness of radiation therapy upon the primary tumor. *Cancer* 22: 64, 1968.
31. Jaffe, B. F., Fox, J. E., and Batsakis, J. G.: Rhabdomyosarcoma of the middle ear and mastoid. *Cancer,* 27:29, 1971.
32. Conte, P. J., and Sagerman, R. H.: Embryonal rhabdomyosarcoma of the middle ear with long-term survival. *New Eng. J. Med.,* 284: 92, 1971.
33. Dido, W. R., and Batsakis, J. G.: Rhabdomyosarcoma of the head and neck. *Arch Surg.,* 84:582, 1962.
34. Conley, J., Stout, A. P., and Healey, W. V.: Clinicopathological analysis of 84 patients with an original diagnosis of fibrosarcoma of the head and neck. *Amer. J. Surg.,* 114: 564, 1967.
35. Stout, A. P.: Fibrosarcoma in infants and children. *Cancer,* 15:1028, 1962.
36. Hays, D. M., Mirabal, V. Q., Karlan, M. S., Patel, H. R., and Landing, B. H.: Fibrosarcoma in infants and children. *J. Ped. Surg.,* 5:176, 1970.
37. Horne, C. H. W., Slavin, G., and McDonald, A. M.: Late recurrence of juvenile fibrosarcoma. *Brit. J. Surg.,* 55:102, 1968.
38. Gross, R. E., Farber, S., and Martin, L. W.: Neuroblastoma sympatheticum. *Pediatrics,* 23:1179, 1959.
39. Beckwith, J. B., and Perrin, E. V.: In situ neuroblastomas: A contribution to the natural history of neural crest tumors. *Amer. J. Path.,* 43:1089, 1963.
40. Conley, J. J.: Neurogenous tumors in the neck. *Arch. Otol.,* 61:167, 1955.
41. Apple, D. J.: Metastatic orbital neuroblastoma originating in the cervical sympathetic ganglionic chain. *Amer. J. Ophthalmol.,* 68:1093, 1969.
42. Fortner, J., Nicastri, A., and Murphy, M. L.: Neuroblastoma: Natural history and results of treating 133 cases. *Ann. Surg.,* 167:132, 1968.
43. Robinson, F., and Solitare, G. B.: Olfactory neuroblastoma. Neurosurgical implications of intranasal tumor. *J. Neurosurg.,* 25:133, 1966.
44. Catlin, D., McNeer, G., and Gupta, T. D.: Melanoma of the skin of the head and neck. *Cancer,* 16:19, 1966.
45. McWhorter, H. E., and Woolner, L. B.: Pigmented nevi, juvenile melanomas and malignant melanomas in children. *Cancer,* 7:564, 1954.
46. Conley, J. J., and Pack, G. T.: Melanoma of the head and neck. *Surg. Gynec. Obstet.,* 116:15, 1963.
47. McCormack, L. J., Dockerty, M. B., and Ghormley, R. K.: Ewing's sarcoma. *Cancer,* 5:85, 1952.
48. Kadin, M. E., and Bensch, K. G.: On the origin of Ewing's tumor. *Cancer,* 27:257, 1971.
49. Kauffman, S. L., and Stout, A. P.: Histiocytic tumors (fibrous xanthoma and histiocytoma) in children. *Cancer,* 14:469, 1961.
50. Kauffman, S. L., and Stout, A. P.: Hemangiopericytoma in children. *Cancer,* 13:695, 1960.
51. Walike, J. W., and Bailey, B. J.: Head and neck hemangiopericytoma. *Arch. Otol.,* 93:345, 1971.
52. Stout, A. P., and Murray, M. R.: Hemangiopericytoma. *Ann. Surg.,* 116:26, 1942.
53. Farr, H. W., Carandang, C. M., and Huvos, A. G.: Malignant vascular tumors of the head and neck. *Amer. J. Surg.,* 120:501, 1970.
54. Kauffman, S. L., and Stout, A. P.: Malignant hemangioendothelium in infants and children. *Cancer,* 14:1186, 1961.
55. Stout, A. P.: Hemangioendothelioma, tumor of blood vessel featuring vascular endothelial cells. *Ann. Surg.,* 118:445, 1943.
56. Case report 30–1971. *New Eng. J. Med.,* 285:279, 1971.
57. Mustard, W., et al.: *Pediatric Surgery.* Chicago, Yearbook Medical Publishers, Inc., 1969, pp. 215–232.
58. Batsakis, J. G., and Farber, E. R.: Teratomas

of the head and neck. *E.E.N.T. Digest,* 30:67, 1968.
59. Hurlbut, H. J., Webb, H. W., and Moseley, T.: Cervical teratoma in infant siblings. *J. Ped. Surg.,* 2:424, 1967.
60. Blair, O. M., and Sanchez, J. E.: Teratoma of the tonsil. *Arch. Otol.,* 89:745, 1969.
61. Henderson, G. P., and Patterson, C. N.: Further experience in the treatment of juvenile nasopharyngeal angiofibroma. *Laryngoscope,* 79:561, 1969.
62. Work, W. P., Boles, R., and Nichols, R. D.: Angiofibromas: Diagnosis and treatment, including cryosurgery. *Trans. Amer. Acad. Ophth. Otol.,* 70:922, 1966.
63. Conley, J., Healey, W. V., Blauground, S. M., and Perzin, K. H.: Nasopharyngeal angiofibroma in the juvenile. *Surg. Gynec. Obstet.,* 126:825, 1968.
64. Gupta, O. P.: Nasopharyngeal fibroma with extrapharyngeal extensions. *Acta. Otol.,* 71:406, 1971.
65. Lichtenstein, L.: Histiocytosis X: Integration of eosinophilic granuloma of bone, "Letterer-Siwe disease," and "Schuller-Christian disease," as related manifestations of a single nosological entity. *Arch. Path.,* 56: 84, 1953.
66. Martin, T. H.: Solitary eosinophilic granuloma of the temporal bone. *Laryngoscope,* 79: 2165, 1969.
67. Hudson, W. R., and Kenan, P. D.: Otologic manifestations of histiocytosis X. *Laryngoscope,* 79:678, 1969.
68. Follette, W. J., and Bell, J. G.: Letterer-Siwe disease or acute histiocytosis X. *Arch. Otol.,* 84:563, 1966.

SECTION XVII

THE LARYNX

Chapter One Hundred One

EMBRYOLOGY, APPLIED ANATOMY AND PHYSIOLOGY

WILLIAM E. LAUPUS, M.D.

EMBRYOLOGY

The laryngeal primordium, of mesodermal origin, appears in the third week of embryologic development as the laryngotracheal groove in an outgrowth from the floor of the pharynx. The fourth and sixth branchial arches contribute significantly to the laryngeal structure, particularly to the cartilages and the intrinsic musculature; the fifth arch is vestigial and does not participate in laryngeal development; the second and third arch cartilages ultimately become the hyoid bone.

As embryogenesis proceeds into the fourth and fifth weeks, the laryngotracheal groove is altered by the growth of the arytenoid eminences and the furcula (later to become the epiglottis), and the laryngeal vestibule is formed. The vocal cords arise from an epithelial and mesodermal mass between the vestibule and the upper trachea; later the development of the laryngeal ventricles and sagittal division of this mass will give rise to both pairs of vocal cords during the tenth embryonic week.

The thyroid cartilage arises from the ventral portions of the fourth branchial arches, which also contribute the lateral glosso-epiglottic folds and probably portions of the epiglottis; the main segment of the epiglottis and the cuneiform cartilages come from the furcular part of the pharyngeal floor. The arytenoid, corniculate and cricoid cartilages are sixth arch derivatives, as are all of the intrinsic muscles of the larynx, except the cricothyroid (fourth arch); the extrinsic muscles are derived from the epicardial ridge. The laryngeal structures are well defined by the twelfth embryonic week.

APPLIED ANATOMY

The larynx has a somewhat triangular funnel shape with the broad opening located superiorly. Structurally, it has a cartilaginous framework which begins with the epiglottis at the base of the tongue and ends in the cricoid ring cartilage at its junction with the upper part of the trachea. The major cartilages are four in number: the thyroid cartilage anteriorly, the two arytenoids superiorly and posteriorly, and the cricoid inferiorly. The epiglottic and the paired cuneiform and corniculate cartilages are termed the accessory group. The cartilages are united by various ligaments and membranes. The mucous membrane of the pharynx and the trachea is continuous and is of the ciliated pseudocolumnar type, except for the stratified squamous epithelium of the vocal cords. The mucous membrane is loosely attached to the areolar tissue of the submucosa; edema of the submucosa tends to be poorly confined and may seriously narrow the airway, causing extensive or complete obstruction. The most constricted area of the laryngeal airway is at the site of approximation of the vocal cords.

The larynx is located at a higher cervical level in infancy, remaining slightly higher in the female at all ages. As the neck elongates with growth, the larynx gradually assumes its adult position approximately two vertebral bodies lower than in infancy. Laryngeal growth is gradual throughout childhood until puberty, when the rate is accelerated in both sexes, especially in the male, in whom voice change and the prominent "Adam's apple" become common.

PHYSIOLOGY

The principal functions of the larynx are protective and phonatory in nature, although the larynx also takes part in respiration, deglutition, coughing and other complex activities. Its phylogenetic oldest and primary role is in safeguarding the lower airway from the aspiration of foreign bodies and liquid substances. Laryngeal participation in phonation and communication is generally considered to be a secondary function.

The valvular closure of the larynx with deglutition is accomplished by strong adduction of the true vocal cords, assisted by approximation of the false vocal cords and of the aryepiglottic folds and by movement of the epiglottis in a posterior and downward direction. Contrary to popular opinion, the epiglottis is not essential to deglutition; other than deflecting the bolus of food and shielding the false vocal cords, closure of the airway by the epiglottis is incomplete and affords limited protection from aspiration.

Infants and children with severe laryngeal disease often appear anxious and apprehensive; cyanosis is unusual unless the airway is greatly constricted. The signs of laryngeal involvement are variable and range from noisy breathing to inspiratory wheezing or stridor with laryngeal "crowing," barking cough, dyspnea and inspiratory retraction in the intercostal, subcostal and supraclavicular spaces. Hoarseness or aphonia may be present. If secretions are abundant, the noisy respirations may have a "gurgling" quality, which is present in both inspiration and expiration. Feeding difficulties, including choking and aspiration, are commonly associated with obstructive laryngeal diseases, and undernutrition may develop in infants with chronic respiratory difficulty. Superimposed respiratory infections usually increase the degree of the pre-existing signs.

REFERENCES

Davies, J.: *Human Developmental Anatomy.* The Ronald Press, New York, 1963.

Hamilton, W. J., Boyd, J. D., and Mossman, H. W.: *Human Embryology.* The Williams and Wilkins Co., Baltimore, 1962.

Chapter One Hundred Two

EXAMINATION OF THE LARYNX

NORMAN M. WOLDORF, M.D., and PETER N. PASTORE, M.D.

Evaluation of the larynx truly begins when one first listens to the patient speak and breathe. Formal examination of the larynx is generally performed during inspection of the entire oral cavity and tongue, the soft palate and tonsils, the nasopharynx and the hypopharynx as well as the larynx. This discussion will be largely confined to the examination of the valleculae, larynx and hypopharynx by indirect laryngoscopy although in the young child such a procedure is often difficult and direct laryngoscopy must frequently be performed. Brief discussions of palpation of the neck and larynx, direct laryngoscopy, and x-ray study of the larynx are included for the sake of completeness.

Instruments for Indirect Laryngoscopy

The examiner should have a 100-watt lamp light source, a head mirror, laryngeal mirrors, a tongue blade, an atomizer, some 4 by 4 squares of gauze, pHisoHex, Pontocaine solution (2 per cent) and Xylocaine solution (2 per cent).*

Indirect Laryngoscopy

Examination of the larynx with a laryngeal mirror and reflected light is known as indirect laryngoscopy. Basic instruments include a 100-watt lamp as a light source, a head mirror and a laryngeal mirror. Generally, the examiner stands comfortably to one side of the seated patient and faces him, with the light source posterior and lateral to the patient's head. The patient should be relaxed and seated with his head, shoulders and trunk adjusted to a suitable and relaxed position, leaning slightly forward from the vertical axis of a straight-backed chair. The arms and shoulders are allowed to droop. The head mirror is used to reflect light into the patient's mouth.

After a brief explanation of what is to follow, the formal examination begins. The patient is requested to open the mouth, protrude the tongue, and breathe slowly and evenly through the mouth. The tongue is grasped firmly with a gauze pad and pulled further forward. The tongue should be protected from the patient's lower teeth. The patient is given time to practice breathing and to phonate "Ah-h-h" and "E-e-e." In some patients the tongue remains in the mouth, and with gentle depression on the anterior two-thirds of the tongue the larynx may readily be visualized.

The largest laryngeal mirror that can be used without contacting any structures should be wiped dry with pHisoHex (or warmed) and inserted into the oral cavity with the reflecting surface toward the larynx. The mirror is advanced posteriorly as far as possible without contacting the oropharyngeal wall while reflected light from the head mirror is focused on the laryngeal mirror (Fig. 1). A formal inspection of the extrinsic and intrinsic larynx may be impeded by several common problems.

The first problem is a small faucial isthmus, which prevents proper placement of the mirror. In such cases, the examiner may touch the middle of the soft palate and uvula, lifting them upward. These areas are less sensitive than the tonsillar pillars. The patient may gag, however, and this is a second problem.

Because some patients have a hyperactive gag reflex, it may be necessary to stop, remove the laryngeal mirror, insert a tongue blade, and anesthetize the oropharynx and soft palate with an atomizer spray, 2 per cent Xylocaine solution. If this does not help, 2 per cent Pontocaine solution may be used, but only a small volume for it is extremely potent. After waiting five to ten minutes, one may again begin the examination. Some patients continue to gag, and are helped by a mucus reduction agent and sedation prior to another attempt at indirect laryngoscopy. An occasional patient still will not allow adequate visualization without general anesthesia.

A third problem is an overhanging epiglottis that prevents inspection of the remaining laryngeal structures. The ultimate solution for patients with this problem, as well as small children, is direct laryngoscopy with either topical or general anesthesia. Before resorting to direct laryngoscopy in the operating room, one should exercise great patience, proceed very slowly and try a different technique.

*The use of any topical anesthetic agent requires extreme care, most especially in children.

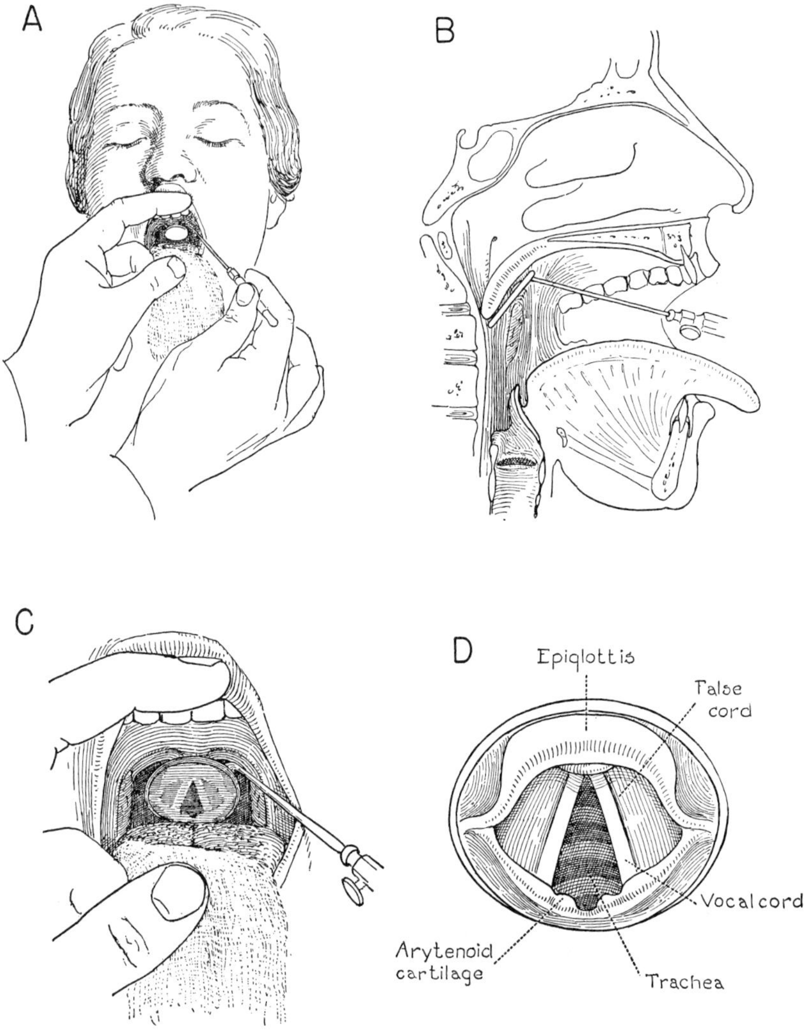

Figure 1. Mirror examination of the larynx. *A*, Note position of the mirror and the manner of holding the tongue. *B*, Side view. Note the relationship of the mirror to the soft palate and the posterior pharyngeal wall. *C*, View of the larynx as seen in the mirror. *D*, Details of mirror image of the larynx. (From Richards, L. G.: *Otolaryngology in General Practice,* Macmillan Co., 1939.)

Instead of having the patient open the mouth and protrude the tongue, just have him open his mouth. Next, insert a tongue blade two-thirds of the way back on the tongue and depress the tongue. The laryngeal mirror is then inserted. By depressing the tongue down and slightly forward and having the patient say "Ah-h-h," the epiglottis may tip forward enough to allow adequate visualization of the larynx. This technique requires considerably more practice than pulling the tongue forward, but it has saved many patients a needless trip to the operating room.

Let us assume that we are dealing with the more typical patient and that the laryngeal mirror has been properly placed for inspection. One should then follow Chevalier Jackson's order of examination, as described by Boies: (1) Free edge of epiglottis. (2) Posterior surface of epiglottis. (3) Right glossoepiglottic fold. (4) Left glossoepiglottic fold. (5) Right arytenoid eminence. (6) Left arytenoid eminence. (7) Right ventricular band. (8) Left ventricular band. (9) Glottic silhouette. (10) Right vocal cord. (11) Left vocal cord. (12) Anterior commissure. (13) Posterior commissure. (14) Anterior wall of trachea.

These structures are examined during quiet respiration. Then the patient is asked to take a deep breath and (15) the glottic chink is inspected. (16) Movement right vocal cord. (17) Movement right arytenoid. (18) Movement left vocal cord. (19) Movement left arytenoid. (20) Patient asked to phonate "E-e-e-e" while preceding four observations are repeated. (21) Repeat during long phonation of "Ah-h-h." (22) Repeat "E-e-e-e" high-pitched. (23) Repeat "Ah-h-h" low-pitched.

Naturally, the hypopharynx and pyriform sinuses are examined at this time.

To the less experienced examiner, the foregoing steps seem difficult to memorize and recall during an actual examination. These steps are quite simple to follow, however, if one stops to analyze what has been described. The examination is simply a step-by-step process whereby one inspects the superior structures first and then logically looks downward one level at a time, noting both the right and left sides. Thus, one examines the free edge of the epiglottis with its laryngeal and lingual surfaces, including the valleculae. Next one follows its folds to the arytenoids, then continues progressively downward to the ventricular bands, true vocal cords and trachea. These same steps are repeated with particular attention to vocal cord and arytenoid movement during deep breathing and low- and high-pitched phonation. Finally, the hypopharynx and pyriform fossae are examined.

Palpation of the Larynx

The larynx is inspected and palpated as part of the general physical examination of the neck. Of course one inspects and palpates for venous distention, arterial pulsation and bruits, masses, glands and areas of tenderness. With particular attention to the larynx, one palpates the hyoid bone, the thyroid and cricoid cartilages, the trachea and the thyroid gland. One examines for tenderness, masses and distortion of contour.

Direct Laryngoscopy

Direct laryngoscopy is an examination of the larynx using a direct lighting source attached to any of a variety of laryngoscopes, with or without the use of a microscope or stroboscopic light. It is performed in an operating room. We will not discuss it in detail. (See Chapter 108.) Suffice it to say that this procedure is employed when indicated to examine difficult patients and small children, to further evaluate suspicious pathology, to obtain biopsy specimens and to remove foreign bodies. It also allows one to inspect the laryngeal ventricles and depths of the pyriform sinuses and hypopharynx, which can not be examined completely by indirect laryngoscopy.

X-ray Studies

Radiologic study of the larynx and hypopharynx is extremely important in selected cases. These studies include soft tissue views of the neck, laminograms of the larynx and contrast medium studies such as laryngograms and pharyngograms.

REFERENCE

Boies, L.: *Fundamentals of Otolaryngology*. Philadelphia, W. B. Saunders Co., 1964.

Chapter One Hundred Three

CONGENITAL MALFORMATIONS

CHARLES F. FERGUSON, M.D., F.A.C.S.

Schaffer and Avery have listed nine factors which may be responsible for congenital malformations.

1. *Gross chromosomal aberrations.*
2. *Defective genes.* Familial and hereditary defects are transmitted as *dominants* (e.g., achondroplasia), as *recessives* (e.g., cleft lip and palate) or as *sex-linked defects* (e.g., hemophilia). Gene mutations may produce entirely new defects.
3. *Fetal radiation.*
4. *Chemical agents.*
5. *Vitamin deficiencies or excesses* (especially vitamin A).
6. *Maternal virus infections* (e.g., rubella).
7. *Faulty implantation of ovum* (in the tube or peritoneal cavity).
8. *Mechanical factors in the uterus* (e.g., faulty position of the embryo or fetus).
9. *Hormonal deprivation or excess.*

The embryologic development of the larynx has been discussed in Chapter 101.

In order to understand *congenital* laryngeal anomalies it is also important to consider the many structural and functional differences between the larynx of the infant and that of the adult.

1. The infant larynx is *higher* in the neck. At birth it is located at C 4, having already descended in the fetal period from a region even above the atlas opposite the basi-occiput. After birth it descends to C 5 by 6 years of age and by puberty to C 6 or C 7, where it remains permanently.
2. It is also *smaller* in size, not only grossly but also in relation to other structures. It is fully developed, however, at birth, but continues to grow larger until puberty when its measurements have just about doubled (except for the infraglottic diameter which has tripled).
3. There is a *more acute angle* between the glottis and the tongue with its attached epiglottis. The larynx tilts downward and anteriorly, allowing the epiglottis to come in closer approximation to the glottic inlet. As the larynx descends, this angle loses its acuteness.
4. The *epiglottis is softer and less rigid* than in the adult and has a much narrower base. (Because of this configuration, it has been called "omega-shaped.") The entire cartilaginous framework of the larynx is also much less rigid, thereby tending to collapse under changing respiratory pressures.
5. The infantile *epiglottis is also longer, narrower and more tubular* and has a deeper anteroposterior gutter than in the adult. Therefore, during inspiration this omega-shaped structure can be more easily sucked into the laryngeal inlet than the wider, more stable and less redundant type of epiglottis seen in the adult.
6. The *aryepiglottic folds are more redundant* and nearer the midline, as they extend posteriorly from the edges of this narrow-based epiglottis. Vibration of these more closely approximated aryepiglottic folds, along with the "exaggerated infantile" structure of the epiglottis itself, is the commonest cause of congenital laryngeal stridor. Constant vibration of these folds may produce edema or thickening which then adds to the respiratory symptoms.
7. The *epithelium and underlying connective tissue* of the larynx and im-

mediate subglottic region (conus elasticus) *are more loosely attached,* predisposing more readily to edema from either infection or instrumentation. Since the subglottic region cannot expand because of the rigid, completely encircling band of the cricoid cartilage, edema in this region may seriously diminish the airway.

8. The *access of entry of air is straighter* in the infant than in the adult.

9. The *lumen* of the larynx in the subglottic area *is funnel-shaped,* and the anteroposterior diameter is proportionately greater in comparison with the trachea during infancy than later in life.

10. The *ventricular air sacs* in infants *are larger.*

The larynx has two primary functions—*respiration* and *phonation.* From an evolutionary point of view the phonatory function is the more recent. Any anatomic abnormality or physiologic disturbance of the larynx may produce symptoms related to either or both of these functions. The larynx also has a *protective* function, and when any foreign material attempts to pass its lumen, sudden closure (spasm), along with the bechic blast (cough), removes the offending substance from the airway before aspiration can occur.

Involvement of the *respiratory* function is obviously the most important, and signs and symptoms of airway obstruction frequently point to an abnormality of the larynx itself, although the entire respiratory tract should be evaluated. These symptoms include stridor, dyspnea, air hunger, cyanotic attacks, increased pulse and respiratory rates, and retractions of the suprasternal, infrasternal, infraclavicular and intercostal regions. Very often the location of the obstruction may be suspected by the quality and type of the accompanying stridor. A high-pitched crow present only during inspiration in most instances indicates an abnormality in the larynx itself—of the epiglottis, the aryepiglottic folds, ventricles, cords or possibly the immediate subglottic region. If the stridor is pitched lower, sounds like snoring, and is heavier and fluttering, and if secretions are excessive, the location may be pharyngeal or occasionally lower, in the large bronchi. A wheezing type of stridor indicates small bronchial or bronchiolar involvement. Stridor which is high-pitched during inspiration and has a prolonged low-pitched expiratory phase (biphasic) suggests main airway obstruction below the larynx, usually in the trachea. In the majority of such cases the cause is narrowing or compression of the tracheal airway from extrinsic pressure, such as a double aortic arch or other congenital malformation of the great vessels. Feeding difficulties, increased salivation and a gurgling type of respiration are common in infants with laryngeal stridor, and nutrition and general development are retarded. The aspiration of saliva, mucus and food material is a recurrent problem, and chronic pneumonitis on this basis is not an infrequent complication. It should be stressed, however, that stridor is merely a *symptom* and never a *diagnosis.* When this term is used, it should always be qualified as to its primary cause and its anatomic location.

When the second primary function of the larynx (*phonation*) is interfered with, there may be a weak feeble cry, a breathy voice, or even aphonia. Such symptoms may suggest a web involving the vocal cords or some neurologic dysfunction. If the cry is hoarse and raspy, tumor or infection must be suspected. An abnormal cry or voice certainly should suggest an abnormal laryngeal condition, but such symptoms may also be noted in subglottic stenosis or even in a central nervous system disturbance.

Direct inspection through a laryngoscope is the most successful and most efficient means of identifying the location and type of any congenital malformation of the larynx. The mirror in infancy is of no value whatever. Direct examination of the larynx with the laryngoscope can be very easily and safely performed without anesthesia by the trained endoscopist who deals with infants, and it is sometimes possible to evaluate the movements of the larynx and cords better than if the patient were asleep. However, general anesthesia has certain advantages, and the greater availability of trained anesthesiologists today makes this procedure now very safe. If the endoscopist is not thoroughly experienced, however, general anesthesia is preferable, since the procedure can be performed with less trauma, and the observer will be given more time to visualize all regions of the larynx and subglottic area as well as the trachea.

The radiologist is an important member of the team in the diagnosis of many laryngeal abnormalities. A lateral radiograph of the neck may give additional information, and cineradiography certainly helps with an evaluation of the swallowing function and with possible aspiration problems. An esophagogram may assist in the correct diagnosis of a vascular ring or other similar abnormality, which often produces symptoms erroneously considered as arising in the larynx itself. Occasionally the esophagogram will demonstrate an unsuspected foreign body in an instance in which all symptoms have pointed to a respiratory problem. Tracheograms or bronchograms, using a contrast medium simply introduced through a laryngoscope without anesthesia, may be of great value in clearly outlining the airway. In infants, however, the airway very often is well delineated by air alone without the introduction of a contrast medium. It should be stressed, however, that if an obvious cause of stridor or other related symptoms is not found in the larynx itself, bronchoscopy must always be performed as a vital part of the investigative procedure.

CLASSIFICATION OF CONGENITAL ANOMALIES OF THE LARYNX

1. *Supraglottic*
   A. Laryngomalacia (the congenitally flaccid or "exaggerated infantile" larynx)
   B. Epiglottic Anomalies (the bifid epiglottis or the overdeveloped, broad-based epiglottis)
   C. Webs
   D. Cysts and laryngoceles
2. *Glottic*
   A. Atresia
   B. Webs
   C. Paralysis (including "cri du chat") (see Chapter 106)
   D. Tumor (papilloma) (see Chapter 104)
   E. Arytenoid displacement (birth trauma)
3. *Subglottic*
   A. Atresia
   B. Stenosis
   C. Webs
   D. Tumors (hemangioma or chondroma) (see Chapter 104)

LARYNGOMALACIA

Laryngomalacia is a term coined by Jackson to emphasize the unusual collapsibility of the laryngeal structures in cases of so-called "congenital stridor." However, this term still suggests to many a pathologic condition similar to osteomalacia or chondromalacia in which there is a true *degenerative* process with abnormal softening or destruction. The term "exaggerated infantile larynx" is cumbersome, but it stresses the fact that this condition is merely a retardation of normal development rather than a true pathologic process. Atkins has termed the condition simply the "flabby larynx," which certainly is an excellent description, although unfortunately it is not accepted by the Committee on Nomenclature!

Although this temporary malfunctioning of the larynx can hardly be regarded as a true anomaly or malformation, it must be discussed here because it comprises well over 75 per cent of all laryngeal problems in infancy. This retardation of development of the larynx results in temporary physiologic dysfunction which subsides with time and further growth. The condition is said to be "outgrown" when the laryngeal framework has become more rigid and shows less collapse during the various phases of respiration. In laryngomalacia the stridor is ordinarily inspiratory in phase. The infant manifests a typically high-pitched crow, more often intermittent than constant, but at times the stridor may be low-pitched and of a vibratory, fluttering nature. Ordinarily, the cry is perfectly clear and strong, so persistent huskiness or true hoarseness should suggest some other condition. Cyanotic attacks are rare, and swallowing in most instances is not compromised unless the stridor is very marked, in which case vomiting and aspiration may occur. The infant usually gains weight and develops satisfactorily. Crying or feeding may increase the stridor temporarily, as do periods of excitement or activity. On occasions the stridor is more noticeable when the infant is lying down, especially if he is placed in a supine position. When lying prone he ordinarily improves. Parental concern may be much greater over simple stridor than over other more serious conditions, and very often a very complete workup is indicated merely to reassure the parents that no other underlying anomaly exists. Congenital stridor is usually not noted immediately at birth but more frequently becomes apparent a few weeks after discharge from the hospital.

Direct examination of the larynx shows a narrow, possibly elongated epiglottis, curled longitudinally on itself so that its entire lateral margins lie in apposition. The aryepiglottic folds, therefore, are closely approximated, appear lax and redundant, and are easily sucked into the glottic inlet during inspiration. On expiration they are blown upward, and this constant motion during both phases of respiration may produce edema, adding to the airway problem. Occasionally, only the mucosa may be redundant and not the entire fold itself. When the epiglottis and aryepiglottic folds are mobilized by the tip of the anterior-commissure laryngoscope, the stridor in such cases immediately ceases, unless there is further obstruction below this level. The use of the anterior-commissure laryngoscope is of great importance to rule out a coexisting subglottic stenosis or an isolated subglottic hemangioma which may otherwise never be suspected if there are no external lesions. Persistence of stridor while the aryepiglottic folds are properly abducted always demands further examination of the entire airway by bronchoscopic examination and possibly a tracheogram. Fluoroscopic studies of the esophagus with contrast-medium evaluation, or possibly angiography, may also be indicated.

If the stridor is due to laryngomalacia alone, the prognosis is excellent, and the symptoms usually subside completely by the end of the first year or within a few months thereafter. If significant symptoms persist much longer than a year, studies as previously noted should be performed. Very occasionally, however, simple stridor will persist longer than this, and the cause is found to be merely unusual redundancy of the mucosa overlying the arytenoids. These folds of mucosa can be easily snipped off with sharp biopsy forceps, but this is the only indication for a surgical procedure in this condition. Great care must be taken to remove very superficially *only* the mucosa and not to damage in any way the underlying arytenoid cartilaginous structures.

CONGENITAL WEBS

Congenital laryngeal webs result from an arrest of development of the larynx around the tenth week of fetal life. Formerly it was considered that fetal inflammation may have played a part in the production of these webs, but this theory generally has been discounted. Formation of a web is probably by the same mechanism which results in atresia of the larynx or congenital subglottic stenosis. There is failure of dissolution of the fused lateral masses at the time the lumen should become re-established.

Holinger in 1967 reported thirty-two congenital webs in his very large series of 866 congenital laryngeal abnormalities. Roughly 75 per cent of webs occur at the level of the vocal cords, about 10 to 15 per cent at the supraglottic level, and the remainder occurs in the subglottic region. If the web occurs in the subglottic region, it is apt to be a thicker and a more fibrous type of structure than the thinner supraglottic or glottic webs. Previous to Holinger's report, supraglottic webs were considered to be very rare and thought to comprise only 1 to 2 per cent of the total.

There is great variation in the thickness of the webs. The larger ones may cover the entire glottic chink and produce great respiratory difficulty, yet the smaller anterior ones may go unrecognized for some time, as the airway is less involved. The appearance of the web varies from a thin transparent membrane over the anterior part of the glottis, with the underlying movements of the cords easily visible, to a thick, fibrous connective tissue obstruction extending far below the glottic level. A typical web is usually concave posteriorly. Its upper surface is covered with squamous epithelium, then a thicker layer of connective tissue, and a layer of tracheal mucosa lies beneath. If the web is at the level of the cords, the anterior two-thirds of the larynx is usually occluded, ordinarily as far back as the vocal processes of the arytenoids. This leaves a small posterior chink in the interarytenoid area. In very rare instances the web, however, may be entirely in the interarytenoid region, leaving a normal anterior commissure.

The infant with a congenital web usually has difficulty from birth in both breathing and in phonating, especially if it is at the glottic level. The degree of stridor depends upon the amount of obstruction to the airway. If the cords are involved, the cry is weak and occasionally hoarse, and sometimes there is true aphonia.

Treatment consists of either direct incision of the web through the laryngoscope or repeated dilatation. If the web is anterior and at the glottic level, it can be separated from the cord by a sharp incision only on one side. The incision is carried up close to, but not immediately involving, the anterior commissure. Dilatation should then be carried out every two to three days to prevent reformation of the web. These dilatations are continued until epithelialization has occurred, which may take about two weeks. Then, if necessary, any remnant which has retracted to the opposite side can easily be removed with sharp biting forceps. By this method, once the operated cord has epithelialized, there will not be the danger of bridging the lumen by reformation of the web. If the web is so thick that it cannot be incised, the only treatment other than tracheotomy is repeated, very gentle, laryngeal dilatation. Even with dilatation tracheotomy usually is necessary in order to avoid serious postoperative edema. McNaught's tantalum keel inserted between the cords through a slot in the thyroid cartilage after the web has been excised is a very satisfactory method of treatment for the older patient, but this has no place in the infant. In an older person such a keel is left in place until complete epithelialization has occurred.

CONGENITAL CYSTS AND LARYNGOCELES

These malformations of the larynx are not as common as the previously discussed anomalies. Suehs in 1967 reported that only twenty-seven cases of laryngeal cysts had been recorded in the entire literature. He added two of his own. He also noted that half of the reported cases had not been diagnosed until postmortem examination. The true cyst secretes fluid and therefore tends to increase in size. It must be differentiated from the laryngocele which is an air-containing sac and does not contain fluid. In Holinger's series of 866 congenital malformations, he reported twelve congenital cysts, half of them involving the ventricles and the other half the aryepiglottic folds. This is certainly the largest group of cases encountered by one observer. The laryngocele may present in the neck as a herniation through the thyrohyoid membrane, and the swelling becomes apparent as the infant cries, strains or coughs. The true cyst may be a simple retention cyst of the mucous membrane, especially in the region of the epiglottis or one of the ventricles, but occasionally it may be an actual anomaly arising from the second or third branchial arches. Cysts of the glottic area have been reported, arising from either the true vocal cord or the false cord or occasionally from the lateral wall of the supraglottic area, the aryepiglottic folds or even the pyriform sinuses. The cyst is sessile and not pedunculated, and its wall ordinarily thin and glistening with prominent blood vessels visible in the epithelium (Fig. 1). It contains a yellow-tinged fluid, which is usually thin, but on occasions may be quite viscid and sticky.

Diagnosis is made by direct laryngoscopy, although the swelling may be easily visualized by a lateral x-ray taken in inspiration. The signs and symptoms are those of ordinary airway obstruction, and the diagnosis cannot be made except by direct examination with the laryngoscope. If the cyst is of good size, there may be dysphagia, as well as dyspnea, cyanotic attacks, retraction of the soft tissues of the chest, and a feeble or even aphonic cry. If the cyst is located at the base of the tongue, an internal thyroglossal duct cyst must always be suspected (see Chapter 100). A thyroglossal duct cyst is proximal to the hyoid bone and may displace the epiglottis backward and downward and may also cause definite airway obstruction.

The best treatment is complete excision of the cyst, since incision and drainage without removal of the cyst wall invites recurrence. Aspiration is of no value except from the diagnostic point of view, and even repeated aspiration is not curative. Glandular elements lining the cyst still continue to secrete fluid. Only in rare instances is an external approach by thyrotomy indicated. Tracheotomy must always be considered if satisfactory management of the cyst is not possible otherwise.

ATRESIA

This condition obviously is incompatible with life unless it is recognized immediately at birth and an adequate airway is promptly established. Tracheotomy is

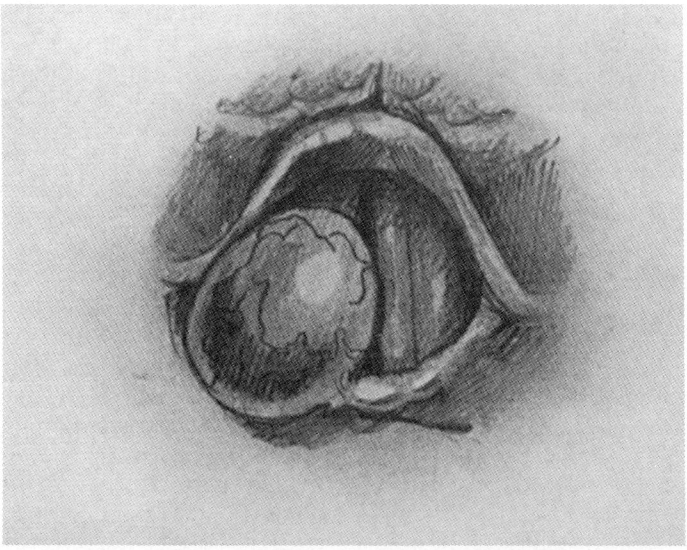

Figure 1. Supraglottic cyst of the larynx, showing prominent blood vessels. (From Suehs, O. W., and Powell, D. B., Jr.: Congenital cyst of the larynx in infants. *Laryngoscope,* 77:654, 1967.)

usually necessary. The term "atresia" literally means *complete* obstruction, although in the literature the term "partial atresia" has been used. Technically, this latter condition should be regarded as marked stenosis as long as there is any opening at all. Because the death of an infant with atresia of the larynx is often recorded simply as a "stillbirth," it is difficult to obtain meaningful statistics as to its incidence. Smith and Bains, from the Hospital for Sick Children in Edinborough, in 1965 reported nine cases of atresia of the larynx and stated at that time only twenty-six others could be found in the literature, but obviously countless cases have never been reported or even diagnosed. In three of their nine patients there was an associated tracheo-esophageal fistula, and in many others there were anomalies of the gastrointestinal tract, genitourinary tract, central nervous system or skeletal system. The presumptive cause of atresia of the larynx dates back to early embryonic life when the laryngeal lumen fails to become re-established after the tenth week of fetal life when the stage of complete epithelial coalescence should have been completed. Wolander has regarded this anomaly as a failure of previous fusion of mesodermal elements, rather than of epithelial derivatives to become obliterated. In the few cases reported there appears to be some hereditary, or at least familial, aspect, since it has occurred in siblings as well as in consecutive generations.

The infant with atresia makes a vigorous effort to breathe if his central nervous system as well as other vital systems are functioning properly. Sometimes these efforts comprise violent respiratory movements, but they fail to admit air into the lungs. These attempts at forceful respiration distinguish the situation from neonatal asphyxia in which the infant never tries to initiate respiration. Cyanosis increases as time elapses even though vigorous respiratory efforts may be maintained for a short time. Within a very few minutes, however, cardiac arrest develops and no further respiratory movements are discernible.

Many years ago the Jacksons reported a case of atresia of the larynx in which direct inspection immediately after delivery showed a simple membranous occlusion of the entire glottis. A 3 mm. bronchoscope was forced into the trachea through this complete glottic web, and this emergency procedure adequately relieved the obstruction. Holinger encountered an infant who had had an emergency tracheotomy performed within a few minutes of delivery when atresia of the larynx fortunately had been promptly recognized. Laryngoscopy on this infant later confirmed the diagnosis. The entire glottis was encased in a thick fibrous sheet of almost cartilaginous material.

Smith and Bains have described three types of congenital atresia of the larynx. *Type I* refers to a situation in which the vestibule is represented by a shallow cleft, flanked by apices of the arytenoid cartilages which are fused in the midline. In such cases the cricoid cartilage is malformed. There is also a fine duct less than 1 mm. which passes through the atretic area into the trachea. In *Type II* the vestibule and laryngeal sinuses are normal, and the arytenoid cartilages are separate, but the glottis is a blind cleft between the vocal folds. The cricoid cartilage is dome-shaped because of a conical cavity in it. This is lined with respiratory epithelium, and its lower end is continuous with the trachea in some cases, or in others the entire trachea may be absent. Cases in which the glottis is occluded by a membrane of fibrous connective tissue and muscle are classified as *Type III*. This membrane is limited posteriorly by a thin base of cartilage behind which is a fine duct which opens into the vestibule just above this membrane.

Obviously, sucessful treatment of congenital atresia of the larynx demands immediate recognition of the problem and establishment of an artificial airway by tracheotomy at the time of delivery, unless a simple membrane can be perforated. Otherwise, cerebral damage from anoxemia results, and death ensues unless an airway is promptly established.

Immediate laryngoscopy should be done, if possible, so that such a membranous occlusion could be discovered and quickly perforated. In such a fortunate case, tracheotomy would not be necessary. Otherwise, immediate tracheotomy should be performed, a 00 or 0 tube inserted, and later on the details of the atresia can be properly assessed. The patient must be kept adequately oxygenated for some time, and effective suctioning of the airway must be employed, constantly removing any obstructing mucus. Only by heroic treatment can the life of an infant with atresia of the larynx be saved.

CONGENITAL SUBGLOTTIC STENOSIS

Congenital subglottic stenosis is a much more common finding in patients with airway obstruction, and the extent of the narrowing determines the severity of symptoms and signs. In Holinger's series of 866 congenital malformations there were fifty-three instances of congenital subglottic stenosis, by far the largest group other than the 650 cases of laryngomalacia. This is a cause of serious neonatal asphyxia, although obviously the clinical picture presented at birth is not as dramatic as that of the infant with atresia of the larynx.

The conus elasticus in the immediate subglottic area is normally the widest portion of the larynx and is even larger than the trachea, since it has an inverted funnel shape. The marked soft tissue narrowing in congenital subglottic stenosis extends from the level of the cords down to the cricoid area. This defect is the result of an arrest of development of the conus elasticus itself, but in other instances occasionally the cricoid cartilage may not be properly developed. Subglottic stenosis is not a web, and the narrowing is ordinarily diffuse and may be very extensive with the point of maximal obstruction ordinarily located 2 to 3 mm. below the glottic level. On some occasions the swelling may be bilateral with a narrow slitlike lumen extending in an anteroposterior direction, or on rare occasions it may be evident simply as a unilateral bulge. In such situations, however, an isolated subglottic hemangioma must be suspected. This area of subglottic stenosis is not inflammatory, nor is it edematous. It is usually an actual structural deformity. The entire larynx is underdeveloped and in some cases is congenitally small, so that frequently it may not give the impression of a truly obstructed lumen. Occasionally, a deformed cricoid cartilage can be seen projecting into the subglottic lumen.

Stridor is usually present from the time of birth, although it is not ordinarily as high-pitched or completely inspiratory as that seen in instances of true laryngomalacia (the "exaggerated infantile larynx"). A history of recurring attacks of croup is common and sometimes the stridor may be noticed only after a respiratory infection. Ordinarily, the cry and voice of the infant are normal, clear and strong, but occasionally the vocal cords are dull and thickened. Holinger reported that congenital absence of the epiglottis was noted in two of his patients with congenital subglottic stenosis. It is difficult to explain this occurrence from the embryologic point of view, since the two areas have different origins of development.

A congenitally small larynx is seen on occasions in which the entire organ is generally underdeveloped but appears perfectly normal otherwise. In 1932 Gabriel Tucker, Sr., made extensive studies of the infant larynx and stated that an anteroposterior diameter less than 6 to 7 mm. or a subglottic region less than 5 mm. was "congenitally small." The average anteroposterior diameter of the larynx of the newborn he considered should be 7 to 9 mm., with a subglottic area usually 1 to 2 mm. less. The length of the cord in the newborn infant is usually 6 to 8 mm. The subglottic area with a diameter of only 4 mm. presents a dangerous situation as far as the airway is concerned.

Over 50 per cent of cases of congenital subglottic stenosis require tracheotomy, and if laryngeal dilatation is to be performed as a therapeutic measure, a previous tracheotomy is almost essential. Otherwise, edema produced by repeated dilatations or infection may pose a serious problem. If dilatation is carried out, it should always be very gentle and not too extensive, but the process may be repeated possibly once a month. Poor results occur from splitting of the tissues if too vigorous or too extensive dilatation is carried out at one time. The indwelling core-mold has been used in an attempt to produce a better airway. This is ordinarily made from some physiologically inert material, such as silastic or teflon, since the old hard rubber core-molds produced severe tissue reaction. If the core-mold is used, obviously such a patient should be tracheotomized previously. Time, however, alleviates this localized obstruction more than any other one factor, even more than repeated dilatations. Growth takes care of the problem satisfactorily in most instances.

LARYNGOTRACHEO-ESOPHAGEAL CLEFT

Laryngotracheo-esophageal cleft is an unusual malformation of the larynx. Many cases, however, must have gone unrecognized and, therefore, have not been reported in the literature. This is a congenital defect due to failure of dorsal fusion of the cricoid lamina, resulting in a cleft extending downward for some distance, even in some cases as far as the carina. A single respiratory-digestive tube is thereby created, and this has been termed an "esophagotrachea." There is always a large interarytenoid cleft, which leaves the larynx open posteriorly, and this fissure extends through the defective cricoid lamina. By the seventh or eighth week of fetal life, the cricoid cartilage should show some chondrification. If, however, such an abnormal cleft develops before chondrification of the cartilage, later on chondrification centers develop laterally on each side of the cleft and the cartilage otherwise develops satisfactorily.

Shapiro and Falla in 1966 reported an eight-month-old infant with this defect in whom this difficult diagnosis was finally made by retrograde esophagoscopy through a previously performed gastrostomy stoma (Fig. 2). Several laryngoscopies had failed to reveal the defect, and this is easy to understand since it is visualized "end on" (and not laterally) so that perspective was distorted. Shapiro repaired the defect successfully through a lateral pharyngotomy incision. Bordley reported having seen two cases of

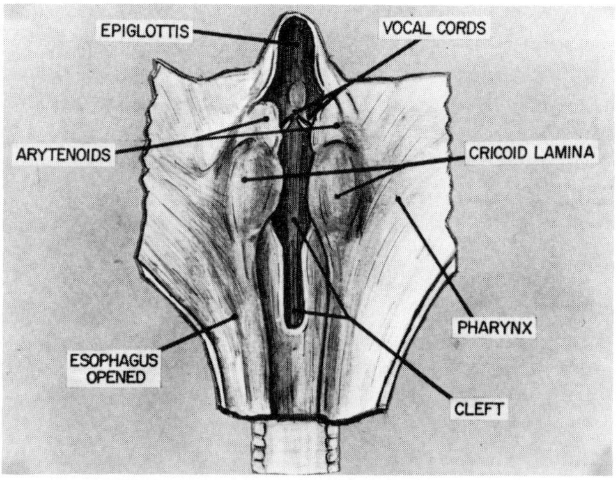

Figure 2. Laryngotracheo-esophageal cleft in an 8-month-old infant. (From Shapiro, M. J., and Falla, A.: Congenital posterior cleft of larynx. *Ann. Otol. Rhin. Laryngol.,* 75:961, 1966.)

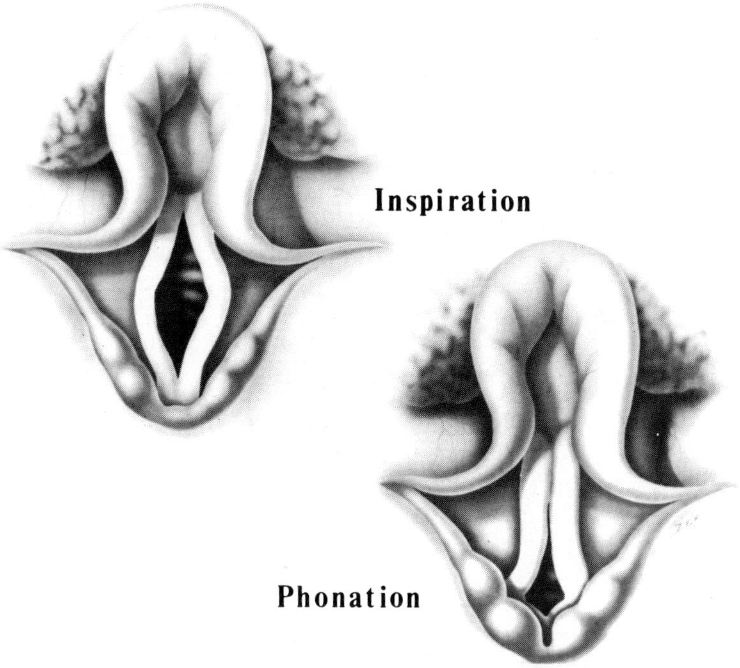

Figure 3. Drawing of the larynx during inspiration in the cri du chat syndrome. Note the long, flaccid epiglottis and the diamond-shaped glottic chink during inspiration. During phonation, the air space remains in the posterior commissure. (From Ward, P. H., Engel, E., and Nance, W. E.: The larynx in the "cri du chat" (cat cry) syndrome. *Laryngoscope,* 78:1716, 1968.)

laryngotracheo-esophageal cleft at Johns Hopkins Hospital; Holinger has also reported two, and Atkins one. Griscom reported one case from the Children's Hospital Medical Center in Boston, and a complete review of the literature by him uncovered only sixteen previous cases, most of which were fatal. Griscom's case was that of a 36-hour-old female who had an extensive cleft extending to within 1 cm. of the carina. Operation was performed, but the patient died on the following day. Postmortem examination showed the long extent of the cleft. In addition there was an exstrophy of the bladder, vaginal and rectal stenosis, a lobulated spleen, and a pseudomonas abscess of the lung.

Diagnosis of this condition is obviously very difficult, even if careful endoscopy and x-ray studies are performed. Radiographic studies suggest an H type of tracheo-esophageal fistula, and the symptoms are similar, although more exaggerated. There is constant difficulty with mucus, and the infant aspirates his own secretions as well as feedings. Since the larynx is split posteriorly, the cry is very weak and feeble and may even be aphonic. Cyanotic attacks and aspiration pneumonitis result, for it is not possible for the infant to swallow either mucus or feedings without entrance into the lungs.

"CRI DU CHAT" SYNDROME

In 1963 LeJeune, a geneticist from Paris, reported three infants who had a weak cry characteristic of the "mewing of a cat," and Ward et al. reported four cases in 1968. Seventy-five cases have been reported since LeJeune's original description, so a definite entity has been established. One of the pictures in Jackson's textbook is labeled "congenital laryngeal stridor" and shows the typical appearance of a larynx as seen in this syndrome, which at the time of the publication of the book obviously was unknown. It is now felt that this condition must be much more common than has been suspected. The larynx is characteristically very narrow with a diamond-shaped glottis noted during inspiration. On phonation (or adduction) the posterior part of the larynx shows an open triangle probably due to paralysis of the arytenoideus muscle (Fig. 3). The epiglottis is ordinarily very long and redundant and somewhat flaccid. There are many other associated abnormalities, including microcephaly, hypertelorism, generalized hypotonia and severe mental retardation. The ears are located very low on the sides of the head, and there are prominent epicanthal folds, strabismus, midline oral clefts and a beaklike profile. The stridor is usually of the inspiratory type and is present from birth; the cry is a typical catlike mew. The nutritional state is always poor, along with

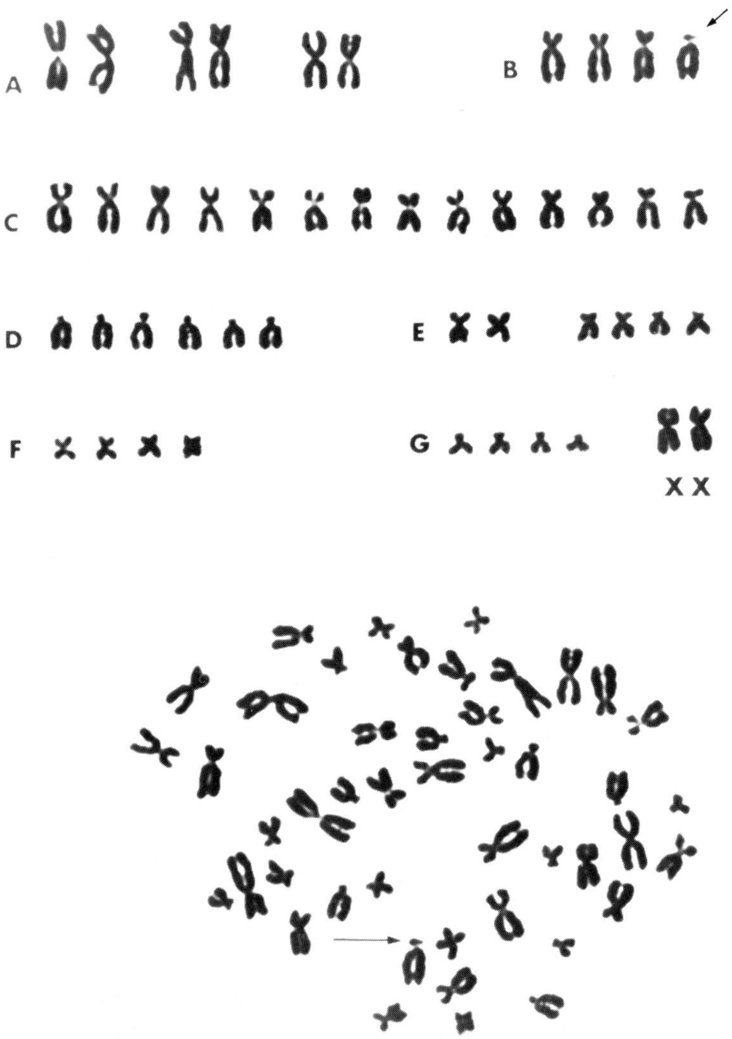

Figure 4. Karyotype of a blood cell preparation showing partial deletion of a short arm of a B group chromosome in cri du chat syndrome. (From Ward, P. H., Engel, E., and Nance, W. E.: The larynx in the "cri du chat" (cat cry) syndrome. *Laryngoscope,* 78:1716, 1968.)

retarded physical and mental development. It is reported that females are more prone to this syndrome than males. The diagnosis must be made on the symptom complex confirmed by chromosome studies, which in every instance show a partial deletion of the short arm of the B 5 chromosome (or one of the B group.) Thus, it is a proven genetic defect. (Fig. 4).

CONGENITAL LARYNGEAL PARALYSIS

Since paralysis of the larynx is not a true congenital *malformation* it will be discussed in detail separately in Chapter 106.

REFERENCES

Baker, D. C., Jr., and Savetsky, L.: Congenital Partial Atresia of Larynx. *Laryngoscope,* 76:616, 1966.

Ferguson, C. F.: Congenital Abnormalities of the Infant Larynx. Otolaryng. Clin. North Amer., 185:185, June 1970.

Ferguson, C. F., and Flake, C. G.: Subglottic Hemangioma as the Cause of Respiratory Obstruction in Infants. *Ann. Otol. Rhinol. Laryng.,* 70:1095, 1961.

Griscom, N. T.: Persistent Esophago-trachea—the Most Severe Degree of Laryngo-tracheoesophageal Cleft. *Amer. J. Roentgen.,* 97:211, 1966.

Holinger, P. H., and Brown, W. T.: Congenital Webs, Cysts, Laryngoceles and Other Anomalies of the Larynx. *Ann. Otol. Rhinol. Laryng.,* 76:744, 1967.

LeJeune, J.: "Cri du Chat" Syndrome—Chromosome Deletion Causes Severe Retardation. *J.A.M.A.,* 197:40, 1966.

Schaffer, A. J., and Avery, M. E.: *Diseases of the Newborn,* 3rd ed. Philadelphia, W. B. Saunders Co., 1971.

Shapiro, M. J., and Falla, A.: Congenital Posterior Cleft of Larynx. *Ann. Otol. Rhinol. Laryng.,* 75: 961, 1966.

Smith, I. I., and Bains, A. D.: Congenital Atresia of the Larynx and Report of 9 Cases. *Ann. Otol. Rhinol. Laryng.,* 74:338, 1965.

Suehs, O. W., and Powell, D. B., Jr.: Congenital Cyst of the Larynx in Infants. *Laryngoscope,* 77:654, 1967.

Ward, P. H., Engel, E., and Nance, W. E.: The Larynx in the "Cri du Chat" (cat cry) Syndrome. *Laryngoscope,* 78:1716, 1968.

Chapter One Hundred Four

TUMORS AND CYSTS OF THE LARYNX

DANIEL C. BAKER, JR., M.D., AND ROBERT M. HUI, M.D.

In the evaluation of disturbance of function of the larynx, mass lesions of the structure must be considered. The size and location of the lesion determine the nature and degree of the changes in the two primary functions of the larynx, namely, respiration and phonation. Changes in respiratory function are manifested by stridor, dyspnea, and apnea in extreme cases. Phonatory abnormalities include aphonia, absent or weak shrill cry, or hoarseness.

The disturbances in phonation may occur when tumors actually involve the vocal cords or put pressure on the vocal cords, interfering with vibration of the cord. The voice may also be modified if the tumor or cyst arises on the epiglottis.

The infant larynx differs from that in the adult in several respects. It is small,

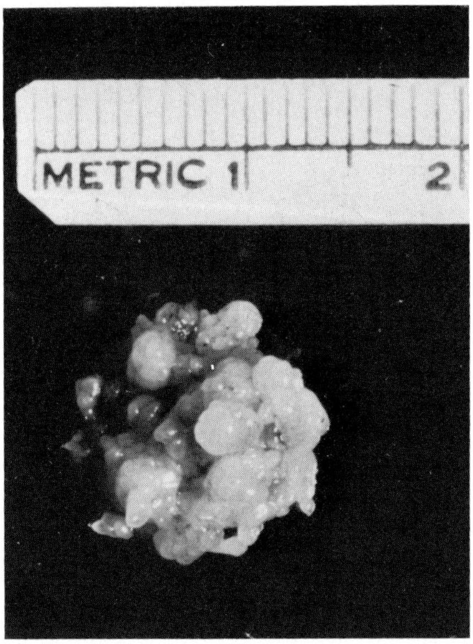

A

Figure 1. Juvenile papilloma of larynx. *A,* Gross specimen. (From Ferguson, C. F., and Scott, H.: Papillomatosis of the larynx. *New Eng. J. Med.,* 230:447, 1941.)

Figure continued on following page.

and it has a lumen that is relatively smaller in relation to the whole body than the adult lumen.[1] The structural framework, including the cartilages and soft tissue, is softer, and therefore likelier to collapse and more likely to cause stridor. The infant larynx is positioned higher in the neck. There is a less rigid, narrower based epiglottis with a more acute angle between the glottis and epiglottis, which contributes to reducing the laryngeal inlet.[2]

Papilloma

The majority of tumors of the larynx in children are benign. The most common neoplasms are papillomas. They are usually multiple in children, whereas adults usually present with a solitary mass. The most common site of origin is the vocal cords, but the tumors may spread to adjacent areas in the tracheobronchial tree and may be implanted at a distance, as in the pharynx or palate. They have been identified in the newborn. In a series reporting 109 patients, 40 per cent had their tumor appearing before age 16 years and 29 per cent had their onset before 5 years of age.[2] There is no significant difference in incidence by sex or by race. In the analysis of another series of 107 children with papilloma, it was reported that most of the patients were from economically disadvantaged families.[4]

The specific etiology of papilloma of the larynx has not been established. There are instances wherein a filterable agent derived from the papilloma has been transplanted to both skin and mucous membrane, suggesting a virus origin.[5] Electron microscopy has failed to demonstrate characteristic inclusion bodies or viruses.[6]

The tumor appears as an irregular warty nodular mass, pink or red in color. The size is variable from small nodules of a few millimeters to masses that occlude the larynx. They are friable and bleed easily. Microscopically, the papillomas are vascular connective tissue cores covered by multiple layers of stratified squamous epithelium (Figs. 1 and 2). There is no invasion of the basement membrane. There is no histologic difference between the adult and childhood tumors. The tumors tend to recur after

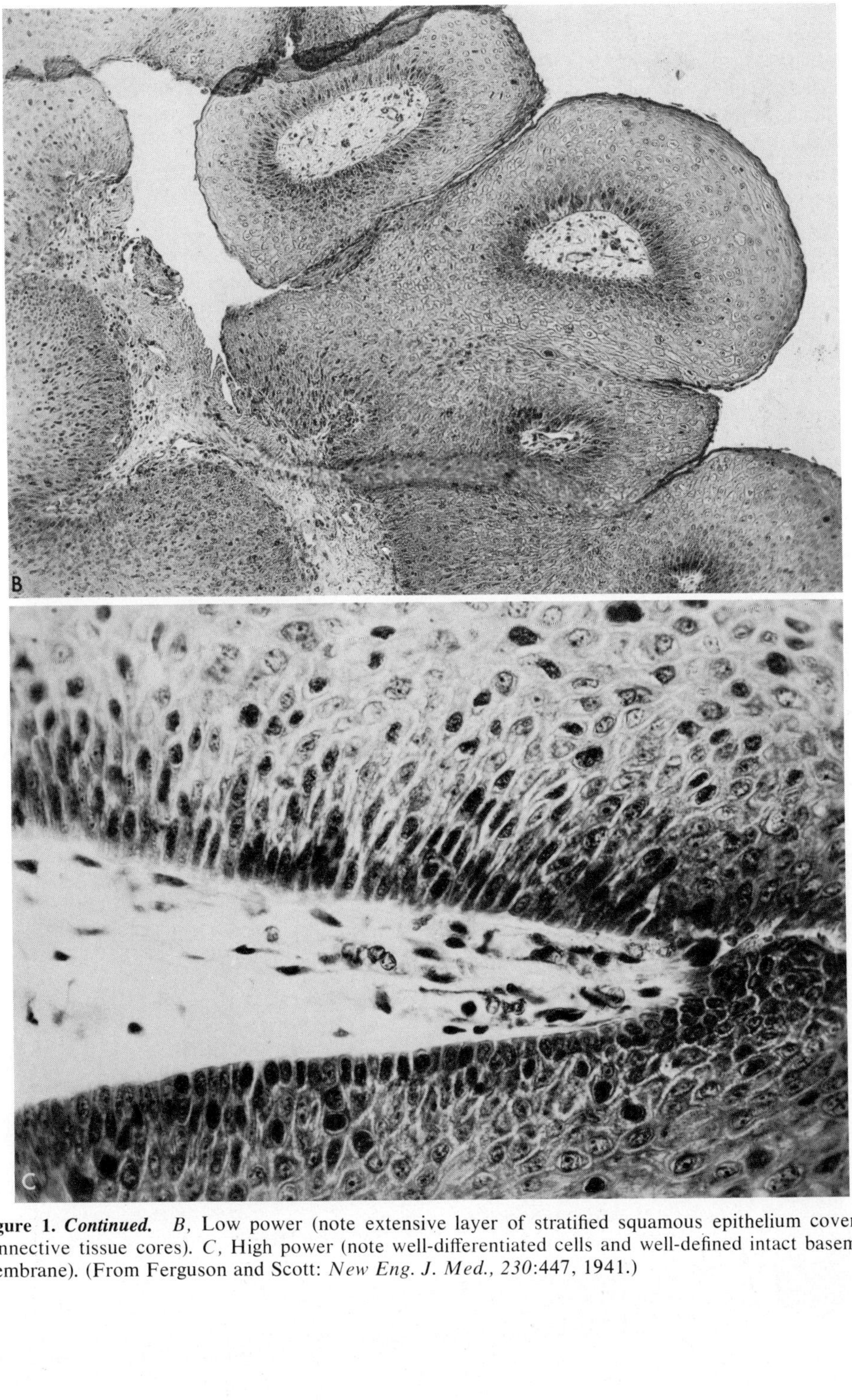

Figure 1. *Continued.* *B,* Low power (note extensive layer of stratified squamous epithelium covering connective tissue cores). *C,* High power (note well-differentiated cells and well-defined intact basement membrane). (From Ferguson and Scott: *New Eng. J. Med., 230*:447, 1941.)

removal, more frequently in children. Gradually, they regress at puberty, suggesting an endocrine influence, and indeed some therapy regimens include hormones.

The papilloma is diagnosed by mirror or direct inspection and by histologic evaluation of tissue.

There are many forms of treatment. Topical agents have included caustics, podophyllin and estrogens. Internal medications that have been tried are heavy metals, arsenic, potassium iodide, bismuth compounds, androgens and tetracyclines. Recently, antimetabolites like methotrexate and alkylating agents have had some success.[3] Surgical measures include forceps removal, cautery, thyrotomy and laryngofissure with vein graft to the denuded cords,[7] and tracheotomy. Irradiation has been used, but these tumors are not radiosensitive, and malignancies have been reported. Recently, ultrasound radiation has been reported to be useful,[8] and cryosurgical application is under trial. Autogenous papilloma vaccines have been tried, as has bovine wart vaccine.[9] The trend of therapy seems to be accurate surgical removal with forceps with maintenance of an adequate airway. Microsurgical approach to the larynx is being developed in many centers for finer control of surgical margins.

In the treatment and management of papilloma of the larynx, the restoration of function should be the goal of the laryngologist. Laryngeal obstruction must be relieved by removal of large masses of papilloma. The phonatory function is restored by very careful removal of the papilloma from the surface and edges of the true vocal cords. Damage to the vocal cords by biting too deeply can result in permanent changes in the voice by causing scar tissue that interferes with vibration of the cords. If the anterior commissure is disturbed, the formation of a web is a possibility.

Chemical or electrocautery should not

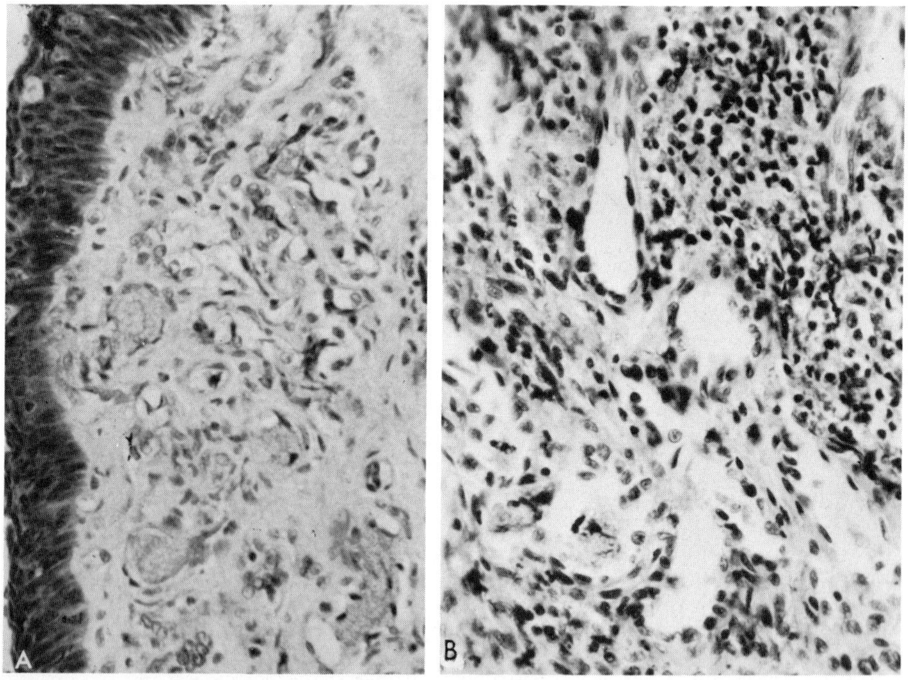

Figure 2. Subglottic hemangioma of the larynx. *A,* Well-defined pseudostratified laryngeal epithelium with large endothelial spaces, containing red blood cells. *B,* Clear endothelial-lined spaces. (From Ferguson, C. F., and Flake, C. G.: Subglottic hemangioma as a cause of respiratory obstruction in infants. *Ann. Otol., 70*:1095, 1961.)

be used because of the difficulty in determining the extent of reaction and destruction caused by the agent. Irradiation therapy has no place in the management of papilloma of the larynx in the infant and child, for it often causes perichondritis, and in several instances, malignant changes in the papilloma.

Tracheotomy is to be avoided if possible. The extension of the papilloma into the trachea and bronchi or even into the tracheal stoma is a possibility in the tracheotomized patient.

Screamer's Nodes

Screamer's nodes are nodules of the vocal cords occurring at the junction of the anterior and middle third of each cord. They result in persistent hoarseness. The gross histologic appearance of a nodule may vary from simple polypoid degeneration of the cord edge to a fibrous aggregate resembling a fibroma. These develop from excessive use of the voice in a child who is undisciplined, a keen competitor in sports, or in a noisy environment in which he has to shout or scream. Voice control therapy is essential. Surgical removal of the lesion is best performed if and when vocal therapy can be carried out successfully.

As a rule, screamer's nodules are not as much a problem in the male child. At puberty, with the greater growth of the larynx and vocal cords, the nodules tend to disappear. In the female, a deep pitch to the voice is apt to persist after puberty.

Hemangiomas

Hemangiomas of the larynx may appear as small multiple swellings in congenital telangiectasia (Osler-Rendu disease) distributed in the mucosa of the lips, nose, tongue, palate, cheeks, epiglottis and interior of the larynx as well as the characteristic skin lesions about the face and neck and fingers. The laryngeal lesions may not produce symptoms other than occasional bleeding.

Subglottic hemangiomas are true angiomas and may produce symptoms of airway obstruction. They frequently escape detection by being deep beneath normal mucosa.[10] They may be part of a distribution of dermal lesions. They become enlarged during stress periods, as in crying. There may be no voice change, as the vocal cords are usually not involved. However, the respiratory distress is such that frequently a tracheotomy is required. Diagnosis may be made by having a high index of suspicion in patients with dermal lesions, plus laryngoscopy, bronchoscopy and radiography.

Though the hemangiomas tend to regress, a high incidence of mortality is reported in untreated cases. Small doses of radiation, 200 to 500 r., have proved helpful.[11] There have been reports of steroid therapy being of promise.

Neurofibromas

Neurofibromas of the larynx may appear as part of von Recklinghausen's disease.[12] Skin nodules and café-au-lait spots are usually present, but not always. Respiratory embarrassment with stridor may develop from the encroachment on the airway by external pressure. The treatment is surgical excision of the lesion.

Cysts

Congenital cysts of the larynx are usually found in the lateral wall of the supraglottic area, and may protrude into the glottis or up into the aryepiglottic fold. Or, the cyst may be a laryngocele and herniate through the thyrohyoid membrane and appear in the neck.[13] Differentiation is made by whether the cyst is air-filled or mucus-filled. The retention cysts have thinner walls, are translucent, and are lined with columnar epithelium. The congenital cyst may arise from a branchial arch or ventricular appendix, or it may be of teratomatous origin. Obstructive dyspnea and stridor are the most common symptoms, along with a weak or absent cry. Diagnosis can be made by laryngoscopy or x-ray.

Endolaryngeal cysts in the infant are usually laryngoceles that arise from the ventricle of the larynx. They may protrude into the cavity of the larynx or extend superiorly to cause swelling of the ventricular band, with narrowing of the aditus to the larynx. They are capable of causing severe obstruction. X-ray is of value in the diagnosis, but a direct laryngoscopy is necessary for a definite diagnosis and for treatment. Therapy consists of opening the laryngocele and removing as much of the presenting walls as possible through the laryngoscope. A tracheotomy may be necessary. Frequent direct laryngoscopies may be necessary to bring the cyst under control. External surgery is seldom necessary to control this cyst in the infant.

Cysts are also found in the aryepiglottic folds. The wall of such a cyst is thicker and less translucent than that of the endolaryngeal cyst. It is more apt to have the appearance of a smooth, rounded tumor mass. An aspirating needle put into the mass will usually establish the diagnosis. In some instances, the cystic contents are so thick that aspiration is not possible and incision is necessary. The cyst should always be entered on its pharyngeal surface and a portion of the wall should be removed. These cysts usually regress or disappear entirely. The anterior surface of the epiglottis is also a frequent location of cysts. The treatment is incision, drainage and removal of a portion of the wall of the cyst. (See Chapter 103.)

Thyroglossal duct cysts may present themselves at the base of the tongue, causing airway obstruction, and are also treated by removal of as much of the wall of the cyst as is possible by pharyngoscopy. (See Chapter 100.)

Cystic hygroma may involve the larynx to the extent that the cystic mass may cause external pressure and distortion of the larynx, or it may actually involve the aryepiglottic folds and the epiglottis. A tracheotomy may be necessary to relieve the airway obstruction. Surgical removal of the cystic hygroma is necessary to relieve pressure on the larynx and pharynx. If the aryepiglottic folds and epiglottis are involved, a part of these structures may require excision, with care being exercised to preserve function. (See Chapter 100.)

Malignant Tumors

Malignancies of the larynx in infants are extremely rare.[14] Their origin is usually of mesodermal tissue, and therefore lymphosarcoma, fibrosarcoma, and rhabdomyosarcoma are the tissue types. The lesion is covered by mucosa and appears as a rounded mass. Epidermoid carcinomas of the larynx have been reported in irradiated papillomas of the larynx.[15]

REFERENCES

1. Wilson, T. G.: *Diseases of the Ear, Nose and Throat in Children,* 2nd ed. London, William Heinemann Medical Books, Ltd., 1962.
2. Holinger, P. H., and Johnston, K. C.: Treatment of benign tumors of the larynx. *Ann. Otol. Rhinol. Laryngol.,* 60:496, 1951.
3. Holinger, P. H., Schild, J. A., and Weprin, L.: Pediatric laryngology. *Otol. Clin. N. Amer.,* 3:625, 1970.
4. Szpurnar, J.: Laryngeal papillomatosis. *Acta Otolaryngol.,* 63:74, 1967.
5. Ullman, E. V.: On the aetiology of the laryngeal papilloma. *Acta Otolaryngol.,* 5: 317, 1923.
6. Svoboda, D. J., Kirshner, F. R., and Proud, G. O.: Electron microscopic study of human laryngeal papillomatosis. *Cancer Res.,* 23:1084, 1963.
7. Tabb, H. G., and Kirk, R. L.: Vein grafts in management of laryngeal papillomas. *Laryngoscope,* 72:1228, 1962.
8. Birck, J., and Mannhart, H.: Ultrasound for juvenile laryngeal papillomatosis. *Arch. Otol.,* 77:603, 1963.
9. Moffitt, O. P., Jr.: Treatment of laryngeal papillomatosis with bovine wart vaccine. *Laryngoscope,* 69:1421, 1959.
10. Campbell, J. S., Wiglesworth, F. W., Latorroca, R., and Wilde, H.: Congenital subglottic hemangiomas of larynx and trachea. *Pediatrics,* 22:727, 1958.
11. Ferguson, C. F.: Congenital abnormalities of the infant larynx. *Otol. Clin. N. Amer.,* 3: 185, 1970.
12. Zobell, D. H.: Massive neurofibroma of the larynx. *Laryngoscope,* 74:233, 1964.
13. Suehs, O. W., and Powell, D. B., Jr.: Congenital cysts of the larynx in infants. *Laryngoscope,* 77:654, 1967.
14. New, G. B., and Hertz, C. S.: Malignant disease of face, mouth, pharynx and larynx in the first three decades of life. *Surg. Gynec. Obstet.,* 70:163, 1940.
15. Walsh, T. E., and Beamer, P. R.: Epidermoid carcinoma of the larynx occurring in two children with papilloma of the larynx. *Laryngoscope,* 60:1110, 1950.

Chapter One Hundred Five

ACUTE AIRWAY OBSTRUCTION

BLAIR FEARON, B.A., M.D., F.R.C.S.(C), F.A.C.S.

ACUTE NONSPECIFIC INFLAMMATORY DISEASES OF THE LARYNX

Of all the diseases or abnormalities involving obstruction of the larynx, by far the most common (at least in the temperate zone of the western world), and the most lethal, if not treated promptly and properly, are (1) acute laryngotracheitis (acute obstructive subglottic laryngitis) and (2) acute supraglottitis (acute obstructive supraglottic laryngitis). At one time these two diseases were considered as one, but in recent years it has been realized that they are entirely different in respect to etiology, signs, symptoms and course. The end-result, however, may be the same in either case—namely, death as a result of airway obstruction.

*INCIDENCE AND MORTALITY**

In 1962 we reported a survey of patients with acute laryngotracheitis and acute supraglottitis admitted to the Hospital for Sick Children, Toronto, from 1952 to 1959 inclusive. In that eight year period 4148 patients were admitted with acute laryngotracheitis, and 78 were diagnosed as having acute supraglottitis (acute laryngotracheitis and supraglottitis were coded as one disease until 1955); 338 tracheotomies were performed in this series, and there were four deaths.[7]

In 1968 we reported a further study of these infections. From 1960 to 1964, inclusive, 3518 patients were admitted with acute laryngotracheitis and 105 with acute supraglottitis. One hundred and three tracheotomies were carried out on patients with severe acute laryngotracheitis; 65 were performed for acute supraglottitis. Three patients failed to survive out of the 3623 admissions.[8]

From 1965 to June 30, 1970, inclusive, 4459 patients were admitted with acute laryngotracheitis. Of these patients, 102 required tracheotomy, and two died—one death occurred when the tracheotomy tube became dislodged from the trachea a few hours after the operation. We believe that too short a tube for the size of the patient was a factor in the child's death, but also, the problem was not recognized and corrected as soon as it should have been. The second patient died twenty-four hours after operation, seemingly because of the development of a tension pneumothorax of uncertain etiology. The likelihood is that in this patient either the tracheotomy tube was plugged or it had slipped out of the trachea into the soft tissues of the neck. In the same period of time, 101 patients were admitted with the diagnosis of acute supraglottitis. Tracheotomies were performed on 51. There was one death in this group—a patient had several cardiac arrests on the operating table while tracheotomy was being performed and could not be resuscitated.

To summarize, in a period of eighteen and one-half years (1952 to June, 1970) 12,125 patients with acute laryngo-

*From the Department of Otolaryngology and Bronchoesophagology of the Hospital for Sick Children, Toronto, and Faculty of Medicine, University of Toronto.

tracheitis and 284 patients with acute supraglottitis were admitted to the Hospital for Sick Children. A total of 659 tracheotomies were performed—489 for acute laryngotracheitis and 170 for acute supraglottitis. There were ten deaths in the total of 12,409 admissions (approximately one in 1200 admissions).

It is noteworthy that none of the 649 patients who survived with tracheotomy had any long-term complications from the tracheotomy nor, in fact, from the disease. Nearly all the patients were extubated within a week—one child required a tracheotomy for four weeks before uneventful decannulation.

Not included in the mortality figures were two patients who arrived in the emergency department in cardiac arrest. Prompt emergency measures restored the heartbeat temporarily, but both patients expired within a few hours. A third patient was transferred from another hospital while being ventilated by an endotracheal tube but was in much the same condition as the first patients. Spontaneous breathing did not return in any of these three patients. In each the duration of symptoms was very brief—from two to four hours from the onset of the illness until arrival at the hospital. There is no record kept of children who have been brought to hospital "D.O.A." with a history indicative of acute supraglottitis or acute laryngotracheitis.

ACUTE LARYNGOTRACHEITIS

Synonyms often used to describe this disease are acute obstructive subglottic laryngitis, "croup," nondiphtheritic croup, pseudocroup, acute stenotic laryngitis and tracheitis. "Acute obstructive subglottic laryngitis" seems to us to be the most descriptive term, but since "acute laryngotracheitis" (or "acute laryngotracheobronchitis") is the most commonly used diagnosis, we will use that term in this text. We dislike particularly the use of the word "croup," since—with the layman especially—croup refers to a number of conditions which have in common a croupy cough. Therefore, the condition may not be taken seriously by the parent (or even the doctor). When such is the case, treatment may not be instituted soon enough to prevent tracheotomy or even death.

Acute laryngotracheitis is a disease occurring in the temperate zone, and it also seems more prevalent in urban areas where there is a high concentration of industrial fumes, or so-called "smog," and seems to be associated with rapid changes in atmospheric humidity.[37]

In the winter months, particularly between October and April, this disease is most prevalent, but nonetheless, it may occur during any month of the year. For example, during the winter months of 1969 and 1970, in two Toronto hospitals (Hospital for Sick Children with over 800 beds and the North York General Hospital with 200 pediatric beds), the number of admissions for acute laryngotracheitis was much less than usual, and no patients needed tracheotomies. In April, May and June of 1970, the admission rate increased and several patients (eleven) had to be tracheotomized. Fortunately, there were no deaths among these patients.

Etiology

The etiology of laryngotracheitis is considered to be of a viral origin, and it is likely that one or more viruses may be implicated. In this regard intensive studies have been carried out at the Hospital for Sick Children, Toronto, and in 1954 Morgan and others[30] isolated a specific virus in a certain number of patients with laryngotracheitis. Subsequently, MacLean and his associates[28] found a high rate of isolation of parainfluenza 1 virus from the respiratory tract of patients admitted to this hospital for laryngotracheitis; parainfluenza 2 and 3 viruses were also isolated from some patients. Usually bacterial cultures show a mixed growth of organisms, including streptococci, pneumococci, staphlylococci and *Haemophilus influenzae*. It is questionable, though difficult to prove, whether antibiotic therapy influences the course of this disease in the early stages, but antibiotic therapy is customary as a part of the treatment and may prevent complications with secondary infections.

Pathology

Acute laryngotracheitis is an inflammation involving particularly the subglottic area of the larynx (conus elasticus), the trachea and the bronchial tree. It is the involvement of the subglottic area that creates the most serious aspect of the disease—namely, airway obstruction. The inflammation results in a firm and indurated swelling of the subglottic tissues, reducing the caliber of the airway at this point to a serious degree (Fig. 1).

The inflammatory involvement of the trachea and the bronchial tree causes swelling of the mucosal lining of these structures, which in itself is relatively unimportant, but a thick, viscous, purulent secretion is also present, which adds another obstructive factor to the disease. The thick and sticky nature of this exudate makes it difficult for the child to expel the material through the already narrowed laryngeal airway by coughing.

On rare occasions we have seen inflammatory swelling of the supraglottic tissues in patients on whom we have performed emergency bronchoscopies and tracheotomies for laryngotracheitis, but the obstruction has been located primarily in the subglottic space.

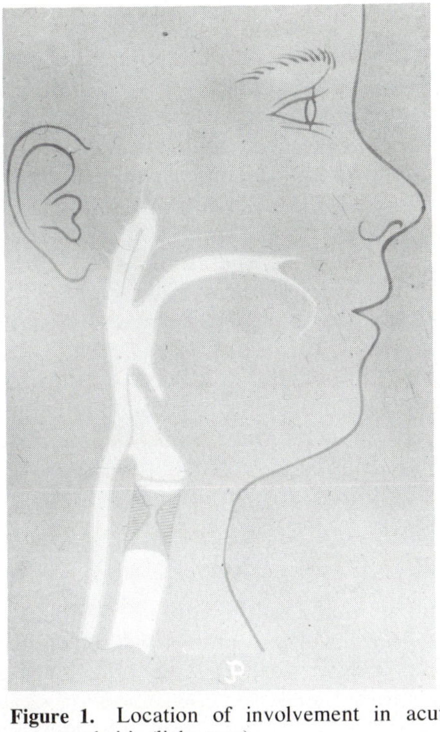

Figure 1. Location of involvement in acute laryngotracheitis (light area).

Clinical Picture

Laryngotracheitis tends to be more common in the young patient (6 months to 3 years) than the supraglottic inflammation, which is more common in the 3- to 6-year age group. In our own experience severe obstructive subglottic laryngitis necessitating tracheotomy has occurred in patients as young as 3 months and as old as 11 years.

The disease is preceded by what appears to be a simple upper respiratory infection or "head cold" for a few days' duration, but in some instances for only a matter of hours. Laryngotracheitis makes itself known when the patient develops a "croupy" cough (like the bark of a seal), stridorous breathing and often, although not necessarily, a hoarse voice.

In the majority of cases the signs and symptoms tend to culminate during the night. Why this should be is not clear, but possibly it is because the child is lying down or because the air in the bedroom has become drier than the rest of the house; perhaps, as Mills[29] has suggested, in "allergic croup" the plasma-cortisol level is at its lowest between midnight and 4:00 A.M.

As the disease progresses, the stridor and the effort to breathe increase, and the child becomes more and more restless because of hypoxia and hypercapnia. The breathing is rapid with a prolongation of the inspiratory phase. Retractions of the chest become more marked. The heart rate increases accordingly and is the most important indication of the degree of hypoxia. Although there is usually an elevation of temperature (and it may become quite high), fever is not an outstanding feature. It is the routine in the two Toronto hospitals previously mentioned to admit all patients with signs and symptoms of obstructive laryngotracheitis for at least twenty-four hours of treatment and observation.

Medical Management

Unless the child is in extremis on arrival at the hospital and emergency tracheotomy is necessary immediately, medical treatment should be instituted with the least possible delay, and all but essential physical and laboratory examinations should be omitted. If the condition of the child permits, a roentgenogram of the chest to include the larynx should be a part of the examination to rule out pneumothorax, pneumonia, radiopaque foreign bodies and the like. Each patient with respiratory difficulty is seen immediately by the resident staff of the Department of Otolaryngology as well as of the Department of Pediatrics.

Some years ago Turner[43] stated that there are three essentials in the medical management of acute laryngotracheitis, and the same dictum holds true today: (1) moist air, (2) *moderate* sedation and (3) antibiotics. To this we would add close observation by expert and experienced personnel.

Moist vapor is best supplied by metered oxygen or compressed air through an electrosonic nebulizer into a croupette. Moist vapor is important not only to allay the irritation of the tissues of the trachea and bronchial tree but to promote liquefaction of the thick secretions generated by the inflammation of the respiratory tract, thus making it easier for the patient to cough up these secretions.

Although sedation may be condemned by some authors, we believe that sedation *in moderation* not only is safe but is beneficial in reducing the child's apprehension. The child is already frightened by this illness and the difficulty in breathing, and the fact that he is in strange hands and in strange surroundings only aggravates the situation. Alleviation of this apprehension allows for more effective and efficient respiration. Seconal 50 mg. per rectum is used for patients over 1 year of age; 15 to 30 mg. of Seconal is given to patients under 1 year of age.

Oversedation must be avoided because of the danger of masking signs of hypoxia. Narcotics must *not* be used to suppress the cough reflex. Accumulation of secretions in the tracheobronchial tree adds to the respiratory distress. It is of greatest importance to avoid the use of atropine or atropine-like drugs, since they make the tracheobronchial secretions even more viscous and more difficult to cough up.

It has become fashionable to carry out blood-gas studies on patients with any type of respiratory or cardiac insufficiency. My personal view is that taking blood samples has on occasion upset some patients to the degree that the respiratory obstruction has worsened and tracheotomy was made necessary. Good clinical judgment is by far the most satisfactory way of determining the child's condition.

Antibiotics or sulfonamides may not affect the immediate course of the disease, since it is usually a viral infection; nevertheless, they may prevent complications by pathogenic organisms, such as *H. influenzae,* pneumococci, streptococci and staphylococci. For many years penicillin and dihydrostreptomycin in combination were given routinely by injection unless there was a penicillin sensitivity. On occasion intravenous chloramphenicol has been used. More recently, unless the patient has a sensitivity to penicillin, ampicillin has been the antibiotic most frequently employed, usually via the intravenous or intramuscular route. Erythromycin and cephaloridine can be used alternatively.

Many of the patients have had insufficient fluid intake prior to hospitalization, and they tend to lose more fluid at a rapid rate because of efforts to breathe; therefore, correction of dehydration is vitally important. The fluid balance usually needs to be controlled by intravenous solutions.

Over the years at the Hospital for Sick Children various corticosteroids have been used, although with dubious or inconclusive results.[30] However, Davison and others have reported such impressively good results in this disease in avoiding tracheotomies by using corticosteroids that we feel they should be given a trial [3,4] Ross recommends an intramuscular dose of 100 mg. of cortisone to be repeated in two hours if improvement is not dramatic. He states that if this medication is to be effective, the improvement will take place in less than four hours.[38] It goes without saying that if a corticosteroid is to be used, it should be given in adequate dosage.

We repeat that it is of utmost importance that the patient receive competent, experienced and continual nursing care from the time of admission to hospital until the danger is past. We emphasize that the pulse rate, especially, and the respiratory rate be checked frequently. Increased pulse rate, restlessness and increasing difficulty in breathing in spite of adequate therapy are indications of worsening of the child's condition and should be reported promptly. Fortunately, most patients with acute laryngotracheitis are out of danger in twenty-four hours, but some may need intensive treatment for several days, and a small percentage requires tracheotomy.

If in spite of adequate therapy the respiratory obstruction progresses, then surgical intervention is clearly indicated. The signs of progressive respiratory obstruction are an increasing pulse rate exceeding and remaining over 160 beats per minute, restlessness, increasing respiratory rate, greater costal, sternal and substernal indrawing, use of the accessory muscles of respiration, suprasternal indrawing, diminishing air entry on auscultation and signs of fatigue. Circumoral pallor and cyanosis, especially gray cyanosis, suggest heart failure and are grave signs.

The degree of indrawing of the chest per se is not a good criterion as to the degree of respiratory distress. Some patients with "soft" rib and sternal structures will show indrawing with little respiratory effort. One must watch for the child in whom the indrawing appears to have stopped. Such a child simply may have become too tired to make sufficient breathing effort to show indrawing; obviously, this patient is in need of urgent relief of airway obstruction.

EMERGENCY RELIEF FOR SEVERE ACUTE RESPIRATORY OBSTRUCTION

In any acute obstructive laryngeal emergency, any method which will help relieve the airway obstruction is justified. This includes the use of blind intubation with the O'Dwyer or Mosher "lifesaver" tubes; direct intubation using the laryngoscope and a semirigid endotracheal "life saver" tube or a conventional endotracheal tube; the use of large bore needles inserted into the trachea; automatic tracheotomes; or by stab tracheotomy. By far the most satisfactory method to relieve laryngeal obstruction is the introduction of a bronchoscope followed by orderly tracheotomy.[7, 8]

Tracheotomy is not an operation to be feared if performed by an experienced laryngologist. As Leegaard[25] has aptly stated, "The main point is not 'a tout prix' to avoid tracheotomy but to avoid the child's dying from respiratory insufficiency." Galloway[20] has pointed out the two most important factors in laryngotracheitis: *first,* the mechanical effects secondary to respiratory infection with associated obstruction and increased negative intrathoracic pressure; and *second*, the effects of hypoxia with associated accumulation of carbon dioxide in the bloodstream. We emphasize this by saying that almost all the deaths in this disease are due to asphyxia or the effects of prolonged hypoxia on the central nervous system and on the heart, even though the airway obstruction may have finally been relieved. Nelson[35] has stated the axiom that "the time to perform a tracheotomy is when one first thinks the operation might be indicated." Keeping this in mind, the operation may be performed in an orderly manner without the risk of complications suggested by some writers on the subject—namely, severe hemorrhage, pneumothorax, subcutaneous and mediastinal emphysema—and without the decannulatory problems that are more likely to result from a hurried procedure.

In recent years, claims have been made by several writers in the medical literature that the laryngeal obstruction of laryngotracheitis can be relieved by the passage of a standard endotracheal tube which may be left in place for the duration of the disease and without the complications of tracheotomy. In the type of disease we have dealt with personally we find it difficult enough to force even a small bronchoscope through the indurated swelling in the subglottic space or through the swelling of the supraglottic area, let alone a flexible endotracheal tube. Prolonged intubation in itself is not without complications, which are likely to be intensified in the presence of acute inflammation.[5,16,22,23] On the other hand, any method is quite justified when someone who is experienced in laryngoscopy and bronchoscopy in the small child is not available.

Unless the surgeon is untrained and unskilled in bronchoscopy in the child or the instruments are not immediately available, we believe most strongly that bronchoscopy preliminary to performing the tracheotomy is mandatory. Even the most experienced and astute clinicians cannot always be certain whether the diagnosis is supraglottitis or laryngotracheitis. From our own experience as well as that of our colleagues, in many instances, although the patient had all the signs and symptoms which indicate one of these diseases, bronchoscopy revealed the obstruction to be due to something entirely different. Some of these causes were foreign bodies in the larynx, trachea or upper esophagus; laryngeal growths or cysts; subglottic stenosis; vascular anomalies compressing the trachea; and congenital tracheal stenosis.

In fact, in some of these patients, although a tracheotomy seemed absolutely necessary before bronchoscopic examination, it was avoided by taking other measures, such as translaryngeal intubation, as determined by the bronchoscopic findings.

ACUTE SUPRAGLOTTITIS (ACUTE EPIGLOTTITIS; ACUTE OBSTRUCTIVE SUPRAGLOTTIC LARYNGITIS)

Acute supraglottitis is an acute inflammatory swelling involving the supraglottic structures of the larynx without involvement of the vocal cords and seldom of the subglottic tissues (Figs. 2 and 3).

We avoid using the term "acute epiglottitis" and prefer the term "acute supraglottitis" because the inflammatory swelling may involve the aryepiglottic folds and ventricular bands without

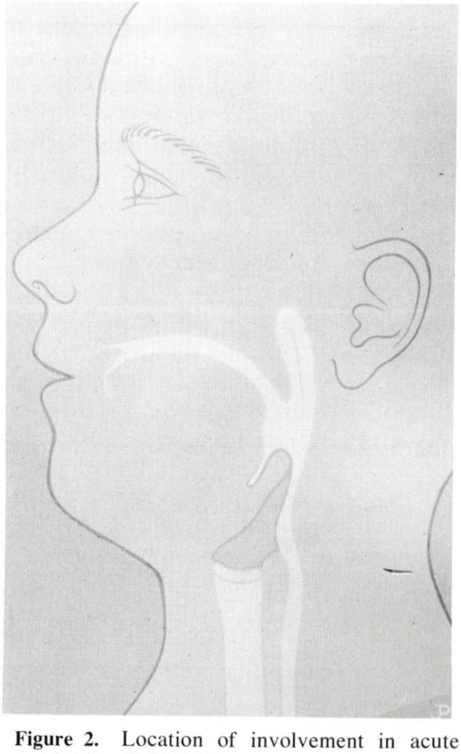

Figure 2. Location of involvement in acute supraglottitis (light area).

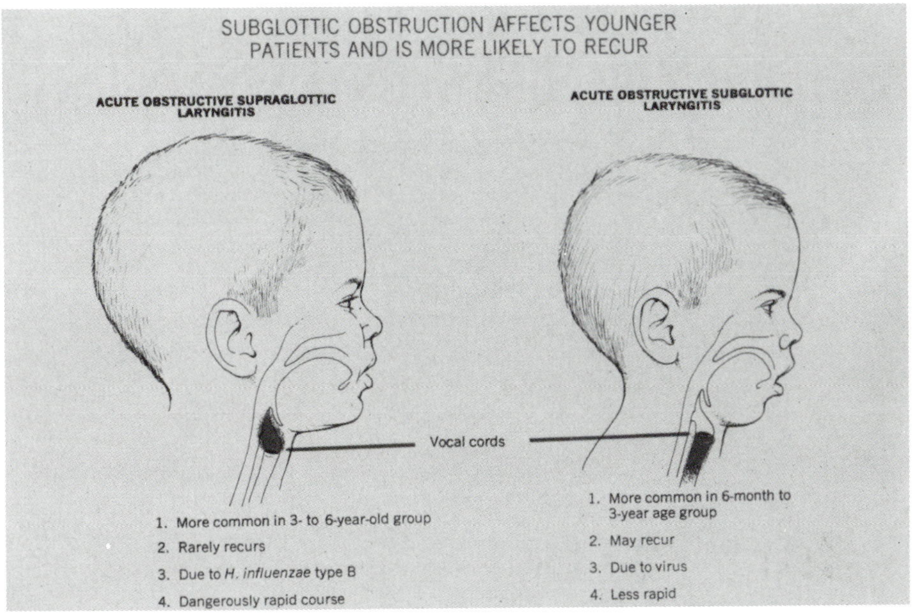

Figure 3. Points of difference between acute supraglottic and acute subglottic obstructive laryngitis. (From *Hospital Medicine,* 4:51, 1968.)

involvement of the epiglottis. The airway obstruction can be just as severe if the epiglottis itself is not involved. We wish to stress this point, since many clinicians expect to see a markedly swollen, inflamed epiglottis, and when they see a rather normal epiglottis instead, the gravity of the patient's condition may not be realized.

Like laryngotracheitis, acute supraglottitis is a disease occurring in the temperate zones and usually is more common in the winter months but may occur in any month of the year. The frequency of this disease is much less than laryngotracheitis in a ratio of approximately 1 to 400 admissions to the hospital. Although other organisms may be etiologic factors, *H. influenzae* type B is the most common organism that is cultured from our patients at the time of tracheotomy. As mentioned earlier, this disease occurs in the age group of 3 to 6 years, but may occur much earlier. We have found it necessary to tracheotomize patients as young as 5 months of age, and one was as old as 14 years.

The most distressing fact is that the course of this disease can be dreadfully rapid in contrast to that of laryngotracheitis. The first complaint may be a sore throat which may proceed quickly to dysphagia and extreme difficulty in breathing in as short a time as two hours from the onset of symptoms to severe airway obstruction. The patient may go to bed with mild signs of a head cold and in two or three hours may be found breathing noisily and actually struggling to breathe. It is especially characteristic of this disease that the patient will not drink or eat, apparently because of painful inflammatory swelling of the supraglottic tissues.

The voice is usually clear, although somewhat muffled at times, and there is little if any cough, in contrast to laryngotracheitis. These patients have a characteristic appearance—they sit up rather than lie down; the chin is forward and the tongue protrudes through the open mouth; and they are usually anxious and frightened (Figs. 4 and 5). It is also characteristic that they breathe slowly and quietly, since they soon learn they can get more air into their lungs this way

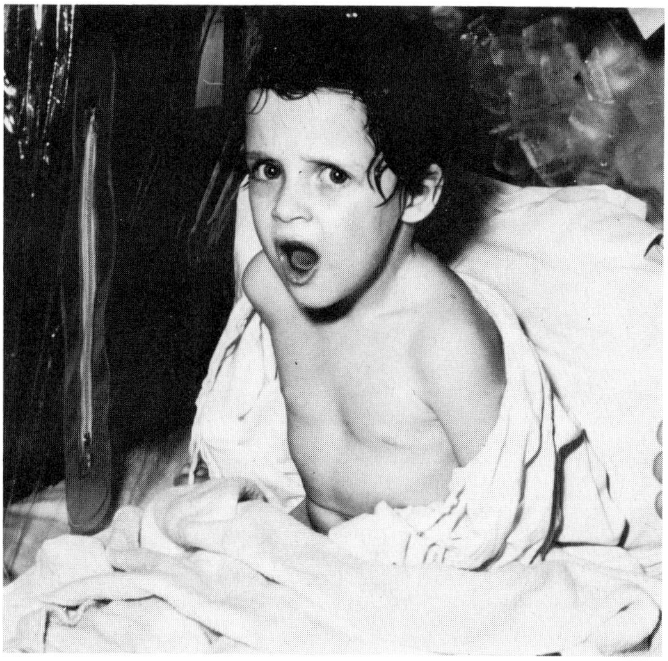

Figure 4. Classic appearance of patient with acute supraglottitis just prior to tracheotomy.

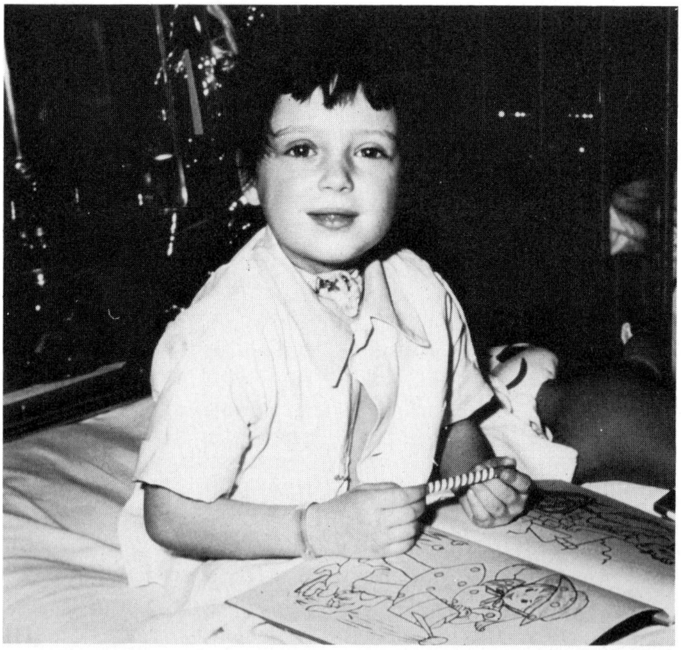

Figure 5. Same patient in Figure 4 two days later.

than if they try to breathe rapidly. Auscultation will reveal exceedingly poor air entry into the lungs.

The temperature is usually elevated, as is the leukocyte count. The degree of prostration and shock is most striking and out of all proportion to the apparent severity of the infection.

The most important single sign of impending disaster is dysphagia. If the child is drooling or there is pooling of saliva in the pharynx, steps should be taken immediately to arrange for a tracheotomy.

Examination of the throat with a tongue depressor can be dangerous as well as unnecessary. One needs only to shine a light into the mouth to see saliva in the pharynx, and, if involved, the epiglottis often can be seen to be a fiery red and swollen mass at the base of the tongue. The forceful depression of the tongue with a tongue depressor may precipitate total airway obstruction. Also, if the epiglottis is badly swollen, it may act like a ball-valve and become impacted in the glottis at the end of a bout of retching or coughing, causing asphyxiation very abruptly.

With increasing respiratory obstruction, hypoxia, hypercapnia and acidosis develop. As with laryngotracheitis and other obstructive airway diseases, hypercapnia produces headache, restlessness, irritability and disorientation. High concentrations of carbon dioxide induce narcosis, respiratory depression and finally circulatory collapse.

Essentially the same medical regimen as for acute laryngotracheitis is instituted on admission. However, tracheotomy is necessary in the majority of patients with acute supraglottitis. Some authorities say that all patients with acute supraglottitis should be tracheotomized, although this has not been necessary in our experience. A few patients, particularly in the older age group, do get by on conservative management alone. Obviously, these patients must be watched very closely, and the laryngologist must be close at hand in case of sudden deterioration of the patient's condition.

ACUTE SPECIFIC INFLAMMATORY DISEASES OF THE LARYNX

DIPHTHERIA

Although Toronto was the first major city in the world to initiate a compulsory diphtheria toxoid program, on rare occasions diphtheria still breaks out in the native population. Never take it for granted that every child in the family has received diphtheria toxoid, even though perhaps all but one may have been immunized. With immigration of large numbers of people from other countries, particularly with today's rapid transportation, one must be on the alert for children who have not had toxoid or who may even have the disease on arrival. Furthermore, the movement of families from one part of the country where immunization may be neglected to another where the immunization against diphtheria is taken for granted may be another source of this infection.

In laryngeal obstruction with diphtheria the indications for tracheotomy and surgical technique are essentially the same as those for other acute inflammatory diseases of the larynx.

In laryngeal diphtheria, the onset of the obstructive phase is relatively slow because the airway obstruction is due largely to the characteristic membrane which forms on the vocal cords rather than the inflammatory swelling of the laryngeal soft tissues as with other laryngeal inflammations. A distinctive sign of this disease is progressive hoarseness over a period of two or three days. There may be patches of membrane on the pharyngeal mucosa and tonsils, and there may or may not be a characteristic odor to the breath. Direct smears should be taken from the involved areas and exudate is cultured specifically for diphtheria. It is of the utmost importance to treat these patients with diphtheria antitoxin (unless there is a sensitivity to horse serum).

The diphtheria organism is sensitive to

penicillin and erythromycin. Even though the airway obstruction is relieved and antibiotics are used, unless the diphtheria antitoxin is used, death may occur from the effects of the toxin on the heart even when the acute inflammatory stage is past. This makes it obvious why it is so important to establish the diagnosis of diphtheria as soon as possible.

MEASLES (RUBEOLA) LARYNGOTRACHEOBRONCHITIS

Measles is another disease that has become relatively uncommon because of immunization with measles vaccine. However, patients with severe airway involvement from measles are seen occasionally. The subglottic tissues may be swollen, as in nonspecific laryngotracheitis, but the involvement of the tracheobronchial tree is more pronounced. The exudate plus the swelling of the tracheobronchial mucosa tend to precipitate pulmonary atelectasis and bronchopneumonia. The bronchopneumonia is often the result of secondary bacterial infection as well.

The treatment in general for measles laryngotracheobronchitis is basically the same as for a nonspecific laryngotracheitis. The indications for tracheotomy are the same and its particular value is that it enables bronchial toilet to be carried out thoroughly, thereby preventing atelectasis and subsequent bronchiectasis due to prolonged endobronchial obstruction by fibrinous exudate.

Whenever atelectasis persists in a specific area for several days, bronchoscopy and aspiration of the involved segment should be carried out. It may be necessary to use forceps to remove fibrinous casts. Other acute exanthemata (rubella, varicella, variola, or scarlatina) rarely, if ever, cause acute airway obstruction. However, in our recent review of the records one patient with scarlet fever (scarlatina) died, and postmortem examination showed inflammatory involvement of the larynx, trachea and tracheobronchial tree. This patient was not seen by our department.

LARYNGEAL TRAUMA

Laryngeal trauma causing acute airway obstruction must be considered from two directions—namely, internal trauma and external trauma.

Internal trauma may be secondary to inhalation of chemicals, steam, intense heat or smoke or the ingestion of caustics, acids or other corrosives and poisons.

In proportion to the number of children who ingest corrosive substances, the number that develop airway obstruction is small; nevertheless, in any child that is known to have ingested a caustic, an acid or solid carbon dioxide snow the possibility of airway obstruction within the first few hours after the accident is always a real one. In our experience, if severe laryngeal edema following ingestion is to occur, it does so within a few hours. Accordingly, it is our policy to admit for at least twenty-four hours all children who have ingested corrosives. When the larynx is involved invariably the child has dysphagia as well, and there should be no hesitation in performing a tracheotomy if obstruction has developed. A tracheotomy not only relieves the airway obstruction due to the swelling of the supraglottic tissues of the larynx but allows the removal by catheter suction of the collected pharyngeal secretions that may be inhaled into the tracheobronchial tree.

THERMAL DAMAGE TO THE LARYNX

Ordinarily the inhalation of heat affects the tracheobronchial tree as well as the larynx. However, on occasion steam may cause severe laryngeal edema alone without tracheobronchial involvement (if, for example, the child puts his mouth over the spout of a teapot). Most commonly the problem is a combination of heat and smoke, affecting the larynx and the tracheobronchial tree.

Heat alone involves the airway if the child takes a deep breath when suddenly exposed to intense heat. For example, a child was standing beside a bonfire when someone foolishly threw a can of gasoline on the fire. The child took a sudden deep breath There was very little burn of the body and face but severe burns of the trachea and major bronchi and little laryngeal involvement. Bronchoscopy showed at first generalized hyperemia without much swelling of the larynx, trachea and bronchial tree. A tracheotomy was performed primarily for bronchial toilet. Patches of ulceration in the trachea and bronchi because of mucosal necrosis later developed, and on occasion masses of debris had to be removed with forceps. Much to our surprise the child eventually recovered without a long-term pulmonary problem from anticipated mucosal obstruction.

These same types of burns may be caused by accidental ignition of clothes made of certain synthetics which are highly flammable and which should not be allowed on the market for clothing material.

When a child is exposed to smoke and fumes, such as in a house fire, marked exudation is frequently the result, causing respiratory difficulty. Tracheotomy helps in carrying out bronchial toilet and the administration of humidified oxygen to the tracheobronchial tree.

INSTRUMENTAL TRAUMA

As a result of improvements in techniques and instrumentarium as well as in materials used for the tubes, serious trauma from intubation for general anesthesia is seldom seen today. It is really quite remarkable—in view of the fact that nearly all general anesthesia administered to children today is given via the endotracheal route—that the complications in routine anesthesia are exceedingly few. Obstructive laryngeal edema is more likely to occur from emergency intubation, but even this is uncommon. Occasionally, laryngeal edema follows intubation for prolonged surgery, especially if the operation is in the vicinity of the neck. The use of corticosteroids very likely helps to prevent obstructive swelling in all but a few cases.

In long-term intubation for the management of respiratory insufficiency from many causes, a varying degree of inflammatory swelling may develop in as little time as twenty-four hours. If the inflammatory swelling follows extubation, then we feel strongly that a tracheotomy should be carried out at this point rather than re-intubation if the airway shows no improvement by conservative measures. Laryngoscopic inspection of the larynx is useless in determining the long-term effects of intubation. Unfortunately, if ulceration of the cord, or more likely the subglottic area, has already occurred, the patient is likely to have a long-term airway problem.[15,21,22]

Digital trauma from clearing the throat of a newborn with gauze on a finger or from attempts to remove a foreign body from the child's throat by digital means may dislocate the arytenoids or cause some inflammatory swelling of the larynx. It is quite unusual to see any significant patho.ogy from either of these maneuvers in today's medical management.

EXTERNAL TRAUMA

Being cartilaginous, more mobile and less prominent, the larynx of the child is much less likely to be affected by external trauma than that of the adult. Nonetheless, injuries to the larynx do occur in auto accidents or falls during which the child is thrown forward or falls with his head extended, striking the laryngeal region on a projecting object. The records at this hospital over the past twenty years, during which time the average annual admission rate has been well over 35,000, have not shown any record of a child with a fracture of the thyroid or cricoid cartilage.

If the thyroid or cricoid cartilage is

fractured, there may not be much sign of injury externally, but laryngeal edema may result quite quickly. Subcutaneous crepitus is an indication that there is most likely a disruption in the internal mucosa and the thyroid or cricoid cartilage. If respiratory distress then develops, tracheotomy should be planned quite promptly At the same time the larynx can be examined endoscopically to determine whether or not corrective surgery is in order.[34,36]

Penetrating wounds in the vicinity of the larynx may not affect the airway directly, but if they are extensive, tracheotomy may be very important in preventing serious airway obstruction subsequent to the repair.

Case History. An 8-year-old boy fell into an excavation with his neck landing on an upright piece of steel embedded in concrete. He was rushed to hospital immediately where examination showed a large gaping laceration extending collarwise from the midline anteriorly to the angle of the jaw on the left. The external carotid artery could be seen pulsating in the depths of the wound, and an avulsed portion of the greater cornu of the hyoid bone was exposed. Examination of the throat showed some fresh blood, and there was a hematoma of the uvula. In spite of the extensive injury the child was not in severe distress and was not bleeding badly, although he was in moderate shock.

He was given standard supportive treatment and taken to the operating room for surgical repair. Direct laryngoscopy showed some laryngeal swelling but no obvious involvement of the intrinsic larynx. A bronchoscope (#4 × 30 mm.) was passed into the trachea, and the patient was anesthetized with diethyl ether via the bronchoscope. Tracheotomy was performed, and the anesthetic was then carried on through the tracheal tube for the remainder of the operation.

The laceration was found to have cut clearly through the lateral 2 cm. of the greater cornu of the hyoid and on into the hypopharynx to the left of the larynx. The opening into the pharynx was large enough to admit two fingers. The soft tissues were closed in layers beginning with the pharyngeal mucosa. The fragment of the hyoid was re-attached in its proper position, and the skin was closed with subcuticular wire, leaving a Penrose drain and Sofratulle in the laceration for drainage. The skin laceration was unusually straight as though it had been made with a sharp knife. The boy made a remarkably good recovery without any sequelae other than the scar (Fig. 6).

In obvious trauma to the larynx, the importance of direct examination of the larynx and trachea cannot be overemphasized. Under what appears to be a minor abrasion of the skin over the larynx may lie not only impending airway obstruction from soft tissue swelling or hematoma but also injury to the intrinsic structures of the larynx, which if corrected at an early stage, might prevent permanent laryngeal deformity. Weaver et al.[44] state that early exploration of all penetrating wounds of the neck will greatly reduce the number of deaths from hemorrhage.

If there is any likelihood at all that the airway might become obstructed, tra-

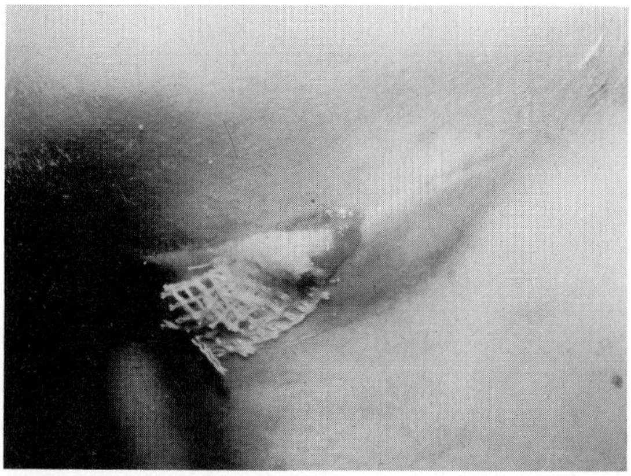

Figure 6. Healing laceration prior to removing drains. Laceration had extended to angle of mandible.

cheotomy should be carried out at the time of the direct examination. If this practice is not followed and obstruction should develop later, sudden emergency measures become necessary; these measures (intubation, stab tracheotomy) under less desirable circumstances could conceivably aggravate the injuries already present or result in the death of the patient.

Complications of an injury are dislocation of the arytenoids, hematoma within the larynx and displaced fractures of the thyroid or cricoid cartilage. As Myerson has pointed out, when the cricoid cartilage is involved by injury, a subglottic stenosis develops. When only the thyroid cartilage is involved, the stenosis and deformity are glottic and supraglottic.[34] When these cartilages are involved a suitable mold should be implanted in the larynx and upper trachea. If there is extensive hematoma involving the vocal cord (or cords), fixation of the vocal cord may be prevented by an external surgical approach as described by Myerson.[34]

Ogura and Biller recently have pointed out that fracture of the epiglottis may be treated satisfactorily by excision of the epiglottis. They describe in detail the surgical management of reconstruction of the larynx and trachea following blunt trauma to these structures.[36]

SUBGLOTTIC STENOSIS

CONGENITAL SUBGLOTTIC STENOSIS

Congenital subglottic stenosis, unless severe, is not always apparent at birth and, in fact, may first present with acute respiratory distress when the child has an acute respiratory infection. On occasion the presence of a stenosis may be detected when the child is being anesthetized for some unrelated surgery. In such a case, when the anesthetist tries to pass an endotracheal tube which is considered to be the correct size for the age of the patient, unusual resistance is encountered in the subglottic space. At this stage the anesthetist is committed to continue the procedure using a smaller endotracheal tube. Usually the anesthetic and surgery can be continued, but a tracheotomy is almost always necessary subsequently, depending to a large degree on the density and the caliber of the stenotic area in the subglottic space (Fig. 7).

The following is a range of endotracheal tube sizes used by the staff of the Department of Anesthesia at the Hospital for Sick Children.[19]

	Magill	*Cole*
Premature	3.0–3.5	10–14
0–3 months	3.5–4.0	14–16
3–6 months	3.5–4.0	16–18
6–12 months	4.0–4.5	18–20
12–18 months	4.5–5.5	18–20

These endotracheal tubes should not fit tightly in the glottic aperture; there should be no resistance at all in the normal subglottic space.

In those patients with congenital subglottic stenosis in whom respiratory distress first becomes manifest during a respiratory infection, there usually has been some degree of stridor for a variable period of time prior to the acute distress. The onset of the stridor may occur at a few days of age or after a year or more. The common time for distress to develop with respiratory infections is from 3 to 6 months of age. Some of the patients have a history of repeated "croup" from which they recover with conservative measures. Some patients with congenital subglottic stenosis are admitted with a diagnosis of acute laryngotracheitis and respond to conventional therapy without obstruction severe enough to warrant emergency tracheotomy; yet, they continue to have a moderate degree of respiratory distress. If the patient's symptoms do not improve after several days of therapy, a relative subglottic stenosis should be suspected. We believe that after several days of treatment without any significant improvement these patients should have a diagnostic laryngoscopy and bronchoscopy, and there is the likelihood that a

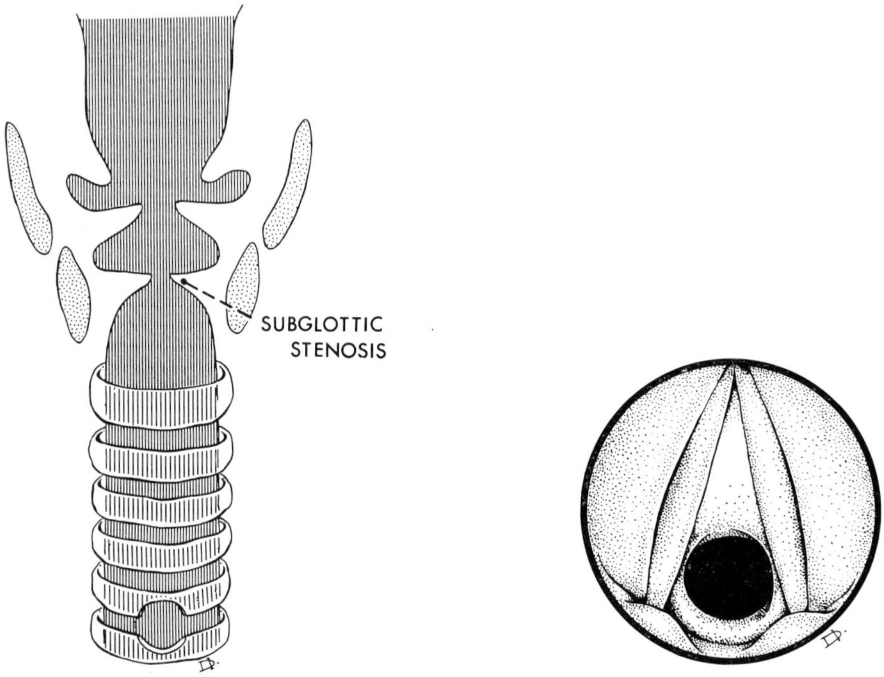

Figure 7. Schematic representation of subglottic stenosis. (From *Ann. Otol., Rhinol. Laryngol.*, 75:975, 1966.)

long-term tracheotomy might be necessary. On the other hand, not all patients with congenital subglottic stenosis require tracheotomy. There is an occasional fortunate patient in whom the subglottic lumen may be quite small but the fibrous narrowing is thin and responds to dilatation very satisfactorily. One dilatation in this type of stenosis may suffice without the need for tracheotomy, and rarely is dilatation necessary more than two or three times.

ACQUIRED SUBGLOTTIC STENOSIS

In the majority of patients in whom tracheotomy has been necessary after prolonged intubation, the operation had to be carried out shortly after extubation. However, in a few patients stenosis developed in a way that is similar to that of corrosive esophageal stricture—that is, some time after the tube had been removed following a period of prolonged intubation. These patients may present with acute respiratory distress three to four weeks after the endotracheal tube has been removed. Such patients are those in whom an endotracheal tube had been in place for several days in the treatment of respiratory insufficiency following such events as major cardiovascular surgery or head injuries and who had little, if any, difficulty following the removal of the endotracheal tube. However, after several days without respiratory embarrassment, signs of obstruction to the airway develop, and this distress may increase rapidly until a tracheotomy is necessary.[16, 26]

Case History. A 10-month-old patient was transferred to our department from another hospital where he had been treated for a period of two weeks by intubation for what was thought to be acute laryngotracheitis. Attempts had been made to extubate the patient, but respiratory distress followed and required re-intubation. The child was admitted to the hospital with the endotracheal tube in place, and bronchoscopy was carried out without a general anesthetic shortly after admission to the hospital.

Direct laryngoscopy on the removal of the endotracheal tube showed the supraglottic and glottic areas to be normal, and very little was seen in the subglottic area except an annular area of ulceration about 2 mm. in extent at the level of the cricoid cartilage. Bronchoscopy showed the actual cause of the distress to be due to a rather severe compression of the trachea by the innominate artery and retention of secretions in the tracheobronchial tree distal to the compression.

The patient was placed in the hands of the cardiovascular surgical department, and a suspension of the innominate artery was carried out. The endotracheal tube was kept in place following the surgery for a period of twenty-four hours and then withdrawn. Following this the patient had no respiratory distress whatsoever and made an excellent recovery from the innominate artery suspension; he was discharged from the hospital ten days after surgery. Four weeks later the child again developed severe respiratory distress rather abruptly and required tracheotomy. At this time direct examination of the larynx showed a moderately severe subglottic stenosis at the level of the annular area of ulceration described at the time of the first diagnostic laryngoscopy and bronchoscopy.

VASCULAR COMPRESSION OF THE TRACHEA

Although compression of the trachea by the innominate artery or by congenital malformations of the great vessels is not ordinarily considered in the category of acute airway emergencies, occasionally a patient will be brought to the hospital (or seen at home by the physician) with what appears to be a sudden onset of acute respiratory infection. Basically, it is a combination of vascular compression of the trachea complicated by an acute respiratory infection (see Fig. 8). Even to the experienced eye a patient in this category will have all the signs and symptoms of acute obstructive laryngotracheitis and appears to need emergency airway relief. The most likely cause of such a problem is compression of the trachea by the innominate artery, although more rarely there is a possibility of tracheal compression by double aortic arch, tumor of the thymus gland or other mediastinal growths.[18, 26] Patients in this category and especially those with innominate artery compression, when in good health, have very little in the way of signs of innominate artery compression

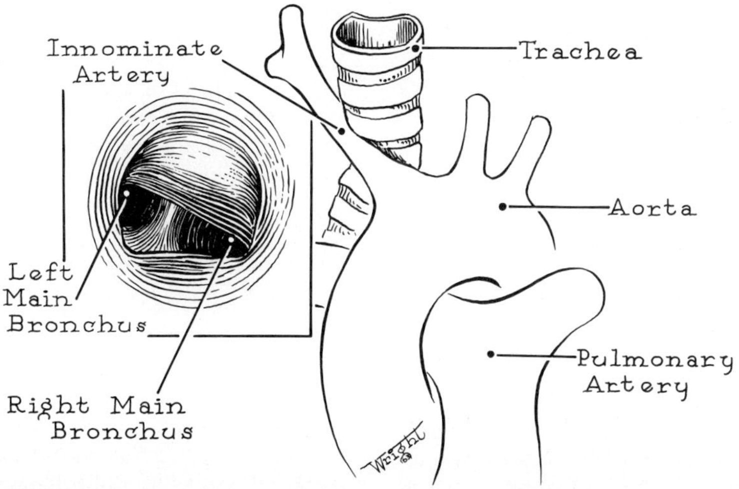

Figure 8. Endoscopic appearance of innominate artery compression of trachea. (From *Ann. Otol., Rhinol. Laryngol.*, 72:949, 1963.)

that are typical of the more severe tracheal compressions. Invariably, though, when asked the mother is likely to say that the child has had "a tendency to croup," meaning that with a mild cough the child has sounded "croupy."

We postulate that a combination of factors may bring on the severe respiratory distress—a rather severe bronchitis, trapping of the secretions by the narrow tracheal lumen at the site of the compression and—as Hilding and Hilding[23] have described—a degree of ciliary paralysis, further retarding the expulsion of the secretions from the tracheobronchial tree.

Case History. A 2½-year-old boy was admitted to the Tracheitis Unit with a history of a head cold for three days. On the day before admission (approximately twelve hours) he developed a croupy cough and late in the evening began to have labored breathing. He was admitted to the hospital in the early hours of the morning with signs and symptoms typical of moderately severe obstructive laryngotracheitis. The past history is rather significant in this particular case. The child was said to be inclined to be croupy, and nine months before this admission he had had an emergency tracheotomy in this hospital in which the diagnosis of acute laryngotracheitis was made. At that time the child had an uneventful recovery from the illness and surgery.

On this admission in spite of intensive conventional therapy the child's condition deteriorated so that the chief of the chest service and this author agreed unequivocally that a tracheotomy was needed. The patient was brought to the operating room in a semi-comatose, restless state, pulse rate approaching 200 beats per minute and poor air entry generally in the chest on auscultation. Sternal, costal and subclavicular indrawing was apparent but not pronounced. On the operating table, without an anesthetic, the larynx was exposed with a standard laryngoscope, and a bronchoscope (#4 × 30 mm.) was introduced into the trachea; no landmarks could be identified because of secretions. In fact, the bronchoscope passed into the trachea with such ease that the immediate thought was that the bronchoscope must have passed inadvertently into the esophagus. The bronchoscope was withdrawn and re-introduced immediately into the trachea without any doubt of its position this second time. (It is this author's practice, if there is any doubt as to the proper location of the bronchoscope in any respiratory emergency, to withdraw and re-insert the instrument rather than waste time looking for landmarks which may be obscured by secretions.) The bronchoscope was advanced to the carina, secretions quickly aspirated, and intermittent positive-pressure ventilation was administered by thumbing the bronchoscope.[17]

When the child's color improved and he was breathing well, more detailed examination of the larynx and tracheobronchial tree was carried out. It was obvious at this time that there was no obstruction of the laryngeal airway, but there was a moderately severe compression of the trachea by the innominate artery. In addition, there was an acute inflammation of the bronchial tree bilaterally, and the aspirated secretions were of a thick purulent nature.

The conclusion was that this patient had in fact a compression of the trachea by the innominate artery, causing the respiratory distress, as was probably the case when the previous tracheotomy had been performed. The trachotomy at that time relieved the problem by providing easy access for tracheobronchial toilet, and when the broncho-pulmonary infection was controlled the tracheotomy was no longer necessary.

In the present situation we decided against tracheotomy but elected to use a nasotracheal tube as a temporary measure until the infection could be treated adequately. The tube was to be removed in forty-eight hours, and if no respiratory difficulty developed, nothing further would be done. However, the patient could not be extubated in forty-eight hours, so at this point a suspension of the innominate artery was performed.[33] The child made an excellent recovery following the cardiovascular surgery and has been well for the past three years.

The principal lesson from this case is that "one sees what one knows." The possibility of innominate artery compression as a cause of acute respiratory distress must not be overlooked. The importance of bronchoscopy in the management of respiratory emergencies is also emphasized.

It is desirable to avoid a tracheotomy when surgery for anomalies of the great vessels is contemplated, but a tracheotomy does not preclude surgery

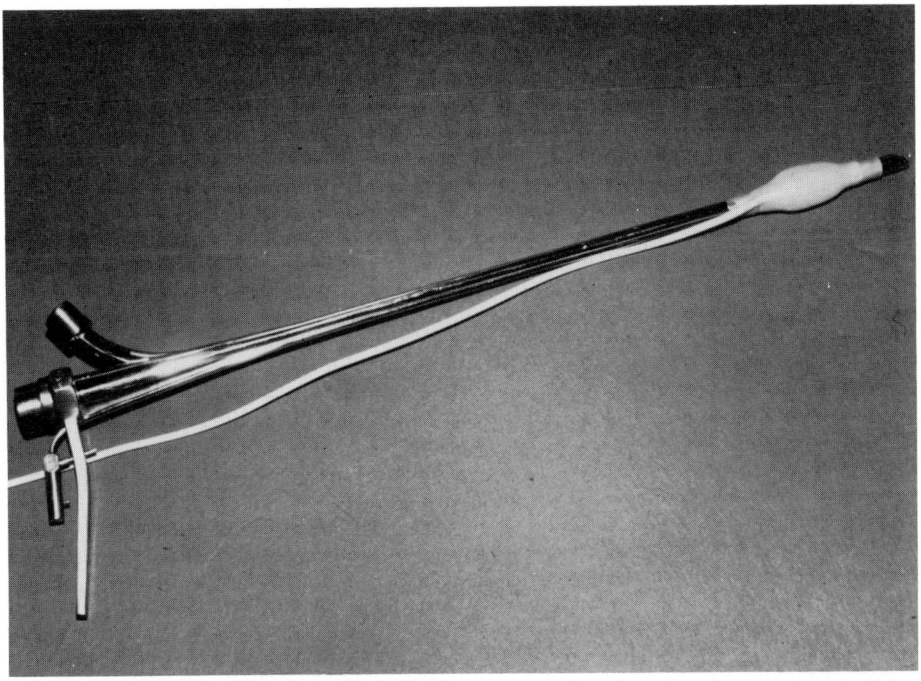

Figure 9. Waters cuff on bronchoscope to ventilate a tracheotomized patient for open chest surgery.

on these vessels. Either a cuffed endotracheal tube to reach beyond the tracheal stoma or a Waters cuff on a bronchoscope permits anesthesia for open chest surgery quite satisfactorily (Fig. 9).

SPONTANEOUS PNEUMOMEDIASTINUM (MEDIASTINAL EMPHYSEMA)

Our concept of a spontaneous pneumomediastinum for the purposes of this text is the development of air in the mediastinum secondary to pulmonary disease (without any *obvious* cause), but we exclude pneumomediastinum from instrumental or other trauma to the esophagus, chest or tracheobronchial tree. Since pneumomediastinum may be a respiratory emergency necessitating emergency surgery, it must be classified along with other acute airway obstructions.

Pneumomediastinum may occur along the fascial planes of the neck following deep wounds of the neck, pharynx or chest; in the retroperitoneal space through the diaphragmatic orifice secondary to a ruptured hollow viscus; or through perforation of the trachea, main bronchus or esophagus. It also may develop secondary to interstitial emphysema of the lung (the most common cause) which, in turn, results from rupture of the pulmonary alveoli.[2]

Air in the mediastinum per se is not a serious matter. It is not unusual to see mediastinal air in chest x-rays after tracheotomy, and it is of little consequence. Indeed, a tracheotomy in itself will relieve a tension pneumomediastinum by opening the fascial planes and allowing air to escape from the anterior mediastinum. Acute respiratory distress will depend on whether or not the disease is as described by Macklin and Macklin – namely, benign or malignant.[27]

It is the malignant form of pneumomediastinum with which we are concerned in respect to surgical management.[15, 42] If a large amount of air is trapped in the mediastinum, there is a "cardiac tamponade"—a collapse of the large veins in the mediastinum obstructing the venous return to the heart. The associated interstitial emphysema causes collapse of pulmonary vessels, resulting in venous stasis, and interferes with the exchange of air on expiration. If this condition progresses, death results. An equally serious alternative is for the air to escape into the pleural spaces, creating a bilateral tension pneumothorax.[15]

The commonest disease in children in which pneumomediastinum is seen is the idiopathic respiratory distress syndrome in which, under these circumstances, survival has been rare, regardless of treatment. Pneumomediastinum is seen occasionally in severe asthmatic attacks, pneumonia, lung abscess and foreign body aspiration. In one of our patients who had aspirated a peanut there was a pneumopericardium as well as pneumomediastinum.

Clinical features of severe pneumomediastinum are complaints of chest pain which may be of a severe precordial type and of subcutaneous emphysema first in the neck and particularly in the suprasternal notch and which may extend over the chest wall. Subcutaneous emphysema may be the first sign of pneumomediastinum in 20 per cent of cases.

Hamman's sign,[21] a clicking sound with systole heard over the precordial area, is diagnostic. Breathing is rapid and labored, with a prolonged expiratory phase along with cyanosis. As the disease progresses, evidence of shock and circulatory failure develop. X-ray examination shows a widening of the superior mediastinum and translucent bands bordering the heart. In the newborn the lateral displacement of the thymus gland by the air creates a so-called "spinnaker sail" sign. Definitive treatment is governed by the underlying cause of the pneumomediastinum. If the cause is asthma, the asthma must be treated; if the cause is pneumonia, the pneumonia is treated.

As Rollins[39] has stressed, positive-pressure therapy is definitely contraindicated and actually magnifies respiratory embarrassment. The hospital records for the past five years show that at least four and possibly more patients being treated for asthma by intubation and intermittent positive-pressure ventilation have died, and at postmortem examination a bilateral tension pneumothorax and pneumomediastinum were found in these cases. If the signs of pneumomediastinum progress in spite of conservative therapy, cervical mediastinotomy can be a dramatic lifesaving measure. Our routine is to perform a bronchoscopy, first to improve the airway and on occasion for diagnosis. If the patient is an asthmatic, ether-oxygen anesthesia is delivered through the bronchoscope.

An anterior mediastinotomy is performed by making a vertical midline incision above the suprasternal notch; the dissection is continued through the fascial layers until the trachea is exposed. The anterior mediastinum is entered by following the anterior tracheal wall by blunt dissection with the curved Kelly forceps or curved scissors to the level of the great vessels providing a passage for the escape of mediastinal air. A one-quarter-inch Penrose drain is introduced into the anterior mediastinum and left in position with the proximal end of the drain retained outside the skin incision. The incision is left open and covered with a light dressing. If there is a question of airway obstruction involving the tracheobronchial tree—e.g., a laryngeal injury—then a tracheotomy may be carried out through the same incision without adding to the morbidity. We are inclined to emphasize this point strongly—if there is any tracheobronchial airway problem at all that can be helped by tracheotomy, then tracheotomy should be carried out along with the mediastinotomy.

Case History. A 6-year-old boy was seen in our emergency department in severe respiratory distress and with obvious subcutaneous emphysema of the neck. The patient had developed an upper respiratory infection five days before arrival which proceeded to a severe cough. Two or three hours before reaching the hospital he had episodes of vomiting and violent coughing as well as labored breathing.

Examination showed a well-nourished and well-developed boy in considerable distress; he appeared to be in shock and was breathing with a prolonged expiratory phase. Further examination revealed a diffuse swelling of the neck, and crepitus was obvious when the neck was palpated. On auscultation there were an asthmatic expiratory wheeze and poor or absent air entry into the right lower chest. X-rays of the chest indicated a consolidation of the right lower lobe of the lung. A tentative diagnosis of right lower lobe pneumonia and pneumomediastinum was made, and in view of the patient's poor condition, it was decided that a bronchoscopy and mediastinotomy should be carried out on an emergency basis. Supportive therapy was instituted, and the patient was taken to the operating room. A bronchoscopy (#4 × 30 mm.) was introduced into the tracheobronchial tree, and a large amount of thick purulent exudate was aspirated from the right lower lobe bronchi. The patient was then anesthetized via the bronchoscope, and a mediastinotomy was performed. Large amounts of air escaped as the fascial planes were opened, and more air was obtained from the anterior mediastinum. A Penrose drain was introduced into the anterior mediastinum. Subsequently, culture from the bronchial tree yielded *Staphylococcus pyogenes*. The patient was treated postoperatively in a croupette, and antimicrobial therapy was administered. All signs of air in the mediastinum and subcutaneous tissues were gone four days after operation. The drain was removed completely on the fifth postoperative day, and the incision was allowed to close without sutures. The chest was perfectly clear on x-ray several days after the admission. On discharge after ten days of hospitalization the boy was quite well.

MISCELLANEOUS CONDITIONS

CONGENITAL SUBGLOTTIC HEMANGIOMA

Charles Ferguson[6] has emphasized the possibility of congenital subglottic hemangioma as a cause of stridor with respiratory obstruction and the importance of making an early diagnosis in order to institute treatment. He has pointed out that a subglottic hemangioma may be present without overt signs of hemangioma elsewhere in or on the body (in 50 per cent of cases).

As with other congenital obstructive lesions involving the larynx and trachea, acute respiratory distress may develop rather suddenly with the onset of a respiratory infection, and the medical management initially is the same as for other obstructive lesions in the presence of respiratory infection. When the obstruction is severe, bronchoscopy and tracheotomy are mandatory. It is at this point that the correct diagnosis should be made. The appearance of the subglottic hemangioma is rather characteristic but not like hemangioma seen elsewhere. It appears as an irregular mass directly below the vocal cords and involves only a part of the circumference of the subglottic space. The color varies from pink to dark bluish pink, and in our experience the mass is quite solid and difficult to compress. Ferguson advises against biopsy because of the possible danger of severe bleeding. We always attempt to do a biopsy in each case; the chief difficulty is to penetrate the rather firm tissue with small biopsy forceps. It is usually necessary to make an incision with the laryngeal knife to enable the forceps to grasp an adequate amount of tissue for biopsy. Hemorrhage in our cases has not been a problem. The treatment of choice is radiotherapy; in this area, radiotherapy is carried out at the Princess Margaret Hospital. For this lesion a single dose of 400 R is administered while the patient is under general anesthesia. As soon as the lesion regresses, which may be from two to six weeks in most cases, the patient is decannulated if direct examination shows the airway to be adequate.

OROPHARYNGEAL LESIONS

Hypertrophy of the adenoid and tonsils is not infrequently the cause of relative obstruction of the airway and particularly that of the nasal airway. Occasionally, such a patient will acquire a bout of acute tonsillitis, causing additional swelling of the adenoid and tonsils so that severe and even total airway obstruction may occur rather suddenly. If such is the case, we advocate emergency bronchoscopy and tracheotomy. As soon as the inflammation has subsided using antimicrobial medication, the adenoid and tonsils should be removed. Decannulation may then be carried out safely.[12]

Fortunately, malignancy of the tonsils in the child is uncommon, but when it does happen the outcome is generally hopeless. The lesions we have encountered have been either lymphosarcoma or reticulum cell sarcoma. Either tumor progresses very rapidly to the point of creating obstruction to the airway and necessitating emergency measures. Generally, these lesions first present as what appears to be an acute inflammation involving a tonsil or the peritonsillar area. The growth is so rapid that it may be necessary to remove the malignant tonsil for the relief of airway obstruction as well as for definitive diagnosis. Blood-borne metastases occur very early, and the treatment is at best palliative.

Retropharyngeal abscesses occur in children 3 years old and under, and although some airway impairment may be a factor, this is corrected by appropriate management of the infection and the abscess. The same holds true (except for age) in peritonsillar and pharyngomaxillary space abscesses, but these must be considered in the differential diagnosis of acute airway obstruction.

Primary abscesses of the larynx are rare but do occur, usually in the aryepiglottic folds. These can be approached and drained by direct laryngoscopy, first by needle aspiration of the abscess and then, as in laryngeal cyst, by removal of enough of the abscess wall to prevent future abscess recurrence.

Foreign bodies in the air and food passages are dealt with in detail in Chapter 109, but one must consider the possibility of a foreign body in the hypopharynx (e.g., "baby-soother"), in the larynx or in the upper esophagus when the child is presented as an acute respiratory emergency. Roentgenograms must include the larynx and upper esophagus as well as the chest, since several patients have been admitted with acute respiratory obstruction in whom x-rays have been said to be negative but in fact had not included the laryngeal area or upper esophagus.

Case History. A 14-month-old boy in severe respiratory distress was rushed from another hospital to the emergency department. He had been treated for acute laryngotracheitis for about twenty-four hours, and x-rays had not shown any abnormality. When his condition worsened he was transferred to our department.

On arrival in the emergency department the child was breathing rapidly with marked respiratory stridor and marked indrawing of the sternum, ribs and supraclavicular areas. Circumoral pallor was apparent, and the pulse rate was approximately 200 beats per minute. The child was taken directly to the operating room for an emergency tracheotomy. The larynx was exposed with a standard laryngoscope preliminary to passing the bronchoscope, but a foreign object was seen in the larynx. It proved to be a safety pin straddling in the larynx; the keeper of the pin was impacted under the left vocal cord, and the point of the pin was projected toward the esophagus. The safety pin was removed forthwith, but because of a rather marked swelling of the subglottic area, a bronchoscope was introduced into the trachea, the patient anesthetized and a tracheotomy was carried out. An uneventful recovery ensued and the patient was decannulated in six days. A review of the original x-rays of the chest showed that they were not high enough in the neck to detect the foreign object.

MULTIPLE PAPILLOMATA OF THE LARYNX

Papillomata of the larynx provide a great challenge to the laryngologist; the chief concern in the management of this pathological entity is directed mainly toward preventing serious obstruction to the airway until such time as the papillomata regress spontaneously. Most often recurrences stop at puberty, but the condition has been reported by Holinger to continue until late adulthood[24] (Fig. 10). Malignant changes have been reported only in those patients who have had irradiation, and irradiation plays no part whatsoever in the treatment of this disease. It is my firm belief that tracheotomy should be avoided if at all possible because of the danger of seeding the tumor in the trachea with subsequent tracheal obstruction or even extension of the growth into the bronchial tree. This routine may result in many worrisome moments for the surgeon, but in the long run we believe it is in the patient's best interest, and so far we personally have had no cases of extension of papillomata beyond the larynx.

The course of this disease is variable. Usually the growth keeps recurring over a period of years; yet, on occasion, it may not recur even after only one resection. In some instances one, two or three resections of the growth over a period of a few months may be all that is necessary to correct the problem, but the parents should be always prepared for the possibility of multiple operations for several years.

This author's approach is to use his own design of laryngoscope retained in position with the Lewy laryngoscope holder (Fig. 11). Resection is performed under microscopic visualization while the patient is under general anesthesia maintained through a connector built into the laryngoscope. A variety of cupped and biting forceps are used to remove the offending tissue while being most careful to avoid damaging normal laryngeal structures and especially not to denude both vocal cords at the anterior commissure in order to avoid the formation of a web at this point. We emphasize that the objective of the procedure is to achieve a good airway and not necessarily a good voice in the early stages of the treatment. The degree of voice involvement will depend on the situation of the tumor in the larynx and even a small amount of abnormal tissue in the anterior commissure will affect the speech quite considerably.

VOCAL CORD PARALYSIS

Vocal cord paralysis which causes obstruction to the airway is not a common problem in children except when associated with generalized neurologic disease, such as the Guillain-Barré syndrome or bulbar poliomyelitis.

Bilateral adductor spasm (or bilateral abductor paralysis) is on occasion a complication of hydrocephalus, and when the airway obstruction is severe, tracheotomy is indicated. On occasion the ad-

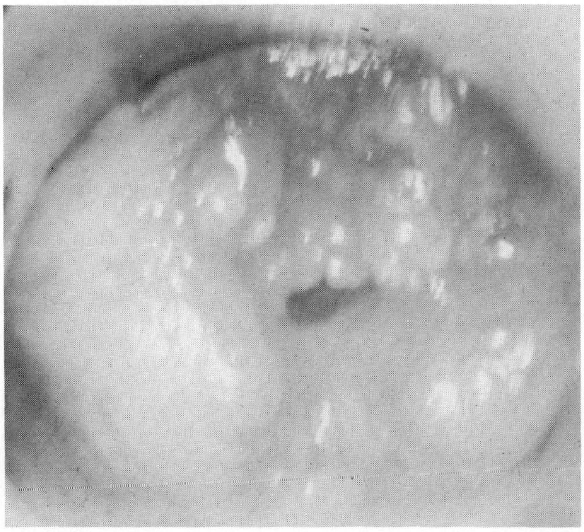

Figure 10. Multiple papillomata of the larynx causing severe obstruction of the laryngeal airway.

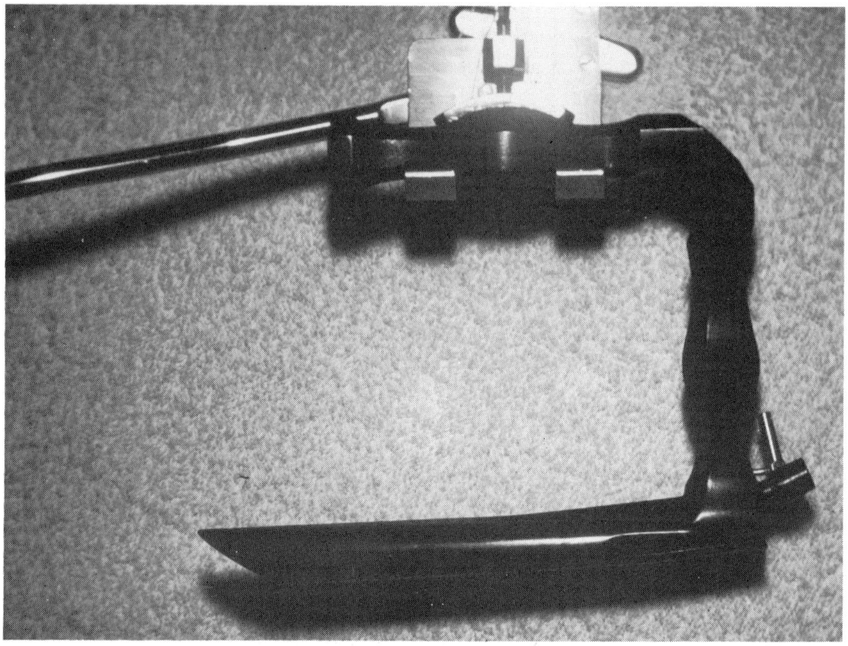

Figure 11. Author's modified laryngoscope for peroral laryngeal surgery. The slot on the left permits easier instrumentation, and it has a tube for insufflation anesthesia.

ductor spasm which is characterized by a very high-pitched sound on inspiration develops when an initially successful shunting procedure to relieve hydrocephalus has become blocked. The problem may, although not always, be relieved by re-instituting the shunt and thus relieving the increased intracranial pressure.

Congenital bilateral abductor paralysis is rare and is said to disappear spontaneously in a few days. The etiology is uncertain, but it would seem logical that it might be due to a pinching of the posterior branch of the recurrent nerve in the cricothyroid joint during delivery. In our experience tracheotomy has been necessary in order to relieve severe hypoxia, and the tracheotomy may have to be maintained for a considerable period of time before the cords regain their function.

CRANIOFACIAL ABNORMALITIES

The Pierre Robin syndrome, Crouzon's syndrome, coronal synostosis, Franconi's syndrome and similar conditions often demonstrate airway obstruction, particularly the Pierre Robin syndrome. This syndrome, which is a triad of micrognathia, cleft palate and microglossia (or glossoptosis), is usually at its worst in early infancy. When the airway obstruction is difficult to control, tracheotomy is justified[8] (Fig. 12). Tracheotomy may be necessary for a year or more and by that time the child's facial structures improve to the degree that the oropharyngeal airway has become quite adequate.

LARYNGOMALACIA (CONGENITAL LARYNGEAL STRIDOR)

Laryngomalacia – or as Atkins[1] describes it, "flabby larynx" – is the commonest cause of stridor in the child but is relatively harmless. The stridor is a coarse rasping sound which is caused by the exaggerated infantile type of epiglottis along with flabby aryepiglottic folds. The epiglottis and its folds tend to be drawn into the laryngeal aperture on inspiration, and the stridor is more pronounced when the child is lying on his back with his head flexed. The obstruction may be severe enough to cause marked sternal and suprasternal indrawing. Usually the stridor can be eliminated by holding the mandible forward while the child's head is extended or by lifting the tongue and epiglottis with a laryngoscope. In extreme cases the obstruction may be severe enough to warrant a tracheotomy. In one such patient under our care recently we were able to eliminate the need for tracheotomy by suturing the epiglottis to the base of the tongue after first resecting the adjacent mucosa of the epiglottis and the base of the tongue.

RESPIRATORY DISTRESS IN THE NEWBORN

We have not dealt with the problems of obstruction to the airway in the newborn because this is a large subject in itself (see Chapter 7 in Volume I). It must be remembered that in the newborn, total obstruction of the nasal airway can cause asphyxia. Accordingly, if the child's breathing becomes obstructed when his mouth is closed, but he is able to cry lustily with a good color, then the cause for the problem should be searched for in the nose[10, 12, 13] (Fig. 13). The commonest cause of nasal obstruction is that of bilateral choanal atresia, but whatever the cause, the immediate procedure is to keep the infant breathing. This may be accomplished by use of the McGovern nipple or by using a suitably sized oral airway retained in the mouth. More definitive measures can be taken electively (see Chapter 86).

PERORAL ENDOSCOPIC AND SURGICAL TECHNIQUES

Peroral examination of the larynx, tracheobronchial tree or esophagus can be performed on the smallest child quite harmlessly with or without general anesthesia if the correct size of instrument is chosen. The endoscopist preferably should be especially experienced in performing the procedure on the small child. Children are not small adults, and therefore their treatment cannot be equated with that of the adult.

A general anesthetic should never be given to the patient with respiratory distress until a bronchoscope is passed and the airway is cleared. Nor is it necessary to give a general anesthetic when the bronchoscope is in place, but this will depend on the patient's condition and the

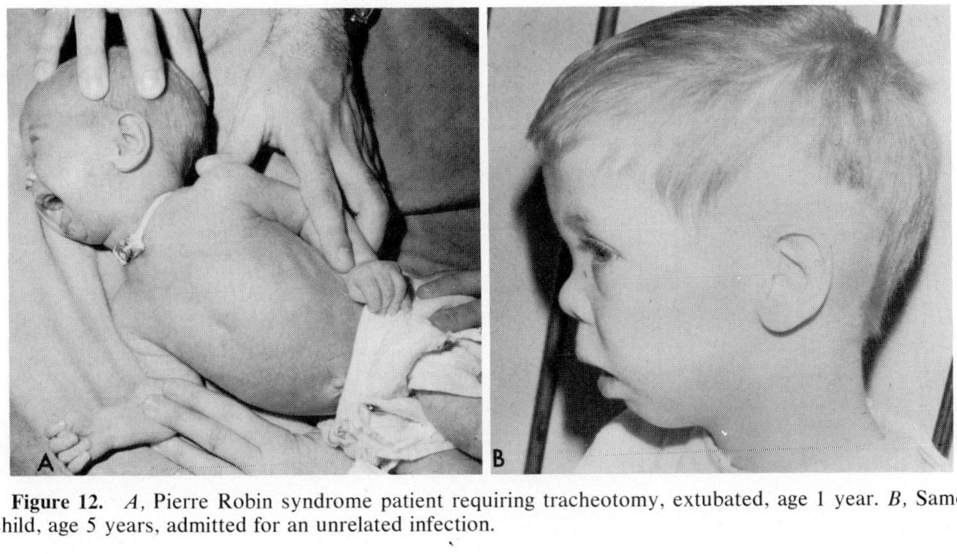

Figure 12. *A*, Pierre Robin syndrome patient requiring tracheotomy, extubated, age 1 year. *B*, Same child, age 5 years, admitted for an unrelated infection.

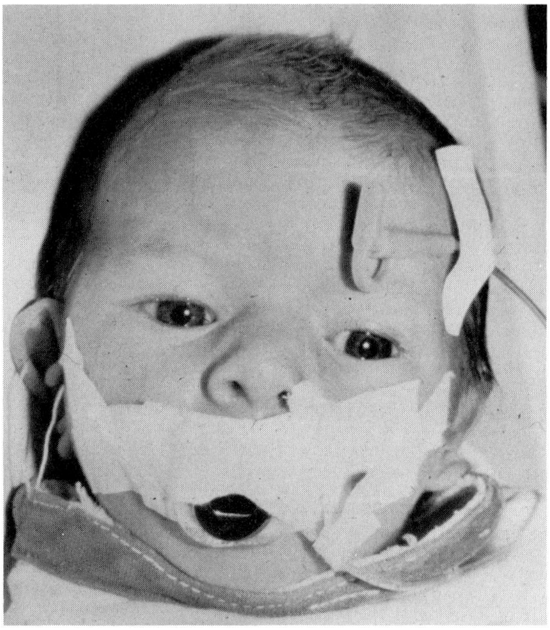

Figure 13. An infant with bilateral choanal atresia must breathe through an oral airway before opening of his nasal airway. (From *Laryngoscope,* 78:1487, 1968.

problem to be dealt with, to say nothing of the skill of the surgeon.

In an acute obstructive emergency, a mouth gag should not be used during the introduction of the bronchoscope. The laryngoscope (or a bite block) can be left in place in the mouth until the child is anesthetized to prevent him from biting the surgeon's fingers or the broncho-scope. In some patients with facial or neck deformities (e.g., the Pierre Robin syndrome) it is sometimes impossible to expose the larynx with the laryngoscope, but a bronchoscope can be passed into the trachea without using the laryngo-scope.

Many different anesthetic techniques for endoscopy are used in the Hospital for Sick Children, but for personal reasons halothane is not administered to our own patients. We prefer the patients to breathe spontaneously, but if necessary, intermittent positive-pressure may be employed by "thumbing" a bronchoscope made especially for this purpose[17] (Fig. 14) or by using the Holinger Fiberoptic bronchoscope with the proximal end covered with a window. The

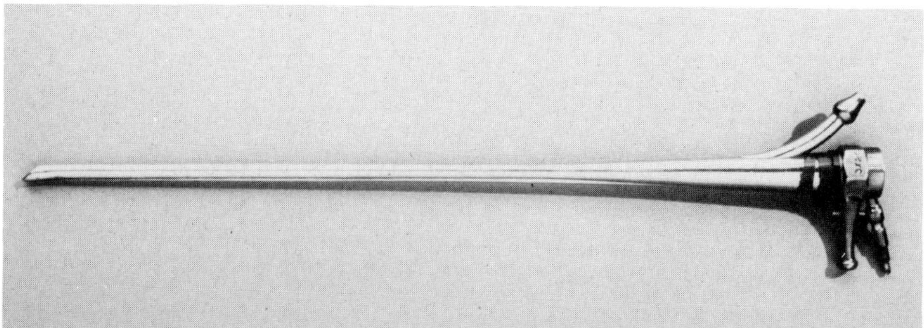

Figure 14. Bronchoscope modified for performing tracheotomies on patients needing assisted ventilation.

Sander's ventilator on the side arm of the Holinger bronchoscope is an alternative method to ventilate the nonbreathing patient.

For patients who present respiratory risks, such as those with asthma, cystic fibrosis or subglottic stenosis, ether-oxygen is the anesthetic of choice. We have found that in patients with long-term airway problems who require repeated anesthetics for treatment, as in subglottic stenosis, the postoperative morbidity is greatly reduced when ether-oxygen is used as the anesthetic agent.

In regard to bronchoscopy in the newborn, a 3-mm. Holinger bronchoscope can be passed through the larynx of any infant who is able to breathe and survive for at least a few hours. In patients with congenital subglottic stenosis, the opening is in a posterior position in the subglottic space, and this must be remembered in attempting to pass a bronchoscope in such a patient. Even when the obstruction is fairly severe the bronchoscope can be advanced by using a spiral movement of the bronchoscope until it is in the trachea. This maneuver with the bronchoscope also serves to dilate the stenotic area.

In patients who are intubated and who require bronchoscopy, instead of removing the endotracheal tube and then using the laryngoscope, the endotracheal tube may be used as a guide for the bronchoscope by following the anterior surface of the tube with the bronchoscope until it reaches the space between the epiglottis and the endotracheal tube. Then the tube may be removed and the bronchoscope advanced into the trachea (Fig. 15).

For the small infant direct laryngoscopy may be best carried out with the Tucker newborn anterior-commissure laryngoscope because the barrel of even the smallest standard laryngoscope may override the upper alveolus of the premature infant, and thus proper visualization of the larynx is obstructed.

Bronchoscopy should be perfectly safe and nontraumatic if the operator uses the instruments gently and properly and if he selects a suitably sized bronchoscope for the size of the patient. Scaroni[40] did an independent review of 430 bronchoscopies carried out in the Department of Otolaryngology and Bronchoesophagology of the Hospital for Sick Children in 1970. He concluded that eight patients had complications from the procedure (1.8 per cent). Two of these patients had subglottic stenosis

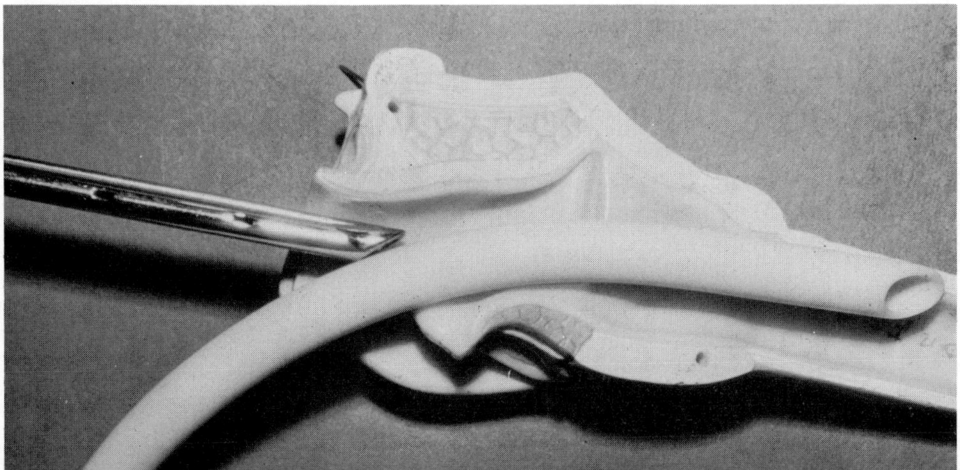

Figure 15. Method of using the endotracheal tube as a guide in passing a bronchoscope in a previously intubated patient. The bronchoscope is advanced as the endotracheal tube is withdrawn.

prior to bronchoscopy and required tracheotomy subsequently, although this was not unexpected. The complications of the remaining six were transient, and there were no deaths. In view of the fact that a large number of the patients bronchoscoped were in the category of poor risks (congenital heart disease, severe asthmatics, cystic fibrosis, newborn prematures), we believe that it is obvious that bronchoscopy need not be detrimental to the patient's welfare (Table 1).

TRACHEOTOMY

Very few significant complications should occur, regardless of the size of the patient, if certain pertinent factors are considered when performing a tracheotomy. With the bronchoscope in place the operation is simplified and the complications are minimized (Fig. 16). A small midline incision provides a rapid, bloodless access to the trachea. It must be emphasized that the tracheal fenestra (or tracheal incision) must be made far enough away from the cricoid so that even the smallest infant need not be a decannulatory problem[16] (Figs. 17 and 18). We have tried all types of tracheotomy tubes that have been available to us, and we still find the Holinger design with our own modification of the inner tube for attaching the ventilator the most generally satisfactory tube (Fig. 19). (Incidentally, a Kistner one-way valve attachment can be used on our modified inner tracheotomy tube so that the patient can breathe in through the tube and out through the larynx.)

In the patients who have had a tracheotomy for acute airway obstruction we believe that it is most important that the tracheotomy tube should be blocked for twenty-four hours before it is removed. However, prior to this, the original tube is removed, and a smaller tube is put into the trachea, depending on the child's progress. If a child can breathe around the tube without distress for a twenty-four-hour period, then it is safe to remove the tracheotomy tube and allow the opening to close (Fig. 20).

TABLE 1. GUIDE FOR SELECTION OF SUITABLE TRACHEOTOMY TUBES AND BRONCHOSCOPES*

Age	Holinger Tracheotomy Tube	Bronchoscope Size	Age
PREMATURE (<4 lbs.)	#000 × 26 mm.	3 mm.	<5 lbs.
PREMATURE (>4 lbs.)	#00 × 26 mm. to 33 mm.		
0–6 mos.	#0 × 33 mm. to 40 mm.	3.5 mm.	0–6 mos.
6–12 mos.	#1 × 40 mm. to 46 mm.	4 mm.	6 mos. ↓ 3 yrs.
12–18 mos.	#1 × 46 mm.		
18 mos. ↓ 4 yrs.–5 yrs.	#1 or #2 × 46 mm. to 50 mm.	5 mm.	3 yrs. ↓ 12 yrs.
4 yrs.–5 yrs. ↓ 10 yrs.	#2 or #3 × 50 mm. to 55 mm.		
10 yrs.+	#3 or #4 or #5 × 50 mm. to 68 mm.	6 mm.	12 yrs.+

*Fearon, B., and Ellis, D.: The Management of the Longterm Airway Problem in Infants and Children. *Ann. Otol. Rhinol. Laryng.*, 669:80 (Oct.), 1971.

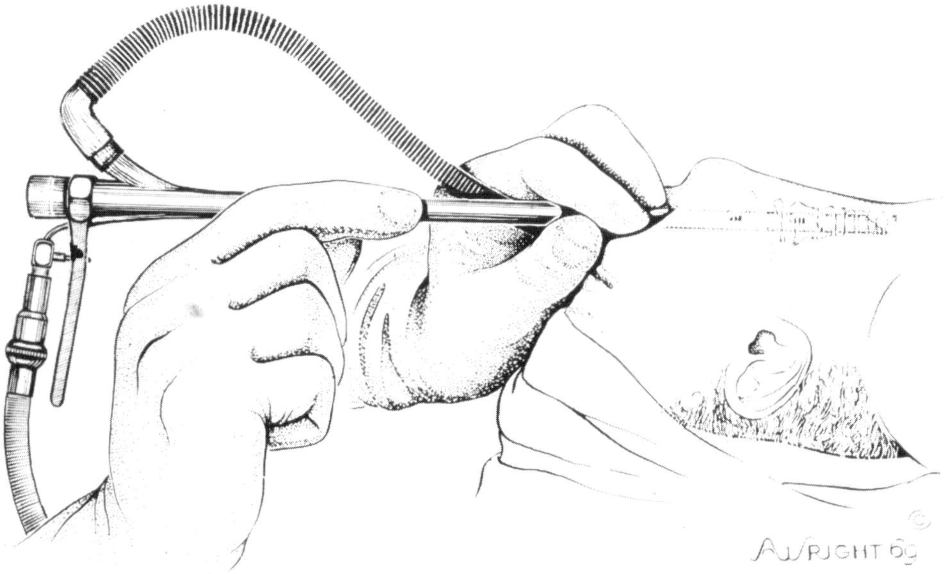

Figure 16. Method of holding bronchoscope while a tracheotomy is being performed.

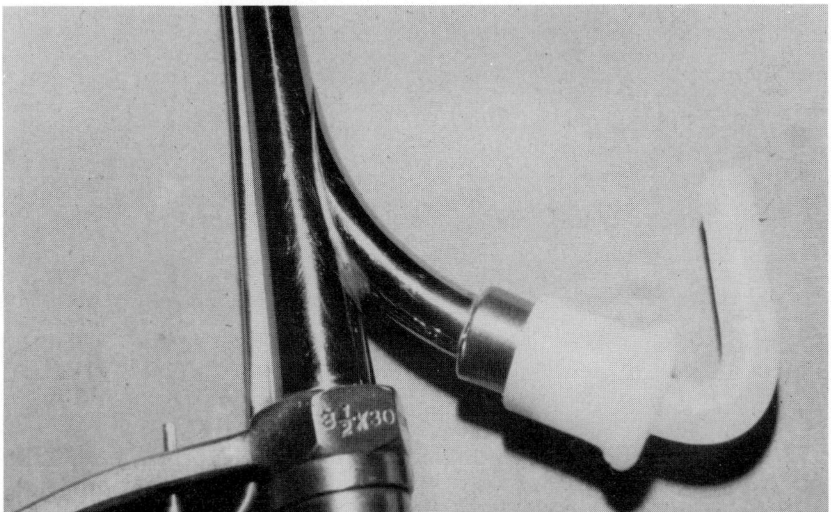

Figure 17. Holinger bronchoscope with an adaptor for the anesthetic tube (or oxygen).

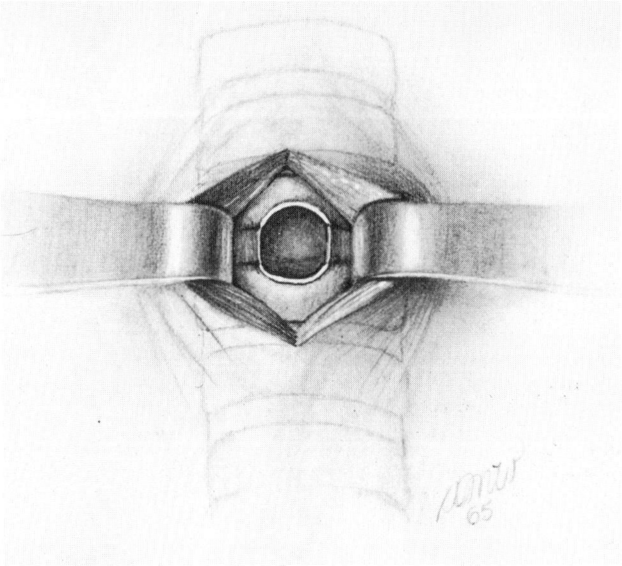

Figure 18. Tracheal fenestra made so that the tracheal ring is not divided.

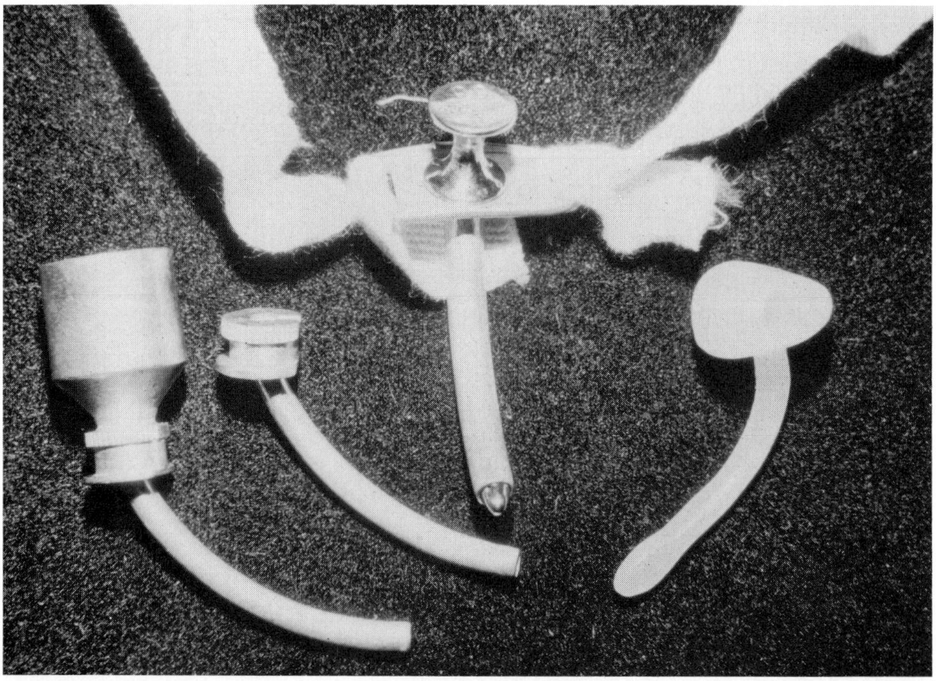

Figure 19. Tracheotomy set used by the author with a 15-mm. adaptor on one inner cannula of the Holinger tracheotomy tube. Also shown is a silicone tracheotomy stent used for long-term airway problems.

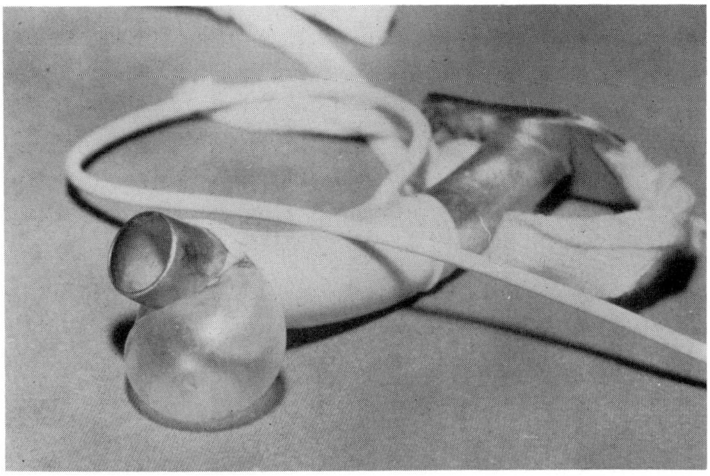

Figure 20. Complication of a cuffed tube. Ballooning of the cuff severely obstructed the airway, but it was removed before serious harm befell the patient. Similar problems can also happen with cuffed endotracheal tubes.

In the long-term tracheotomy problems—especially those with subglottic stenosis—we maintain a tracheal stoma by the use of a plastic stent (Fig. 19) for at least three months, and if the patient has had no significant respiratory distress in that three-month period, we consider it safe to decannulate.[14] This ensures that the patient will be able to manage without a tracheotomy. In the long-term cases the stoma usually closes quite quickly; there may be some leak of air through the stoma on forced expulsion of air, but this in itself is not important. When a tracheotomy tube has been worn for a long period of time considerable scar formation develops around the tube so that when it is removed there is an unsightly identation in the neck; this does not happen with the short-term tracheotomies. The deformity can be corrected by excising the scar tissue, but this should not be carried out until the patient is 5 or 6 years of age. Furthermore, thorough examination of the larynx and the tracheobronchial tree by peroral endoscopy should be routine before excising the scar. If the airway is compromised to any significant degree, the procedure should be delayed until postoperative airway problems are not likely to occur.

In conclusion, we wish to add a word of caution to those surgeons and operating room personnel who are repeatedly exposed to certain anesthetic agents, such as halothane, methoxyflurane and trichlorethylene, in the operating room and in particular while performing bronchoscopies. Evidence seems to be accumulating to the effect that repeated exposure to one or more of these anesthetic gases over a period of time may result in permanent damage to the liver, kidneys, pancreas or even the central nervous system. We advocate strongly that some means should be taken to avoid the inhalation of these anesthetic agents. We use a plastic oxygen mask into which is introduced a constant flow of compressed air (15 liters per min.) with a Kistner valve cemented in the mask on either side of the nose to vent out the air and to prevent the inhalation of the gas or the air in the operating room. This makeshift device, although far from perfect, does help to prevent the inhalation of much of the volatile anesthetic agents to which we are exposed while operating.

REFERENCES

1. Atkins, J. P.: Laryngeal Problems of Infancy and Childhood. *Pediat. Clin. North Amer.*, 9:1125 (November), 1962.

2. Banyai, A. L.: *Nontuberculous Diseases of the Chest.* Charles C Thomas, Publisher, Springfield, Ill., 1954, p. 930.
3. Davison, F. W.: Acute Laryngotracheal Infections in Children. *Otolaryng. Clin. North Amer.* (Bronchoesophagology), 69 (June), 1968.
4. Davison, F. W.: Inflammatory Diseases of the Larynx; in *Otolaryngology,* Vol. IV. Chap. 15. Harper & Row, Publishers, Inc., Hagerstown, Maryland, 1971.
5. Downs, J. J., Striker, T. W., and Stool, S.: Complications of Nasotracheal Intubation in Children. Letter to editor. *New Eng. J. Med.,* 274:226, 1966.
6. Ferguson, C. F., and Flake, C. G.: Subglottic Hemangioma as a Cause of Respiratory Obstruction in Children. *Ann. Otol. Rhinol. Laryng.,* 1095:60 (December), 1961.
7. Fearon, B.: Acute Laryngotracheobronchitis in Infancy and Childhood. *Pediat. Clin. North Amer.,* 9:1095 (December), 1962.
8. Fearon, B.: Acute Obstructive Laryngitis in Infants and Children. *Hosp. Med.,* 4:51 (December), 1968.
9. Fearon, B.: Anesthesia in Pediatric Peroral Endoscopy. *Ann. Otol. Rhinol. Laryng.,* 78:469 (June), 1969.
10. Fearon, B.: The Endoscopic Management of Congenital Atresia of the Esophagus with or without Tracheo-esophageal Fistula. *Ann. Otol., Rhinol. Laryng.,* 68:1047 (December), 1959.
11. Fearon, B.: Respiratory Distress in the Newborn. *Otolaryng. Clin. North Amer.* (Bronchoesophagology), 147 (June), 1968.
12. Fearon, B.: Pediatric Adenoidectomy and Tonsillectomy—Divergent Views. *Proceed. Canad. Otolaryng. Soc.,* 17:32 (June), 1965.
13. Fearon, B., and Dickson, J.: Bilateral Choanal Atresia in the Newborn—Plan of Action. *Laryngoscope,* 9:1487 (June), 1968.
14. Fearon, B., and Ellis, D.: The Management of the Longterm Airway Problem in Infants and Children. *Ann. Otol. Rhinol. Laryng.,* 669:80 (October), 1971.
15. Fearon, B., and MacDonald, R. E.: The Surgical Management of Spontaneous Pneumomediastinum in Children. *Proceed. Canad. Otolaryng. Soc.,* 17:32 (June), 1963.
16. Fearon, B., MacDonald, R. E., Smith, C., and Mitchell, D.: Airway Problems in Children Following Prolonged Endotracheal Intubation. *Ann. Otol. Rhinol. Laryng.,* 75:964 (December), 1966.
17. Fearon, B., Smith, C., et al : The Idiopathic Respiratory Distress Syndrome in the Newborn. *Ann. Otol. Rhinol. Laryng.,* 73:1082 (December), 1964.
18. Fearon, B., and Shortreed, R.: Tracheal Compression by Cardiovascular Anomalies in Children. *Ann. Otol. Rhinol. Laryng.,* 72:949 (December), 1963.
19. Fearon, B., and Whalen, J. S.: Tracheal Dimensions in the Living Infant. *Ann. Otol. Rhinol. Laryng.,* 76:964 (December), 1967.
20. Galloway, T. C.: *Treatment of Respiratory Emergencies Including Bulbar Poliomyelitis.* Charles C Thomas, Publishers, Springfield, Ill., 1953.
21. Hamman, L.: Spontaneous Mediastinal Emphysema of the Lungs and Mediastinum. *Bull. Johns Hopkins Hosp.,* 44:1 (January), 1931.
22. Hilding, A. C.: Tracheal Damage During Intratracheal Anesthesia. *Ann. Otol. Rhinol. Laryng.,* 565:80 (August), 1971.
23. Hilding, A. C., and Hilding, D.: Tolerance of the Respiratory Mucous Membrane to Trauma: Surgical Swabs and Endotracheal Tubes. *Ann. Otol. Rhinol. Laryng.,* 71:455, 1962.
24. Holinger, P. H.: Benign Tumors of the Trachea and Bronchi. *Otolaryng. Clin. North Amer.* (Bronchoesophagology), 219 (June), 1968.
25. Leegaard, T.: Pseudocroup. *Acta Otolaryng.* (Suppl.), 158:10, 1960.
26. MacDonald, R. E., and Fearon, B.: Innominate Artery Compression Syndrome. *Ann. Otol. Rhinol. Laryng.,* 80:535 (August), 1971.
27. Macklin, M. T., and Macklin, C. G.: Malignant Interstitial Emphysema of the Lungs and Mediastinum. *Medicine,* 23:281, 1944.
28. MacLean, D. M., et al.: Para-Influenzal Viruses in Association with Acute Laryngotracheitis—Toronto 1960–1961. *Canad. Med. Ass. J.,* 85:290, 1961.
29. Mills, I. C.: *Clinical Aspects of Adrenal Function.* Philadelphia, F. A. Davis Co., 1964.
30. Morgan, E. A., et al.: Observations on the Etiology of Acute Laryngotracheobronchitis—Toronto 1953–1954. *Canad. Med. Ass. J.,* 75:638, 1956.
31. McGovern, F. H., FitzHugh, G. S., and Edgemon, L. J.: The Hazards of Endotracheal Intubation. *Ann. Otol. Rhinol. Laryng.,* 80:556 (August), 1971.
32. Moseley, J. E.: Loculated Pneumomediastinum in the Newborn—a Thymic "Spinnaker Sail" Sign. *J. Radiol.,* 75:788, 1960.
33. Mustard, W. T., Bayliss, C. E., Fearon, B., Pelton, D., and Trusler, G. A.: Tracheal Compression by the Innominate Artery. *Ann. Thorac. Surg.,* 8:312 (October), 1969.
34. Myerson, M. C.: *The Human Larynx.* Charles C Thomas, Publishers, Springfield, Ill., 1964, Chapt. 6, p. 61.
35. Nelson, T. G.: *Tracheotomy.* Williams and Wilkins Co., Baltimore, 1958, pp. 60–69.
36. Ogura, J. H., and Biller, H. F.: Reconstruction of the Larynx Following Blunt Trauma. *Ann. Otol. Rhinol. Laryng.,* 80:492 (August), 1971.
37. Peach, A., and Zaiman, E.: Acute Laryngotracheitis. *Brit. Med. J.,* 1:416, 1959.
38. Ross, J. A. T.: Special Problems in Acute Laryngotracheobronchitis. *Laryngoscope,* 79:1218, 1969.
39. Rollins, L. R.: Mediastinal Emphysema and

Bilateral Pneumothorax Following Surgery of the Neck. *Amer. Surg.*, 22:567 (June), 1956.
40. Scaroni, V.: Dept. Surgery, Hospital for Sick Children. Personal communication.
41. Silverthorne, N.: Personal communication.
42. Thaler, M., Krieger, E., McKee, J., and Fearon, B.: Surgical Treatment of Subcutaneous and Mediastinal Emphysema Complicating Asthma in Children. *J. Pediat.*, 65:75 (July), 1964.
43. Turner, J. A.: Present-day Aspects of Laryngotracheitis. *Canad. Med. Ass. J.*, 70:401, 1954.
44. Weaver, A. W., et al.: The Management of Penetrating Wounds of the Neck. *Surg. Gynec. Obstet.*, 49:133 (July), 1971.

Chapter One Hundred Six

LARYNGEAL PARALYSIS

CHARLES F. FERGUSON, M.D., F.A.C.S.

Laryngeal paralysis is not common in pediatric otolaryngology, but its causes should be better understood. Paralysis of the larynx is ordinarily seen as a motor involvement rather than a sensory one. *Sensory paralysis*, however, may occur under extremely rare circumstances, usually related to pathology in the central nervous system. The sensory nerve supply to the larynx is through the internal branch of the superior laryngeal nerve from the vagus (tenth cranial nerve) on each side. It also supplies the mucous membrane of the upper trachea and hypopharynx as well as the larynx. Sensation, however, extends beyond the midline, so both nerves must be involved if there is true anesthesia of the larynx. In such a case, there is no cough reflex until food, fluid, saliva or foreign material has passed down the trachea and reached the bronchi. Aspiration under such circumstances is frequent.

Motor paralysis is the much more common type, yet this also is rare in infants and children as compared with adults. The motor nerve supply to the larynx is through the recurrent laryngeal nerves and from the vagus (except for the cricothyroid muscle, which is supplied by the external branch of the superior laryngeal nerve). The left recurrent nerve has the longer course, as it runs down into the chest under the arch of the aorta and ascends in the groove between the trachea and the esophagus. Therefore, it is subject to much more pressure from thoracic lesions, so paralysis of the left vocal cord is much more common than of the right. The right recurrent laryngeal nerve passes under the subclavian artery. Motor paralysis is usually due to involvement of the peripheral nerve itself, as there is a bilateral cortical innervation to each side of the larynx. Therefore, in cases of bilateral paralysis, a lesion of the cortex would of necessity be perfectly symmetrical, or comprise a mass lesion covering a very large area. However, in the region of the nucleus ambiguus and just above it, the fibers decussate, so a lesion in that location could involve both sides at the same time.

Paralysis of the larynx may involve three muscle groups, abductors, adductors and tensors.

Unilateral Abductor Paralysis

Unilateral abductor (midline) paralysis is the slightly more common type, and in most instances it is a peripheral paralysis. The cord lies in the midline and cannot be abducted even on enforced deep inspiration. It is "paralyzed shut" (Fig. 1). It may not be suspected until the infant is 3 or 4 days of age when he is better able to move air in and out of his lower respiratory tract and pulmonary aeration has improved. Sometimes is is not even noted until he develops a respiratory infection. The cry and voice are clear and may be fairly strong as long as the cords can approximate adequately.

Because of its long and devious course, the left recurrent laryngeal nerve is much more often involved. In the infant, pressure of an enlarged heart or conus, intrinsic congenital cardiac defects, abnormal great vessels or a dilated aorta are the commonest causes. Since congenital cardiovascular malformations also produce cyanosis, attention is often misdirected to the more obvious cardiac problem, and the airway obstruction may be neglected if direct laryngoscopy is not carried out. Other causes of laryngeal paralysis are intrathoracic masses, such as tumors or cysts of the mediastinum or tracheobronchial tree malformations. Esophageal malformations, such as duplications or cysts, should also be considered as mass lesions producing pressure on the left recurrent nerve and giving rise to this peripheral type of paralysis. Occasionally, a cystic hygroma or other external lesion in the neck causes sufficient pressure on the nerve to produce paralysis. Transient paresis lasting for only a few weeks after birth is usually caused by traction on the nerve during a difficult breech delivery, or by some other type of trauma to the neck, which may also produce a visible hematoma or torticollis.

In older children, pulmonary lesions or enlarged lymph nodes, apical adhesions from tuberculosis, and pulmonary or bronchial tumors have to be considered as causes. Mitral stenosis following rheumatic fever, thyroid swellings, trauma to the neck or virus infections may also produce a paralyzed cord, as well as lead poisoning and diphtheria, which cause a toxic neuritis. Paralysis is not always complete, because the arytenoideus muscle has bilateral innervation, and a persistent functioning of this muscle allows the posterior commissure to close adequately. The paralyzed cord appears to be concave and not straight, preventing complete approximation, which results in audible air waste. Usually no treatment is necessary for unilateral paralysis of the larynx, but on occasion tracheotomy has been indicated.

Bilateral Abductor Paralysis

Bilateral abductor (midline) paralysis of the larynx is nearly as common in infants as the unilateral type, but it ordinarily suggests a central nervous system lesion. It may not be suspected for a few days after birth, until the infant is stronger and has developed better respiratory exchange. The cry may be weak, but it is not particularly hoarse or otherwise abnormal, even though the airway may be seriously obstructed. Stridor is apparent on exertion, and may also occur at rest. Central nervous system pathology is probably the most common causative factor in bilateral abductor paralysis, and this includes cerebral agen-

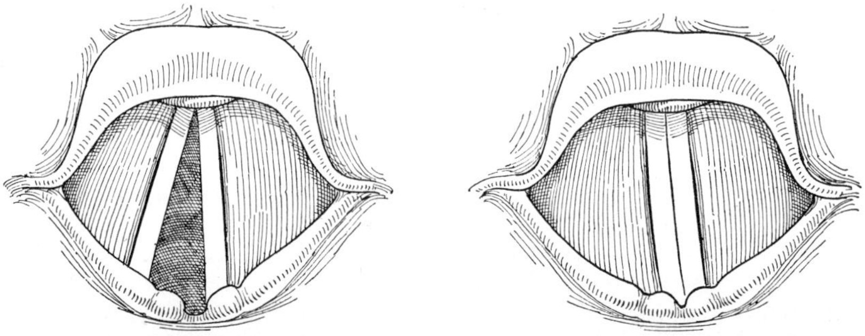

Figure 1. Unilateral abductor paralysis of the larynx. Note that the left cord in this mirror view remains in the midline. (From Richards, L. G.: *Otolaryngology in General Practice,* Macmillan, 1939.)

esis or cerebral (or cerebellar) meningocele or myelomeningocele. Cases have also been reported of Arnold-Chiari malformations with bilateral abductor paralysis of the larynx. In these cases a tongue of cerebellum herniates into the foramen magnum and may extend down as far as the sixth cervical vertebra. Birth injury to the brainstem, or hemorrhage either from trauma or from an underlying blood dyscrasia, especially in the region of the nucleus ambiguus, is probably the commonest causative factor. If paralysis is the result of cerebral hemorrhage, but the hemorrhage is not marked, and has been brought promptly under control, such laryngeal paralysis of the newborn may be only transient. However, in most instances the prognosis is not good.

In 1964, Plott reported three unusual cases of congenital laryngeal paralysis in three brothers, all of whom showed congenital abductor paralysis. One other sibling had died 15 hours after birth with severe respiratory distress. He also may have had the same lesion. The causes obviously are difficult to determine. It is well known that the motor neurones innervating the intrinsic laryngeal muscles are located in the nucleus ambiguus in the inferior portion of the reticular formation of the medulla. It was felt, therefore, that since all three brothers had the same signs, symptoms and clinical findings, there was a good possibility of a genetically determined dysgenesis of the abductor portion of the nucleus ambiguus at the level where the bilateral fibers decussate. It is hard to explain three such identical lesions as mere coincidence. All three of these patients also showed marked retardation of mental development and were considered to have some organic cerebral dysfunction.

In the chest, extensive cardiovascular malformations may on occasion produce even a bilateral involvement. In older children, surgery in the neck has to be considered as a cause of paralysis, along with simple postoperative edema or later scar formation. (Such paralyses, however, are usually temporary.) Cricoarytenoid joint fixation must always be ruled out by the "passive mobility" test, using closed forceps to determine whether gentle pressure on the arytenoid or cords produces satisfactory passive movement. The arytenoideus is not involved, so paralysis usually is not complete, and the cords may remain halfway between abduction and adduction, with concave edges that produce both air waste and aspiration. This position has wrongly been called "cadaveric."

Bilateral abductor paralysis produces serious interference with air exchange, and in well over half of the cases emergency tracheotomy is indicated to relieve the obstruction caused by the paralyzed cords, which lie as curtains drawn across the airway (Fig. 2). The patient may have to wear the tracheotomy tube until the larynx grows and develops sufficiently to allow a satisfactory external operation, such as arytenoidectomy and lateral fixation of the cord. The tube may be fenestrated to allow some vocal function. The advantage of such an operation as arytenoidectomy is that sat-

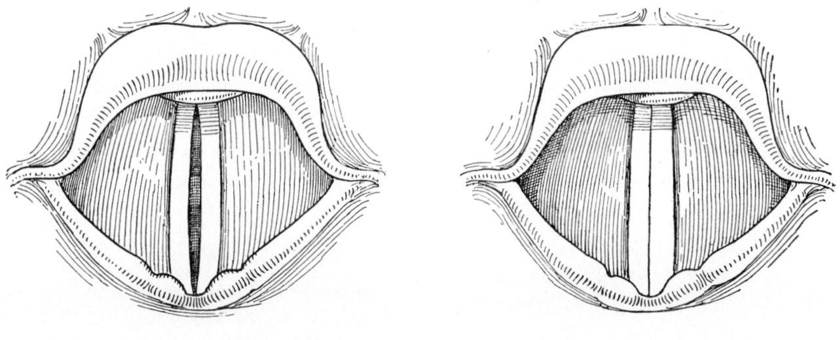

Figure 2. Bilateral abductor paralysis of the larynx. Note that both cords remain in the midline position. (From Richards, L. G.: *Otolaryngology in General Practice,* Macmillan, 1939.)

isfactory phonation is retained and at the same time the obstruction is relieved.

In 1960, Priest et al. reported three cases in childhood (or adolescence) who were relieved of their tracheotomy tubes by this operation. It consists of a slight modification of the Woodman technique, performing a partial arytenoidectomy through an external approach, and retaining the vocal process. The operated cord is fixed to the inferior cornu of the thyroid cartilage. This leaves a satisfactory airway posteriorly, and allows the cord to remain in adduction, but with an audible voice. In children this approach is probably better than the intralaryngeal method advocated for adults by Thornell and Havens. Transplantation of the omohyoid muscle and other similar procedures have not been as satisfactory.

Adductor Paralysis

Adductor paralysis is very rare at any age, and in older individuals it is usually suspected as being on a functional or hysterical basis. The larynx is "paralyzed open." There is, therefore, no obstruction to the airway in this condition, but the patient is aphonic and shows a marked air waste. If the paralysis is bilateral and on an organic basis, fibers from both sides must be involved by a lesion in the central nervous system located above the nucleus. The glottis, however, may still close posteriorly, as long as the arytenoideus muscle is not involved.

Cricothyroid Tensor Paralysis

This muscle is supplied by the superior laryngeal nerve, which is the sensory nerve to the larynx, and not by the recurrent laryngeal nerve. In such paralysis, the cords move satisfactorily, if all else is normal, but show wavy edges, as it is not possible to tense them. If there is bilateral involvement of the superior laryngeal nerve, there may also be anesthesia, which results in aspiration of secretions, choking attacks and a weak, slightly rough voice. This is a rare condition at any age, especially in childhood.

Obviously, direct laryngoscopy is the only method of diagnosis of laryngeal paralyses in the newborn. This should always be done whenever paralysis is suspected, or when a weak, husky cry or stridor is noted, or the airway is impaired. The procedure preferably should be performed without anesthesia in order to study the various movements of the cords throughout several phases of both respiration and phonation. If general anesthesia is employed, the patient is best evaluated as he is coming out of the anesthesia. It should always be remembered that intubation or even tracheotomy may become necessary as an emergency procedure and oxygen must always be readily at hand. In performing the laryngoscopy, great care must be taken not to fix one cord by pressure of the tip of the laryngoscope. Movements of the cords may be evaluated with the tip of the laryngoscope held only in the vallecula. The laryngoscope should be inserted first through one side of the mouth and then through the other, and moved about in order that paralysis can be accurately diagnosed. The tongue should be lifted forward with the tip of the laryngoscope and movements of the cords studied before the epiglottis is even elevated. The subglottic area should also be carefully examined with the anterior commissure laryngoscope.

If paralysis is found, x-rays of the chest, fluoroscopic studies and possibly a tracheogram or bronchogram ought to be considered. A barium swallow may give further valuable information. Angiography may also be indicated to ascertain an obscure intrathoracic cause for the cordal paralysis. Satisfactory evaluation of the central nervous system should also be completed before the true cause is definitely diagnosed.

REFERENCES

Priest, R. E., Ulvestad, H. S., Van de Water, F., and Richardson, R. L.: Arytenoidectomy in children. *Ann. Otol.,* 69:869: 1960.

Plott, D.: Congenital laryngeal abductor paralysis due to nucleus ambiguus dysgenesis in three brothers. *New Eng. J. Med.,* 27:593: 1964.

Snow, J. B., Jr., and Rogers, K. A.: Bilateral abductor paralysis of vocal cords secondary to Arnold-Chiari malformations and its management. *Laryngoscope,* 25:316, 1965.

SECTION XVIII

THE TRACHEA

Chapter One Hundred Seven

TRACHEOTOMY

JOHN A. TUCKER, M.D. and HARVEY D. SILBERMAN, M.D.

INTRODUCTION

Although tracheotomy is one of the oldest recognized surgical procedures, dating back into the second century, it was not until 1766 that the first successful pediatric tracheotomy was published in the world literature by Caron at St. Germain. It was performed on a 7-year-old boy for removal of a foreign body, a bean.[34]

The formerly prevalent attitudes of intense opposition to pediatric surgery have now largely disappeared. Nevertheless, despite the widespread acceptance of even major cardiac pediatric surgery, both the physician and the patient's family are often reluctant to accept surgical management of the pediatric airway. Therefore, intense efforts are often made to use drugs, humidity, oxygenating devices and endotracheal tubes in order to avoid tracheotomy in children.

ANATOMICAL CONSIDERATIONS

The small size of the patient is only one of the obvious unique differences in pediatric tracheotomy. Fundamentally, the infant tissues are softer, and the tissue planes are looser and more compressible than in the adult. The skin is not only smoother and without hair but contains the subcutaneous baby fat, which is particularly prominent in the pre-tracheal area. The high location of the infant larynx is well appreciated. In embryonic development the larynx—in fact, the entire respiratory primordium—is at the level of the base of the skull. At birth the epiglottis of the larynx is at the first cervical vertebra (C 1); the cricoid is at C 3. There is a gradual descent of the larynx during childhood and adolescence to the level of C 5 or C 6. With the attainment of adulthood, the larynx may finally rest opposite C 7. The larynx and carina descend two to three additional vertebrae during life.

In the infant the hyoid bone is in close approximation to the larynx, for the thyrohyoid membrane is extremely short. In contrast to the adult, the mid-hyoid is more ventral than the thyroid notch. The most prominent ventral structure in the infant larynx as well as in the female adult larynx is the cricoid arch. The thyroid notch, of course, does not begin to develop in males until adolescence. The cricothyroid membrane is not readily identified in the infant. Cricothyroidotomy, therefore, is not really feasible in the infant and is not a procedure of choice, even under emergency situations.

The tracheal diameter varies from 3 mm. in the premature infant to 25 mm. in the adult.[15a] The tracheal rings are 2 mm. in width, and there are approximately four rings per 10 mm.[36] The total number of tracheal rings varies from 18 to 20. The average laryngeal glottis to tracheal bifurcation distance endoscopically measured in a live infant ranges from 5.7 cm. at birth to 3 months to 8.1 cm. at 12 to 18 months.[27] The length of the trachea in the "living dynamic state" is significantly longer than in the cadaver.[27]

The relationship of the skin to the trachea is not a parallel one but is angulated at a 65° angle.[44] Hyperextension of the neck not only makes the larynx and trachea more prominent against the cervical spine, but it also elevates two or more additional rings out of the chest.[61] With flexing of the neck the tracheotomy site will then assume a lower position in the neck or mediastinum. Therefore, an excessively low tracheotomy might possibly lead to mediastinal emphysema.[44]

The normal anatomical relationship of the innominate artery to the trachea in the infant is variable and not well documented. It is not uncommon to be able to palpate the innominate artery in the suprasternal notch of the adult. Infrequently, this artery may actually cross the trachea above the level of the suprasternal notch in the patient whose neck is extended for tracheotomy.

Clinical tracheal compression by the anomalous innominate artery in the infant is noted endoscopically (with the head extended) to be about 2 cm. above the carina.[28] With the neck flexed, the innominate artery would be placed at the level of the middle third of the trachea, i.e., 3 to 4 cm. above the carina.

Placement of the tracheal fenestration has been recommended at various levels: second, third and fourth rings,[2] not lower than the third ring;[59] the third and fourth rings,[44] preferably not higher than the fifth ring; and the sixth and seventh rings.[21, 23] The rationale for the level of the tracheotomy is determined by several factors. The inflammatory and edematous reaction of the subglottic larynx, with the subsequent formation of laryngeal stenosis and therefore delayed decannulation, encourages lowering of the tracheal fenestration site away from the larynx. The problems associated with creation of mediastinal emphysema, pneumothorax and major vascular erosion encourage a higher tracheal location for tracheotomy. Certainly, in the adult, tracheotomy at the sixth ring or below when the head and neck are not extended places the tracheotomy tube in direct contact with the innominate artery. Such a situation may have catastrophic complications of vascular erosion and hemorrhage.

TECHNIQUE

In the approach to the patient for tracheotomy some principles do not change. The procedure should be done with as absolute control over airway and ventilation as possible. A tracheotomy should not be done for *airway obstruction*. The obstruction should first be relieved with either a bronchoscope or an endotracheal tube, preferably the former. Only in extreme cases, when intubating facilities are not available, should tracheotomy be performed in children without complete control of the airway. Statistically, this should amount to less than 1 per cent of all tracheotomies done.

The use of the bronchoscope to achieve an orderly tracheotomy technique has been pointed out by many more than are listed in our references.[23, 31, 33, 44, 74] The specific advantages of a bronchoscope over an endotracheal tube are (1) that the rigid instrument is more capable of introduction in the presence of laryngeal tissue obstruction; and (2) that laryngeal, tracheal, or bronchial examination can be accomplished by one who is trained in the pathology of these areas and not only one who is technically proficient in intubation. In some instances, this examination may prove to be not only diagnostic but also therapeutic. The light from the bronchoscope is valuable in tissue transillumination and is a great aid in identifying the exact laryngeal tracheal ring for fenestration.[21] Finally, in mass obstructive lesions of the neck, a needle may be passed through the skin and mass and can be visualized via the bronchoscope within the trachea. This identifies a plane of dissection into the true tracheal lumen.

Once the airway has been established, transbronchoscopic general anesthesia may now be easily delivered as desired. Such excellent ventilating bronchoscopes as the Holinger system provide a safe and a reliable means for transbronchoscopic anesthesia.

The endotracheal tube and the bronchoscope both provide an adequate mechanical airway and a firm support to the larynx and yield more exacting palpation. In addition, these tubes provide protection from injury to the soft posterior tracheo-esophageal wall at the time of tracheal incision.[44a]

After the airway has been secured and aspirated and adequate ventilation has been achieved, the patient is positioned with the neck extended and the head in the midline. Digital examination of the anterior neck identifies superiorly to inferiorly the hyoid, the flat thyroid cartilage and the prominent cricoid arch. As mentioned previously, cricothyroidotomy is not feasible in the infant, since the cricothyroid membrane is only 3 mm. long, and insertion of an adequate airway would undoubtedly create injury to the cricoid cartilage. The thyroid isthmus is usually easily palpable. The suprasternal notch is then palpated for the presence of the innominate artery.

A vertical incision one fingerbreadth in length (about 3/4 inch) is made just below the thyroid isthmus. The ultimate cosmetic result of tracheotomy depends not so much on the plane of the incision (horizontal or vertical) but on the length of the incision and the duration of the tracheotomy. The transverse incision may create a pocket in its inferior aspect that collects secretions and increases local infection.[44] Further, with such an incision extension of the neck may actually lift the shorter pediatric tube up and out of the tracheal stoma.

Dissection is then performed with a small curved hemostat in a blunt mid-vertical plane at right angles to the trachea. Dissection with alternate retraction of the strap muscles and tissue layers is accomplished. Great care is taken to keep a narrow field and to avoid needless wide paratracheal dissection.[30a] The vasculature of the median raphe is sparse but easily identified.

The anterior jugular arch and the inferior thyroid veins are readily retracted laterally. Dissection is below the thyroid isthmus, and in 10 per cent of the patients the lowest thyroid artery may be present. If there is a need, the isthmus may be clamped, divided and ligated with chromic sutures. These sutures are then tagged and make an excellent aid in retraction and exposure of the trachea. A vertical incision is then made through the fourth and fifth tracheal rings. No tracheal cartilage is removed. The tracheal edge may be grasped with mosquito hemostats. A loop of silk sutures introduced through each divided ring permits retraction and serves as a guide for tube replacement.[29a] This is particularly valuable when introducing plastic tubes that are relatively large and do not have an obturator. In our experience, the Trousseau dilator is too large for aiding insertion of the tube in children.

With the tracheotomy open, the endotracheal tube or bronchoscope is visualized and is withdrawn to the level of the subglottic larynx. The tracheotomy tube is then inserted. We prefer to use Holinger pediatric tubes. Once the tube is proved to be within the true tracheal lumen, and to be properly seated, the bronchoscope is then removed. A small amount of packing, if desired, may be placed under the flange of the tracheotomy tube for hemostasis and to pack the wound open and assist in preventing mediastinal emphysema. Skin sutures are not necessary and, indeed, are contraindicated.[59] With the tube securely held by an assistant, the neck is then flexed, and the tapes tied to the neck with three square knots. If two fingers can fit underneath the tracheotomy tape, the tube is not too tight and venous distention is avoided. A small square of Telfa pad makes an excellent tracheotomy dressing and helps prevent maceration of the skin by secretions.

TYPES OF TRACHEOTOMY TUBES

There are many satisfactory tracheotomy tubes available today. Fundamentally, these tubes vary in size, length, angulation and types of material (metal or plastic). We prefer the Holinger tracheotomy tube because it provides the proper size flange that does not cut into the neck of the child and has an obturator. The skin-trachea angle seems appropriate, and the tube utilizes an inner cannula. The Fearon adaptation of this tube is excellent in cases in which controlled ventilation is necessary. Cuffed tracheotomy tubes are seldom used for children, as an adequate seal can be obtained to lift the chest wall and provide satisfactory ventilation without the use of a cuff. Table 1 in Chapter 105 illustrates the recommended selection of tracheotomy tubes and bronchoscopes in infants and children as compiled by Fearon. Specific factors that should be taken into consideration in determining tube length are the thickness of the neck, the level of the tracheotomy site within the trachea and the distance from this site to the carina.

POSTOPERATIVE CARE

Since the nose and throat are now bypassed, adequate tracheal humidification must be provided.[14, 39, 44, 59] In the immediate postoperative period there is a tendency toward relaxation in the care of the patient. It is the responsibility of the physician to be sure that nursing personnel are made aware of the need for constant careful supervision of the infant.

Frequent tracheal aspiration is performed as necessary, at least every 30 minutes, until a schedule for aspiration can be established, according to the patient's needs. A small amount of saline may be necessary to assist in aspiration. Gentle nasopharyngeal aspiration should also be performed. Chest physiotherapy every three hours, turning of the child from one side to the other every hour, and auscultation of breath sounds before and after tracheal aspiration are all important points in maintenance of the tracheotomy.

The tracheotomy tube is first changed 48 hours after the tracheotomy and daily thereafter. During the changing of the tracheotomy tube the patient is placed with his neck extended over a pillow while he is in the tracheotomy position. This provides proper tissue alignment and facilitates changing of the tube. The new tube is fully prepared and ready for insertion before the old tube is removed. A child's tracheotomy tube is never changed without adequate assistance. An additional tube is always kept available at the patient's bedside.

HOME CARE OF THE TRACHEOTOMY PATIENT

The key to proper care and maintenance of the patient with a tracheotomy in the home environment is thorough instruction of the parents. Instruction is provided by the physician and the nursing staff in the hospital. The parents should become competent in aspirating, cleaning, maintaining and changing the tube before the patient is discharged. If a plastic tube has been used in the hospital, the patient must be sent home with a metal tube that has an obturator, for this greatly facilitates placement of the tube in a small tracheal stoma, which has the potential to close within ten minutes. The visiting nurse may aid in checking on the home facilities for aspiration and tube care. Effective continuing communication between the physician, the parents and the visiting nurse is essential.

DECANNULATION

The obvious time for decannulation, or permanent removal of the tracheotomy tube, is when it is no longer needed. That is, when the patient can ventilate properly through the major conducting airway, and when the patient has the capacity to maintain an airway free of secretions. It is usually best to perform a direct bronchoscopic examination prior to the intended time of decannulation. This allows for complete inspection of the conducting airway, and granulations, if present, can at that time be excised.

Our routine for decannulation is to reduce the size of the tube daily until reaching the smallest tube the patient can tolerate – that is, 0 or 00. The tube is then plugged, and if the patient can tolerate this for 48 hours without running a temperature, indicating retained secretions, and if he can ventilate properly around the tube, then he is extubated. Extubation is always done early in the day and in an area where the patient can be observed closely. In the statistical review, there were four deaths attributed to improper decannulation of the patient. The total number of patients in the series of 350 that sustained decannulation amounted to 79. The vast majority of these were originally tracheotomized for laryngotracheobronchitis. Decannulation was delayed in one-third of this group. Fearon has recommended placement of the tracheotomy tube at the level of the seventh tracheal ring to avoid excessive laryngeal subglottic reaction and delayed decannulation.

STATISTICAL ANALYSIS

This analysis[74b] includes a review of 350 tracheotomies from one specific study and a comparison with 4000 pediatric tracheotomies from 30 articles in the world literature (Fig. 1). Over 208,000 pediatric admissions to five Philadelphia hospitals are covered in this study. A total of sixty-five hospital admission years were surveyed during this period of time, ending December, 1970. The age group studied included newborns to children aged 12 years. The hospitals reviewed in this survey are so distributed that the study has a fairly realistic cross section of all socioeconomic and racial groups in the Philadelphia area (Table 1).

This survey confirms a significant increase in the total number of pediatric tracheotomies, a finding which is in

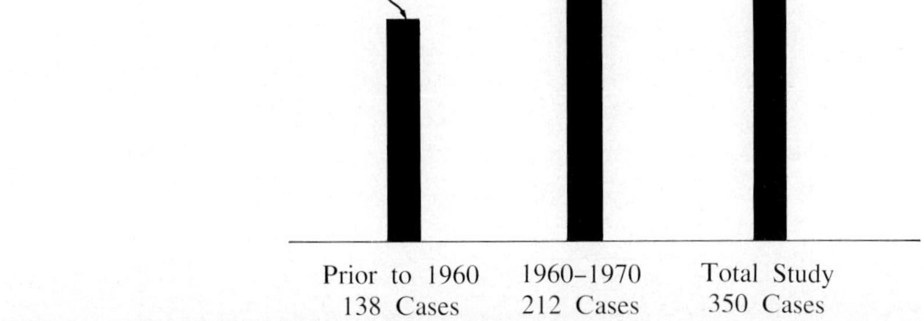

Figure 1. Over-all incidence before and after 1960 in series of 350 tracheotomies.

TABLE 1. NUMBER OF PEDIATRIC ADMISSIONS

Hospital	Number of Admission Years	Total Admissions
Children's Hospital of Philadelphia	24.5	160,000
Hospital of the University of Pennsylvania	15.5	18,000
Bryn Mawr Hospital	5	10,000
Philadelphia General Hospital	7	16,000
Graduate Hospital of the University of Pennsylvania	13	4,000

agreement with McGovern's study in 1968[49a] but which is contrary to a study of Beatrous, also made in 1968.[8a] In the years prior to 1960 the incidence of tracheotomy in children was 1 per 1000 pediatric admissions. Since 1960 the incidence has increased to 2.7 per 1000 pediatric admissions. It is interesting to note that the period prior to 1960 covered 46 hospital admission years while that after 1960 covered only 16 admission years. In the earlier period 138 tracheotomies were performed, but in the last decade there were only 215. The age distribution revealed that 30 per cent of the tracheotomies were performed in the age group of the newborn to 1 year. In the 1- to 5-year age group 50 per cent of the tracheotomies were performed. The remaining 20 per cent occurred in those from 5 to 12 years of age (Fig. 2).

An enigma of this study and that of Oliver et al. (1962) and Holinger et al. (1965) is the sex incidence of tracheotomy (Table 2). In all series the ratio of approximately 2 males to 1 female has remained almost constant. This further substantiates the observation that males have a greater susceptibility to congenital problems necessitating tracheotomy and also to acquired diseases requiring tracheotomy[44,57] (see Fig. 2).

Because of the variations in classifica-

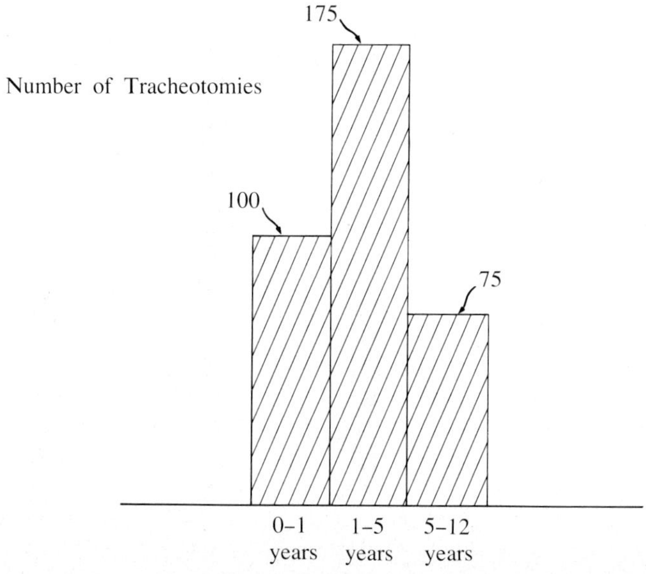

Figure 2. Age incidence of tracheotomy in series of 350 tracheotomies.

TABLE 2. SEX INCIDENCE

Hospital	Male*	Female
Children's Hospital of Philadelphia	146	80
Hospital of the University of Pennsylvania	55	27
Philadelphia General Hospital	11	6
Bryn Mawr Hospital	10	6
Graduate Hospital of the University of Pennsylvania	6	3
Totals	228	122

*Approximately two-thirds of all tracheotomies were performed on males.

tion of indications for tracheotomy and its complications, it was impossible to specifically compare each series with this study. The specific studies which were comparable include those of Holinger (1965), Jaffee (1962), Oliver (1962), Bigler (1953) and Fitz-Hugh (1941). The largest single indication for tracheotomy in this series (36 per cent) was laryngotracheobronchitis and epiglottitis. Indeed, these diseases represent over one-third of the tracheotomies performed in the 4000 tracheotomies surveyed. Historically, the decline of diphtheria as an indication for tracheotomy is noted in the review. Further, in this specific series, tracheotomies performed for epiglottitis and laryngotracheobronchitis has decreased rather sharply since 1960. One may conjecture on the cause of this decline, but undoubtedly, therapy with steroids and racemic epinephrine has played an important role.[74c] In Fearon's review in 1964, 385 tracheotomies were performed on 7 per cent of the patients treated for laryngotracheobronchitis. Our comparative figure is a 6 per cent incidence of tracheotomy in laryngotracheobronchitis. It should be specifically pointed out that the incidence of tracheotomy in epiglottitis in this study was 100 per cent. This also compares with Fearon's figure, which approximates 90 per cent[23] (Table 3).

Historically, the use of tracheotomy in the extraction of foreign bodies of the tracheobronchial tree has been documented by Figi (1934), 12 cases; Neffson (1943), 4 cases; Fitz-Hugh (1953), 26 cases; Oliver (1962), 17 cases; Holinger (1965), 3 cases; and this study, 2 cases. However, this technique is no longer encouraged. Congenital malformations accounted for only 49 cases of tracheotomies, one-seventh of the total series. Conglomerate laryngeal anomalies were the largest congenital indication, and this is in keeping with Holinger's 1965 experience. Tracheoesophageal fistulas were the second most common indication. This confirms a definitive trend in tracheotomy as a prophylactic measure in the more aggressive surgical management of congenital disease. This is further illustrated in Aberdeen's series[2] in which 105 tracheotomies were performed in the management of congenital cardiac disease (Table 4).

TABLE 3. INDICATIONS FOR TRACHEOTOMY–ACQUIRED LESIONS

Disorder	Number
Tonsillitis	7
Laryngotracheobronchitis	91
Epiglottitis	36
Pneumonia (primary)	15
Retropharyngeal abscess	1
Pneumonia (secondary to other causes)	30
Laryngeal edema (from trauma, etc.)	10
Laryngeal spasm	1
Foreign body (tracheobronchial)	2
Tracheal edema (from trauma)	3
Asthma	1
Hyaline membrane disease	3
Cystic fibrosis	1
Atelectasis	2
Cardiac arrest	8
Pulmonary edema	3
Tracheal stenosis	2
Total	216

TABLE 4. INDICATIONS FOR TRACHEOTOMY – CONGENITAL MALFORMATIONS

Disorder	Number
Choanal atresia	1
Pierre Robin syndrome	9
Unfolding of epiglottis	2
Laryngeal paralysis	3
Laryngeal cyst	1
Laryngomalacia	2
Subglottic stenosis	6
Redundant laryngeal mucosa	1
Congenitally small larynx	1
Tracheal stenosis	6
Tracheo-esophageal fistula	12
Vascular ring	2
Laryngeal web	3
Total	49

Other significant congenital anomalies included the Pierre Robin syndrome (9 cases and 12 additional cases in the literature reviewed). Subglottic stenosis is the second most frequent congenital laryngeal anomaly and occurred in 6 cases requiring tracheotomy. An additional 39 cases of subglottic stenosis requiring tracheotomy were recognized in the literature reviewed.

Tracheotomies performed for central nervous system disorders accounted for only 39 procedures. Almost all of these patients died from the primary disease (Table 5). Ten deaths alone were caused by brain tumors.

TABLE 5. INDICATIONS FOR TRACHEOTOMY – DISEASES OF THE CENTRAL NERVOUS SYSTEM

Disorder	Number
Bulbar poliomyelitis	1
Head injuries	3
Tumors	10
Transverse myelitis	1
Meningitis or encephalitis	2
Cerebral palsy	1
Guillain Barré syndrome	4
Multiple sclerosis	1
Meningocele	4
Hydrocephalus	9
CVA	1
CNS depression (neurological diseases)	2
Total	39

TABLE 6. INDICATIONS FOR TRACHEOTOMY

Disorder	Number
NEOPLASMS	
Hemangioma	4
Papillomata of larynx	4
Teratoma	4
Granuloma (after tracheotomy)	1
Total	13
MISCELLANEOUS	
Prophylactic (after surgery, etc.)	31
Tetanus	1
Burns (lye)	1
Total	33
GRAND TOTAL FROM TABLES 3, 4, 5 and 6	350

Neoplasms other than those of the central nervous system totaled 13. There were 4 hemangiomas out of a total of 21 in the reviewed world literature. Multiple papilloma required tracheotomy in 4 cases as compared to a total of 19 cases reviewed in the literature (see Table 6).

COMPLICATIONS

The total number of complications in this series of 350 tracheotomies was 163. This amounted to an over-all complication rate of 46.5 per cent. However, this figure is misleading, since often there were multiple complications in the same patient. For example, one patient with cardiac arrest also had subcutaneous emphysema and a pneumothorax. The largest single complication was delayed decannulation. This was defined as any tracheotomy that was still in place 30 days after the procedure. Table 7 lists the specific complications that occurred in this series. The single, most fatal complication was pneumothorax (Table 8). Out of 201 reported pneumothoraces there were 27 deaths. In decreasing order it will be seen that in 17 cases of

TABLE 7. TOTAL COMPLICATIONS ENCOUNTERED IN PEDIATRIC TRACHEOTOMY

Complication	Number	Complication	Number
Pneumothorax	15	Tracheocutaneous fistula	2
Subcutaneous emphysema	6	Tracheal granuloma	3
Excessive bleeding	1	Obstruction by chin	2
Tracheal stenosis	4	Deaths due to tracheotomy	5
Traumatic tracheotomy	1	Total	163
Cardiac arrest	1		
Accidental extubation	5	Over-all complication rate	46.5%
Mediastinal emphysema	1	Deaths due to primary disease	83
Delayed decannulation	117	Tracheotomy mortality rate	1.4%

TABLE 8. FATAL COMPLICATIONS IN PEDIATRIC TRACHEOTOMY

Complications	Number	Deaths	Complication	Number	Deaths
Pneumothorax	201	27	Tracheal granuloma	18	2
Delayed decannulation	163	4	Plugged tracheotomy tube	17	8
Mediastinal emphysema	59	3	Cardiac arrest (circulatory collapse)	16	4
Accidental extubation	51	4	Misplaced incision	1	1
Postoperative bleeding	36	5			

tracheotomy tube plugging there were 8 deaths, and in 36 reported cases of hemorrhage there were 5 deaths. Cardiac arrest (16 cases), accidental extubation (51 cases) and delayed decannulation (163 cases) each resulted in 4 deaths. The formation of tracheal granuloma, which occurred in 18 patients, accounted for 2 deaths. Table 9 is a specific listing of the deaths due to airway obstruction that occurred in our series; these 5 deaths accounted for a mortality rate of 1.4 per cent secondary to tracheotomy.

CONCLUSION

In conclusion, two fundamental changes in the pattern of pediatric tracheotomy have been recognized (see Table 10):

1. The incidence of tracheotomy in children has increased and continues to increase.

2. The indications for tracheotomy are changing.[49a] Tracheotomy for acute airway obstruction is still the prime indication, but it occupies a significantly

TABLE 9. DEATHS DUE TO AIRWAY OBSTRUCTION IN PATIENTS WITH TRACHEOTOMY

Causes	Number of Cases
Plugged	2
Displacement	2
Aspiration	1
Total	5

TABLE 10. RESULTS OF STUDY

	Number of Cases
Total number of tracheotomies	350
Deaths due to primary disease	83
Deaths due to improper tracheotomy care	5
Decannulation without delay	150
Delayed decannulation (longer than 30 days)	117

smaller percentage of the total tracheotomies performed in accordance with new objectives and modalities of pediatric medical and surgical therapy.

REFERENCES

1. Abbott, O.: Recommended Principles Relative to the Use of Bronchoscopy and Tracheotomy in Infants and Children. *Dis. Chest,* 52:117–123, 1967.
2. Aberdeen, E.: Tracheotomy and Tracheotomy Care in Infants. *Proc. Roy. Soc. Med.,* 58:900, 1965.
3. Allen, T. H., and Steven, I. M.: Prolonged Endotracheal Intubation in Infants and Children. *Brit. J. Anaesth.,* 37:566, 1965.
4. Atkins, J. P.: Current Utilization of Tracheotomy as a Therapeutic Measure. *Laryngoscope,* 70:1672–1690, 1960.
5. Atkins, J. P.: Tracheal Reactions Following the Use of Cuffed Tracheotomy Tubes. *Ann. Otol.,* 73:1124, 1964.
6. Atkins, J. P.: Tracheotomy for Prevention of Pulmonary Complications in Post-Operative and Severely Debilitated Patients. *J.A.M.A.,* 146:241–243, 1951.
7. Avery, M. E., March, E., and Benson, D.: Critically Crushed Chest—A New Treatment. *J. Thorac. Surg.,* 32:291, 1956.
8. Baxter, J. D.: Acute Epiglottitis in Children. *Laryngoscope,* Vol. 79, February, 1968.

8a. Beatrous, W.: Tracheostomy (Tracheotomy), Its Expanded Indications and Its Present Statistics. *Laryngoscope,* 78:3, 1968.

9. Bergstrom, J., and Morley, A.: On the Pathogenesis of Laryngeal Injuries Following Prolonged Intubation. *Acta Otolaryng.,* 55:342, 1962.
10. Bergstrom, O., and Diamant, H.: Mediastinal Emphysema Complicating Tracheotomy. *Arch. Otlaryng.,* 71:628–734, 1960.
11. Berenberg, W., and Kevy, S.: Acute Epiglottitis in Childhood. *New Eng. J. Med.,* 258:870, 1958.
12. Bigler, J. A., Holinger, P., Johnston, K. C., and Schiller, F.: Tracheotomy in Infancy. *Pediatrics,* 13:5, 1954.

12a. Bridges, C., Ryan, R., Longenecker, C., and Vincent, R.: Tracheostomy in Children: A 20 Year Study—Plastic and Reconstructive Surgery. 37:117–120, 1966.

13. Blumenthal, S., and Revitch, M.: Seminar on Aortic Vascular Rings and Other Anomalies of the Aortic Arch. *Pediatrics,* 20:896, 1957.
14. Bradham, R., Randolph, H., and Paul, J.: Tracheotomy for Respiratory Muscle Failure in Infants and Children. *Amer. J. Surg.,* 25:242, 1959.
15. Carter, N., and Geuseffe, J.: Tracheotomy as a Useful Procedure with Special Reference to Chest Trauma. *J. Thorac. Surg.,* 21:495, 1951.

15a. Croteau, J. R., and Cook, C. D.: Volume-Pressure and Length-Tension Measurements in Human Tracheal and Bronchial Segments. *J. Appl. Physiol.,* 16:170–172, 1961.

16. Davis, H. S., Kretchmer, H. E., and Bryce-Smith, R.: Advantages and Complications of Tracheotomy. *J.A.M.A.,* 153:1156, 1953.
17. Dwyer, C. S., Kronenberg, S., and Sakland, M.: Endotracheal Tube: Consideration of its Traumatic Effects with Suggestions of Modifications Thereof. *Anesthesiology,* 10:74, 1949.
18. Diamant, H., Kinnman, J., et al.: Decannulation in Children. *Laryngoscope,* 71:404–414, 1961.
19. Epstein, B. S., et al.: Comparison of Orotracheal Intubation with Tracheostomy for Anesthesia in Patients with Face and Neck Burns. *Anesth. Analg.,* 45:352, 1966.
20. Everett, A.: Acute Laryngotracheobronchitis —Analysis of 1175 Cases with 98 Tracheotomies. *Laryngoscope,* 61:113–123, 1951.
21. Fearon, B.: Acute Laryngotracheobronchitis in Infancy and Childhood. *Pediat. Clin. North Amer.,* 9:1095, November, 1962.
22. Fearon, B.: Airway Problems in Children Following Prolonged Endotracheal Intubation. *Ann. Otol.,* Volume 75, No. 4, December, 1966.
23. Fearon, B., Smith, C., Delivoria-Papadoulos, M., Levinson, H., and Sawyer, P.: The Idiopathic Respiratory Distress Syndrome in the Newborn. *Trans. Amer. Bronchoesoph. Ass.,* 44:90–105, 1964.
24. Fearon, B., and MacDonald, H.: The Surgical Management of Spontaneous Pneumomediastinum in Children. *Proc. Canad. Otolaryng. Soc.,* 1963.
25. Fearon, B.: Respiratory Distress in the Newborn. *Otolaryng. Clin. North Amer.,* June, 1968.
26. Fearon, B.: Acute Obstructive Laryngitis in Infants and Children. *Hosp. Med.,* December, 1968.
27. Fearon, B., and Whalen, J.: Tracheal Dimensions in the Living Infants. *Ann. Otol.,* 76:964, December, 1967.
28. Fearon, B., and Shortreed, R.: Tracheobronchial Compression by Congenital Cardiovascular Anomalies in Children. *Ann. Otol.,* 72:949, 1963.
29. Ferguson, C. F.: Respiratory Obstruction in the Role of Tracheotomy (in Changing Concepts of Otolaryngology). *Pediatrics,* 25:1043, 1960.

29a. Figi, F.: Tracheotomy: A Study of 200 Consecutive Cases. *Ann. Otol.,* 43:178–192, 1934.

30. Fitz-Hugh, G. S., and McLean, W. C.: Tracheotomy, Indications and Comments. *J. Michigan State Med. Soc.,* 56:1400, 1957.

30a. Fitz-Hugh, G. S.: Tracheotomy, A Study of 100 Consecutive Cases. *Southern Med. J.,* 34:1116–1121, 1941.

31. Forbes, G., Salmon, G., and Herweg, J.: Further Observations on Post-Tracheotomy Mediastinal Emphysema and Pneumothorax. *J. Pediat.*, 31:172–194, 1947.
32. Georgiade, N., et al.: Practical Considerations Regarding Tracheotomy; Surgical Errors and Safeguards. *J.A.M.A.*, 160:940, 1956.
33. Goldberg, J. D., and Mitchell, N.: Mediastinal Emphysema and Pneumothorax Following Tracheotomy for Croup. *Amer. J. Surg.*, 56:448–454, 1942.
34. Goodall, E. W.: The Story of Tracheotomy. *Brit. J. Child. Dis.*, 31:167, 1934.
35. Gotsman, M. S., and Whitby, C.: Respiratory Infection Following Tracheotomy. *Thorax*, 19:89, 1964.
36. Gray, L. P.: Infant Tracheostomy. *J. Laryng.*, 74:145–54, 1960.
37. Green, N. M.: Fatal Cardiovascular and Respiratory Failure Associated with Tracheotomy. *New Eng. J. Med.*, 261:846, 1959.
38. Hamilton, R. D.: Fatal Hemorrhage During Tracheotomy. *J.A.M.A.*, 174:530, 1960.
38a. Hatch, D.: Prolonged Nasotracheal Intubation in Infants and Children. *Lancet*, 1:1272, 1968.
39. Hatcher, C., Abbott, O., Logan, W., and Patterson, J.: Tracheostomy in Infancy and Childhood. *Southern Med. J.*, 60:411, 1967.
40. Head, J. M.: Tracheostomy in Management of Respiratory Problems. *New Eng. J. Med.*, 264:587–591, 1961.
41. Hilding, A. C., and Hilding, J. A.: Tolerance of the Respiratory Mucous Membrane to Trauma. *Ann. Otol.*, 71:455, 1962.
42. Holinger, P., and Johnston, K.: Factors Responsible for Laryngeal Obstruction in Infants. *J.A.M.A.*, 143:1229, 1950.
43. Holinger, P.: A New Infant Tracheotomy Tube. *Ann. Otol.*, 65:239, 1956.
44. Holinger, P., Brown, T., and Maurizi, D.: Tracheostomy in the Newborn. *Amer. J. Surg.*, 109:771–779, 1965.
44a. Jackson, C., and Jackson, C. L.: *Diseases of the Nose, Throat and Ear.* 2nd edition. Philadelphia, W. B. Saunders Co., 1959.
45. Jackson, B.: Management of Tracheotomy in Cases of Tetanus Neonatorum. *J. Laryng.*, Volume 77, July, 1963.
46. Jaffee, I. S.: Tracheostomy in Infancy. *Laryngoscope*, 73:1336, 1963.
47. Koedick, J. M.: The Place and Management of Tracheostomy in Respiratory Insufficiency. *J. Laryngol.*, 74:891, 1961.
48. Lampe, I., et al.: Management of Hemangiomas in Infants. *Pediat. Clin. North Amer.*, 6:511–528, 1959.
49. Meade, J. W.: Tracheotomy, Its Complications and Their Management. Study of 212 Cases. *New Eng. J. Med.*, 265:519–523, 1961.
49a. McGovern, F., and Link, N.: The Hazards of Tracheostomy. *Virginia Med. Monthly*, 96:133–141, 1969.
50. Neffson, A. H.: Tension Pneumothorax, and Mediastinal Emphysema After Tracheotomy. *Arch. Otolaryng.*, 37:23–39, 1943.
51. Negus, V.: Tracheostomy. *Laryngoscope*, 67:1098–1112, 1957.
52. Nelson, T. G.: Tracheotomy: A Clinical and Experimental Study, Part I. *Amer. J. Surg.*, Vol. 22, July, 1957.
53. Nelson, T. G.: Tracheotomy: Clinical and Experimental Study, Part II. *Amer. J. Surg.*, 23:750, 1957.
54. Nelson, T. G., and Bowers, W. F.: Tracheotomy, Indications, Advantages, Techniques, Complications and Results. Analysis of 310 Operations. *J.A.M.A.*, 164: 1530–1534, 1957.
55. Nicholas, T. H., and Rummer, R.: Emergency Airway—A Plan of Action. *J.A.M.A.*, 174:98, 1960.
56. Norris, C. M.: The Role of Tracheostomy in Major Surgery. *Trans. Penn. Acad. Ophthal.*, 71:61–65, 1964.
57. Oliver, P., Richardson, J., Clubb, R., and Flake, C.: Tracheotomy in Children. *New Eng. J. Med.*, 267:631, 1962.
58. Pearce, D. J., and Walsh, R. S.: Respiratory Obstruction Due to Tracheal Granuloma After Tracheotomy. *Lancet*, 2:135–136, July, 1961.
59. Putney, F. J.: Complications and Postoperative Care After Tracheotomy. *AMA Arch. Otolaryng.*, 62:272, 1955.
60. Ravenel, S.: New Techniques of Humidification in Pediatrics. *J.A.M.A.*, 151:707, 1953.
61. Reading, P.: Some Post-operative Hazards in Tracheostomy in Infants. *J. Laryng.*, 72:785, 1958.
62. Shepard, R.: Indications, Technique and After Care of Tracheotomy. *J. Oklahoma State Med. Ass.*, 49:6, 1956.
63. Skolinik, E. M., and Fornatto, E. J.: Tracheotomy—Its Present Day Application. *Laryngoscope*, 68:32, 1958.
64. Snow, W. J., and Withers, B.: A Study of 42 Tracheotomy Cases Including Review of the Literature Regarding Complications. *Med. Rec. Ann.*, 42:503–506, 1948.
65. Sophocles, A., and Atkins, J. P.: The Widening Scope of Tracheotomy. *J. Med. Soc. New Jersey*, 57:23, 1960.
66. Spencer, W. A.: *Treatment of Acute Poliomyelitis*, 3rd edition. Charles C Thomas, Publishers, Springfield, Ill., 1956.
67. Stool, S., Campbell, J., and Johnson, D.: Tracheostomy in Children. The Use of Plastic Tubes. *Pediat. Surg.*, 3:402, 1968.
68. Stool, S., and Groff, D.: Disposable Plastic Tracheotomy Tubes. *Laryngoscope*, 79: 1088, 1968.
69. Stool, S., and Tucker, J.: *Larynx, Trachea and Endoscopy, Brennan's. Proceedings of Pediatrics.* Vol. IV. New York, Harper and Row, 1968, Chapter 48.
70. Taber, R.: A Tracheotomy Program. *J. Michigan State Med. Soc.*, 61:327, 1962.

71. Teplitz, C., et al.: Pathology of Low Tracheostomy in Children. *Amer. J. Clin. Path.,* 42:58, 1964.
72. Toremalm, N. G.: Postoperative Care and Complications after Tracheotomy in Infants and Children. *Acta Anaesth. Scand.,* 4:105, 1960.
73. Tucker, G.: Infant Larynx – Direct Laryngoscopic Observation. *J.A.M.A.,* 99:1899–1902, 1932.
74. Tucker, G.: An Infant Bronchoscope and Infant Tracheotomy Tube. *Trans. Section on Laryng. Otol. Rhinol.,* American Medical Association, 1932.
74a. Tucker, J. A.: The Endoscopic Aspects of the Infant Larynx. Amer. Acad. Ophthalmol. Otolaryng., Instruction Section, Course 551, 1971.
74b. Tucker, J. A., and Silberman, H. D.: Tracheotomy in Pediatrics. *Trans. Amer. Bronchoesoph.,* 1972.
74c. Turtz, M. G., and Tucker, G. F.: The Current Spectrum of Pediatric Bronchoesophagology. *Laryngoscope,* June, 1972.
75. Venables, A. W.: Tracheostomy in Childhood. *Med. J. Aust.,* 2:141, 1959.
76. Ver Meulen, V., and Brick, H.: Prolonged Intubation vs. Tracheostomy in Children. *Arch. Otolaryng.,* 87:56, 1968.
77. Von Leden, H.: Newer Indications for Tracheotomy. *Trans. Amer. Acad. Ophthalmol. Otolaryng.,* 56:52, 1952.
78. Weseman, C.: Tracheotomy in Children; A Controlled, Planned Emergency Procedure. *California Med. J.,* 93:269, 1960.
79. Weseman, C.: Tracheotomy in the Newborn. *Amer. J. Dis. Child.,* 100:881, 1960.
80. Wittenborg, M. H., Gyepes, M. T., and Crocker, D.: Tracheal Dynamics in Infants with Respiratory Distress, Stridor and Collapsing Trachea. *Radiology,* 88:653–662, 1967.
81. Yanagisawa, E., and Kirchner, J. A.: The Cuffed Tracheotomy Tube. *Arch. Otolaryng.,* 79:80–87, 1964.

SECTION XIX

PERORAL ENDOSCOPY

Chapter One Hundred Eight

BRONCHOLOGY: ANATOMIC CONSIDERATIONS AND OPERATIVE TECHNIQUES

CHARLES F. FERGUSON, M.D., F.A.C.S.

Immediately below the vocal cords is the subglottic region of the larynx, an area of loose areolar connective tissue. In infants and young children, this area promptly becomes edematous when traumatized or infected. The lumen here is narrow and wedge-shaped and the region is known as the conus elasticus.

The trachea is the direct continuation of the larynx and its measurements have always been a source of considerable disagreement. In 1955, Hall published a study of tracheal lengths and diameters based on post-mortem findings. His tabulation is shown in Table 1. In 1967, Fearon and Whalen made an attempt to develop better scientific principles for the use of proper-sized endotracheal and tracheotomy tubes. They conducted a very important study on the living infant and discovered a surprising discrepancy between such measurements on the living patient and the results obtained at autopsy. After 3 months of age, the tracheal lengths as determined by a calibrated bronchoscope were found to be nearly twice as great as those stated for the cadaver (Table 2). They believed that this marked difference was due in great part to vertical movements of the diaphragm, which becomes displaced from 1.5 to 7 cm., depending on the depth of respiration. The length of the trachea increases greatly during inspiration, extension of the neck and swallowing.

In a classic and scholarly radiologic study of tracheal dynamics in the infant, Wittenborg et al. have shown that changes in diameter of the trachea during ordinary quiet breathing are not as marked as was formerly believed. There is only slight expansion of the trachea during inspiration, and some narrowing during expiration, but there is a marked collapse on coughing or on execution of the Valsalva maneuver. Crying, breath-holding or struggling reduces the caliber of the lumen anywhere from 25 to 50 per cent. Wittenborg believed that the tracheal diameter at any time was determined by a balance between the inherent structural rigidity of the tracheal wall (*compliance*) and the deforming force (*transmural pressure*).

The trachea bifurcates in young children at the third costal cartilage about

TABLE 1

Age	Tracheal length (cm.)	Tracheal diameter (mm.)
Birth	4.0	6.0
3 months	3.8	6.8
6 months	4.2	7.2
12 months	4.3	7.8
18 months	4.5	8.8

TABLE 2

Age	Length (cm.)	Range (cm.)
Birth to 3 months	5.7	5.0–7.5
3 to 6 months	6.7	5.5–8.0
6 to 12 months	7.2	5.0–9.0
12 to 18 months	8.1	7.0–9.0

the level of the fourth or fifth thoracic vertebra. It is slightly flattened at the aortic crossing, but not as significantly as in older patients. The right main bronchus is said to deviate only 25 degrees from the midline (the carina being just to the left of the midline), but the left main bronchus shows an angle of deviation of about 75 degrees. However, Fearon and Whalen have demonstrated that these angles of bifurcation in the dynamic trachea of the living infant are considerably smaller than those seen at post-mortem examination.

The right main bronchus is shorter, straighter and of greater caliber, as it is simply a continuation of the trachea. There is an upper lobe bronchus laterally at the carinal level (eparterial), a middle lobe bronchus directly anteriorly, and a lower lobe bronchus with its various subdivisions. On the left side, the main bronchus is much longer before the upper lobe orifice originates laterally. Various subdivisions of the lower lobe bronchus on the left are noted and are somewhat similar to those on the right. The bronchi elongate and also dilate during inspiration, then contract, and shorten or may even kink during a forced expiratory phase.

In 1943, Jackson and Huber developed a nomenclature of bronchopulmonary segments that now has become standard throughout the world (Fig. 1). This classification has been of tremendous advantage in producing a better universal understanding of the exact location of a pathologic lesion of the tracheobronchial tree.

OPERATIVE TECHNIQUES

Endoscopic examination of the tracheobronchial tree can be successfully and safely performed at any age (even in the premature infant) if certain important considerations are heeded. Extreme gentleness is always most essential, whether or not the patient is under general anesthesia. It is vital that the bronchoscope should be small enough so that subglottic edema and other untoward effects of trauma are not precipitated. The length

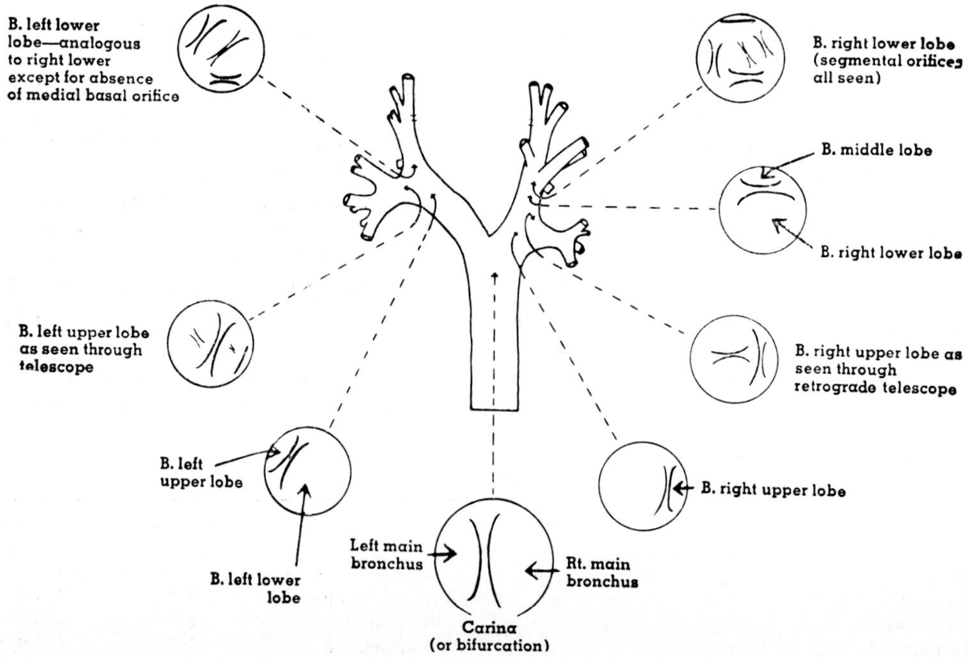

Figure 1. The lobar bronchi and their segmental branches. (From Jackson, C., and Jackson, C. L.: *Diseases of the Nose, Throat and Ear.* W. B. Saunders, 1945.)

of time the instrument remains in the airway must also be seriously considered; it should be left in place not longer than five minutes in a tiny infant. A 2.5 cm. bronchoscope has been manufactured for premature infants, but this tiny instrument is not widely available. Ordinarily, a 3 mm. size is used in the normal infant up to 6 months of age, a 3.5 mm. scope from 6 to 18 months, a 4 mm. scope from 18 months to 5 years of age, and a 5 mm. one up to 12 years of age. (These measurements refer to the internal diameter of the bronchoscope.) These ranges are only suggestive, however, as the degree of airway obstruction, the size of the patient, and the purpose of the bronchoscopy (whether diagnostic or therapeutic) must also be considered when deciding upon the particular bronchoscope to use.

The value of general anesthesia in bronchoscopic work is still debated. Since anesthetic agents and techniques have improved so markedly in the past several years, and since better training in the administration of these agents is now available, there has been a tendency toward more widespread use of general anesthesia for all pediatric patients. Its safety has been dramatically increased. If the anesthesiologist happens to be more experienced in his field than the endoscopist is in his, general anesthesia obviously is preferable. On the other hand, if the endoscopist is well trained and has a competently functioning team, or if safe general anesthesia, including good constant postoperative care, is not available, then not using anesthesia is preferred. As stated so wisely by Dr. Paul Holinger in his Wherry Lecture a few years ago, anesthesia is never a substitute for endoscopic skill or good teamwork.

Local anesthesia by itself has little place in the very young patient. The advocates of "no anesthesia" describe it as "vocal anesthesia," which means that the patient is constantly and quietly given much-needed reassurance. The procedure is performed in a quiet, efficiently run operating room, with the patient carefully but securely mummified in a blanket, his arms pinned to his sides, but his chest uncovered so as not to restrict his respiratory movements. A better functioning, efficient team is necessary when no anesthesia is used, as cooperation of the very young patient cannot be taken for granted. When general anesthesia is used, it must always be borne in mind that two physicians are constantly competing for the same vital airway.

Over the years, diethyl ether has stood the test of time as the anesthetic agent with the greatest margin of safety, especially in the hands of the relatively less experienced or less well-trained anesthetist. Longer relaxation can be obtained with ether, allowing more time for better visualization or treatment of the open tracheobronchial tree, even after administration of the anesthetic agent has been discontinued. However, its flammability is a hazard, and present-day fears of legal complications have greatly diminished its general use. It still may have a place in foreign body removal and in endoscopic procedures on cystic fibrosis patients or severe asthmatics, as it relaxes bronchospasm and may minimize postoperative complications.

Today, however, halothane is the most commonly and widely employed anesthetic agent, but its shorter period of action, together with its inability to produce or retain prolonged relaxation without cardiac irregularities are disadvantages. It usually must be supplemented by spraying the larynx and trachea with a local anesthetic, such as a 2 to 4 per cent lidocaine solution. The patient is then re-oxygenated for a few minutes while the topical agent is allowed to work. The general anesthetic agent can then be continued throughout the operative procedure by attaching tubing from the machine to the sidearm of the bronchoscope. Frequently, a short-acting muscle relaxant such as succinyl-choline must be administered, especially during foreign body removal, when operative conditions should be as ideal as possible, and the patient should be completely immobile with the bronchial lumen dilated. Thumbing the proximal end of the bronchoscope gives the patient a few breaths, or a glass window, as in the ventilating-bronchoscope, may be inserted if longer time is needed. If the patient is very young and is under general anesthesia, a headholder is not necessary. If the left thumb and forefinger of the operator are used to steady the bronchoscope and protect the lips of the patient, the other fingers can easily manipulate the head and maintain it constantly in the desired position. In the older child, a headholder is important, and the head should be extended only after the neck has been flexed (Fig. 2).

Before beginning the bronchoscopic procedure, equipment, lights and cords should be carefully checked, and the table should be adjusted to the proper height for the surgeon. Teeth must also be carefully examined and a dangerously loose tooth should always be carefully removed preoperatively. A gauze sponge over the upper teeth is added protection, even though pressure should never be applied to the teeth. The teeth must

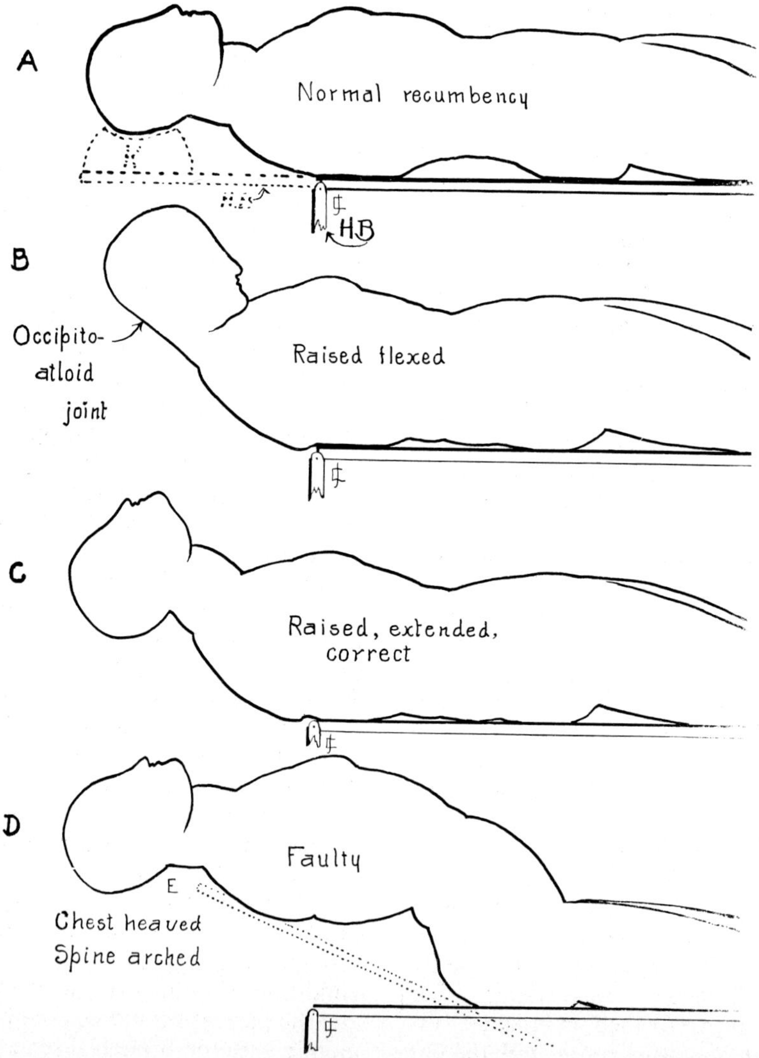

Figure 2. Position for laryngoscopy or bronchoscopy (*C* is the best position). (From Jackson, C., and Jackson, C. L.: *Bronchoesophagology*. W. B. Saunders, 1950.)

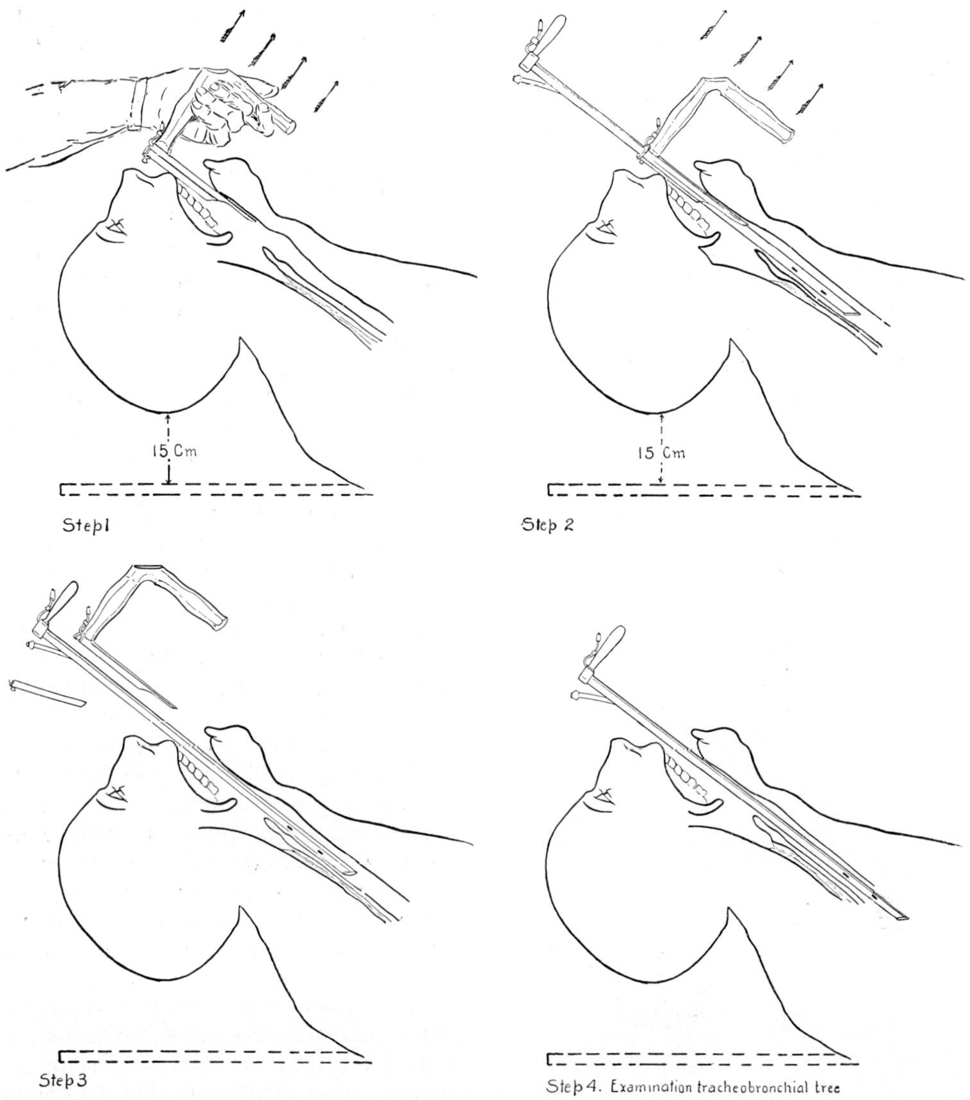

Figure 3. Technique of introduction of the bronchoscope through the laryngoscope. Head is lifted in direction of darts. (From Jackson, C., and Jackson, C. L.: *Bronchoesophagology*. W. B. Saunders, 1950.)

never be used as a fulcrum. A bronchoscope in a young child, especially an infant, should always be introduced through a laryngoscope with a removable slide, as it makes the procedure much quicker and less traumatic, particularly if the endoscopist does not feel at home with a pediatric patient. The laryngoscope merely lifts the head of the patient nearly off the table and is never used to hyperextend the head (Fig. 3). It should be inserted along the side of the tongue, allowing that large muscular organ to be displaced to the opposite side of the mouth. The glottis then is exposed by picking up the epiglottis with the tip of the laryngoscope and holding it elevated. The proper-sized bronchoscope is then moistened with saline solution for lubrication and gently passed through the glottis to the level of the second or third tracheal ring, with the bevel gently separating the vocal cords (handle of the instrument held horizontally to the right) (Fig. 4).

The bronchoscope is never forced through the larynx, but is gently guided with very little pressure. Atkins has described this maneuver as simply allowing the patient to "inhale the tube." Jackson describes it as "insinuation of the glottis." The trachea must be lined up in the same axial plane as the bronchoscope by properly moving the head of the patient and keeping his shoulders firmly

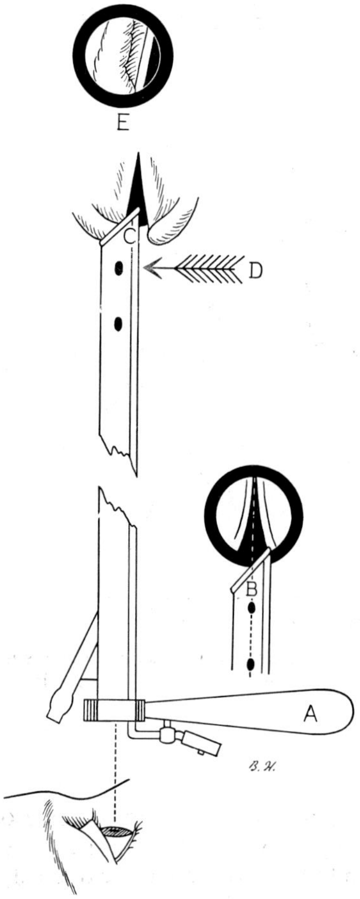

Figure 4. Introduction of bronchoscope through the glottis. *A*, The handle is on the right. *B*, Locate scope centrally. *C*, The tip of the scope is inserted during inspiration between the cords by moving slightly to left. *D*, Giving a glottic view. *E*, The glottic view. (From Jackson, C., and Jackson, C. L.: *Bronchoesophagology*. W. B. Saunders, 1950.)

down on the table. The head is pulled back off the edge of the table, and if the head is not properly extended on the flexed neck (see Fig. 2), only the posterior portion of the larynx will come into view. The position must then be corrected before proceeding further. The laryngoscope is turned 90 degrees, with the handle to the left, and then discarded once the slide has been carefully removed. The teeth and lips must not be traumatized. The head may then be lowered and the tracheobronchial tree carefully examined systematically, always using the same routine in order not to miss any positive finding. The bronchoscope should pass up and down the trachea freely, unless there is obvious obstruction ahead, the jaws are too tightly closed, the lips are caught between the scope and the teeth, or the angle of the head and neck is incorrect.

A specific routine should be developed and used in every procedure or pathological findings will go undetected. The endoscopist should know the exact area he is visualizing at all times, and this can be done only if a systematic examination is carried out one step at a time, proceeding all the way from the subglottic region to the lowermost segmental bronchus. The subglottic region should be examined first, noting any narrowing (stenosis or edema) or localized swelling (i.e., subglottic hemangioma or cyst). The color of the mucous membrane is observed, as well as the character and amount of any secretion. Secretions are then aspirated. Any region of constriction or pulsation, as well as general displacement of the trachea, is also noted.

Tracheal movements should be visualized, especially noting any abnormal collapsibility, either generalized or localized. The carina should be seen normally as a vertical spur, slightly to the left of the midline, and any widening, displacement, ulceration or difference in the caliber of the main bronchial orifices should be recorded (Figs. 5 and 6). The bronchoscope is turned at the carina so that the handle is again horizontal, putting the bevel in proper position to allow the bronchoscope to slip easily to one

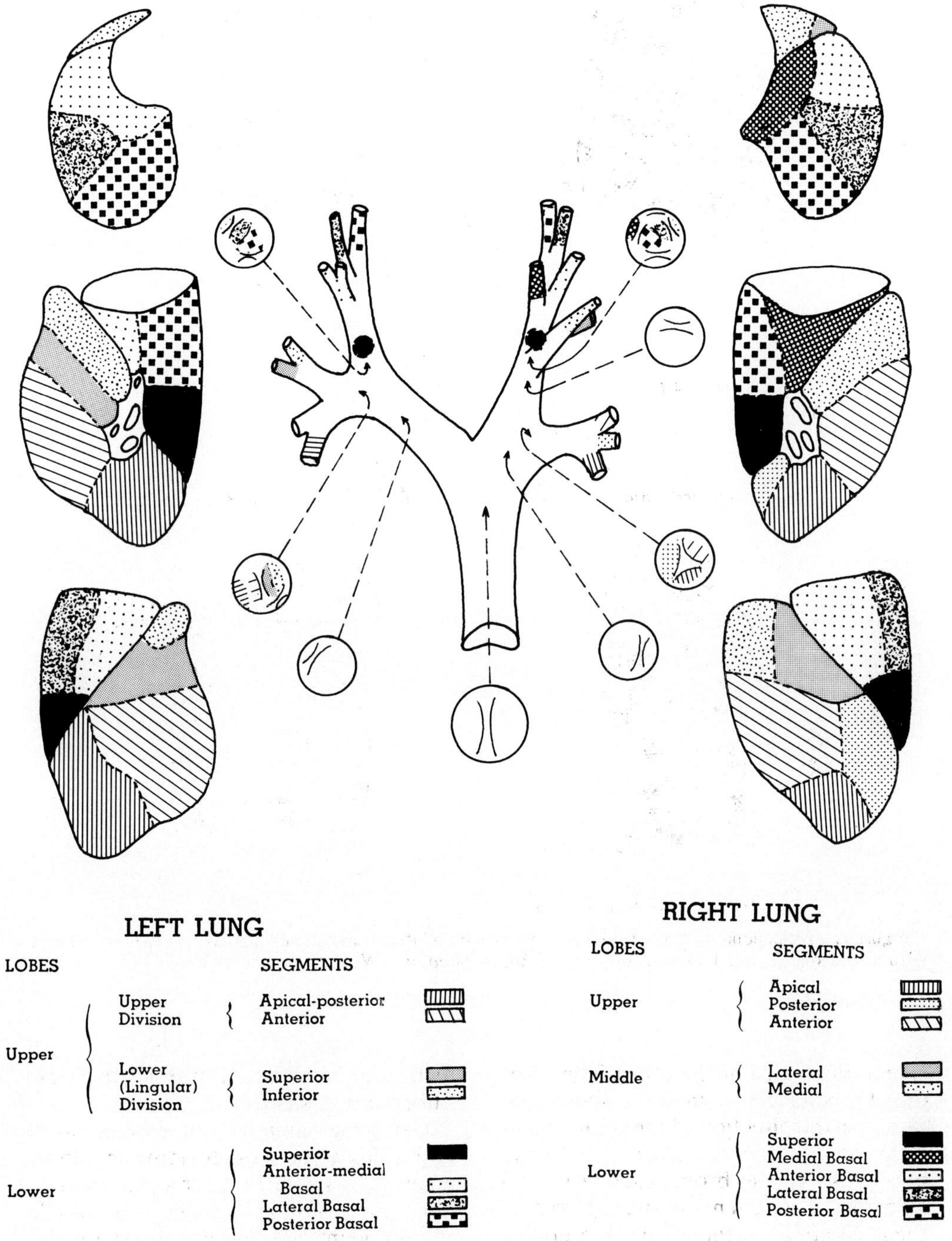

Figure 5. Schematic drawing of subdivision of lobes into bronchopulmonary segments. (From Jackson, C., and Jackson, C. L.: *Bronchoesophagology*. W. B. Saunders, 1950.)

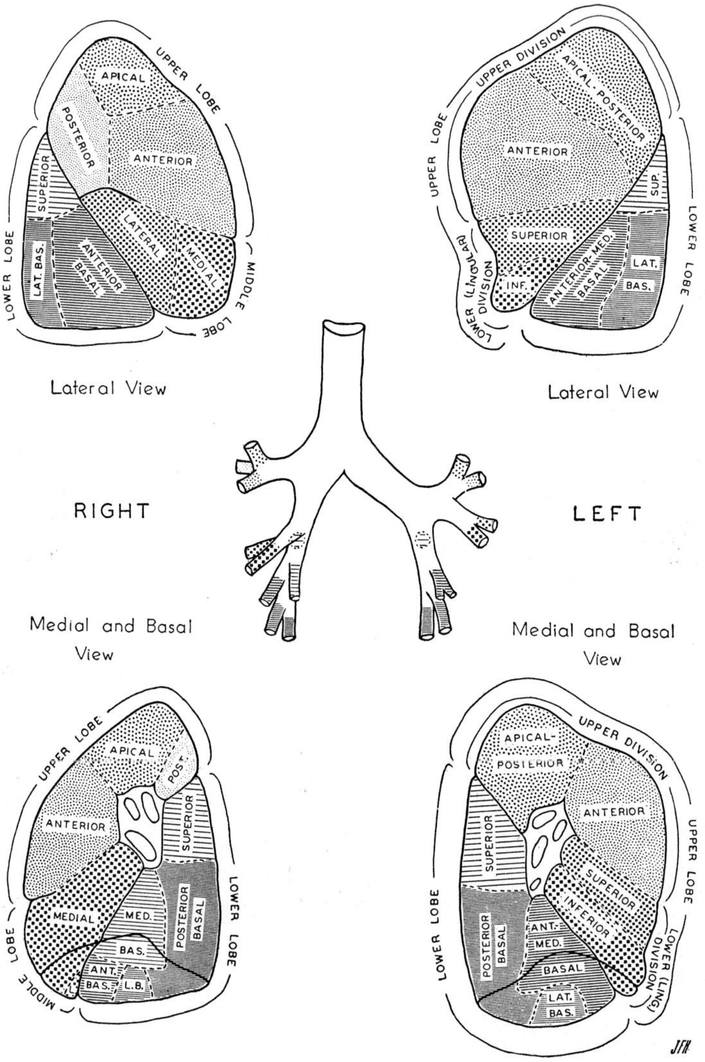

Jackson Huber Nomenclature

Figure 6. Bronchopulmonary segments shown on both lateral (above) and mediastinal (below) aspects. (From Jackson, C., and Jackson, C. L.: *Bronchoesophagology*. W. B. Saunders, 1950.)

side of the carina or the other. The lip of the bronchoscope should always be turned in the direction of the bronchus to be examined and the axes of both the bronchus and the bronchoscope should coincide. The tracheobronchial tree is then carefully cleaned of secretions, which are aspirated into a sterile glass Lukens collecting tube (Fig. 7). The aspirate is then sent to the laboratory for bacteriologic cultures, including sensitivity tests, smears, search for a fungus infection or inoculation into a guinea pig (tuberculosis suspect).

Using the same factors, evaluation of both sides of the bronchial tree should be made as was done in the trachea. In addition, the various orifices should be serially identified and examined for patency, narrowing, foreign body, exudate or mucus plug. Occasionally, absence of the right upper lobe orifice or an extraneous orifice is noted, or in agenesis of the lung the entire main bronchus as well as the carina may be absent. It must be remembered that the right main bronchus is actually a continuation of the trachea, deviating only 25 degrees or so from the midline, but that the left main bronchus deviates about 75 degrees. Therefore, positioning of the head must always be correct. The right upper lobe orifice with its vertical spur will be seen at the level of the carina at 3 o'clock with the patient recumbent on the table. Occasionally, an accessory right upper lobe bronchus is found arising from the trachea well above the carina with or without the normal orifice below.

The middle lobe orifice, indicating the largest of all the anterior branches, is seen directly anteriorly at 12 o'clock just beyond the upper lobe opening. The head must be dropped to a lower position for examination of the middle lobe bronchus, and the handle of the bronchoscope should be kept in a vertical position to allow the tip of the bronchoscope to slide into this orifice. The segmental bronchi of the right lower lobe are then identified as far as possible (obviously, this is limited by the size of the bronchoscope in relation to the size of the bronchus, as well as the age and size of the patient). On the left side, the upper lobe bronchial orifice is found much further down from the carina, and the head must be bent markedly from the midline well onto the right shoulder. The spur of the left upper lobe orifice runs from about 2 o'clock to 8 o'clock, and the orifice itself is seen around 9 or 10 o'clock.

Segmental bronchi of the left lower lobe are then examined as far as possible. If the head is placed firmly on the right shoulder, it may be possible to see the lingular division of the left upper lobe bronchus. This is better visualized with the telescope.

Two very important additions to the original armamentarium of the Jacksons have been the telescope of Broyles of Johns Hopkins University and the flexible fiber-bronchoscope of Ikeda of Tokyo. These two newer instruments, however, are of much more value in adults, for neoplasms are more common in them than in children. The telescope, either the right-angled or the foroblique type, is passed through the standard bronchoscope, and gives much better visualization of the upper lobe bronchi as well as the segmental bronchi. The flexible fiber-bronchoscope is similarly used and is also best for the upper lobes and the subsegmental bronchi, not only facilitating visualization, but also enhancing the possibility of a satisfactory biopsy in

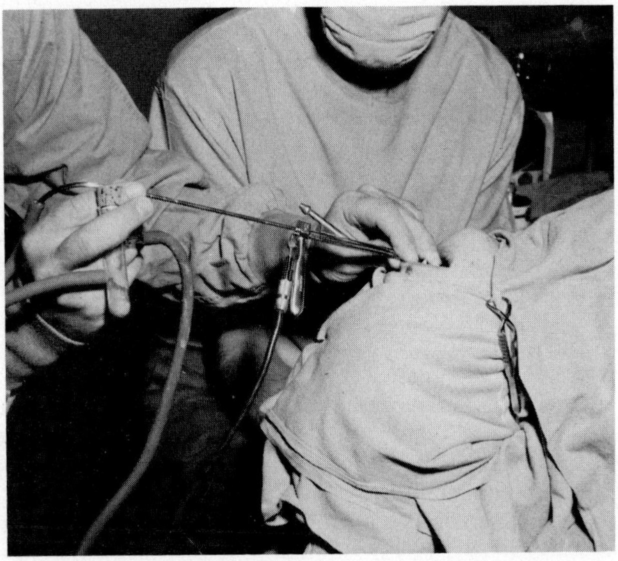

Figure 7. Bronchoscopic aspiration of secretions for culture (Lukens tube).

areas that were previously totally inaccessible.

In recent years, brighter and more constant illumination has been provided by the fiberoptic bronchoscope, laryngoscope and esophagoscope. Here there is no tiny "grain-of-wheat" bulb to burn out at the wrong moment! The source of illumination is kept several feet from the operating table and from the anesthetic agents, and intense illumination is conducted thence deep into the dark tracheobronchial tree by millions of light-carrying optical fibers encased in a flexible cable.

Bronchoscopy is performed for various reasons, both diagnostic and therapeutic. *Diagnostic* uses include direct inspection, culture, biopsy and bronchography. *Therapeutic* uses include aspiration of secretions to clear airway, removal of foreign bodies, removal of tumors, preparation for performing tracheotomy, dilatation of a stricture and bronchial lavage.

There is no contraindication to bronchoscopy at any age or at any time, if it is felt that valuable information may thereby be obtained to assist in a more accurate diagnosis, or to initiate more effective therapy.

REFERENCES

Fearon, B., and Whalen, J. S.: Tracheal dimensions in the living infant. *Ann. Otol. Rhinol. Laryng.,* 76:964, 1967.

Hall, J. E.: The physiology of respiration in infants and young children. *Proc. Royal Soc. Med.,* 48:761, 1955.

Hagens, E.: Anatomy of the tracheobronchial tree from the bronchoscopic standpoint. *Arch. Otology,* 38:469, 1943.

Jackson, C., and Jackson, C. L.: Bronchoesophagology. Philadelphia, W. B. Saunders, Co., 1950.

Jackson, C. L., and Huber, J.: Correlated applied anatomy of bronchial tree and lung with a system of nomenclature. *Dis. Chest,* 9:319, 1943.

Wittenborg, M. H., Gyepes, M. T., and Crocker, D.: Tracheal dynamics in infants with respiratory distress, stridor and collapsing trachea. *Radiology,* 88:653, 1967.

Chapter One Hundred Nine

FOREIGN BODIES IN THE AIR AND FOOD PASSAGES

GABRIEL F. TUCKER, JR., M.D., and MYLES G. TURTZ, M.D.

INTRODUCTION

The clinical problem presented by ingestion of foreign objects into the air or food passages ranges from the urgent, often fatal, lodgement in the larynx to the more subtle symptomatology of those objects which cause only partial esophageal obstruction or which lodge in a peripheral bronchus.

The pediatric endoscopic aspects of such problems are characterized by the frequent lack of any history of ingestion and the increased technical challenge of retrieving such objects from patients who are not only physically smaller, but also more at risk from the mechanical effects of the presence of the object or its manipulation. The same few millimeters of laryngeal edema which would make an adult hoarse could well prove fatal to an infant.

Techniques of manipulation and extraction of foreign objects and preoccupation with technical expertise have often overshadowed the broader clinical aspects of foreign body management. The current size of the foreign body collection at the Chevalier Jackson Clinic at Temple University Medical Center now approaches 6000 foreign objects. This is impressive but perhaps can be viewed more realistically if one realizes this figure was reached over a period of more than 50 years. The National Safety Council tells us that there are approximately 1000 foreign body deaths a year in this country. The discrepancy, of course, lies in the fact that those foreign bodies which cause death usually do so quickly. Such patients are often examined by no physician other than the coroner or medical examiner. Recent writings by forensic pathologists have pointed out the part that undiagnosed foreign bodies may play in the production of sudden death.

It is a common misconception that all patients who have "choked" on something will be coughing or sputtering. However, it should take very little logic to realize that the more complete the patient's obstruction the less air he can move and, therefore, the less sound he will produce.[12]

Patients who are in imminent danger of death may require emergency tracheotomy. Only in situations in which the patient is in extremis may such measures of desperation as probing the pharynx with a finger, turning the patient upside down or pounding him between the shoulder blades be condoned (see Fig. 2).

Those foreign objects which do not immediately cause complete obstruction but which present with gagging, coughing, sputtering or wheezing place the physician in a position to inadvertently make the patient worse. In such situations, probing the hypopharynx with the finger may (1) impact a loose hypopharyngeal foreign body tightly into the larynx, thus transforming partial obstruction into complete obstruction; (2) force the foreign body into the esophagus where it may compress the trachea against the upper sternum, thus causing an obstruction which cannot be relieved even by tracheotomy; and (3) either remove the foreign body to the mouth or allow it to be carried harmlessly through the alimentary tract.

Turning the patient upside down and pounding him on the back may well dislodge an aspirated foreign body. The question then becomes, Where will the aspirated foreign object go? If the foreign object was initially impacted in the glottis, it is quite possible that such

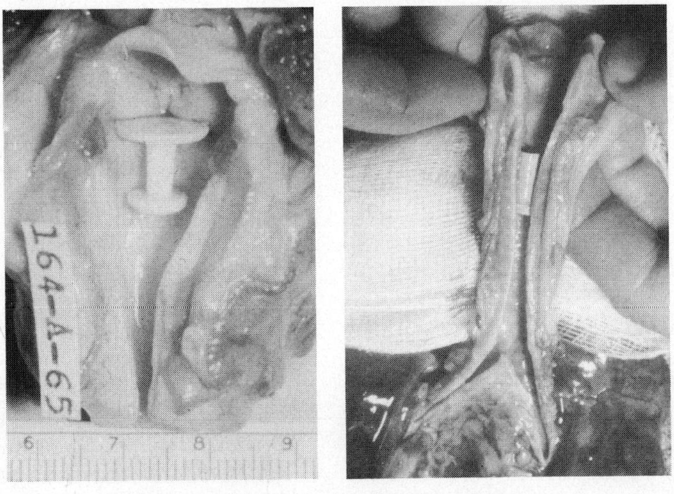

Figure 1. Foreign bodies found at autopsy.

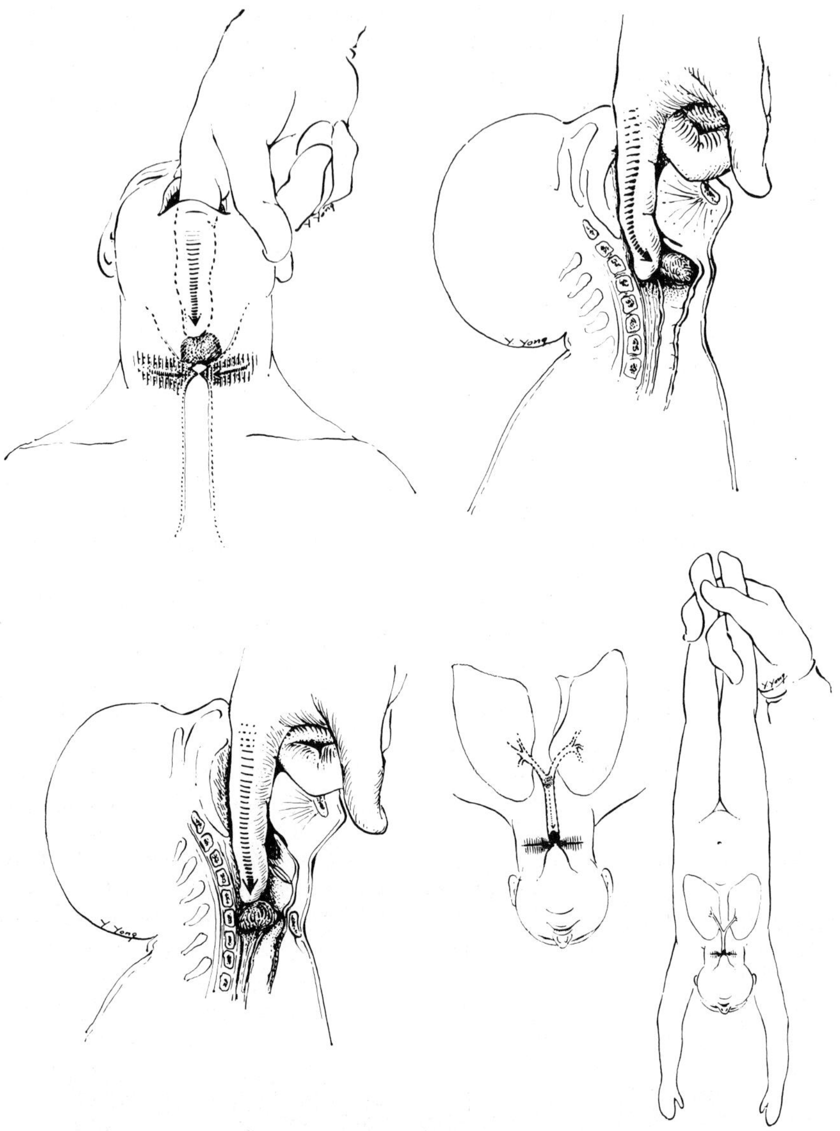

Figure 2. Possible methods of impaction of a foreign body by ill-advised first aid. (From Tucker, G. F., Jr.: Report of the committee for the prevention of foreign body accidents. *Trans. Amer. Bronch-Esoph. Ass.*, 49:181, 1969.)

treatment will cause its expulsion. However, if the foreign body has passed the glottis and is in the lower trachea, such treatment may cause the foreign object to impact in the glottis from below and thus precipitate complete obstruction. If the foreign object has already traveled to a bronchus, it is probably initially located in one of the lower lobe bronchi where it may be most readily approached endoscopically. If such a patient is, however, turned upside down, such a foreign body may well migrate to an upper lobe bronchus where anatomic factors usually imply much greater difficulty in removal. In recent years attempts have been made to return to the treatment of airway foreign bodies that was proposed in the

1850's, namely that of physiotherapy to retrieve a foreign body.[1] The advent of bronchodilators in no way diminishes the potential dangers of this type of treatment.[2]

It is difficult to estimate when dealing with death statistics how many cases were initially truly obstructed and how many were actually made fatal by ill-advised attempts at first aid.

The majority of foreign body problems which come to the otolaryngologist have already survived the acute phase. Problems in which there is no urgent danger to the patient's existence should be approached with full and thoughtful consideration of the physiological and mechanical factors involved, i.e., contemplative management.

ETIOLOGY

The tendency of many small children to put whatever comes into their grasp into their mouths is well known. To this is added the tendency to imitate an adult; the mother who holds an open safety pin in her mouth while she diapers her child should not be at all surprised when the infant puts an open safety pin in his own mouth at the first available opportunity.

Carelessness may contribute to foreign body ingestion in many ways: improper preparation of food, hasty eating and drinking, permitting children to play while eating, talking with food in the mouth, giving food such as peanuts to children who do not have the proper molar teeth to chew them and improper supervision of small children in the vicinity of infants. On a number of occasions, a definite history is found in which small children have been seen to deliberately feed an object they know to be dangerous (such as a safety pin) to their infant sibling. Such primitive solutions to the problem of sibling rivalry can be eliminated only by careful supervision.

An equally dangerous threat lies in the desire of some children to share, and thus place in the reach of infant siblings, treasures such as coins, marbles and lapel buttons.[15]

Special Properties of the Foreign Body Itself

Of current note here are light slippery, plastic imitation lipsticks and doll bottle caps which not only are physically easy to ingest but psychologically are made to imitate objects which would normally be put in or near the mouth.

The Incorrect Use of Objects Designed to Be in or Near the Mouth

Included in this category would be inhaled beans from beanshooters and darts from plastic blowguns, dental instruments dropped during surgery, toy plastic lipsticks and broken rattles and pacifiers.

INCIDENCE

Today foreign body removal accounts for about 5 per cent of all pediatric peroral endoscopic procedures; more than half of these are esophageal foreign bodies. The children most at risk are those between the ages of 14 months (the inquisitive, orally oriented toddler) and 6 years (the appearance of back molars).[14] Obstructive foreign bodies in children who are under 1 year of age are unusual and suggest deliberate feeding; a variant of the "battered child." Potential foreign bodies are so ubiquitous that the wonder is that the problem is not encountered more frequently.

PATHOPHYSIOLOGY

Initial contact of the foreign object with the respiratory mucosa classically produces choking, gagging, coughing or wheezing, depending on the exact location.[3] As the stimulated mucosa accommodates to the presence of the foreign object a symptomless interval often follows such manifestations. If the initial reaction caused either the expulsion of the offending foreign object or its passage into the lower gastrointestinal tract, the episode may be quickly forgotten by the patient without further sequelae. The initial symptomatology may have been unrecognized or forgotten if the foreign object is retained. The occurrence of late symptoms depends on patient reaction to the foreign object. This may have occurred in a variety of ways, depending on whether the object ingested caused chemical or mechanical irritation or interfered with physiological functions such as the passage of air or food. Persistent pain is not common in the esophagus or tracheobronchial tree. Intermittent pain in association with attempts to swallow in the presence of an esophageal foreign body is, of course, not unusual.

Late symptomatology may also include that due to infection occasioned by the long-standing presence of a foreign object, especially in the bronchial tree where the object may interfere with normal bronchial toilet.

Current radiological techniques provide often invaluable assistance to the endoscopist not only in the establishment of the diagnosis of foreign body but as an actual aid to the process of removal. Incomplete studies may lead to errors in diagnosis. It should be remembered that an ingested object may lodge anywhere between the floor of the perineum and the base of the skull. Although many foreign bodies are radiolucent, special techniques such as inspiration-expiration films and fluoroscopy, with or without contrast material, may help to establish the diagnosis.

Accurate localization of the foreign body is also enhanced by proper x-ray studies. It is necessary to understand the relation of the foreign object to surrounding tissues in order to properly plan the endoscopic procedure. Newer fluoroscopic techniques with television-type monitoring may add a second or even a third dimension of perspective to the endoscopic image if employed during the procedure.[8]

Neck

The lateral soft tissue film taken of the neck during inspiration is one of the most useful single films available to the endoscopist. Even without supplementary contrast material the caliber of the airway is often readily appreciated. Holinger has suggested an "endoscopic" lateral film in which the arms are held backward. A profile of the air column in the larynx and trachea is thus visible in a single film.

Chest

In addition to the usual posteroanterior, anteroposterior and lateral films of the chest normally taken during inspiration, similar films taken at the end of expiration are often most helpful. Such studies are especially useful to delineate obstructive emphysema, since the air trapping behind the foreign object and the failure of the trapped air to empty on expiration will be most apparent on this type of film. An even more dynamic demonstration of this phenomenon can, of course, be obtained by fluoroscopy, wherein the motion of the chest throughout the entire respiratory cycle may be continuously observed.

Contrast Studies

Contrast material such as barium should be used with great caution and only after plain films have been found to be inadequate to meet the specific problem. An object such as a chicken or pork bone may be apparent in the lateral soft tissue film of the neck. Administration of contrast material in such a situation normally tends to delay the performance of the endoscopic procedure until such material has passed beyond the stomach. If retained above an obstructive foreign body, contrast material would not only complicate the attempt at the removal of the foreign object but also would most likely be aspirated into the respiratory tract. Bronchography has occasionally been useful to demonstrate the relation of a given foreign object to the bronchial tree or even to localize an otherwise radiolucent plastic foreign object.

GENERAL CONSIDERATIONS

Once the presence of a foreign object is established as a working clinical impression, the next question to be decided is whether intervention is necessary or whether it can be assumed that natural processes will safely eliminate the foreign object.

Hypopharyngeal foreign objects imply the danger of downward descent into the respiratory or gastrointestinal tract and thus should be removed before such migration occurs.

Foreign bodies in the larynx and trachea, even if nonobstructive, present an eventual threat to the airway via the mechanisms of the tissue reaction that their presence engenders.

Foreign bodies in the bronchial tree are seldom expelled spontaneously. Unless the sojourn of the object has been so prolonged as to cause enough tissue destruction, thoracotomy is rarely warranted. Grasses such as Timothy[3] may migrate by a rachet-like action which precludes their endoscopic removal. However, even among those cases referred after an unsuccessful attempt at endoscopy had impacted the object in a position peripheral to its original lodgment, thoracotomy was seldom required.

PLANNING THE PROCEDURE

When Should Foreign Bodies Be Removed?

Foreign bodies should be regarded as true emergencies only when the airway is embarrassed, when there is imminent danger of perforation or if it is felt that the foreign body may readily migrate to a more dangerous position.

The suspicion of "foreign body" carries with it the unreasoning connotation that haste is always necessary. Deliberate speed is, of course, desirable in those emergent situations enumerated in the previous paragraph. A properly trained endoscopic team with a full selection of instruments to meet the mechanical problems is of inestimable value in rising to the challenge presented by the true acute emergency. The experienced endoscopist also appreciates the value of careful preparation of himself, the patient and the team. *A minimal morbidity and mortality will depend on the adequate preparation of the patient, the instrumentarium and the endoscopic team before starting the procedure. If two hours are spent in such preparation, the safe endoscopic removal of the foreign body may take only two minutes. But if only two minutes are taken for preparation, the endoscopist may find himself attempting makeshift, ineffective procedures for the next frustrating two hours.*[3]

An unsuccessful attempt—for whatever reason—may well imply that repeated instrumentation should not be undertaken again for several days. This is especially true when a second procedure will require the reintubation of a child's larynx with either a bronchoscope or an endotracheal tube. In this day and age of air transport, the lack of local endoscopic facilities is no excuse for the performance of a bronchotomy.

The majority of foreign bodies that reach the stomach unassisted go on through natural passages, provided that the natural functions are not impaired by the administration of laxatives or changes in diet. This, however, does not mean that esophageal foreign bodies should be pushed into the stomach by blind methods, which are always dangerous, or even by esophagoscopy, because a swallowed object lodged in the esophagus can practically always be removed through the mouth. In the case of a nontraumatizing foreign body in the stomach it may be wise, if the pylorus is of normal size, to wait as long as several weeks. The passage of a heavy object, such as a quarter, may be assisted by encouraging the patient to sleep on his right side. If it is determined by radiographic studies that the presence of a pyloric stenosis will prevent the passage of the foreign body, it should be removed by peroral gastroscopy or by the use of a fluoroscopically guided flexible gastric forceps.[8a]

The most dangerous foreign body to be allowed to pass through the pylorus is one that is too long to pass the turns of the duodenum. As a criterion it may be stated that a foreign body 2 inches long, or longer, is likely to lodge at the turn of the duodenum in a child 2 years old. A large safety pin will lodge at the same point, and a small one may stick anywhere in trying to turn over; a pin of medium size that cannot turn over has the best chance of going through, usually spring end first. The danger of administering cathartics which cause the intestine to cramp should be obvious here. About 25 per cent of safety pins lodge. Ferrous foreign bodies can be removed from the stomach with an Alnico magnet.[1]

Recent experience with steroids would seem to suggest that such an interval might well be utilized under steroid-antibiotic coverage to lessen not only laryngeal reaction but also bronchial reaction at the site of lodgment of the foreign object. Steroids should be withheld if there seems to be danger of esophageal perforation.

Time is also required to permit the stomach to empty of residual barium or food. Ideally, endoscopic procedures should be undertaken in the forenoon when the team is at its best and a full range of ancillary services (anesthesia and radiology) is available. Children especially should be treated early in the day so that any untoward laryngeal reaction can be diagnosed and treated with expediency.

Where Should Foreign Bodies Be Removed?

Only in the most desperate emergency should removal be attempted at the scene of ingestion. As has been pointed out, ill-advised attempts at first aid may precipitate a fatal respiratory obstruction. Few doctors' offices are equipped to meet the need for tracheotomy or to provide proper x-ray studies.

Most community hospital emergency rooms are equipped to provide basic x-rays and such lifesaving procedures as tracheotomy; however, few are staffed around the clock with personnel who are experienced in handling more than the most urgent problems.

Hospitals large enough to generate a sufficient endoscopic experience should concentrate this experience in the hands of those who are to handle the foreign body problems. To request a doctor to remove foreign bodies and at the same time deny him the full range of endoscopic practice is a disservice to the patient. Even in the most specialized clinics foreign bodies constitute less than 10 per cent of the over-all endoscopic experience.

Those hospitals which presume to offer this service to the patient must have available not only an experienced endoscopist but also a full team of nurse assistants, anesthesiologists and radiologists, fully equipped to meet not only the apparent problems but also the "unplanned" complications.

Method of Removal

The selection of a specific approach to an endoscopic procedure depends not only upon the patient and the problem he brings but also upon the team and its particular capabilities to best meet the challenge.

The reader is referred to the general discussion on anesthesia in Chapter 108. There are, however, several points which should be emphasized in considering foreign body removal.[6, 7, 11, 13] The endoscopic team should be capable of working safely with the awake patient wherever general anesthesia would increase the risk of the procedure. This is especially true in those situations in which the anesthesiologist and the endoscopist must share a respiratory tract which is not functioning optimally. If anesthesia is to be used for endoscopy, the closest possible teamwork between the endoscopist and the anesthesiologist is mandatory. In foreign body situations the induction of anesthesia should be begun in the endoscopic operating room after the endoscopic team is fully prepared to proceed. This is required because the induction of anesthesia may precipitate coughing or retching, which may in turn cause the foreign object to shift into an obstructive position and thus require the immediate availability of the endoscopic team to preserve the patient's airway.

The specific problems of bronchial foreign body removal under general anesthesia are discussed in detail elsewhere in this chapter. In general they revolve about the fact that the requirements for instrumentation prevent the anesthesiologist from working with a closed system. The loss of normal bronchial tone in a flaccid thoracic cage encourages the migration of the foreign object into the more peripheral bronchi if the operator pushes on the foreign body with his forceps.[10] The presence of a foreign body does not lessen the normal patient requirements for safe anesthesia—i.e., empty stomach, proper hydration, hemoglobin level, renal function.

Anesthesia is in no way a substitute for an inadequate team or instrumentation. In many ways it increases the challenge, since it adds another member (the anesthesiologist) who must work smoothly as part of the team which has elected to suppress many of the patient's vital functions and reflexes.

MECHANICAL PROBLEMS OF FOREIGN BODY EXTRACTION

Preliminary Study

The first step in the solution of the mechanical problem presented by any case of foreign body is the study of the roentgenograms made in at least three planes: (1) anteroposterior, (2) lateral and (3) the plane corresponding to the greatest plane of the foreign body. The next step is to put a duplicate of the foreign body into the open manikin, or simple piece of rubber tubing, and to try to simulate the probable position shown by the roentgenograms in order to get an idea of the endoscopic appearance of the probable presentation. Since shifting may change the presentation of the duplicate foreign body, it is turned into as many different positions as possible, in order to educate the eye to assist in the comprehension of the largest possible number of presentations that may be encountered during bronchoscopy on that particular patient. For each of these presentations a method of disimpaction, disengagement, disentanglement, or version and seizure is worked out according to the kind of foreign body.

Selection and Use of Forceps

It cannot be too strongly stated that preliminary selection and test of forceps with a duplicate of the foreign body should be made in every case. It has often been a sad sight to see a child arrive at our clinic very ill or moribund from prolonged efforts, performed elsewhere, to remove a foreign body with forceps the utter uselessness of which could have been determined in a moment by testing on a duplicate. It is necessary, in some cases, to have different forceps ready for different presentations. Forceps jaws must expand sufficiently to take in the foreign body, if not in every diameter, at least in the diameter of the selected presentation.

Prepared by this practice and the radiographic study, the endoscopist introduces the endoscope into the patient. The location of the foreign body is approached *slowly* and *carefully* to avoid overriding or displacement. A study of the presentation is as necessary for the endoscopist as it is for the obstetrician, and it should determine the following points: (1) the relation of the presenting part to the surrounding tissues and (2) the probable position of the unseen portion, as determined by the appearance of the presenting part taken in connection with the knowledge obtained by the previous roentgen ray study and by inspection of the films upside down on the view box.

The standard forceps have a powerful grasp and are used on dense foreign bodies which require a very firm grasp on the object to prevent the forceps from slipping off. For more delicate manipulation, and particularly for friable foreign bodies, the lighter forceps, such as the fenestrated peanut forceps, are best. Forceps are held in the right hand, the thumb in one ring, and the third, or ring, finger in the other ring. These fingers are used to open and close the forceps; all traction and pulsion are to be made by the right index finger, which is positioned on the forceps handle near the stylet, as shown in Figures 3 and 4. The impulse to seize the foreign body as soon as it is discovered must be strongly resisted. A careful study of its size, shape, position and relation to surrounding structures must be made before any attempt at extraction. Thc most favorablc point and position for grasping having been determined, the closed forceps are inserted through the scope; the light reflex is noted as the forceps pass the distal lamp and emerge from the distal end. The forceps are then advanced until they lightly touch the foreign body; they are then allowed to expand and are further advanced far enough to get a secure grasp on the intruder. If there are no potentially traumatizing points on the foreign body, it is held until the tube mouth is advanced against it. If it is too large to come out through the tube, it is held against the tube mouth, the grasp of the forceps being firmly maintained by the fingers of the right hand while all traction for withdrawal is made with the left hand, which firmly clamps forceps and bronchoscope as one piece. Thus, the three units are brought out as one, the bronchoscope keeping the cords apart until the foreign body has entered the glottis. Coins require a flatwise grasp. They should be kept close against the tube mouth and turned sagittally before reaching the glottis. If in the esophagus, they should be rotated to the frontal plane.

Pins, needles, and similar long pointed objects are classified in two groups: (1) bendable pins and (2) breakable pins and needles. It is often desirable to bend a pin; it is less desirable to break it. When searching for such objects as pins and needles special care must be taken not to

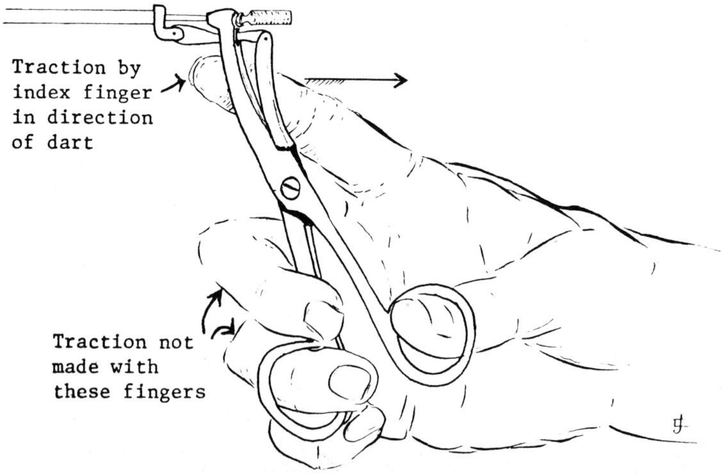

Figure 3. Proper grasp of forceps. The right thumb and third finger are inserted into the rings while the right index finger has its place high on the handle. All traction is made with the index finger, the ring finger being used only to open and close the forceps. If any pushing is deemed safe it may be done by placing the index finger back of the thumb-nut on the stylet. (From Jackson, C., and Jackson, C. L.: *Diseases of the Nose, Throat, and Ear,* 2nd ed. Philadelphia, W. B. Saunders Co., 1959.)

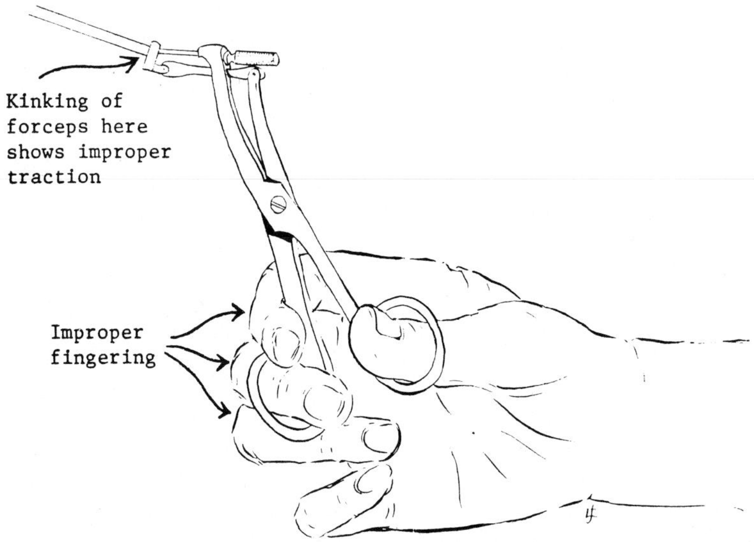

Figure 4. Improper grasp of forceps. Forceps can be so constructed as not to bend as here shown; but the delicacy of touch essential to safe and efficient work would be thus destroyed. (From Jackson, C., and Jackson, C. L.: *Diseases of the Nose, Throat, and Ear,* 2nd ed. Philadelphia, W. B. Saunders Co., 1959.)

override them. Pins are almost always found point upward, and the dictum can therefore be invented: "Search not for the pin, but for the point of the pin." If the point be found free, it should be worked into the lumen of the bronchoscope by manipulation with forceps and the lip of the tube. It may be then seized with the forceps and withdrawn. Should the pin be grasped by the shaft, it is almost certain to turn crosswise of the tube mouth, where one pull may cause the point to perforate, enormously increasing the difficulties of removal, and perhaps resulting in serious trauma. Pins in the costophrenic angle, or elsewhere in the periphery of the lung, require costophrenic bronchoscopy under fluoroscopic guidance.

The sheathing and protective methods for the removal of pins apply also to the removal of tacks. Double-pointed tacks and staples require the special staple bronchoscope and forceps. Hollow metallic objects are best held with one of the forceps jaws inside and one outside. Hard, smooth globular objects, such as ball bearings, are best held with the ball forceps. The same is true of globular glass beads. Oval beads and marbles are securely held with the Gordon bead forceps. They require extremely gentle and careful use for safety. The forceps should not be allowed to expand until they have touched the bead. If gentle traction meets with resistance, the bead must be released and a fresh grasp made.

The subject of exogenous foreign bodies in both the air passage and the food passage lends itself to one chapter because (1) the route of entry is the same, (2) the initial symptoms are frequently similar and (3) their removal is effected by way of peroral endoscopy (usually with forceps). They have many mechanical problems in common. The obvious differences in anatomy and function between the air passage and the food passage, however, require each to be treated separately.

FOREIGN BODY IN THE AIR PASSAGE

Initial Symptoms

All airway foreign bodies either lodge in or pass through the larynx. Initial symptoms, therefore, will be of laryngeal mucosal irritation (coughing, choking, stridor). Large foreign bodies aspirated at the end of an inspiration without enough reserve to develop a bechic blast are seen more frequently by medical examiners than by endoscopists (see Fig. 1). This laryngeal irritation phase will last briefly. Subsequent signs and symptoms will be a reflection of tracheobronchial responses.

Delayed Signs and Symptoms

Shortly after the initial mucosal stimulation there ensues a "silent period," which is characteristic of most airway foreign bodies. This symptomless interval lasts a variable period of time—from hours to years. The signs and symptoms that subsequently develop will be a function of the condition of the airway before aspiration, the shape and size of the foreign body, the nature of the foreign body and the mucosal reaction it will cause, and the subsequent alteration in airway dynamics.

Current medical practice in which antibiotics and steroids are used to treat "asthmatic" or "croupy" children may well obscure signs and symptoms which would normally be expected with a retained foreign object. Clearing of symptoms with these agents cannot be assumed to be diagnostic of a specific disease process. The fact that a wheeze disappears or that a pneumonic process clears may merely mean that the patient's reaction to the presence of the foreign object has been temporarily controlled. The recurrence of "asthma" after the withdrawal of therapy should heighten the physician's suspicion of a foreign object as the possible underlying cause.[10]

The Condition of the Airway Preaspiration

It is curious to note the inordinately high incidence of upper respiratory infections in children at the time of aspiration of airway foreign bodies. Whether this is a function of the frequency with which children get upper respiratory infections or whether the obstructive rhinorrhea and associated inflammation disturbs the oropharyngeal reflexes is not clear. Frequently, the fact that the problem is caused by an airway foreign body is obscured by the cough and associated symptoms of the upper respiratory infection. The state of the tracheobronchial mucosa at the time of aspiration will affect the subsequent presentation of the problem; e.g., presence of edema, excessive secretions and pathogens will alter events. A peanut bathed in the suppuration of the child with cystic fibrosis is considerably different from the same peanut in an otherwise healthy child. Similarly, developmental narrowed airways (stenosis, aplasia, vascular compression, repaired esophageal atresia) (Fig. 5) will function to determine the position of the foreign body and perhaps the degree of severity.

Relative Size of the Foreign Body

Obviously, the smaller the foreign body, the more peripherally it will lodge. From the immediate subglottic space downward the tracheobronchial tree narrows. The branching of the right main bronchus from the trachea is straighter and more accessible than the left; in the smaller child the orifice of the right main bronchus occasionally seems almost in direct line with the trachea when viewed endoscopically. The majority of bronchial foreign bodies therefore descend on the right side. The infant aspirating a foreign body while on his belly will frequently present with middle lobe involvement (because of anterior branching of the middle-lobe bronchus). The presentation of a foreign body is also a function of weight, shape and balance of the object; open safety pins (see Fig. 25) descend spring downward, common pins (see Fig. 20) head downward, wooden screws head up. Details of the "anatomy" of the foreign body are frequently as critical to successful endoscopic extraction as knowledge of the anatomy of the infant airway itself.

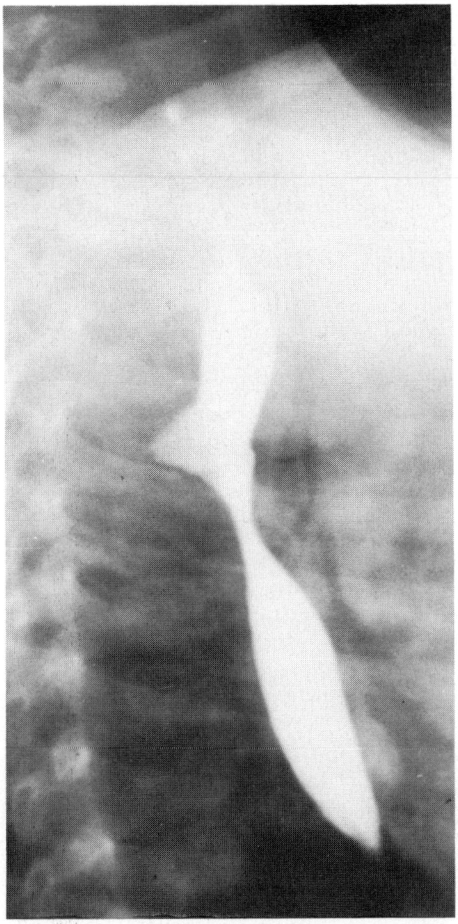

Figure 5. Esophageal abnormalities years after repair of esophageal atresia with fistula. There is repeated foreign body impaction proximal to stenosis.

Nature of the Foreign Body

A distinction is made between vegetal and nonvegetal foreign bodies. By vegetal is meant those materials that either are plants themselves or behave as plants—i.e., those which swell in the presence of water. The classic example is the dry bean. A moderately large bean in the trachea of a child is of more immediate concern than a nonreactive gold button. Of technical interest to the endoscopist is the relative difficulty in grasp of slippery-smooth plastics[10] and irregularly hollowed toys. The oil of commercially prepared peanuts can create severe mucosal reaction.

Disturbances in Aeration

All the above considerations will affect where, when and how the foreign body will situate itself in the airway. A loose foreign body will create a confusing picture clinically but most foreign bodies will usually descend in the airway and seat proximal to a slightly smaller opening. Tracheal foreign bodies may be visualized by x-ray or by expiratory wheeze coupled with the "auditory thud," i.e., the foreign body striking the undersurface of the vocal cords. The explanation for the wheeze is described best by the "check-valve" mechanism first defined by Dr. Chevalier Jackson. If the foreign body lodges in a bronchus and allows air to enter by virtue of normal bronchial widening and lengthening on inspiration but not exit because of similar physiologic narrowing on expiration, an obstructive emphysema will develop. Normal toilet will be interfered with, obstructing that portion of the lung distal to the foreign body, and suppurative bronchitis eventually involving parenchyma and pneumonitis will develop (see Fig. 18). If total block of the bronchus and "corking" obtain, the absorption of the air will lead to collapse of the distal parts, i.e., atelectasis (Fig. 6). Another finding is pneumothorax secondary to airway foreign body (see Fig. 19); a strong Valsalva maneuver (i.e., cough) against an obstructed bronchus may create critical pressures peripheral to the obstruction, and a microtear in either bronchiole or alveolus may occur with subsequent dissection of air along vascular sheaths to the hilus.

Diagnosis

Since fewer than half of the children with airway foreign bodies will give a positive history, all the above points must be considered in evaluating disturbances in aeration in infants and children. There must be a high index of suspicion of airway foreign bodies in any noncystic, fibrotic, nonasthmatic, nonallergic child with spontaneous pneumothorax, atelectasis, obstructive emphy-

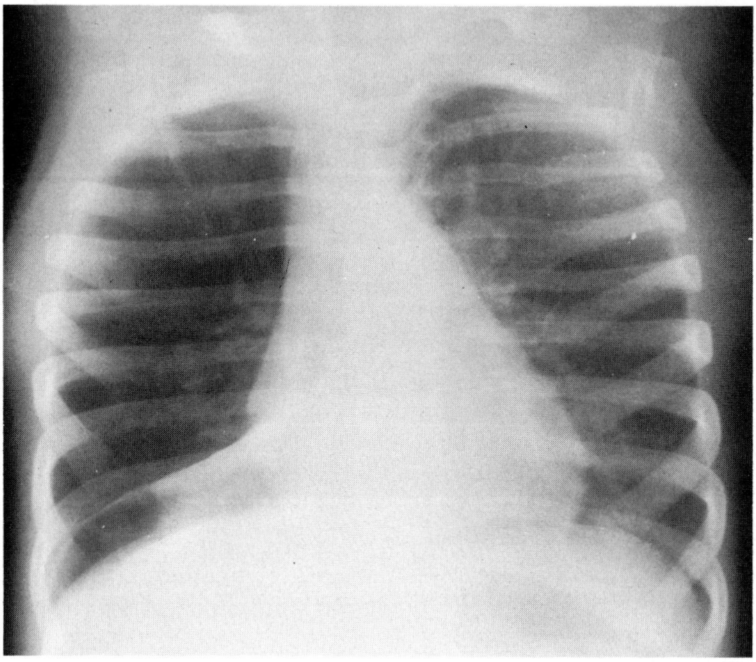

Figure 6. Atelectasis in right lower lobe secondary to "corking" of the bronchus with a pretzel.

sema, persistent or recurrent pneumonia, "atypical" asthma and unilateral wheeze.

X-Ray Studies

LATERAL VIEW OF NECK TAKEN DURING INSPIRATION. Expiratory films of the neck usually give more false (positive) information because the tissues are soft and pliable and usually fold, giving false shadows. Radiopaque foreign bodies will be apparent (Fig. 7).

ANTEROPOSTERIOR VIEW OF CHEST USING INSPIRATION-EXPIRATION FILMS. The classic approach is to look for obstructive emphysema and mediastinal shift, the Holznecht sign. Any lung that will fill with air, but incompletely empty unilaterally, will, on expiration, push the mediastinum toward the side which empties. The smaller the child, the more difficult it is to time this study correctly and, therefore, fluoroscopy is most helpful. If, for some reason, fluoroscopy is unavailable, then similar information requiring less timing may be obtained by taking decubitus films in the frontal projection; the dependent side should empty; if it does not, there is an obstructive emphysema (see Fig. 16).

LATERAL VIEW OF CHEST. The lateral chest x-ray is taken to help identify which segments are involved (see Fig. 17).

Technique

The general rule is to "make haste slowly." Deliberate measurements of the foreign body, selection of the appropriate bronchoscope and forceps, and formation of a preoperative plan are essential. For all but the most common foreign bodies preoperative trials at the practice board with a duplicate foreign body are most helpful and can frequently spell the difference between success and failure. Because the concentration of the operator is on the mechanical problem, there is a tendency to minimize or overlook subtleties in the child's general condition, such as his state of fluid and electrolytes, any existing abnormalities or underlying disease processes. With few exceptions—for example, vegetal foreign bodies in the trachea—most foreign bodies in the air passages will allow hours before endoscopy to carefully design the operation and manage associated medical problems. The use of aerosols, postural drainage and physiotherapy in an attempt to retrieve the airway foreign body should be reserved for those situations in which either experienced endoscopy is unavailable or the child is too sick for reasons other than the foreign body to allow for bronchoscopy.

Choice of Anesthesia

Whether or not general anesthesia is used depends on the nature of the foreign body, its location, the skill and experience of the endoscopist, the confidence of the holding team and the experience of the anesthesiologist. As a rule, all laryngeal or hypopharyngeal foreign bodies are most safely managed while the patient is awake. Certainly any child whose anatomy suggests possible difficulty in intubation (e.g., micrognathia) should be awake for the procedure.

The advantages of not using an inhalation anesthesia are a safe airway protected by all its reflexes, only one man dealing with the airway, the opening of the airway on deep inspiration and the possibility of the patient coughing up the foreign body through the bronchoscope without the need for forceps manipulation, the usually shorter duration of the procedure, the avoidance of inhalation anesthetics, and a wide-awake safe patient with active laryngeal and hypopharyngeal reflexes at the end of the procedure. The advantages of using general anesthesia are a quiet "cooperative" patient, the absence of patient anxiety, somewhat more time available for manipulation, the ability to employ larger bronchoscopes, and the expertise of the anesthesiologists brought to bear in an active participation in the care of the patient.

Administration of Anesthesia

Anesthesia is induced with nitrous oxide, oxygen and halothane by mask. An

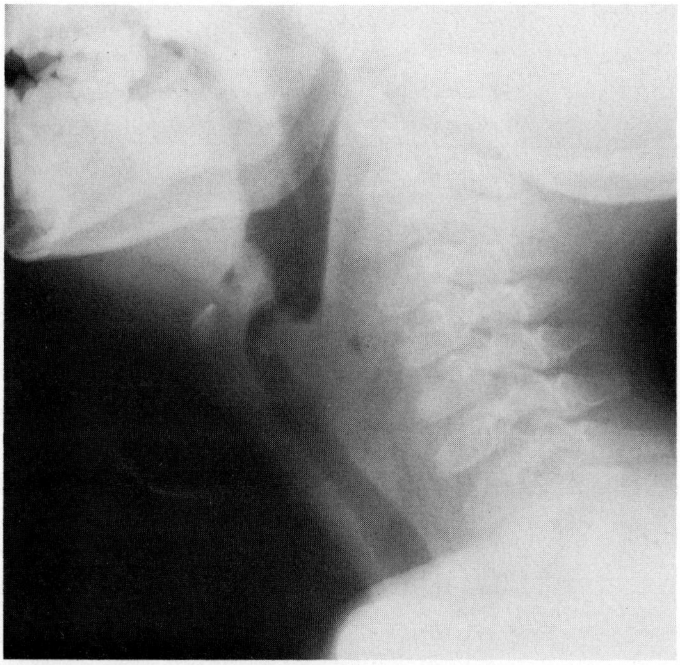

Figure 7. Lateral neck x-ray taken in inspiration. Note air in the esophagus. Esophagoscopy revealed impacted meat proximal to an esophageal stenosis.

intravenous infusion is started. Laryngoscopy is done to insure ease of bronchoscopic intubation and assure normal function. After the initial laryngoscopy, the patient is given halothane and oxygen by mask, and succinylcholine (1/2 to 1 mg. per pound) is administered intravenously; the bronchoscope is then introduced. Our preference in apparatus is the Sanders ventilating attachment or the Holinger ventilating bronchoscope.

An alternate method is to use either Penthrane or ether with the endoscopic manipulation done during the recovery phase. Apnea techniques have not been used in our clinics since the advent of halothane. For infants under 1 year of age oxygen alone is insufflated through the side arm of a Holinger ventilating bronchoscope.

Cooperation between the endoscopist and the anesthesiologist, with a constant flow of information between them, is critical. Ventilation of the patient with a Holinger apparatus is effected either by sealing the proximal end of the bronchoscope with a glass window or by intermittent "thumbing" of the proximal end of the bronchoscope.[11] Bradycardia suggests hypoventilation and priority is given to the anesthesiologist. The patient is monitored with a precordial stethoscope; occasionally a cardioscope is used.

When the grasp of the foreign body seems acceptable, the patient is allowed to recover spontaneous respirations, and the foreign body is removed.

The greater majority of the foreign body removals are done in a general operating room. Occasionally, a foreign body that has lodged peripherally will require, for its extraction, the use of x-ray guidance. These procedures are then performed under biplane fluoroscopy in the X-ray Department (Fig. 8).

ESOPHAGEAL FOREIGN BODIES

Much of the previous discussion regarding airway foreign bodies applies

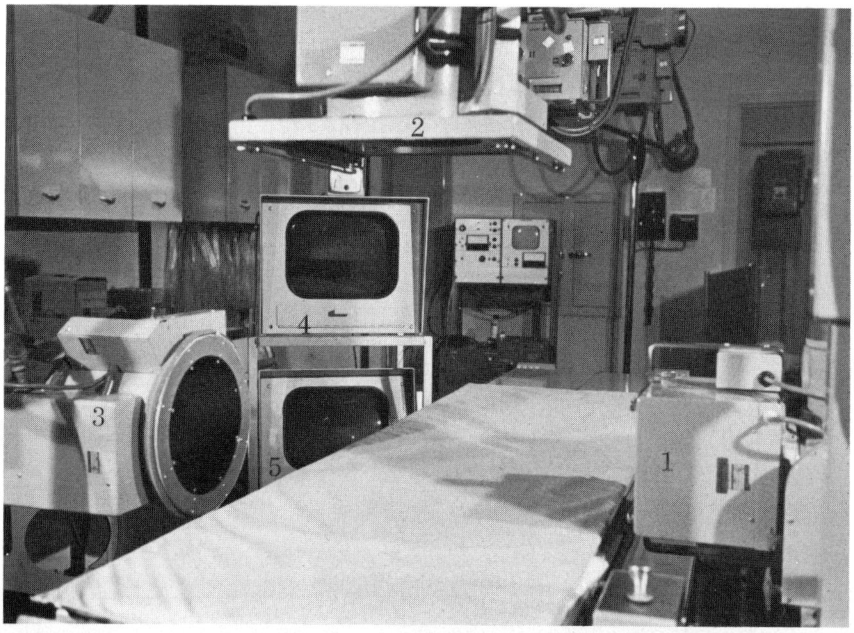

Figure 8. Biplane fluoroscope. (1) Tube for horizontal beam, (2) and (3) dual field 6"-9" image intensifiers for vertical and horizontal beam projections, (4) and (5) television monitors for horizontal and vertical beam projections. (From Norris, C. M., Tucker, G. F., Jr., and Woloshin, H. J.: Bronchoesophagologic application of recent advances in fluoroscopy. *Ann. Otol.*, 80:528, 1971.)

to foreign bodies of the swallowing passages: the group most at risk, the frequently negative history, the reliance on signs rather than symptoms, the need for complete x-ray study and the attention to minutia in technique. Because of the common wall between the upper airway and the upper esophagus, the initial symptoms are frequently laryngeal.

Subsequent signs and symptoms will, as with the airway foreign body, be a function of the pre-existing status of the esophagus, the relative size of the foreign body, the nature of the foreign body and disturbances in deglutition.

Pre-existing Status

In general, abnormalities of the esophagus frequently affect the site where the foreign body will arrest in its passage. Normally there are three areas of physiologic narrowing: the cricopharyngeus, the crossing of the aortic arch and the distal cardioesophageal sphincter. Such conditions as congenital stenosis, vascular compressions, repaired esophageal atresias, duplications, colon interpositions, strictures secondary to caustic esophagitis, ectopic gastric mucosa with inflammation or external compressions from mediastinal masses may all function to determine the level of the foreign body arrest.

Nature of the Foreign Body

Larger objects with irregular surfaces (bones, jacks) may arrest in their descent in the normal esophagus. In our experience in children, the hypopharynx and cervical esophagus are the most common sites. Open safety pins frequently lodge distally and, as with all sharp esophageal foreign bodies, create a sense of urgency. Smooth plastic objects of reasonable size appear to be able to negotiate the tract; however, some may create problems (see Fig. 24).

Disturbances of Deglutition

Obviously, if a foreign body completely obstructs the esophagus, excessive salivation and upper airway distress will eventually occur. But most esophageal foreign bodies do not completely obstruct; some enjoy a prolonged sojourn with minimal signs or symptoms for a considerable period of time (see Fig. 23).

Diagnosis

As with airway foreign bodies, the younger the child the more a negative history will obtain. The parent will usually present the child with a feeding problem. Older children frequently deny foreign body ingestion. Occasionally, hypopharyngeal and cervical esophageal foreign bodies will present as upper airway obstructions.

X-Ray Studies

Neck and chest x-rays will determine radiopaque foreign bodies. The films should be in both the lateral and anteroposterior planes. If positive, an x-ray should be taken in the plane of the largest diameter of the foreign body because of the ease of identification, (especially of flat bones and plates of metal which are seen best on end); the need for the endoscopist to have a three-dimensional concept of the foreign body; and the appreciation of rouleaux in the problem of multiple coins. If, in spite of negative plain x-rays, the clinical evidence for an esophageal foreign body is compelling, if the esophagus is widened on lateral x-ray of the neck, or if there is air in the upper esophagus (see Fig. 7), then a barium esophagram is done. The danger that the child will aspirate in such cases is real, but the information must be obtained. Techniques of barium esophagram using things such as cotton pledgets have been of no help to us and frequently confuse the endoscopic picture.

Choice of Anesthesia

As stated before, any child with an acute airway problem caused by a laryngeal or hypopharyngeal foreign body is, in our opinion, best managed

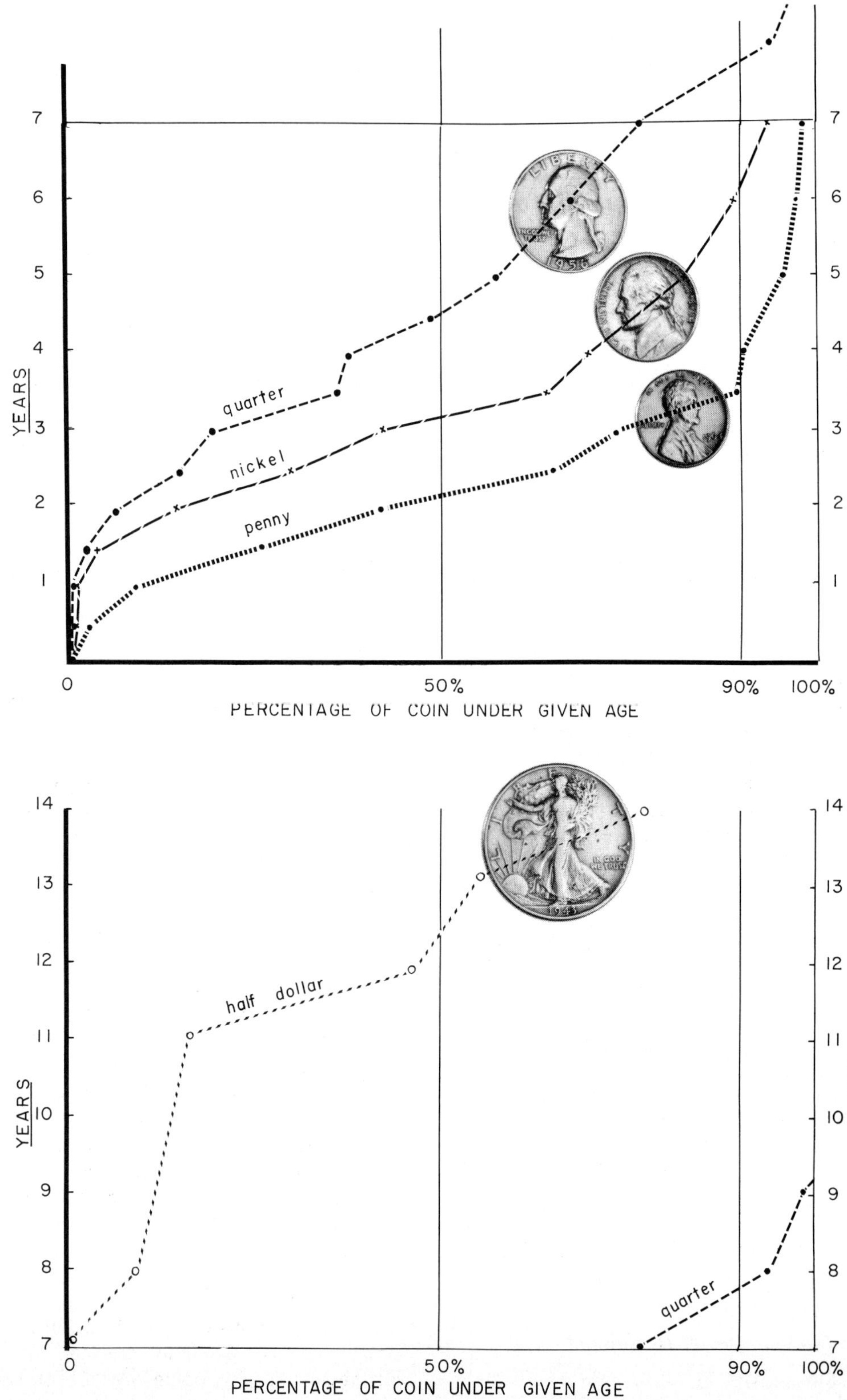

7
6
5
4
3
2
1
YEARS
quarter
nickel
penny
0
50%
90%
100%
PERCENTAGE OF COIN UNDER GIVEN AGE
14
13
12
11
10
9
8
7
YEARS
half dollar
quarter
0
50%
90%
100%
PERCENTAGE OF COIN UNDER GIVEN AGE

Figure 9.

while he is awake. In general, all esophageal foreign bodies below the cricopharyngeus are removed endoscopically under general anesthesia delivered through an endotracheal tube.

The orotracheal tube must not enter the esophagus during intubation if the foreign body is in the cervical esophagus. Anesthesiologists often pass a nasogastric tube to decompress the stomach; this is, of course, contraindicated in the presence of an esophageal foreign body. With endotracheal intubation it is common practice to breathe for the patient by having the anesthesiologist squeeze the inflatable bag. In such a system inspiration is obtained by creating an endothoracic pressure which is greater than atmospheric pressure. When such pressure is present around it the esophagus tends to collapse around the foreign object, since the esophagoscope keeps the endoesophageal pressure at atmospheric level. A bulky foreign body, such as a jackstone, in the cervical esophagus may displace the posterior tracheal wall anteriorly and thus make intubation difficult.

A coin lodged in the esophagus may well pass into the stomach when anesthesia is induced or even after sedation is administered. Review of the relationship between coin denomination (i.e., size) and age of the patient suggests that the likelihood of a coin passing on can be estimated,[9] and this estimate is then used in selecting management (Fig. 9 *A* and *B*).

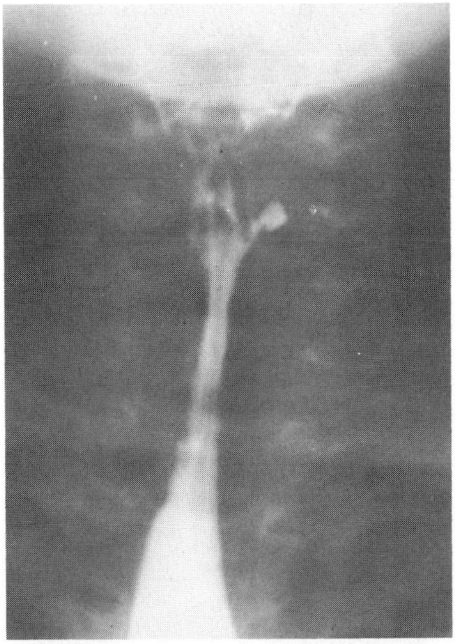

Figure 10. Sinus following removal of jackstone.

COMPLICATIONS

Complications from peroral endoscopy in infants and children should be uncommon. The complications seen as a result of endoscopic removal of foreign bodies therefore are largely a result of the foreign body itself, the peculiarities of its presentation and the length of time that has elapsed from ingestion or aspiration to removal. Most complications occur *before* the attempt at removal; the most common complications are pneumothorax, mediastinitis, pneumomediastinum, croup, pneumonia, airway obstruction, dysphagia or odynophagia or death. In general, complications occur in less than 2 per cent of procedures (Figs. 10, 11 and 12).

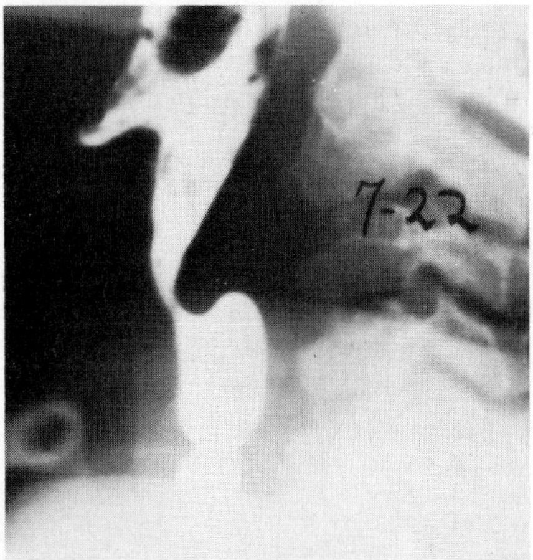

Figure 11. Granulations and stenosis following toy extraction.

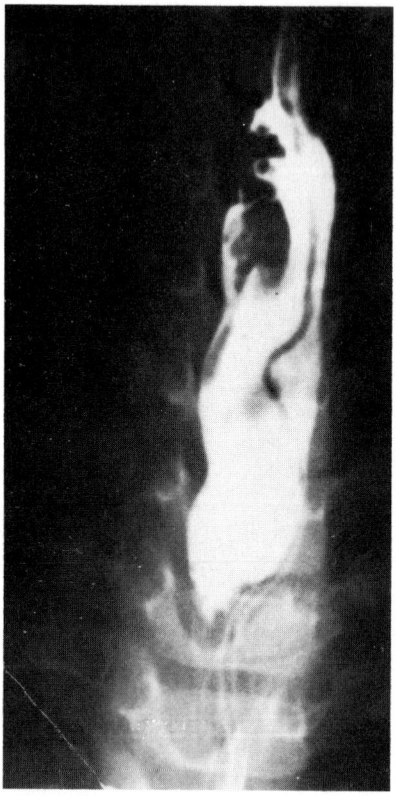

Figure 12. Granulations following spring extraction.

ILLUSTRATIVE CASES

General Discussion

The technique of endoscopic foreign body removal in infants and children requires meticulous preoperative attention to detail. As with all pediatric bronchoesophagological operations, selection of the proper size of endoscope is critical. Too large an instrument will unnecessarily traumatize tissues; one which is too small will limit the operator's ability to manipulate the foreign body. Rigid rules regarding appropriate sizes of endoscopes should be avoided, but Table 1 may serve as a general guide. The forceps and aspirators selected must be tested preoperatively for fit as well as function.

More than 60 per cent of all pediatric foreign bodies are esophageal and, of them, about two-thirds are located at or just below the pyriform apex (Figs. 13, 14 and 15). The Forbes esophageal speculum allows easy access to these "high" foreign bodies and permits the use of laryngeal forceps; the shorter working distance simplifies the extraction considerably. Coins in the esophagus are the most common pediatric foreign body.

Peanuts have been our most common foreign body in the air passage (see Fig. 16). Almost all other airway foreign bodies have been problems unique to themselves, requiring considerable preoperative planning. The value of a duplicate foreign body for preoperative practice with a manikin, of selection of appropriate forceps, of practicing point of grasp and of consideration of problems of rotation, endoscopic anatomy and sharp-edge protection cannot be overemphasized.

Bronchial Peanut

Figure 16 shows a 2-year-old male who aspirated a peanut. Presenting complaint: "swallowed a peanut and choked." Auscultation: expiratory

TABLE 1

	Laryngoscope*	Bronchoscope**	Esophagoscope**
Newborn	7, 9	2½, 3	3
10–20 lbs.	9	3, 3½	4
20–30 lbs.	9, 10½	3½, 3¾, 4	4, 5
30–40 lbs.	10½	4	5
50–70 lbs.	10½, 11, 12	4, 5	5

*Numbers refer to working length in centimeters.
**Numbers refer to internal diameter in millimeters.

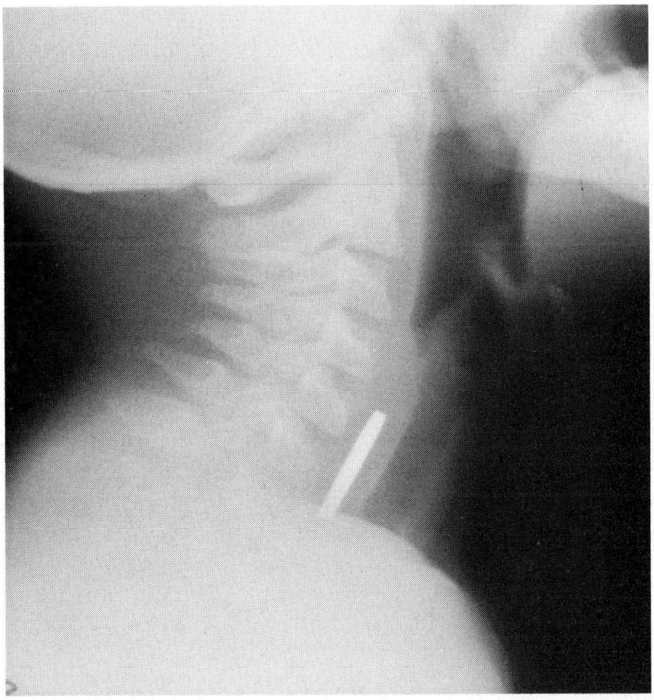

Figure 13. Common presentation for esophageal coin.

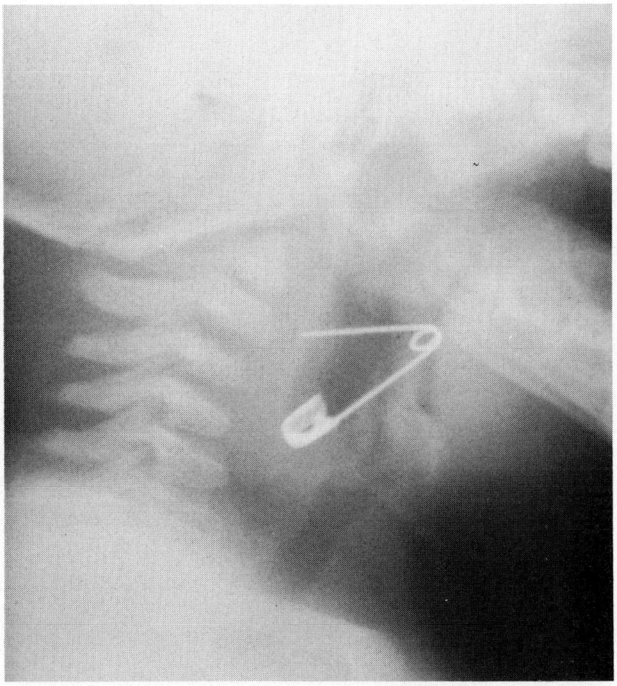

Figure 14. Hypopharyngeal presentation of open safety pin.

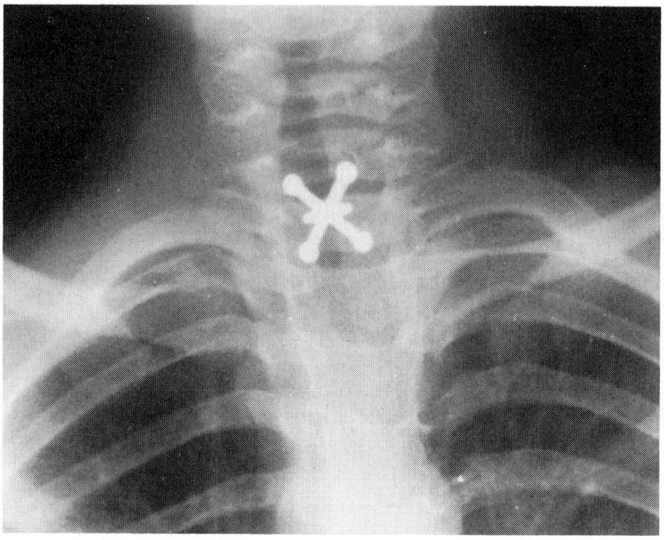

Figure 15. Usual position for jackstone.

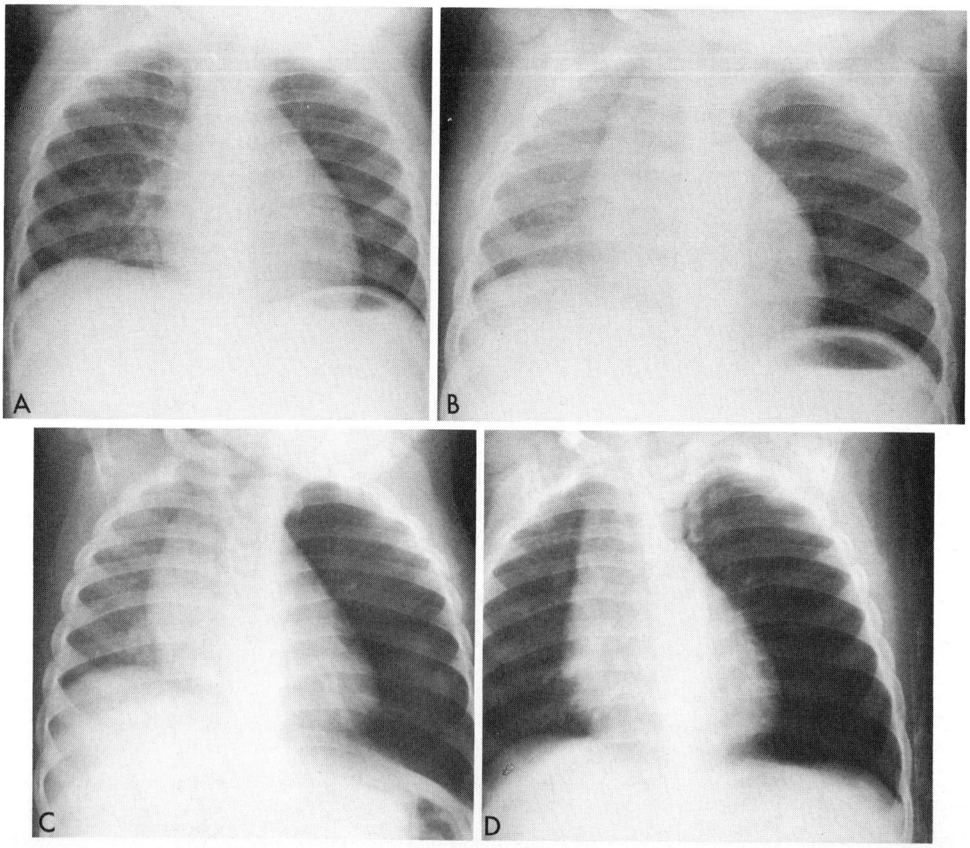

Figure 16. Bronchial peanut present during inspiration (*A*) and expiration (*B*). *C*, Lateral decubitus film taken with right side down; right side empties. *D*, Lateral decubitus film taken with left side down; left side does not empty.

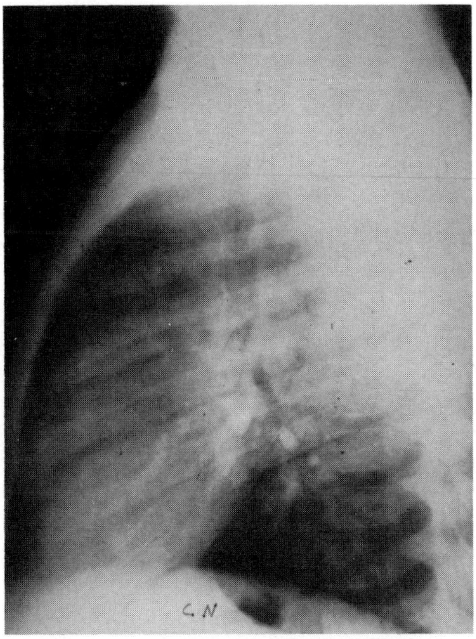

Figure 17. Glass in multiple bronchi.

wheeze over entire left chest. X-rays lateral: obstructive emphysema. Bronchoscope: 4 × 30 Holinger. Presenting part: one-half peanut in left main bronchus. Forceps: Jackson fenestrated peanut. Complications: none.

COMMENT. This case represents a fairly typical sequence of events for patients who have aspirated peanuts.

Glass

Figure 17 shows a 20-month-old male who aspirated multiple fragments of glass. Presenting complaint: cough. Hx: negative for foreign body. X-ray: multiple radiopaque 1/2-cm. squares throughout lungs. Anesthesia: general. Bronchoscope: 4 × 30. Presenting part: edges of glass. Forceps: Jesberg fenestrated peanut. Complications: none.

COMMENT. This child aspirated multiple safety glass fragments when thrown through the windshield during an auto accident.

Rubber Bottle Stopper

Figure 18 shows a 6-year-old boy who aspirated a rubber bottle stopper. Presenting complaint: recurrent left lower lobe pneumonia for eight months. Hx: negative for foreign body. Anesthesia: general. Bronchoscope: 4 × 30 Holinger ventilating. Presenting part: granulations over edge of rubber bottle stopper. Forceps: Jesberg fenestrated peanut. Grasp: edge of foreign body. Complications: required several subsequent bronchoscopies to remove exuberant granulations.

COMMENT. Unsuspected foreign body presenting as recurrent pneumonia.

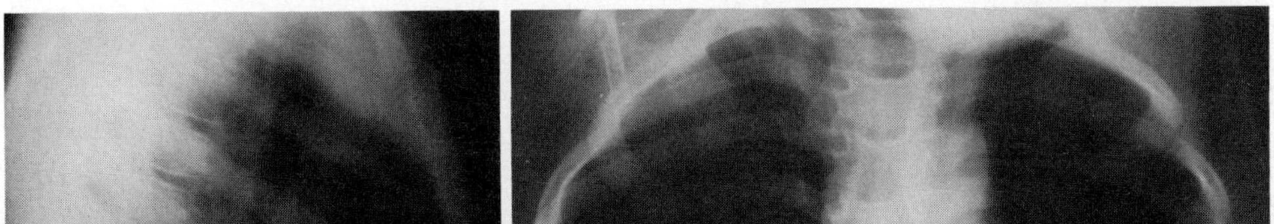

Figure 18. Lateral (*A*) and anteroposterior (*B*) views of bronchial rubber stopper.

Styrofoam

Figure 19 shows styrofoam present in a 17-month-old male. Presenting complaint: "fever and fast breathing." Hx: negative for foreign body. X-rays: infiltration, atelectasis and pneumothorax. Anesthesia: general. Bronchoscope: 4 × 30. Presenting part: white, wet, soft material in bronchial orifices of right middle lobe, right lower lobe and left lower lobe. Forceps: Jackson forward grasping. Complications: required two separate bronchoscopies for extraction cure.

COMMENT. This youngster presenting with pulmonary infiltrates, atelectasis and pneumothorax was, in spite of a firm negative history, an excellent candidate for an airway foreign body.

Common Pin

A 20-month-old female is seen in Figure 20. Presenting complaint: cough. X-ray: pin. Anesthesia: none. Laryngoscope: $10^1/_2$ side slide Jackson. Presenting part: pin shaft. Forceps: laryngeal grasping. Extraction: disempaction caudally and removal. Complications: none.

COMMENT. The assumption here is that the child aspirated the foreign body and coughed it up, imbedding the point into the anterior tracheal mucosa.

Coin

Figure 21 illustrates a 2-year-old girl who swallowed two coins. Presenting complaint: parents saw the child "swallow a nickel." Child asymptomatic. X-ray: showed "coin." Anesthesia: none. Esophagoscope: Forbes esophageal speculum. Presenting part: edges of two nickels in rouleaux. Forceps: laryngeal grasping. Complications: none.

COMMENT. A case of two foreign bodies in the esophagus. The child subsequently recalled swallowing the other coin two weeks prior to this one.

Jackstone

Figure 22 shows a jackstone in the esophagus of a 4-year-old boy. Present-

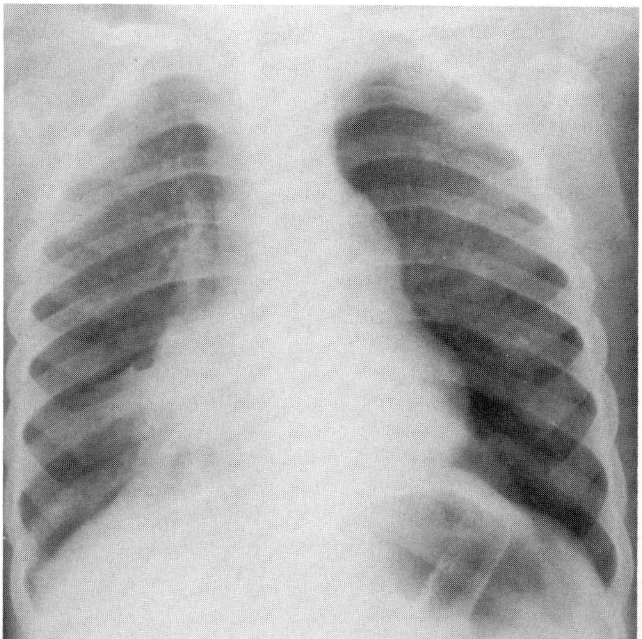

Figure 19. Bronchial styrofoam.

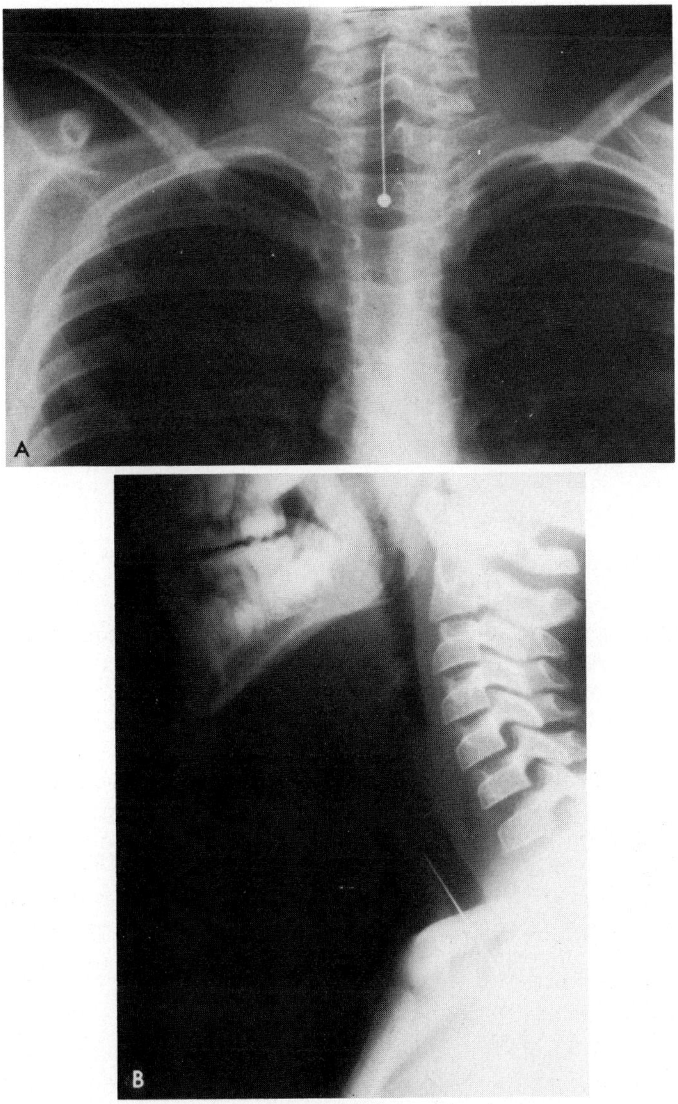

Figure 20. Anteroposterior (*A*) and lateral (*B*) views of a hat pin in the trachea.

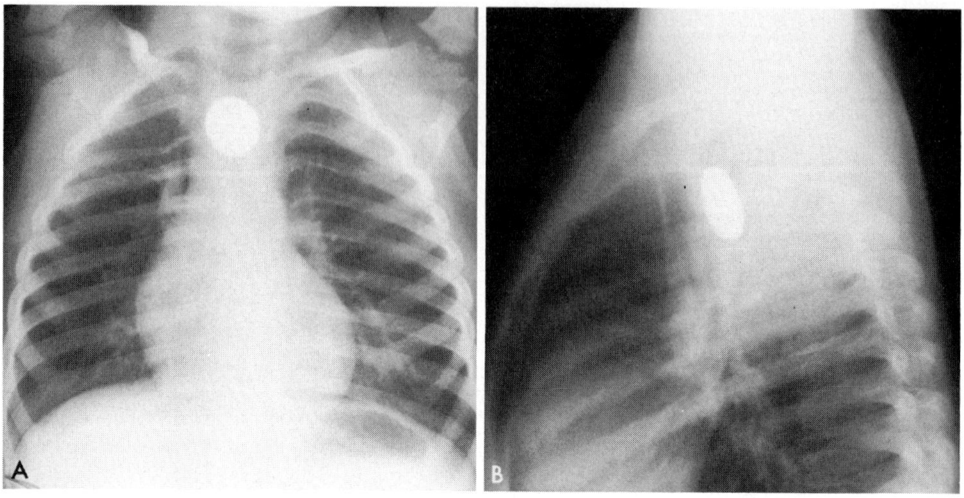

Figure 21. Esophageal coins (rouleaux) shown in anteroposterior (*A*) and lateral (*B*) views.

ing complaint: dysphagia. Hx: negative for foreign body. Anesthesia: general. Esophagoscope: Forbes esophageal speculum. Presenting part: ball. Forceps: ball. Complications: required tracheotomy ten hours after esophagoscopy.

COMMENT. Jackstones are a fairly common foreign body of the older child. Even with positive x-ray the children frequently deny ingestion. Because of the irregular shape, large size, rigidity and high level of presentation some airway distress occurs in about one-third of cases.

Wire Spring

Figure 23 shows a wire spring in the esophagus of a 14-month-old male. Presenting complaint: recurrent croup, bronchitis and cough for six months. Hx: negative for foreign body. X-ray: spring in midthorax. Barium swallow: barium column narrowed; not in contact with coils of spring. Anesthesia: general, via woodbridge. Esophagoscope: 6 × 20 Holinger. Presenting part: granulation. Forceps: laryngeal grasping. Complications: manipulation of spring dislodged endotracheal tube; bronchoscope was required to establish airway.

COMMENT. Long-standing esophageal foreign body presenting with respiratory complaints. Foreign body so completely embedded as to be invisible endoscopically. Symmetrical periluminal object required biplane fluoroscopic guidance. Final result: extraction cure.

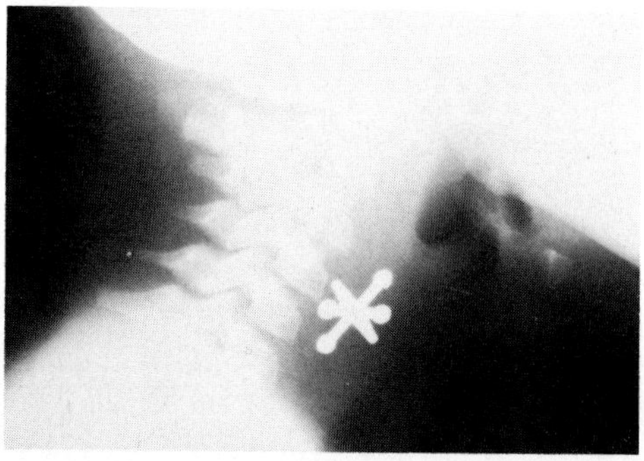

Figure 22. Jackstone present in esophagus.

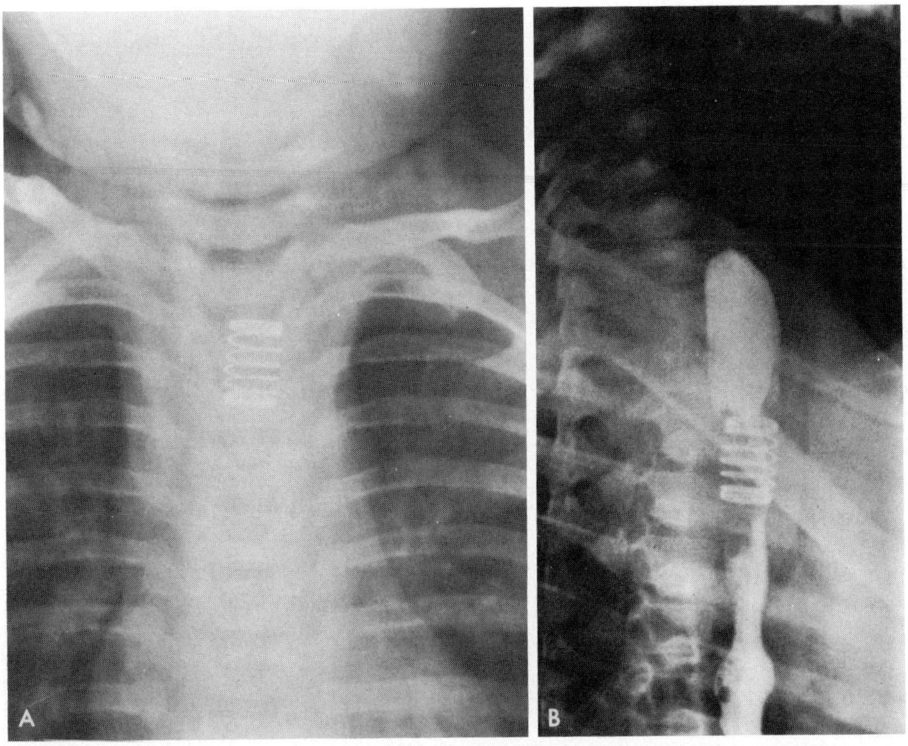

Figure 23. *A*, Spring in esophagus. *B*, Spring seen during barium study.

Plastic Wheels and Axle

Figure 24 shows a 3-year-old girl with a plastic toy in the esophagus. Presenting complaint: parents saw the child swallow and gag on foreign body ten months prior to admission. Child cachectic. Could only swallow liquids. X-ray: confirmed foreign body with barium coating. Anesthesia: general. Esophagoscope: Forbes esophageal speculum. Presenting part: upper wheel. Forceps: laryngeal rotation. Complications: tracheotomy, gastrostomy for retrograde dilatations of esophageal stenosis.

COMMENT. The parents of this child saw many physicians over the ten-month period. Plain x-rays of neck and chest were done repeatedly. Finally an otolaryngologist saw the foreign body during mirror laryngoscopy. A barium swallow confirmed the foreign body.

Open Safety Pin

Figure 25 shows a 16-month-old male who swallowed an open safety pin. Presenting complaint: "won't eat and irritable." X-ray: showed "open safety pin." Anesthesia: general. Esophagoscope: 4 Jackson. Presenting part: keeper. Forceps: ring rotation. Grasp: spring. Extraction by version. Complications: none.

COMMENT. Jackson described sixteen methods to remove open safety pins from the esophagus. Basically there are three techniques: (1) advancing into the stomach, turning and removing with a dangling "trailing point," i.e., version; (2) point protection, usually by sheathing the point in the esophagoscope with direct removal; and (3) closing techniques (most difficult and definitely not for the novice).

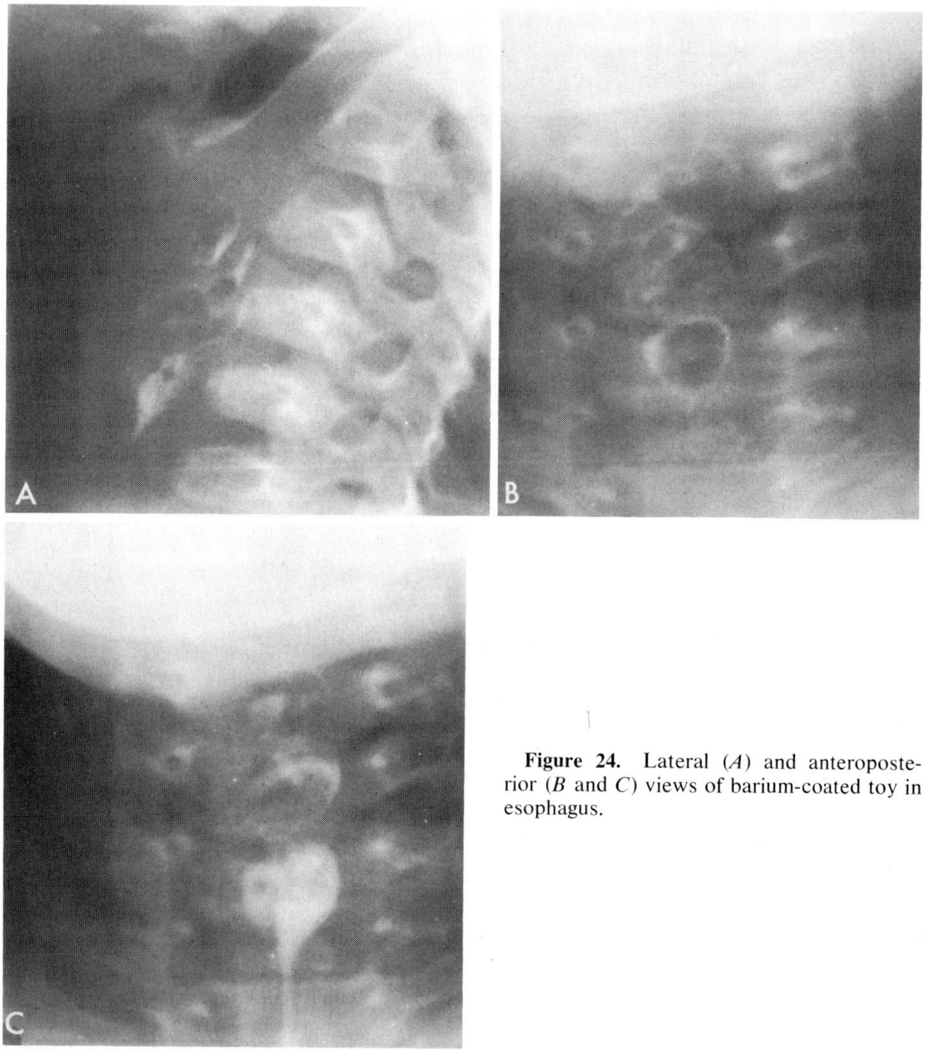

Figure 24. Lateral (*A*) and anteroposterior (*B* and *C*) views of barium-coated toy in esophagus.

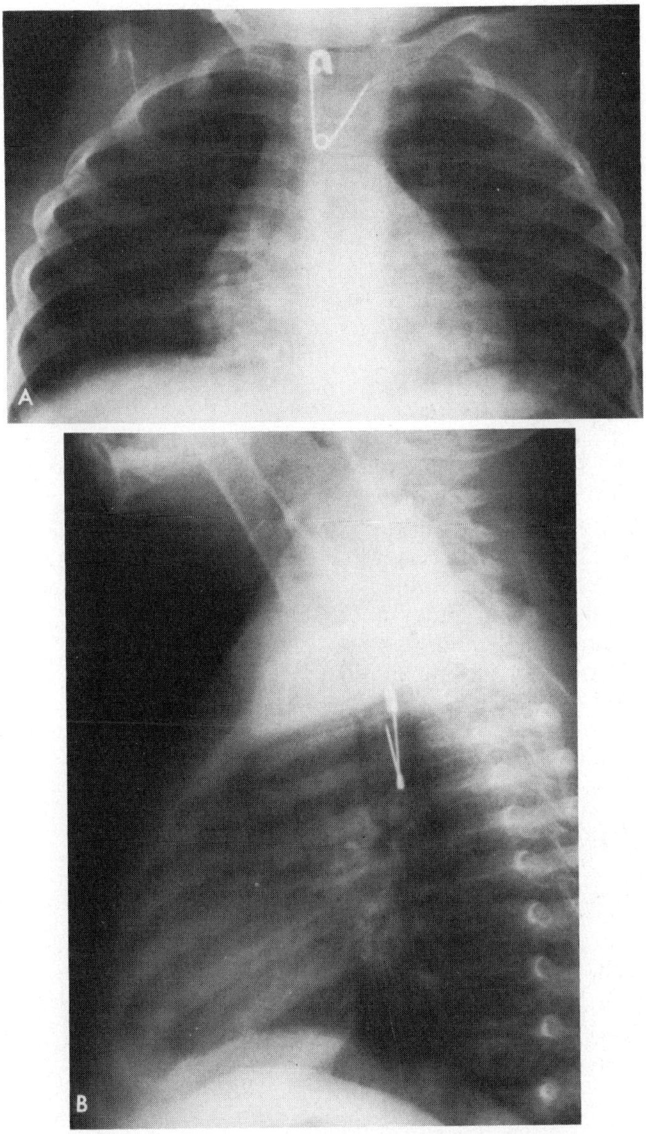

Figure 25. Anteroposterior (*A*) and lateral (*B*) views of an open safety pin.

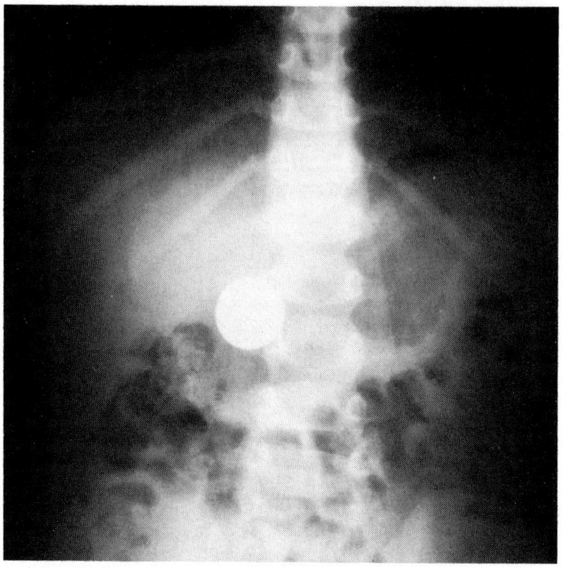

Figure 26. Coin in stomach.

Gastric Coin

Figure 26 shows a 3-year-old male who swallowed a coin. Presenting complaint: "swallowed quarter." X-ray: coin in stomach. Anesthesia: general. Esophagoscope: 5 Jackson. Presenting part: edge of coin in stomach. Forceps: forward grasping under fluoroscopic guidance. Complications: none.

COMMENT. The coin had been in the stomach for at least nine weeks. The child had a repair of a pyloric stenosis as an infant with subsequent scarring.

REFERENCES

1. Equen, M.: *Magnetic Removal of Foreign Bodies.* Springfield, Ill. Charles C Thomas, Publishers, 1951.
2. Gross, S.: *A Practical Treatise on Foreign Bodies in the Air-Passages.* Philadelphia, Blanchard & Lea, XVI, 468, 1854.
3. Holinger, P. H.: Foreign Bodies in the Air and Food Passages. XVII Wherry Memorial Lecture. *Trans. Amer. Acad. Ophthal. Otolaryng.,* 66:210, 1962.
4. Jackson, C., and Jackson, C. L.: *Diseases of the Air and Food Passages of Foreign-Body Origin.* Philadelphia, W. B. Saunders Co., 1936.
5. Jackson, C., and Jackson, C. L.: *Diseases of the Nose, Throat, and Ear.* 2nd ed. Philadelphia, W. B. Saunders Co., 1959, pp. 842–855.
6. Krumperman, L., Tucker, G. F., Jr., and Norris, C. M.: Adaptation of the Sanders Ventilating Attachment to the Side Arm of the Holinger Bronchoscope. *Ann. Otol.,* 79:958, 1970.
7. Morse, H. R., and Hartman, M. M.: General Anesthesia for Peroral Endoscopy, Apneic Technique. *Ann. Otol.,* 75:1040, 1966.
8. Norris, C. M., Tucker, G. F., and Woloshin, H. J.: Bronchoesophagologic Application of Recent Advances in Fluoroscopy. *Ann. Otol.,* 80:528, 1971.

8a. Tucker, G.: A New Method of Removal of Foreign Bodies from the Stomach with the Author's Sheathed Flexible Gastroscopic Forceps. *J.A.M.A.,* 105:1596–1597, Nov. 16, 1935.

9. Tucker, G. F., Jr.: The Age Incidence of Lodgement of Single Coins in the Esophagus. *Trans. Amer. Broncho-Esoph. Assn.,* 44:145, 1964.
10. Tucker, G. F., Jr.: Laryngeal and Tracheobronchial Foreign Bodies. *Trans. Penn. Acad. Ophthal.,* 19:12, 1966.
11. Tucker, G. F., Jr.: Anesthesia in Peroral Endoscopy. *Otolaryng. Clin. N. Amer.,* 1:37, 1968.
12. Tucker, G. F., Jr.: Report of the Committee for the Prevention of Foreign Body Accidents. *Trans. Amer. Broncho-Esoph. Assn.,* 49:181, 1969.
13. Tucker, G. F., Jr., Adriani, J., Atkins, J., Fearon, B., and Benson, D. W.: Symposium: Anesthesia in Peroral Endoscopy. *Trans. Amer. Broncho-Esoph. Assn.,* 49:116, 1969.
14. Turtz, M. G., and Tucker, G. F., Jr.: The Present Day Spectrum of Pediatric Bronchoesophagology. *Laryngoscope.* June 1972.
15. Weston, J. T.: Airway Foreign Body Fatalities in Children. *Trans. Amer. Broncho-Esoph. Assn.,* 45:105, 1965.

Chapter One Hundred Ten

BRONCHOGRAPHY IN INFANTS AND CHILDREN

CHARLES F. FERGUSON, M.D., F.A.C.S.

Frequently it is desirable, and sometimes even necessary, to obtain more information regarding the tracheobronchial tree than can be detected by a simple roentgenographic study or a bronchoscopic examination. This is especially true when an underlying congenital malformation is suspected, or when the presence or extent of a suspected bronchiectatic process should be determined. Although endoscopic examination should always be performed first, bronchographic studies virtually extend the range of visualization directly into the more peripheral, and therefore more inaccessible, recesses of the lower bronchopulmonary segments.

HISTORICAL DEVELOPMENT OF CONTRAST MEDIA

In 1918, Jackson described the use of bismuth subcarbonate powder insufflated through a bronchoscope, a technique he had been using for 11 years to delineate foreign bodies or to attempt to outline abscess cavities. It was difficult, however, to visualize much beyond the carina or portions of the main bronchi. In 1922, Sicard and Forestier introduced Lipiodol, a 40 per cent freely flowing iodized poppyseed oil that was in continuous and universal use for well over 30 years. Its main disadvantage was that it frequently flowed too readily into the alveolar spaces, and troublesome overfilling resulted. It also persisted in the lung too long after instillation, with a theoretical danger of iodism. It was, however, a very satisfactory contrast medium, and today it still has its place in bronchography in infants, in whom the other media tend sometimes to cause severe untoward reactions. In order to make it less freely flowing, the Fougera Company later added sulfanilamide to Lipiodol (Visciodol), but the oil then became too thick, and the added drug was found undesirable in many allergic individuals.

Three years later, the first aqueous contrast medium was developed in England by the Glaxo Company. This was Dionosil (propyliodine), an aqueous suspension of 30 per cent iodine compounds, but it caused considerable local irritation, as well as frequent febrile reactions. So, in 1956 Dionosil Oily was produced. This obviated the use of a thickening agent necessary for aqueous products (carboxymethyl-cellulose), which tended to obstruct the smaller bronchi and bronchioles, thereby producing hypoxia. It was less irritating and its 4 per cent greater iodine content gave better contrast. However, it had the disadvantage of all oily preparations in that it tended to produce more alveolarization than is desirable.

In 1961, the Fougera Company came out with Hytrast, a 50 per cent aqueous suspension of various small-sized particles of iodine compounds, with a minimum of carboxymethyl-cellulose. This preparation was at first considered nearly ideal, but later was found to produce areas of focal pneumonitis with deposition of crystals, persisting for as long as a month, as well as considerable local and systemic reaction, and was removed from the market. The iodine compounds were too slowly eliminated. If absorbed, iodine compounds in general are systemically toxic, and absorption can take place through the gastrointestinal tract as well as through the respiratory tract. Oily or aqueous preparations have limited radiopacity, and in addition require a larger volume, which fills and even partially obstructs the airway, rather than merely coating it.

More recently, microbarium (barium sulfate in saline solution, with a little carboxymethyl-cellulose added) has been employed as a radiopaque medium, but in this country it has not been obtainable, as it has not been licensed by the Federal Drug Administration. Because it consists of very minute particles, it is not too dangerous in the respiratory tract. It is rapidly eliminated systemically (although not from the bronchi), and it is nontoxic and nonirritating.

Since 1968, the most hopeful agent, used as yet only experimentally and not at present approved otherwise by the FDA, is tantalum powder. Nadel and others from the University of California, who began the use of this agent, feel that it is nontoxic, 25 times more radiopaque than iodine compounds, and that it adheres much better to the mucosa than do liquid media. It is not dispersed by respiratory movements or by coughing. Since smaller amounts are used, it does not interfere with pulmonary function. The powder is blown by compressed air from a grounded flask through a catheter introduced into the tracheobronchial tree. Because the powder merely coats the mucosal lining of the airway and does not flood the lumen, better physiologic studies of dynamic behavior can be obtained. The appearance and behavior of the tracheobronchial tree can be permanently recorded on cineradiographic film, and a beautiful demonstration, literally in 3 dimensions, is produced. The tantalum particles measure 2.5 mμ. in diameter, and only 0.5 mgm. is needed even in an adult. This medium clears rapidly from the airway, and is usually not visible 24 to 48 hours after insufflation. Microscopic examination of bronchial and pulmonary tissues after its use has shown no abnormal histologic changes, and if a few particles happen to be retained, there is no surrounding inflammatory reaction. Unfortunately, the FDA has not as yet licensed this very promising agent for general use, but clearance is anticipated soon.

Thus, bronchography has come a full cycle during the past 50 years, from Jackson's bismuth powder through oily preparations, then to aqueous media, and now back to powder again. The completely ideal agent is still not available, but such a preparation should have the following specifications if it is truly ideal: good ability to adhere to the tracheobronchial mucosal surfaces, and not fill the lumen of the bronchi; good radiopacity and contrast visualization; no alveolarization to obscure finer details; nontoxic and nonobstructive; and prompt and safe elimination.

INDICATIONS FOR BRONCHOGRAPHY

It is impossible to describe all indications for this valuable diagnostic procedure, as each patient always presents a special, individual problem. When there is airway obstruction, or when a more accurate evaluation of pulmonary disease cannot otherwise be made, bronchography is most valuable, and a very important addition to our diagnostic armamentarium. Confronted with a specific problem, the physician should consider the following possible indications.

Chronic Cough Not Otherwise Satisfactorily Explained. X-ray studies of the chest may be normal, and clinical examination of the patient may show very little to account for persistent symptoms. Endoscopic examination followed by contrast medium studies may show minimal bronchiectasis, stenosis of a bronchus, compression of the trachea from nodes, a cyst, a tumor, or commonly from vascular anomalies of the aortic arch or great vessels, tracheoesophageal fistula without atresia of the esophagus, or possibly a nonopaque foreign body that does not obstruct the airway sufficiently to produce the usual signs of emphysema, atelectasis or chronic pneumonitis.

CHRONIC PULMONARY CHANGES DEMONSTRABLE BY ROUTINE X-RAY STUDIES. When localized emphysema or atelectasis is present, further investigation of the cause is always indicated, unless it has already been discovered by bronchoscopy. Constant increased lung markings or persistent evidence of unresolved pneumonia is another indication. Occasionally, unsuspected agenesis of the lung is found after the contrast medium is injected into the tracheobronchial tree.

PERSISTENT WHEEZING. Wheezing, especially when localized to one particular area of the chest, may be associated with or independent of recurrent respiratory infections. Such cases may show an unrecognized bronchial stenosis, a nonopaque foreign body, external compression from without, due to mediastinal masses or large lymph nodes, or vascular anomalies producing such compression. Asthma is sometimes erroneously diagnosed in such cases, but rhonchi and wheezing localized to only one particular area of the chest are most unusual findings in true asthma. One must always recall the famous aphorism of Jackson that "all that wheezes is not asthma."

RECURRENT ATTACKS OF PNEUMONITIS IN THE SAME AREA OF THE LUNG. Here only the past history gives a diagnostic lead, because between attacks there are no symptoms, such as chronic cough, and no signs or pulmonary changes are detected on physical examination or by the usual x-ray studies. There is a history, however, of many prior admissions to the hospital for pneumonitis, always localized in one particular area of the chest (as for example in the right upper or right middle lobe). Congenital malformation of the supplying bronchus must always be considered as a cause. The right upper lobe bronchus is the most anomalous bronchus, and frequently has an abnormal origin just *above* the carina. Such a bronchus may be angulated, twisted or stenosed, and therefore is frequently the cause of recurrent or unresolved pneumonitis, persistent emphysema or atelectasis in that lobe. The middle lobe syndrome of Brock with chronic cough, productive sputum, occasional hemoptysis, and recurrent middle lobe pneumonitis, is very difficult to diagnose unless bronchographic studies are performed.

HEMOPTYSIS. In the younger age group, this is a rare symptom as compared with adults, but when it does occur it always suggests serious underlying disease. Bronchiectasis usually caused by cystic fibrosis is the commonest source of hemoptysis in the young, but occasionally a foreign body is the responsible agent. Bronchial tumors are rare in the younger age group, but nearly 20 bronchial adenomas have been reported in the literature (Vawter and Ferguson, 1958).

CHRONIC STRIDOR. Stridor that is not explained by careful laryngoscopic examination must be considered an indication for bronchographic studies. The typical patient with laryngomalacia ordinarily has simply an inspiratory type of stridor. If, however, the stridor is expiratory or biphasic, compression of the trachea or main bronchi must be suspected. Sometimes this is not apparent even on endoscopic examination, or on the ordinary chest film, but further studies are necessary. Tracheal or bronchial stenosis may be due to malformation of the anatomic wall, but in most instances the obstruction is due to compression from without, and frequently it is produced by an anomaly of the aortic arch or great vessels. Unless there is a true vascular ring going all the way around the esophagus, as is seen with a double aortic arch or a right aortic arch with a left ligamentum arteriosum, esophagoscopy and barium studies may be negative, even if severe signs of airway obstruction are present.

CONTRAINDICATIONS TO BRONCHOGRAPHY

There are very few contraindications to bronchographic studies in infants or children of any age, if it is felt that information so obtained would be of value either diagnostically or therapeutically. Such an indication would in most cases warrant the very slight risk involved. However, these studies should not be performed during the acute stage of a febrile infection or immediately following an episode of acute pulmonary disease. When this infection has been properly controlled, and the patient is still maintained on antibiotic therapy, there should be no increased risk. If the patient has asthma and an investigation of the tracheobronchial tree is also indicated, especially if there is a suspicion of bronchiectasis or a foreign body, the acute asthmatic attack can first be treated by the use of antihistamines or steroids. When the acute stage has been brought under control, bronchography can be safely performed.

Tuberculosis was formerly considered a contraindication to bronchography. With more effective drug therapy, however, there is very little chance of dissemination of the disease or reactivation of a tuberculosis infection if the patient is properly controlled by long-term antituberculosis therapy, such as Isoniazid. Obviously, this procedure should not be performed until the disease has been adequately stabilized. Cardiac failure or serious heart disease in the past has been suggested as contraindication to bronchography, but sometimes such studies in infants and young children will be of great value in the treatment of the underlying cardiac situation. Here again, the heart disease must be properly controlled beforehand, and the patient should be protected preoperatively with antibiotics. If general anesthesia is used for the bronchoscopy and contrast medium studies, extra oxygen is employed during the induction stage of the anesthesia. The dye is then aspirated *immediately* following the films in order to minimize the possibility of hypoxia.

Fortunately, iodine sensitivity in children is relatively rare as compared to adults. In 1967, the Committee on Bronchoesophagology of The American College of Chest Physicians sent out a questionnaire to 108 doctors. Iodine sensitivity was reported to be the most frequent contraindication to bronchography in adults. Since Dionosil, which today is the most commonly used radiopaque preparation, does not free iodine, there is less chance of iodism than with some of the other contrast media. If iodism is a concern, the stomach may be washed out following the procedure or starch may be given to absorb the iodine, because there is more danger when the dye is coughed up and then swallowed into the stomach than there is from direct absorption through the mucosa of the tracheobronchial tree. If iodine sensitivity is suspected, preoperative skin tests could be employed. When tantalum powder or microbarium can be used on a wider scale than at present, such possibilities of iodism will be eliminated.

COMPLICATIONS OF BRONCHOGRAPHY

Complications are infrequent when it is considered how commonly bronchographic studies are performed today. Frequently these procedures are done under difficult circumstances, often by physicians with little background, training, or experience, and such men may have had little exposure to bronchoesophagology. In the report of the Committee of the American College of Chest Physicians, it was estimated that the combined experience of 108 participants (39 radiologists, 33 thoracic surgeons, 20 otolaryngologists, and 16 chest physicians) who answered the questionnaire entailed about 100,000 bronchograms. In this entire group, 18 deaths were reported, three of them due to cardiac arrest, but most of the others were in children (or adults) with limited respiratory reserve who from the beginning were poor risks for the procedure.

If bronchographic studies are definitely indicated in patients with poor pulmonary function, both lungs should not be filled at once, but examination should be directed only to the suspected area. If local anesthesia is used, toxic reaction to the anesthetic drug has to be considered as a possible cause of death. The usual methods must be employed to counteract any toxic or sensitivity reaction. If general anesthesia is used, it is essential that the patient be kept well-oxygenated throughout the procedure, and that the contrast medium remain in the airway only long enough to obtain necessary films. If the patient shows signs of hypoxia or other untoward reaction, obviously the dye must be aspirated immediately, even before films can be taken.

Occasionally, acute attacks of asthma have been precipitated by the use of contrast media in the tracheobronchial tree, but these have been reported mostly in adults and are very rare in children, as are other sensitivity reactions to the various media. Temporary febrile reactions may occur in infants and children, but they occur more frequently after the use of the aqueous media. Nausea and vomiting are relatively rare, and the incidence is usually no greater than that seen after general anesthesia for any purpose. Following bronchographic studies in adults, symptoms of iodism may appear, with occasional evidence of acute parotitis. Preoperative skin tests could be performed in an adult suspected of being iodine-sensitive, but such a procedure is rarely indicated in children.

TECHNIQUE

Bronchography or tracheography in infants and children should be performed as a hospital procedure, except under very unusual circumstances. Laryngeal edema may occur whenever instruments of any type have been passed through the infant larynx, and several hours will elapse before serious edema becomes apparent. Such untoward reactions following bronchography are very uncommon, although most of the time these studies are performed on patients who have some type of airway obstruction to begin with, and therefore, further respiratory embarrassment is to be avoided. Age is no contraindication to bronchographic studies, and such procedures can be carried out perfectly safely even in newborn infants if indications should arise, providing the proper precautions are taken. A very tiny amount of contrast medium will sometimes be all that is necessary to give valuable information that is not obtainable otherwise.

Preoperative Preparation

The patient should be given nothing by mouth for at least six to eight hours preoperatively. The procedure is usually done in the morning. If the patient is over 1 year of age, an appropriate dose of pentobarbital is used one hour preoperatively, and atropine given one-half hour beforehand to reduce vagal stimulation. These doses are regulated by the age, weight and general condition of the patient. If bronchiectasis is present, as it so frequently is in cystic fibrosis, postural drainage an hour or two before the operation may help clear the lower respiratory tract of obstructing tenacious secretions. Anesthesia can then be more safely administered, and better filling of the desired areas obtained. If there has been recent acute infection or if significant chronic infection persists, preoperative broad-spectrum antibiotics are used, and patients with cystic fibrosis are constantly on such a regime. Atropine may be omitted if the secretions are very thick and tenacious. Bronchial dilators, mucolytic agents and steroids are used preoperatively in some clinics, but we have not considered them to be generally indicated.

Anesthesia

Over the past several years, general anesthesia has become much more widely used than it was 10 or 15 years ago, and this is especially true in children. In 1967, the Committee of Bronchoesophagology of the American College of Chest Physicians reported that general anesthesia in children is now "almost universally employed" for bronchography. Ether is still probably the safest anesthetic agent for general use in the pediatric age group, and entails very little, if any, increased risk over local anesthesia, which is usually employed in adults. However, it has some drawbacks. The greatest is its potential explosiveness or flammability, which is a very important consideration, especially when working in a radiology department.

Today, halothane is the most commonly employed anesthetic agent, but it has some disadvantages in endoscopic work, since it produces less relaxation than ether, is too short-acting, and necessitates a closed system for maintenance of adequate concentration. Methoxyflurane can be used in the same manner as ether, but induction takes much longer, and it is excreted more slowly. There is also more postoperative nausea and vomiting with methoxyflurane. The advantage of both of these agents is their nonflammability. A combination of nitrous oxide and halothane has been used effectively with little danger of respiratory irritation. When an adequate stage of anesthesia has been established, the glottis, trachea and carina are sprayed with a 4 per cent lidocaine solution. The patient is then reoxygenated and the general anesthetic agent continued through the sidearm of the bronchoscope. Succinylcholine may be administered for its short relaxant effect to produce complete apnea if this is necessary while films are being taken. Intravenous morphine will reduce activity of the patient without abolishing spontaneous respiration.

Operative Procedure

Teamwork is essential for good bronchographic studies, and this entails the utmost general cooperation of anesthesiologist, radiologist, bronchoscopist and radiologic technician. If the patient is in too deep a stage of anesthesia, a "dead tree" effect is obtained, with little contrast medium visible in the smaller bronchi. If the anesthesia is too light, coughing may fill the alveoli and produce a "snowstorm" appearance, obscuring finer details. Frequently, the radiologist is so intent on good pictures that he may unconsciously subject the patient to further risk as he requests the injection of more contrast medium, or too frequent changes in position while the patient is still under anesthesia. The use of the image-intensifier reduces radiation exposure and produces better films. On the television screen, the action of the heart and lungs can be easily monitored while the procedure is being carried out in a somewhat lighted room, which also insures the safety of the patient. Cineradiographic studies give a permanent record that can later be studied more carefully from the physiologic point of view.

A preoperative x-ray of the chest is usually taken to check exposure time and delineate the normal lung markings. A bronchoscopic procedure should be carried out first and any obstructing secretions removed. This assists in better gaseous exchange to maintain a proper level of anesthesia and to permit better filling by the contrast medium. Cultures can be obtained for bacteriologic studies, including sensitivity tests, fungus studies in obscure pulmonary infections, and occasionally smears for tuberculosis or injection of secretions into a guinea-pig. After the endoscopic examination has been completed, the bronchoscope is withdrawn and an endotracheal tube inserted. From then on, a closed system for anesthesia can be maintained. A tiny opening has already been cut in a stopper that rests in the side port of the gas-machine. Through this tiny hole, a small flexible catheter can be inserted, through which the contrast medium can be injected. (When using Dionosil, a red rubber catheter is better than the silastic or polyethylene tube, since chemical changes in the medium develop when it is in contact with some synthetic materials.) The catheter must be long enough to reach the lower bronchi. If the contrast medium is allowed to fill the catheter right to its tip before injection begins, its exact location can at all times be seen on the fluoroscopic screen of the image-intensifier. The anesthesiologist can assist the patient at any necessary time, and the presence of the endotracheal tube prevents laryngospasm. If the patient has received a relaxant, the anesthesiologist can keep him breathing adequately and permit excellent oxygenation throughout the entire procedure.

Ordinarily, the affected side of the chest is filled under the direction of the radiologist, who may position the patient as desired to obtain adequate filling. The right middle lobe can be filled more easily when the patient is tipped face down, and the right upper lobe better filled when he is lying on his right side. The left upper lobe is best filled with the patient turned 180 degrees. Since cardiac monitors on the chest would interfere with the films, the patient is constantly monitored by watching the television screen. Spot films are usually taken with the patient's arms held up over his head. Ordinarily, anteroposterior, lateral, oblique and posteroanterior films are taken (Fig. 1). The amount of the dye injected depends upon the age of the patient, his physiologic state, the depth of anesthesia and the amount of filling necessary.

Ordinarily, a general working rule is to use 1 ml. of contrast medium per year of age, and 10 ml. are rarely exceeded. It has been found in studies on adults that when more than 20 ml. of a contrast medium is used, greater alveolarization follows and untoward reactions may develop. The dye is aspirated as completely as possible just as soon as the films are obtained, and the mouth, pharynx and nose are also cleared by catheter suction. The endotracheal tube is then removed by the anesthesiologist and replaced by a pharyngeal airway. When the patient is transferred to the recovery room, he is kept in a prone position with the head kept low for drainage and one shoulder slightly elevated over a sandbag. If he is under 2 or 3 years of age, he is always kept in a vapor room,

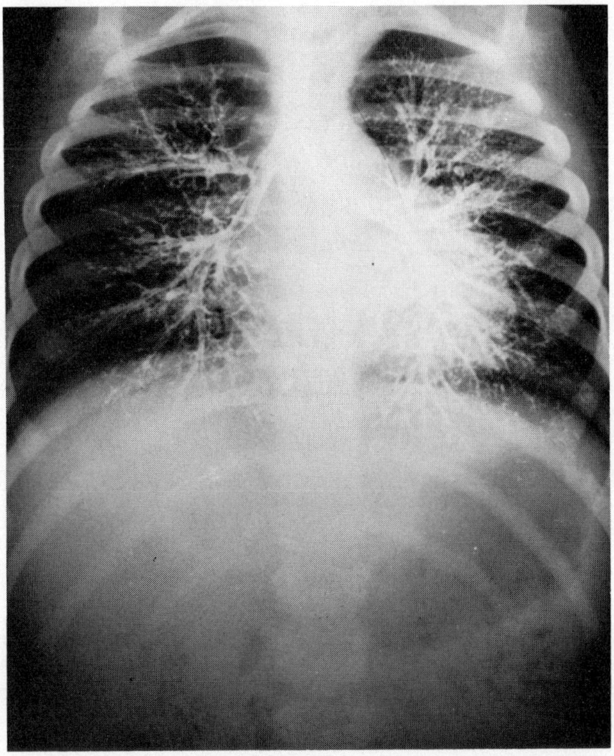

Figure 1. Normal Lipiodol bronchogram of a 1-year-old infant, showing adequate filling (posteroanterior view).

mist tent or croupette for the first 24 hours. Suctioning is carried out as necessary. Postoperative sedation is not necessary, and is generally undesirable, as the patient is encouraged to wake up as quickly as possible and to cough out any remaining contrast medium or secretions. Continued postural drainage is not necessary.

Occasionally, a slight febrile disturbance may be manifested for 24 to 36 hours, and sometimes nausea and vomiting are encountered. Laryngeal edema is rare, but has been observed on occasions. Such symptoms are minimized if care and gentleness are used throughout the procedure. The patient is discharged 24 hours after bronchography unless further studies or operative procedures are indicated. If laryngeal edema develops, one or two doses of a corticosteroid may be given. We prefer Decadron given in a single intramuscular dose (1 mgm. per 10 lbs. of body weight), but this is necessary only in very rare instances.

REFERENCES

Bronchography: A Report of the Committee on Bronchoesophagology. *Dis. Chest,* 51:663, 1967.

Ferguson, C. F.: Bronchography in children. *Otolaryng. Clin. N. Amer.,* 91, 1968.

Ferguson, C. F., and Flake, C. G.: Tracheographic and bronchographic studies as aids in the diagnosis of congenital malformations of the tracheobronchial tree and aortic arch in infants and children. *Ann. Otol.,* 63:1056, 1954.

Ferguson, C. F.: Congenital tracheoesophageal fistula not associated with atresia of the esophagus. *Laryngoscope,* 61:718, 1951.

Ferguson, C. F., and Neuhauser, E. B. D.: Congenital absence of the lung (agenesis) and other anomalies of the tracheobronchial tree. *Amer. J. Roentgen.,* 52:459, 1944.

Flake, C. G., and Ferguson, C. F.: Tracheography and bronchography in infants and children. *Ped. Clin. N. Amer.,* 2:279, 1955.

Greenberg, S. D., Hallman, G. L., Jr., and Spjut, N. J.: Pulmonary tissue reaction following hytrast bronchograms. *Ann. Otol.,* 73:1095, 1964.

Jackson, C.: The bronchial tree - its study by insufflation of opaque substances in the living. *Amer. J. Roentgen.,* 5:454, 1918.

Nadel, J. A., et al.: Powdered tantalum. *New Eng. J. Med.,* 283:281, 1970.

Nadel, J. A., Wolfe, W. G., and Graf, P. D.: Powdered tantalum as a medium for bronchography in canine and human lungs. *Invest. Radiol.,* 3:229, 1968.

Rayl, J. E.: Clinical reactions following bronchography. *Ann. Otol.,* 74:1120, 1965.

Rose, R. M., Cardona, J., and Daly, J. F.: Bronchographic sequelae of endobronchial tuberculosis. *Ann. Otol.,* 74:1133, 1965.

Sicard, J. A., and Forestier, J.: Methode generale d'exploration radiologique par l'huile iodée (Lipiodol). *Bull. Soc. Med. Hop. Paris,* 46:463, 1922.

Vawter, G. F., and Ferguson, C. F.: Bronchial adenoma in childhood. *Ann. Otol.,* 67:1113, 1958.

Chapter One Hundred Eleven

TRACHEOBRONCHIAL TREE MALFORMATIONS

PAUL H. HOLINGER, M.D., ARNOLD A. ZIMMERMANN, Dr. ès Sc., and JOYCE A. SCHILD, M.D.

EMBRYOLOGY

Correlation of normal tracheobronchial developmental events with observed congenital malformations of the lung is of value in interpreting unusual clinical findings.[1] Human lung development progresses through the embryonic and fetal periods and continues in postnatal life. The embryonic phase lasts to the end of the second month; both major divisions of the bronchial tree as well as the differentiation of the main pulmonary lobes are apparent by the end of this period. During the fetal period, beginning with the third month, these primordia grow and elaborate. The first true alveoli are established with birth and the intake of air, but the process of gradual transformation of the prenatal lung parenchyma and further differentiation of the terminal branches of the bronchial tree continues well into childhood.

In tracheal and pulmonary development, the general form and even the differentiation of the bronchopulmonary segments are attained at six to seven weeks of ovulation age. In sections of embryonic lungs, the earliest signs of fissuration are recognizable in 10 mm. human embryos; the fissures and developing lobes are clearly marked in embryos 15 to 20 mm. long (six to seven weeks of development). Once these major developmental events in the primal lung tissues have occurred, the basic ground plan is definitely established and the time for the development of marked anomalies has passed at that early stage. This has been called the teratogenic termination period. In regard to lung development, most dangerous growth interference and production of aberrance occur prior to eight weeks of embryonic development.

The normal development of the trachea and lungs proceeds from two major constituent parts. The entodermal primordium arises as a ventral outgrowth from the primitive foregut at three and a half weeks when the embryo measures only a few millimeters in length. It forms the epithelial lining of the entire tracheobronchial tree and of the glandular derivatives. This is the primal lung tissue and constitutes the mold for the developing lower respiratory tract, determining the trachea, bronchi and all their subdivisions. This entodermal primordium is surrounded by the mesodermal constituent part, which forms the connective tissue, septa, smooth muscle, cartilaginous plates, the vascular stroma and the visceral pleura. Streeter has shown that part of that early visceral mesenchyma is derived from cells of the primary coelomic epithelium which invest the esophagus and lung primordium.[2]

The midventral zone in the entoderm of the primitive foregut, at which the laryngotracheopulmonary primordium arises as a sprouting bud, represents the "pulmonary field" of the foregut. It lies directly caudal to the mesobranchial area of the visceral arches and is early recognized as the laryngotracheal groove. The manner of its partial separation from the foregut is most important in the development of the respiratory tract, normally leading to the establishment of the future laryngeal inlet and of the originally unpaired primary lung bud. Developmental disturbances in this area produce severe anomalies, such as tracheoesophageal fistulae.

Streeter confirmed and further established the important fact that the basic pattern of the tracheobronchial tree, with secondary and tertiary bronchial branches, differentiates early and relatively quickly between the fourth and sixth weeks of human development. Wells' and Boyden's studies indicate that all anomalies of the pulmonary segments appear no later than the fortieth day after ovulation.[3]

Figures 1, 2 and 3 give a general idea of the bronchopulmonary development in human embryos. The fast rate of development of the bronchial tree is striking, and it becomes obvious that the time for the development of bronchial and segmental anomalies lies between 33 and 39 days, ovulation age.

Certain further details of lung differentiation are relevant for the consideration of abnormal development. Already in the fourth week of human development (5 mm. embryo), the lung primordium becomes bifid, and this event is followed by the caudal growth of the trachea and the appearance of the two primary bronchi. The latter rapidly become asymmetrical, the right stem bronchus growing somewhat faster and the left assuming a more transverse direction. Their free tips are

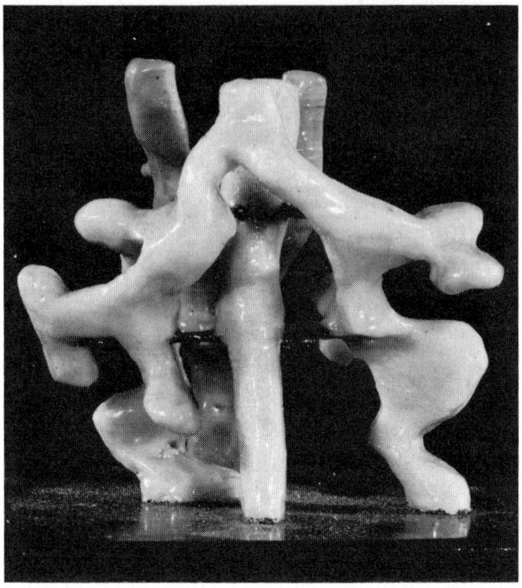

Figure 1. Wax reconstruction of bronchopulmonary development in an 8 mm. human embryo, ovulation age 33 days, plus or minus one day. (Courtesy of Dr. O. F. Kampmeier, Dept. of Anatomy, University of Illinois.)

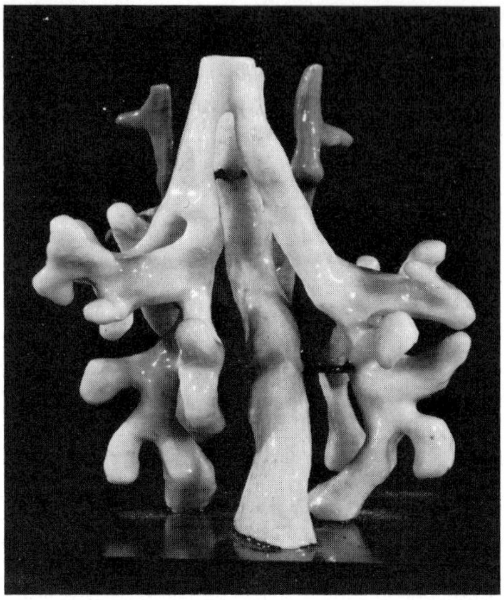

Figure 2. Similar reconstruction of bronchopulmonary development in human embryo, 13 mm. in length. Ovulation age 35 days, plus or minus one day. (Courtesy of Dr. O. F. Kampmeier, Dept. of Anatomy, University of Illinois.)

bulging and constitute growth foci. In 7 to 8 mm. embryos (31 to 32 days), there are as yet no distinct secondary bronchi, but focal swellings are recognizable where such secondary bronchial buds will arise. At 33 days of development (8 to 11 mm. embryos), the right primary bronchial tube has formed two secondary epithelial outgrowths that represent the segmental stem buds for the future right upper and middle lobes. The left primary bronchus has only one such evagination, developing into the left upper lobe.

The conditions portrayed in Figure 1 are slightly further advanced, since the monopodal segmental bronchial tubes already have further divided. At this early stage (8 mm. embryo), a tubular outgrowth developing into the future apical segment of the lower lobe already is present.

The recognition of these early events makes it obvious that agenesis of an entire lung must be due to a developmental interference at this early stage (teratogenic termination period). It is not possible that a secondary degeneration

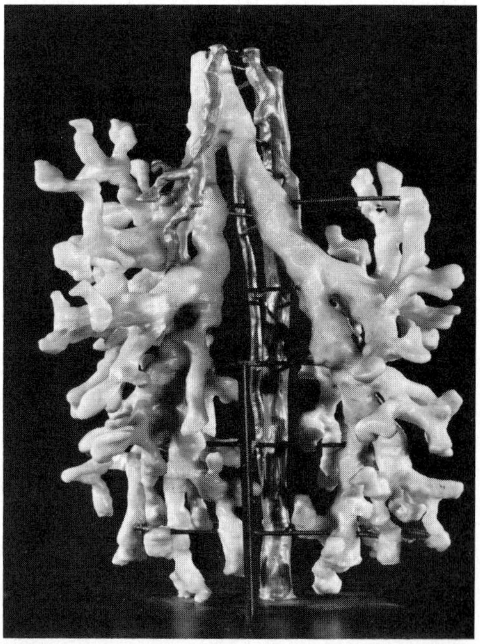

Figure 3. Bronchopulmonary development in human embryo, 18 mm. in length. Ovulation age 39 days, plus or minus one day. (Courtesy of Dr. O. F. Kampmeier, Dept. of Anatomy, University of Illinois.)

in toto of a once established lung anlage could occur to account for such an agenesis. It is a fact that the earlier the damaging disturbance occurs, the more severe will be the result.

Figure 4 shows a photomicrograph of the distended lung buds, capped by their mesodermal investment, and bulging into the common pleuroperitoneal cavity in an 8 mm. human embryo. Since the secondary evaginations from the primary bronchial tubes occur at this time, the future subdivisions of the lungs are already foreshadowed by three monopodal sprouts on the right lung primordium (one terminal and two lateral) and by two secondary bronchial stems on the left primordium (one terminal and one ventrolateral).

These progressing events of pulmonary differentiation are revealed in Figures 5 and 6. One of the subdivisions of the right bronchial stem bud is shown in an embryo that measured 9.5 mm., ovulation age 33 days plus or minus one day. The further division into tertiary bronchial tubes during normal pulmonary development is illustrated by Figure 6 (15 mm. embryo; estimated ovulation age 36 days). In both stages the beginning lobation and fissuration are clearly indicated, the capping mesenchyme reflecting the successive dichotomous divisions of the bronchial secondary tubes. This early developmental period and its characteristic events evidently mark the time at which aberrations in supernumerary or subnumerary lobes may occur.

In referring to Figure 2 (13 mm. embryo), it will be noted that apical development has not yet occurred, although the secondary bronchi for the upper, middle and lower lobes on the right and for the upper and lower lobes on the left are well established. Several of these secondary bronchi have sub-bronchial buds which lead to the differentiation of

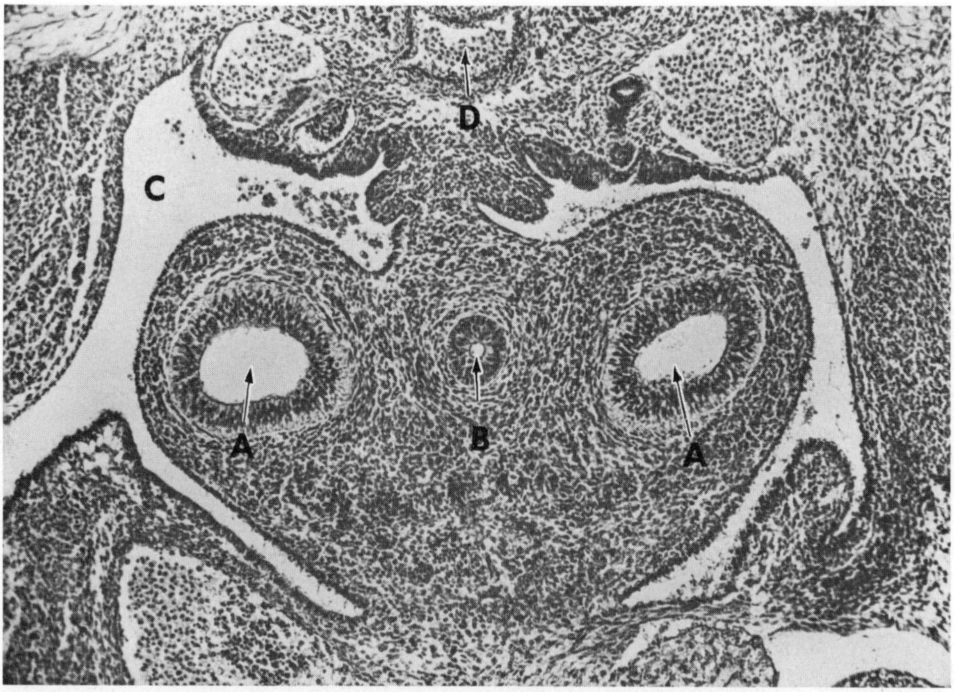

Figure 4. Bronchopulmonary development in an 8 mm. human embryo, ovulation age 31–32 days. (A) Dilated ends of primary bronchial stem buds. (B) Esophagus. (C) Common pleuroperitoneal cavity. (D) Aorta. (From the collection of serially sectioned human embryos, Dept. of Anatomy, University of Illinois, A. Zimmermann.)

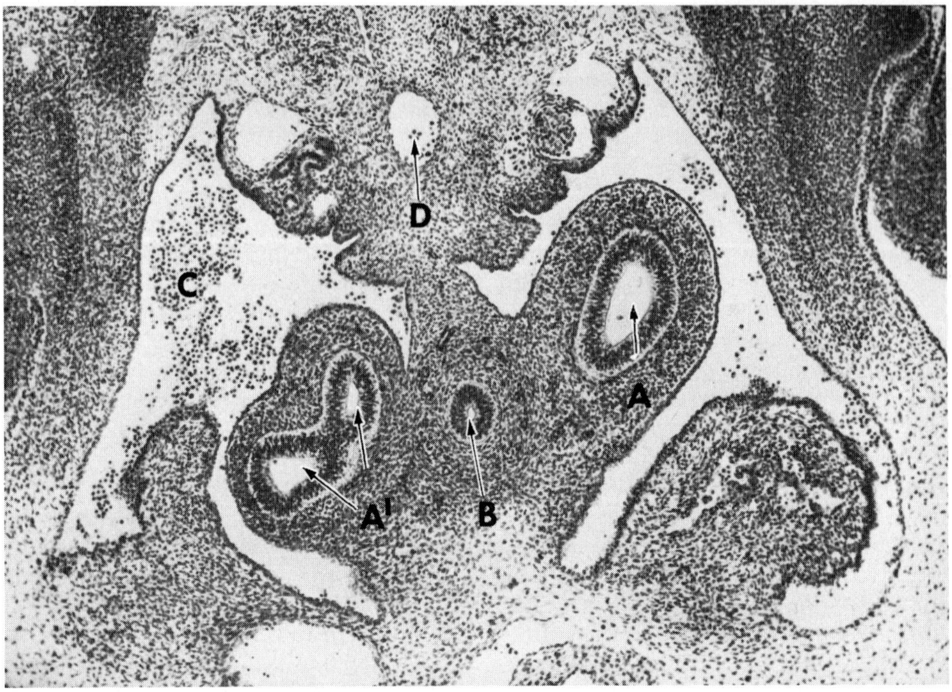

Figure 5. A 9.5 mm. human embryo, ovulation age 33 days plus or minus one day, (a) Left bronchus. (a′) Right bronchus. (b) Esophagus. (c) Pleuroperitoneal cavity. (d) Aorta. (From the collection of serially sectioned human embryos. Dept. of Anatomy, University of Illinois, A. Zimmermann.)

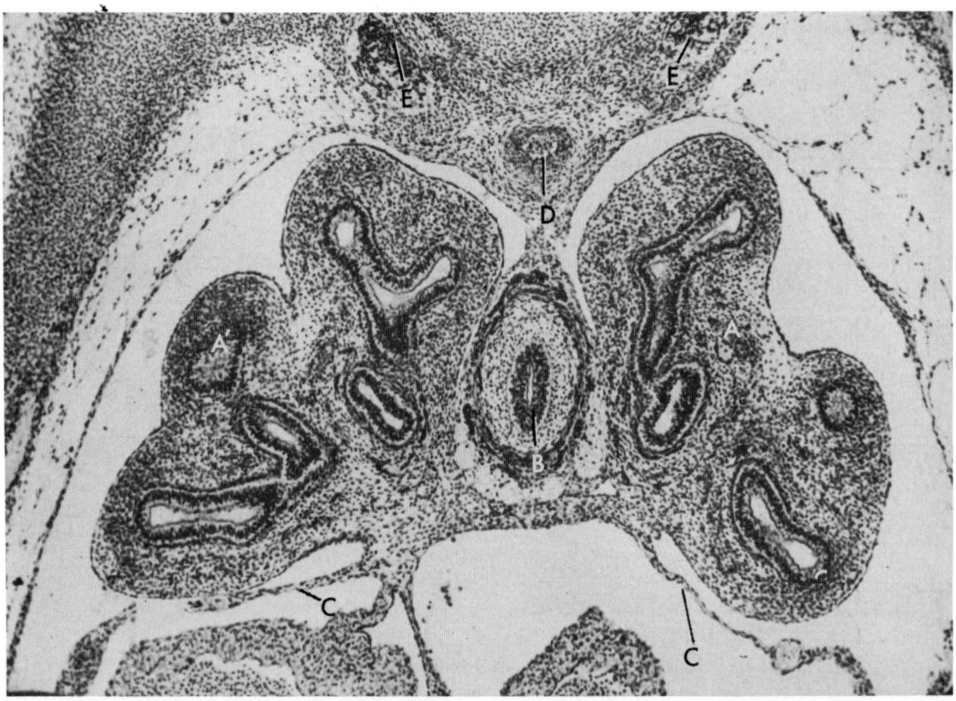

Figure 6. A 15 mm. embryo, estimated ovulation age 36 days, showing beginning lobulation and fissuration. (a) Left lung with two lobes. (a′) Right lung with three lobes. (b) Esophagus. (c) Pleuropericardial membrane. (d) Aorta. (e) Sympathetic trunks. (From the collection of serially sectioned human embryos, Dept. of Anatomy, University of Illinois, A. Zimmermann.)

lobar segments. Their definite identification is difficult at this early stage. The bronchial tubes of the future right and left superior lobes already are subdivided into two segmental buds. The bronchial stem (secondary bronchus) for the right middle lobe has three tertiary evaginations, and on the bronchus of the right inferior lobe there are subdivisions for the future apical (dorsal), medial, posterior and lateral basal segments. The bronchial tube of the left inferior lobe presents sub-bronchial evaginations that are tentatively identified as apical, anterior and posterior basal buds.

Figure 3 shows the bronchopulmonary differentiation in an 18 mm. human embryo. It is apparent that here, in the sixth week, apical development is well under way. Furthermore, it is of special interest that at this early stage all segmental bronchial buds can be recognized. Thus, each bronchus may be identified in the sixth week of development.

All subsequent subdivisions of the monopodal secondary bronchial tubes are dichotomous and often unequal. This manner of growth of the bronchial tree continues throughout the further development of the lungs. Broman counted 18 generations of divisions in the middle lobe of the right lung in the newborn.[4] As there are 23 to 25 generations of divisions in the same lobe of the adult lung, it is evident that the formation of bronchial subdivisions does not terminate at birth.

The progressive branching of the epithelial bronchial tree is illustrated in Figure 7, which also shows the corresponding lobation of the lungs (31 mm. embryo; seven and a half weeks of development).

Due to the continued pulmonary differentiation through the end of the second and early in the third month, the lung assumes more and more the form of a multilobed glandular primordium (tubulo-acinar type). Figure 8 illustrates this condition in a 36 mm. embryo in the ninth week of development. Tracheal and bronchial cartilages are well established at this time. Such cartilages

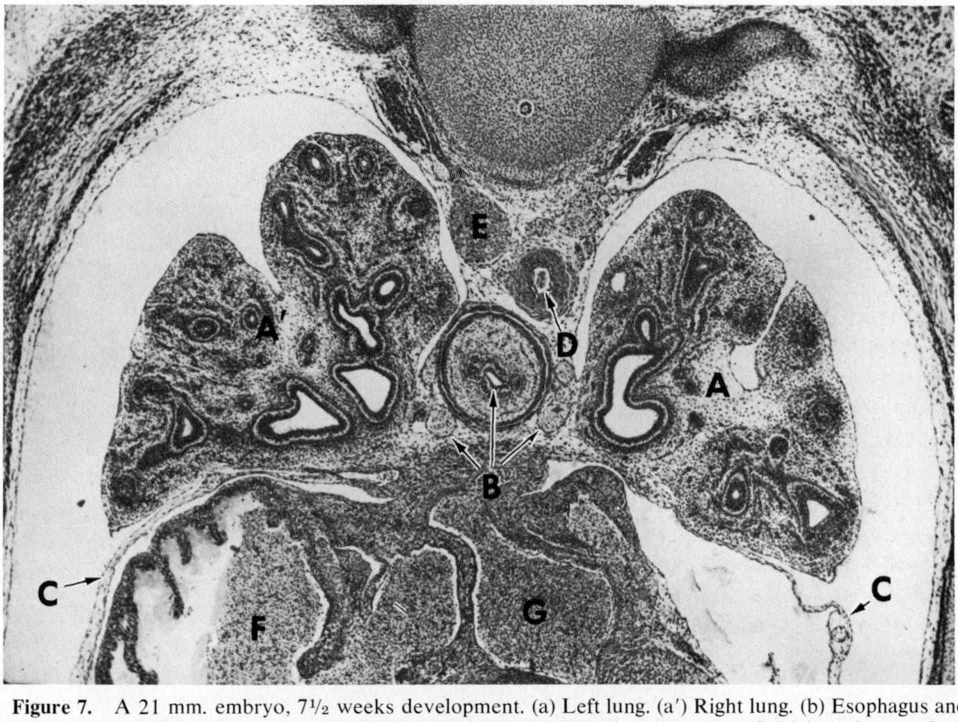

Figure 7. A 21 mm. embryo, 7½ weeks development. (a) Left lung. (a′) Right lung. (b) Esophagus and vagus nerves. (c) Pleuropericardial membrane. (d) Aorta. (e) Superior vena cava. (f) Right atrium. (g) Left atrium. (From the collection of serially sectioned human embryos, Dept. of Anatomy, University of Illinois, A. Zimmermann.)

will be noticed in Figure 8. They invest the stem bronchi, which were encountered in the section directly below the bifurcation of the trachea (carina).

It has long been established that during the process of arborization the main bronchial evaginations follow a fairly definite schedule and appear in a predictable sequence and in definite locations. Temporarily present supernumerary lobes, developed from the dorsal or the infracardiac evagination, usually become fused with the inferior lobes.

THE DEVELOPMENT OF THE TOTAL FORM OF THE LUNGS

Although the main branches of the bronchial arborization arise early and the overlying mesenchyma follows its subdivisions, marking them off as lobes and fissures, the general form of the embryonic lung remains rounded and mulberry-shaped. For a short time there is neither an apex nor a well-defined base, and the directions of the primary fissures are quite different from those in the adult. Toward the end of the second month (18 to 20 mm. embryo), the superior lobes expand craniad and form definite pulmonary apices. This leads to a relative shift in the position of the root, or hilus, which at first appears to lie near the cranial end of the lung primordium. Consequently, a greater caudal portion of the embryonic lung hangs freely into the pleural cavity.

During the latter part of the second month the inferior lobes likewise expand, particularly on their dorsal aspects. These expansions change the

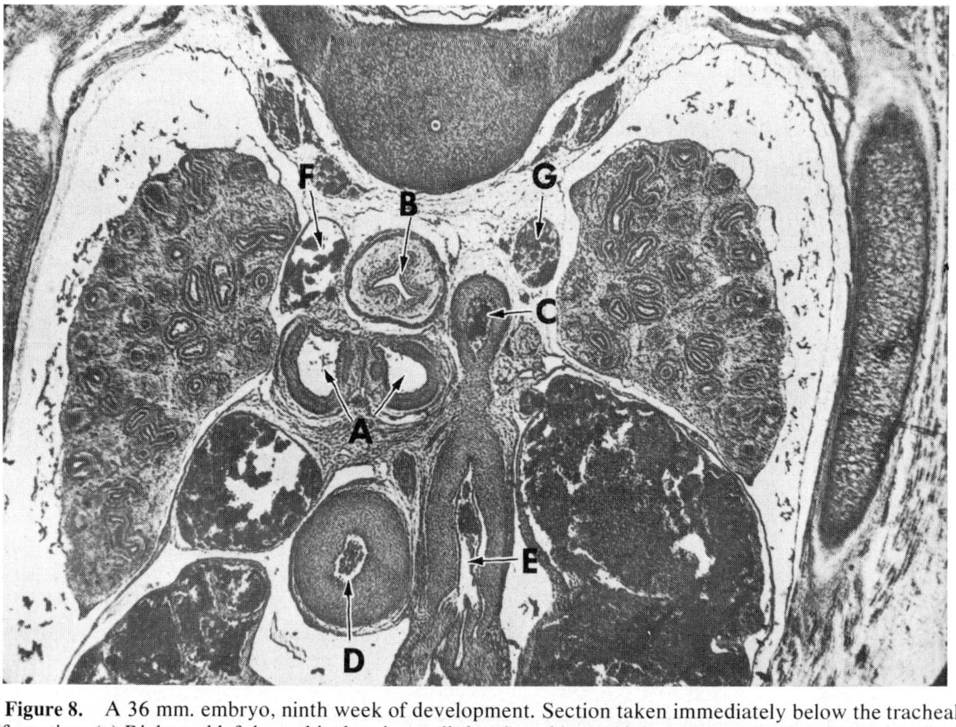

Figure 8. A 36 mm. embryo, ninth week of development. Section taken immediately below the tracheal bifurcation. (a) Right and left bronchi, showing well-developed bronchial cartilages. (b) Esophagus. (c) Descending aorta. (d) Ascending aorta. (e) Pulmonary artery. (f) Superior vena cava. (g) Accessory hemiazygos vein. (From the collection of serially sectioned human embryos. Dept. of Anatomy, University of Illinois, A. Zimmermann.)

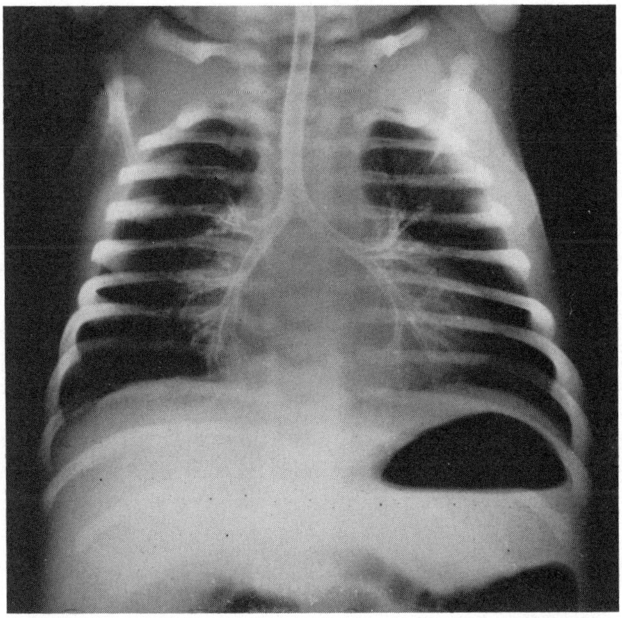

Figure 9. Bronchogram of a newborn infant showing the normal distribution of the segmental bronchi.

course of the primary fissures. Between the developing broncho-pulmonary segments of the major lobes accessory fissures may be retained. They follow the planes of separation between such segments. Some accessory lobes may become sequestrated at this time, most frequently observed in relation to the base of the left lung. Such "lower accessory lungs" may develop without any apparent bronchial communication with the normal lung, and with their vascular components arising from below the diaphragm. Completely detached lung tissue may be encountered below the diaphragm (so-called "abdominal lungs"), usually in the neighborhood of the left kidney. Such an occurrence is undoubtedly due to a sequestration by the developing pleuro-peritoneal membrane, which is a constituent element of the diaphragm and permanently seals off the pleural from the peritoneal cavity in the 20 mm. embryo (seven and a half weeks). This event indicates the last possible time when lung primordia may become dislocated (sequestrated) into the abdominal cavity.

Concurrent with the growth of the major pulmonary lobes, secondary shaping factors exert their influence on the developing form of the lungs. The enlarging liver primordium bulges the diaphragm upward and flattens the inferior lobes to form the pulmonary base. The relatively large embryonic heart likewise contributes to the establishment of the external form of the lungs. Thus, *a definite form of the lungs is attained early in the third month of intrauterine development* (3 cm. fetus), which is beyond the point in time for the occurrence of embryonic and truly congenital malformations. It is apparent that the phase of most active differentiation of the primary ground plan of an organ corresponds to the time when the primordium is most vulnerable to noxious influences. Viral toxins, oxygen deficiency, and interferences with the normal chemical constituents of cells during this early formation may severely affect mitotic activity and phenotypic development of the lungs. Little is known as yet of genetic (hereditary) aberrations in lung development. (A.Z).

CLASSIFICATION OF TRACHEAL AND BRONCHOPULMONARY MALFORMATIONS

The correlation of pulmonary malformations with normal development is based mainly on the time sequences at which the malformations may occur. A simplified, practical classification that includes all recognized anomalies, except those of monster and conjoint twins, is given in Table 1.

Anomalies of the Trachea

Tracheal Agenesis. Tracheal agenesis must be ascribed to growth-inhibitory influences effective in the fourth week of human development. Such an early arrest of differentiation naturally prohibits the formation of all subsequent bronchopulmonary structures and it is therefore incompatible with life, although it has been described frequently.[7]

TRACHEAL CONSTRICTIONS OR STENOSES. These occur in numerous forms

TABLE 1. CLASSIFICATION OF CONGENITAL ANOMALIES OF THE TRACHEOBRONCHIAL TREE[5,6]

- I. Anomalies of the trachea
  - A. Agenesis or atresia
  - B. Constriction
    - 1. Fibrous strictures
      - a. Webs
      - b. Fibrous stenosis of tracheal segments
      - c. Stenoses associated with tracheoesophageal fistula
    - 2. Absence or deformity of tracheal cartilages
      - a. Tracheomalacia
      - b. Deformity due to vascular anomalies
      - c. Individual cartilage deformity
      - d. Tracheopathia osteoplastica
  - C. Tracheal enlargement (congenital trachiectasis)
  - D. Tracheal evaginations or outgrowths
    - 1. Tracheoceles, diverticula, cysts
    - 2. Fistulas
    - 3. Tracheal lobe
  - E. Abnormal bifurcation or deviation
  - F. Other anomalies of gross morphology
- II. Anomalies of bronchi and lungs
  - A. Agenesis or atresia
  - B. Constriction
    - 1. Fibrous strictures
      - a. Webs
      - b. Fibrous stenoses of bronchial segments
    - 2. Absence or deformity of bronchial cartilages
      - a. Bronchomalacia
      - b. Bronchial hypoplasia
      - c. Compression due to cardiovascular anomalies
  - C. Bronchial enlargement (congenital bronchiectasis)
  - D. Bronchial evaginations or outgrowths
    - 1. Bronchoceles, diverticula, cysts
    - 2. Fistulas
  - E. Abnormal bifurcation
    - 1. Subnumerary bronchi, lobes, fissures
    - 2. Supernumerary bronchi, lobes, fissures
  - F. Anomalous bronchial and lung tissue attached to some part of the respiratory system
  - G. Anomalous bronchial and lung tissue attached to tissues other than those of the respiratory system (sequestrated lung)
  - H. Situs inversus
    - 1. Thoracic
      - a. Kartagener's syndrome
    - 2. Complete

and have variable origins and periods of formation. They include (1) congenital fibrous strictures, consisting of webs, stenoses of lengthy segments of the trachea, and stenoses associated with tracheoesophageal fistula, and (2) stenosis due to absence or deformity of tracheal cartilages, such as tracheomalacia, individual cartilage deformity, including posterior fusion of the cartilaginous rings,[9] and stenosis associated with anomalous vascular or thymic compression. Congenital webs (Fig. 10) and fibrous strictures of the trachea may occur as a definite membranous web or as an hourglass-shaped constriction. These are identified with the bronchoscope when a small, central opening through the web is seen. Careful dilatation gradually increases the lumen to relieve continuous chronic respiratory obstruction. Fibrous tracheal stenosis may be associated with congenital esophageal atresia and tracheoesophageal fistula. In these infants, the tracheal stenosis is at the level of the fistula and becomes a serious clinical problem. It may be difficult to ascertain whether this stenosis is a developmental anomaly or is caused by the tightness of the surgical closure of the tracheal fistula.

Absence or Deformity of Tracheal Cartilages. These conditions are responsible for many clinical problems of respiratory obstruction. *Congenital tracheomalacia,* a common form of congenital stridor, may or may not be associated with the similar anomaly of laryngomalacia. Its symptoms are those of varying degrees of stridor, dyspnea and periods of cyanosis, all manifestations of marked obstruction. X-ray and bronchoscopic evidence of a flaccid trachea indicate the presence of retarded development of the tracheal wall. Flaccidity is more pronounced than that seen in allergic infants, and there is usually no evidence of allergy. Lateral x-rays of the neck and chest on inspiration and expiration may demonstrate the anteroposterior collapse that is visible during bronchoscopy. In extreme cases, postmortem examination shows complete absence or only islands of rudimentary cartilages in the trachea or bronchial walls.

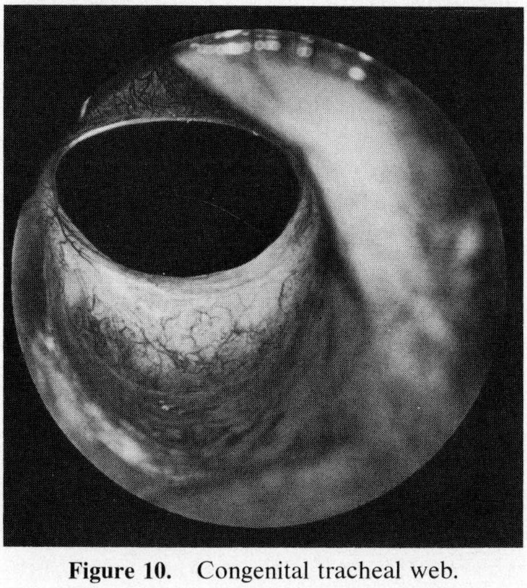

Figure 10. Congenital tracheal web.

Vascular Anomalies. Deformity due to vascular anomalies, particularly anomalies of the aortic arch and its main branches that cause tracheal or bronchial obstruction, has long been recognized as a cause of tracheal stenosis. The tracheal obstruction is usually, but not always, associated with esophageal constriction. Such deformities as the result of faulty differentiation of the tracheal wall with absence of tracheal cartilages would be true teratogenic events in the embryonic period, occurring most likely during the fifth and sixth weeks of development. Definite cartilages are differentiated after the fifth or sixth week of development (15 mm. embryo) and are well established at the end of the embryonic period. Deformities of tracheal cartilages may also arise during that time. In either case, the tracheal wall may be more flaccid than normal, and varying degrees of obstruction would be likely to result.

However, when compression stenoses are a secondary result due to the proximity and pressure of the vascular anomaly, the differentiation, or the deformity of tracheal cartilages, would then have arisen at a later period, possibly during the third fetal month. The recognition that this developmental deformity exists apart from the pressure factor alone is of great clinical significance. It is apparent that the constricting deformity of the trachea, for example, will persist even after the vascular anomaly that caused it is severed, although clinical improvement is obtained by relief of pressure. Postsurgical endoscopic dilatation may be necessary to obtain a satisfactory lumen in tracheal and bronchial obstruction caused by the congenital cardiovascular anomalies of double aortic arch or an anomalous subclavian vessel.

The possible compression effects of abnormal blood vessels in front of the lower trachea, perhaps, should not be entirely excluded in attempts to explain the mode of origin of tracheoesophageal fistulae. In such cases, the fistular opening usually occurs at a caudal level of the trachea, and the larynx is normally differentiated. A middle segment of the esophagus may be atretic. According to Gruenwald, the atretic portion of the esophagus contributes a strip of tissue in the dorsal wall of the trachea and the genesis of the tracheoesophageal fistula is based entirely on a failure of the laryngotracheal tube to properly separate from the esophagus.[9]

TRACHEAL ENLARGEMENT. This is also called congenital trachiectasis. It has been described by Mounier-Kuhn.[10] It is rare and usually is associated with congenital bronchiectasis.

TRACHEAL EVAGINATIONS OR OUTGROWTHS. These may develop as tracheal cysts (tracheoceles) or as tracheal lungs in the form of abnormal pulmonary segments or lobes. The cysts most likely arise subsequent to disturbances in the chondrogenic phase of the trachea. If some tracheal cartilages are malformed or absent, the tracheal mucosa may evaginate in areas of the corresponding weakened wall. The further development of such evaginations into tracheal cysts of considerable size probably is a pathological process and may continue throughout the later fetal life. Examples of such outgrowths are not uncommon, causing increasing respiratory obstruction manifested by a wheeze, a brassy cough and considerable dysphagia. Fluoroscopy and films demonstrate a mass compressing the trachea, above the aortic arch or as far caudad as the bifurcation. Bronchoscopy and esophagoscopy show the obstructing lesion to be entirely extraluminal. On exploratory thoracotomy, a cyst is found attached to the trachea; when it is resected, symptoms are completely relieved. Histologic examination of the walls demonstrates respiratory epithelium. Similar cysts that do not differ from tracheal cysts are found attached to the bronchi and are designated as bronchogenic or bronchial cysts.

The formation of *tracheal lobes and segments* is a true teratogenic event that must occur early in embryonic life, before the end of the second month. These processes are related to abnormal bifurcation of the trachea. They reveal the high potentiality of the caudal end of the trachea for division by focal swellings that normally establish the stem bronchi. Abnormal conditions found in this area give the impression of having been established by trial and error. Obviously they are the opposite of inhibitory effects, and the specific causes remain unknown. However, it is quite apparent that an abnormally arising right upper lobe is the most frequent occurrence.[11,12] It may take origin from the trachea and substitute the absent upper lobe of the right lung or it may duplicate it in its entirety. In some cases the tracheal evagination forms only an apical segment; this segment may be duplicated in the normal right upper lobe, or the right upper lobe bronchus may give rise to only the anterior and posterior bronchi and segments.

The possibilities of aberrations at the tracheal bifurcation evidently are multiple and varied. The time of their genesis must lie between the thirtieth and fortieth day of ovulation age. The variability in the origin of the eparterial bronchi in vertebrates and especially in mammals is well known. In some instances, in the pig's lung, the eparterial bronchus is shifted back on to the trachea, and there is a right tracheal (eparterial) bronchus in sheep embryos. However, in almost all mammals this is an unpaired element and occurs only on the right side. One would hardly be justified, therefore, to assume that the rare case of bilateral tracheal bronchi represents an atavistic reversal to ancestral characteristics.

Anomalies of the Bronchi and Lungs

COMPLETE AGENESIS OF AN ENTIRE LUNG. Complete agenesis is a major anomaly that occurs fairly frequently and that often accompanies anomalies of other systems.[13] This indicates that the teratogenic agent was effective during a considerable time of the embryonic period. Since the human lung primordium becomes bifid when the embryo is 4 to 5 mm. in length, and has an ovulation age of 28 days plus or minus one day, this is the most likely time for complete arrest in development of one lung to occur. At that time, the primary bronchi begin to diverge from the lung anlage, before there is marked caudal growth of the trachea. The condition appears to affect the right and left lungs with approximately equal frequency, although it much more commonly affects females than males. Schneider divided these malformations into three classes.[14] Class 1 consists of cases in which no trace of a bronchus or lung is found. In Class 2 there is some trace of a bronchus, but no lung tissue is present. In Class 3, the main bronchus is incompletely developed, and there is marked hypoplasia of one or both lungs. Apparent atelectasis of an entire lung in the newborn often is found to be an agenesis rather than an actual atelectasis due to an obstructed bronchus. Infants are generally referred by the pediatrician or obstetrician after tracheal catheterization attempts fail to remove the suspected mucus plug.

A clinical diagnosis for these patients can usually be made on the basis of the physical examination, the x-ray and fluoroscopic findings indicating the displacement of the mediastinum and of the heart toward the affected side, especially if associated skeletal anomalies of the spine and of the ribs and other anomalies are also present. Bronchoscopic examination, a bronchogram, and angiocardiography may be necessary in some cases to establish the diagnosis.[15] The condition is not incompatible with life,

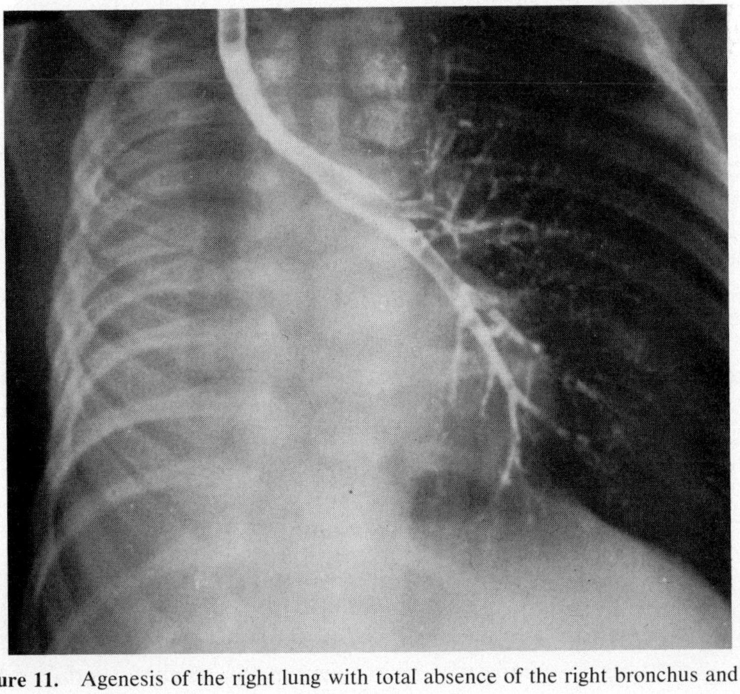

Figure 11. Agenesis of the right lung with total absence of the right bronchus and lung.

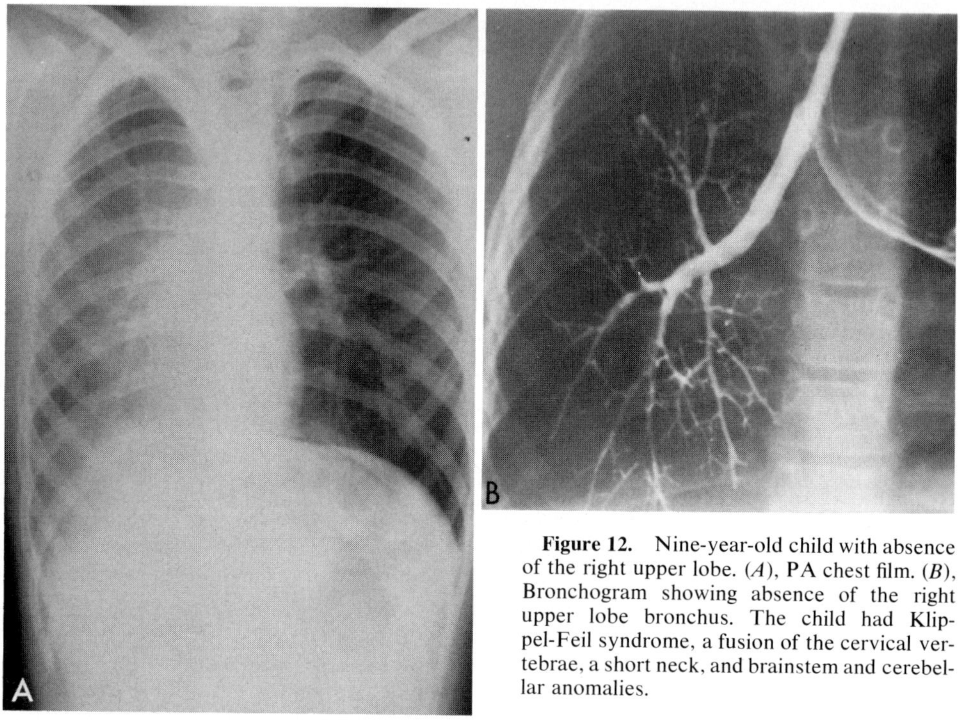

Figure 12. Nine-year-old child with absence of the right upper lobe. (*A*), PA chest film. (*B*), Bronchogram showing absence of the right upper lobe bronchus. The child had Klippel-Feil syndrome, a fusion of the cervical vertebrae, a short neck, and brainstem and cerebellar anomalies.

although often one such severe anomaly is associated with others of equal severity in other systems.

Types of anomalies of the bronchial tree are numerous and complex. In many cases it is difficult to determine whether they are teratogenic, pathologic or mixed in their mode of development. As far as the truly embryonic malformations are concerned, it can be definitely stated that they originate before the fortieth day of ovulation age. It has been pointed out that the lobar and segmental bronchi become established during the fifth to sixth week of development (18 mm. embryo) and that the basic bronchopulmonary pattern is completed at that early stage.

CONSTRICTIONS OF THE BRONCHIAL TREE. These follow the pattern of similar anomalies of the trachea. Congenital webs appear as membranes partially or completely obstructing the bronchial lumen to produce obstructive emphysema or atelectasis. Dilatation of a pinpoint opening through the web may relieve such symptoms by deflating an overexpanded lung to allow the heart and mediastinum to return to their normal positions.

BRONCHOMALACIA. This is common and is of unusual clinical interest. A flaccid bronchial wall may give rise to rapidly progressive respiratory distress, necessitating emergency thoracotomy and lobectomy to relieve progressive obstructive emphysema. On thoracotomy, an absence of cartilage in part of the wall of a bronchus may be found responsible for the emphysema through a check-valve mechanism. However, this is not invariably the etiology of so-called idiopathic lobar emphysema, which appears more likely to be due to a deformity of elastic tissue development.

BRONCHIAL HYPOPLASIA. This is seen in association with Class 3 agenesis leading to a rudimentary lung, or involving a segment of bronchus with complete or partial stenosis.

BRONCHIAL COMPRESSION. Either partial or complete bronchial compression corresponds to the similar condition seen in the trachea produced by anoma-

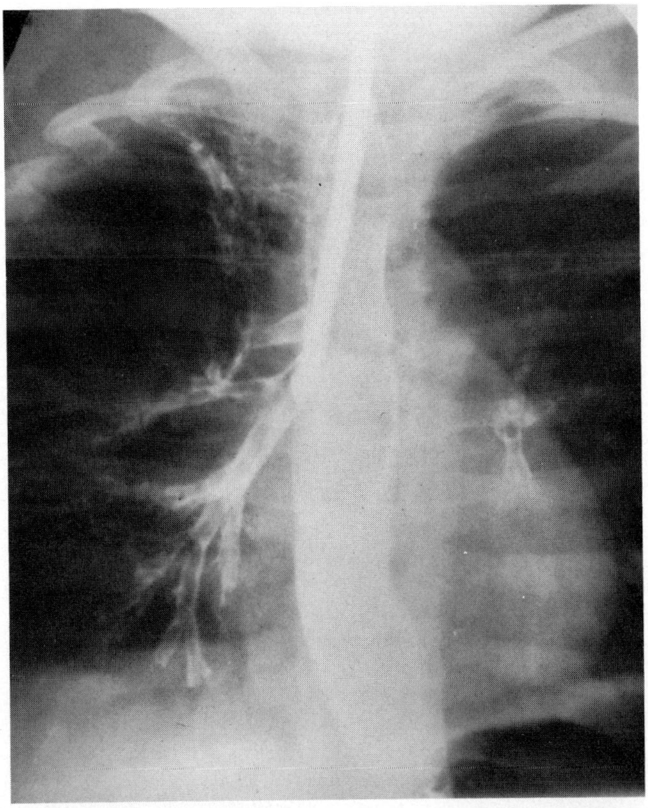

Figure 13. Tracheal right upper lobe bronchus with duplication of the bronchus. The anomalous bronchus leads to a congenital cystic accessory right upper lobe.

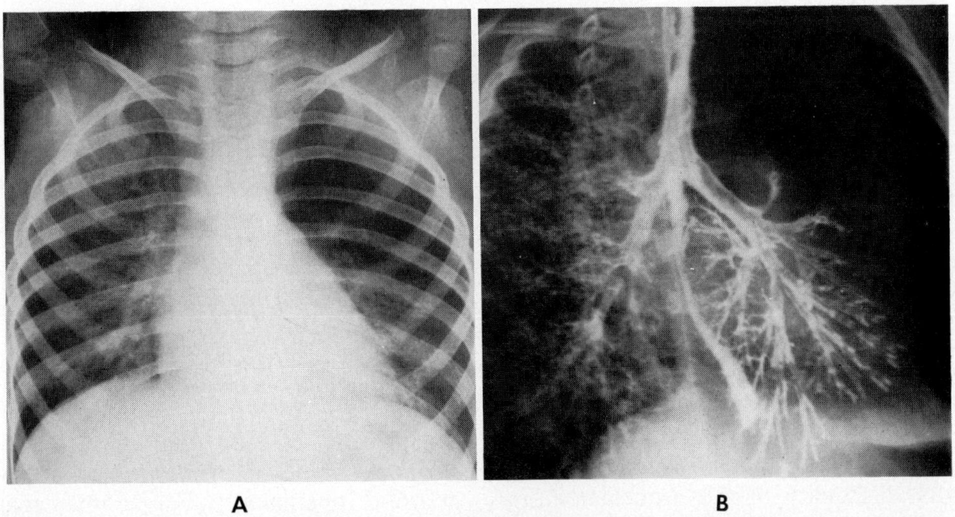

Figure 14. Duplication of the left upper lobe bronchus leading to an emphysematous anomalous left upper lobe. *A*, Left upper lobe emphysema. *B*, Bronchogram with accessory bronchus.

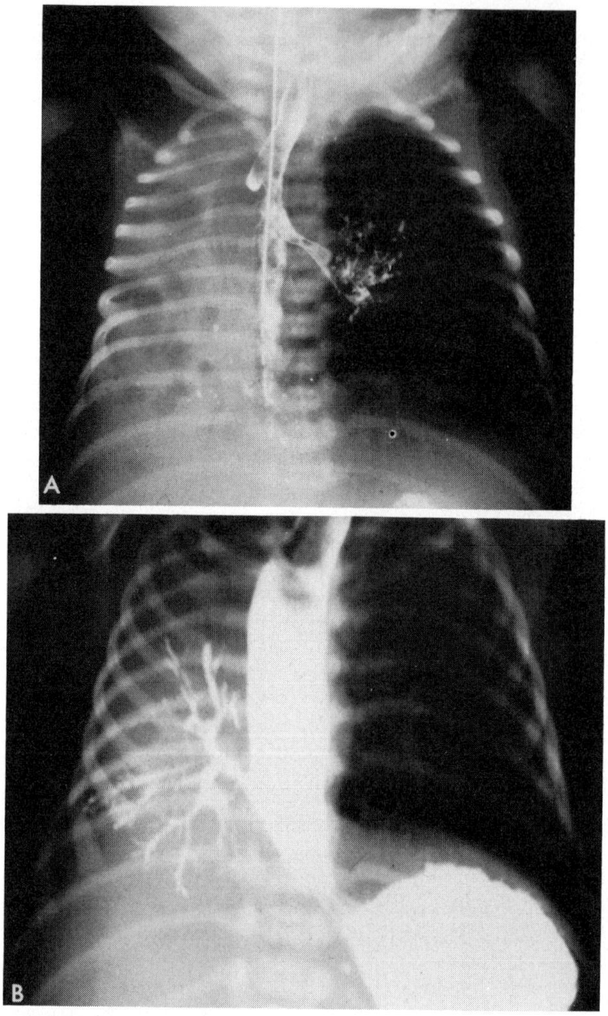

Figure 15. *A*, Bronchogram of 9-day-old infant demonstrating agenesis of right lung with rudimentary right bronchus. Ingested Lipiodol in the esophagus is overflow from the tracheobronchial tree. Spots of Lipiodol are seen in radiolucent areas of the right lower hemithorax. *B*, Esophagram demonstrating anomalous bronchus originating from the esophagus and leading to sequestrated lobes.

lies of the heart and great vessels. Such constrictions may cause extreme respiratory emergencies and always enter into the differential diagnosis of respiratory obstruction in infants. Cardiac anomalies may compress the left main bronchus, whereas anomalies of great vessels may be responsible for compression of either the left or right main bronchus. As was noted in similar conditions in the trachea, examination of the bronchi in these cases demonstrates not only compression stenosis but also an absence or gross deformity of the bronchial cartilages in the segment of the bronchus involved. This deformity, which most likely occurred during embryonic development as the result of the shaping influence of the constricting vessel, persists to some degree after the vessel is severed. This is significant, since it explains a failure of complete relief of symptoms in some cases following surgery.

CONGENITAL BRONCHIECTASIS. Congenital bronchiectasis and various other forms of cystic disease do not appear to be anomalies of a teratogenic nature. It is probable that prenatal and postnatal inflammations may interfere with the normal differentiation of pulmonary parenchyma and are responsible for such conditions. Kartagener's syndrome,[16] a triad of bronchiectasis, situs inversus and sinusitis, must be considered in this category.

Many conditions of enlargement, constriction or compression of segments of the bronchial tree undoubtedly are pathological in nature, as are many forms of congenital bronchial webs, cysts and fistulae. Most of these probably arise during fetal life. It is possible that some conditions of bronchomalacia with hypoplasia or absence of cartilaginous plates in certain bronchi are of embryonic origin. However, these anomalies, similar to those of the trachea, are found most frequently to be associated with cardiovascular anomalies that had caused bronchial compression.

BRONCHIAL EVAGINATIONS OR OUTGROWTHS. Outgrowths consist primarily of fistulae, bronchogenic cysts, diverticula and bronchoceles, which are relatively rare, and the more numerous congenital cystic malformations of the lungs. The bronchogenic cysts manifest themselves by varying degrees of localized bronchial obstruction. These cystic formations are usually found to lie in the posterior mediastinum. They contain a clear, thick, viscid fluid that puts pressure on both the airway and the esophagus. However, since the walls are lined with ciliated pseudostratified columnar epithelium containing mucous glands and occasionally plaques of cartilage, it is possible that they are the result of a pinched off pulmonary bud. The final diagnosis is dependent upon the resection of the cyst and the histologic study of its walls.

Congenital cystic malformations constitute a large variety of lesions that present many symptoms and gross and microscopic findings. A differential diagnosis between congenital and acquired cysts is of clinical as well as academic importance, although the differentiation is not always a simple one. The diagnosis between congenital cystic disease and other types of congenital anomalies often depends upon bronchoscopic examination, particularly in the newborn, since similar physical and x-ray findings are

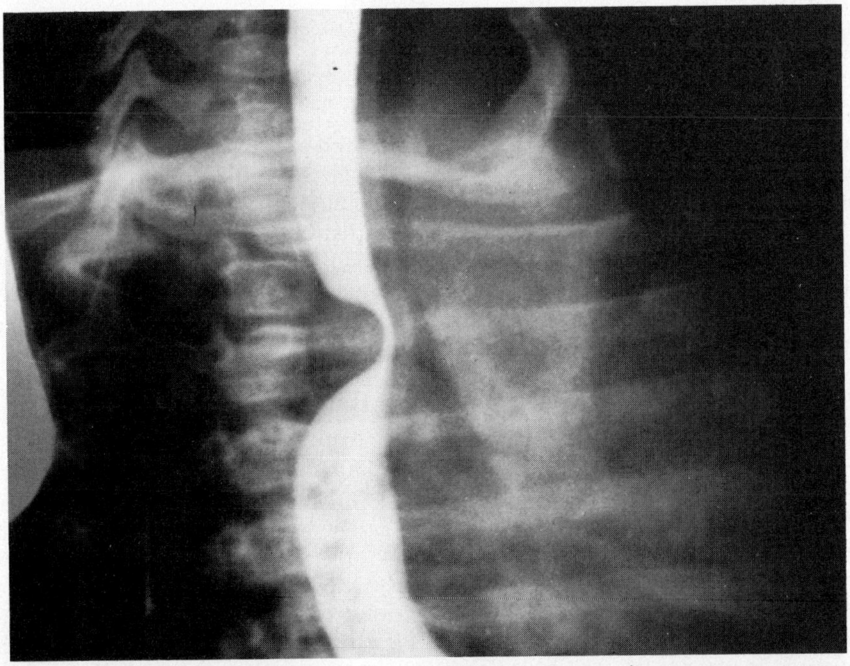

Figure 16. Esophagram of an infant with a large posterior arch of a vascular ring. Both tracheal and esophageal constrictions are seen.

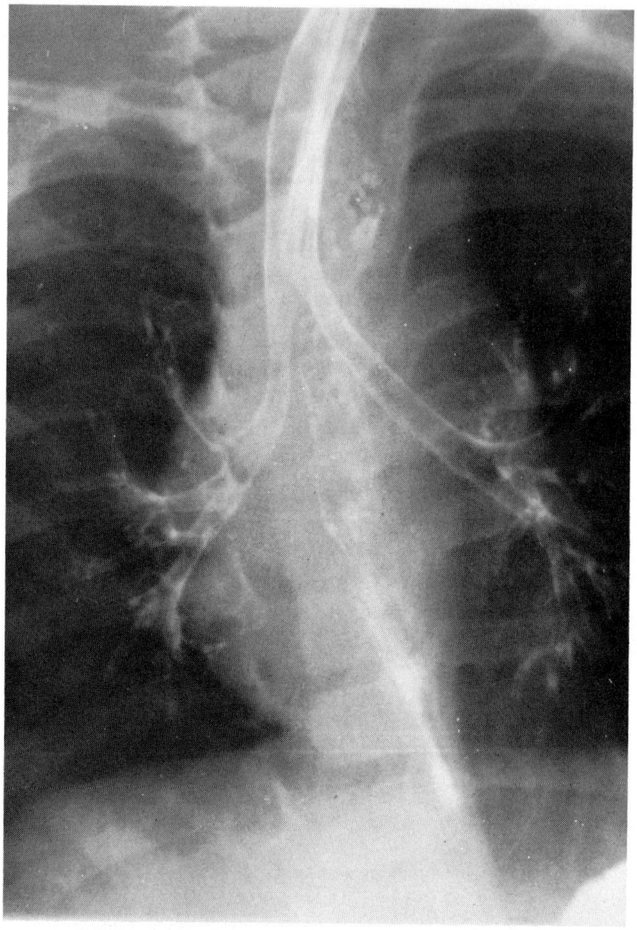

Figure 17. Distortion of the right bronchus of an infant with a right aortic arch, characterized by the long right main bronchus and an unusually low take-off of the right upper lobe bronchus.

seen in infants with congenital bronchial stenosis, tension cysts, cardiac or vascular anomalies compressing the bronchus, spontaneous tension pneumothorax and even the acquired cysts due to staphylococcus pneumonia.

The final differential diagnosis between congenital and acquired lung cysts cannot be made with absolute certainty without the histologic examination of the walls of the cyst itself. Lung cysts that are apparent during the first few days after birth probably are congenital. Cysts due to staphylococcus pneumonia, however, are truly acquired cysts. They develop in the immediate postnatal period and may simulate the conditions of congenital cysts. The majority of the cysts are dilated branches of the bronchial tree. Histologically, the congenital cyst is lined with ciliated columnar epithelium, whereas the inflammatory acquired cyst is lined with epithelium of a squamous character or merely with inflammatory exudates. The diagnosis is more difficult in older individuals when the congenital cyst may have become infected or may have been drained externally. This occurs frequently and may be erroneously diagnosed as an encapsulated empyema.

Congenital Bronchial Fistulae. These are unusual but of considerable clinical significance. They may prove to be the cause of spontaneous pneumothorax in the newborn, with bronchial mucosa fusing directly with the pleura at the site of the fistula. However, fistulae that result from bronchial evaginations are relatively common if one includes those cases of esophageal atresia in which the lower esophageal segment is connected with the left main bronchus rather than with the trachea. Distinguishing this type of secondary connection from the connection with the lower portion of the posterior wall of the trachea is of relatively little clinical significance.

SUBNUMERARY BRONCHI, LOBES AND FISSURES. These conditions are rarely reported in the literature. Although the most accurate method of determining the presence of these anomalies is the postmortem examination, the descriptions of the fissures, vessels and bronchi are usually inadequate or entirely lacking in most autopsy reports. However, where these reports describe subnumerary variations of lobation, it is found that they seldom coincide with bronchial variations. Nevertheless, it appears that there are varying degrees of pulmonary hypoplasia in conjunction with subnumerary lobes.[17] Absence of fissures is found not uncommonly during surgical procedures, more often on the right than the left.

SUPERNUMERARY LOBES, BRONCHI AND FISSURES. These may be grouped as tracheal accessory lobes, already described, and as lower accessory lobes. Supernumerary fissures dividing the right lung into as many as five lobes and, less frequently, a third lobe on the left, are generally not associated with bronchial anomalies. Supernumerary fissures without additional bronchi or lobes are common surgical observations and are of little practical importance. The additional fissures, which appear to be the most frequent type of pulmonary abnormality, are those that separate the medial basal and the superior basal segments from the remainder of the lower lobes. The azygous lobe, of course, is not a true supernumerary structure. The common variations of subnumerary anomalies (bilobation of the right lung) and of supernumerary fissures (trilobation of the left lung) do not necessarily reflect basic aberrations in the pattern of the bronchopulmonary tree, but may be quite secondary in origin. In such cases the bronchial tree usually is normal.

SEQUESTRATED LUNGS. The sequestration of a "lower accessory lobe" and the existence of abdominal lung tissue are related to the development of the pleuro-peritoneal membrane, which contributes to the formation of the diaphragm. The anomaly is usually associated with anomalous arteries from the aorta,[18] most often arising in the region of the pulmonary ligament but sometimes arising from below the level of the diaphragm.

A most interesting and rare anomaly is produced by *lung tissue originating* from the esophagus.[19,20] There appears to be an esophageal diverticulum arising at (or more caudad to) the level of the bifurcation of the trachea and extending as a soft mass into the pleural cavity. The mass is covered by parietal pleura, which excludes the possibility of an aberrant pulmonary segment having made a secondary connection with the esophagus, and in reported cases the mass contains bronchus-like structures lined with pseudostratified columnar epithelium. Vascular supply varies and the ectopic and atelectatic lung tissue generally produces compression effects on the normal bronchi and lung tissue, and the aberrant lung itself appears to be cystic in part.

Previous explanations of the possible origin of this type of anomaly are unsatisfactory. It had been postulated that a group of cells representing the anlage of a lung lobe was somehow mislocated in the wall of the early gut and proceeded to evaginate and develop in a manner similar to that of a normal lobe, but retaining its embryonic connection with the gastrointestinal tract. By such speculation it would be easy, of course, to "explain" almost any ectopic and baffling condition. Factual evidence is lacking, and an explanation of the teratogenic events remains entirely hypothetical.

REFERENCES

1. Holinger, P. H., Zimmermann, A. A., Parchet, V. N., and Johnston, K. C.: A correlation of the embryonic development of the trachea and lungs with congenital malformations. In Ruedi, L. (Ed.):*Fortschritte der Hals-*

Nasen-Ohrenheilkunde Progres en Oto-Rhinolaryngologia. Zurich Bibliotheca Oto-Rhino-Laryngologica, Vol. 3. Basel, S. Karger Publisher, 1956.
2. Streeter, G. L.: Developmental horizons in human embryos. *Contr. Embryol. Carneg. Inst.*, 31:27, 1945, and 32:133, 1948.
3. Wells, L. J., and Boyden, E. A.: The development of the bronchopulmonary segments in human embryos of horizons XVII-XIX. *Amer. J. Anat.*, 95:163, 1954.
4. Broman, I.: *Die Entwicklung des Menschen vor der Geburt.* Munich, J. F. Bergmann, 1927.
5. Jordan, H.: Anomalies of the human respiratory system; a proposed classification. *Amer. Rev. Tuberc.*, 40:517, 1939.
6. Holinger, P. H.: Congenital anomalies of the tracheobronchial tree. *Postgrad. Med.*, 36:5, 1964.
7. Oyamada, A., Gasul, B. M., and Holinger, P. H.: Agenesis of the lung. *Amer. J. Dis. Child.*, 85:182, 1953.
8. Cantrell, J. R., and Guild, H. G.: Congenital stenosis of the trachea. *Amer. J. Surg.*, 108:297, 1964.
9. Gruenwald, P.: A case of atresia of the esophagus combined with tracheoesophageal fistula in a nine mm. embryo, and its embryological explanation. *Anat. Rec.*, 78:293, 1940.
10. Soules, A., and Mounier-Kuhn, P. L.: *Bronchologie.* Paris, Messon et Cie, 1956.
11. Huizinga, E., and Smelt, G. J.: *Bronchography.* Assen, Van Gorcum, 1949.
12. Atwell, S. W.: Major anomalies of the tracheobronchial tree with a list of the minor anomalies. *Dis. Chest,* 52:5, 1967.
13. Ferguson, C. F., and Neuhauser, E. B. D.: Congenital absence of the lung (agenesis) and other anomalies of the tracheobronchial tree. *Amer. J. Roentgenol. Rad. Therapy,* 52:5, 1944.
14. Schneider, L.: Bronchopulmonary hypogenesis. *Amer. J. Med. Sci.*, 215:665, 1948.
15. Ferguson, C. F., and Flake, C. G.: Tracheographic and bronchographic studies as aids in the diagnosis of congenital malformations of the tracheobronchial tree and aortic arch in infants and children. *Ann. Otol., Rhinol. Laryngol.*, 63:4, 1954.
16. Kartagener, M.: Zur Pathogenese der Bronchiektasien bei Situs Viscereum Inversus. *Beitr. Z. Klin. Tuberk.*, 83, 1933.
17. Strupler, W.: Missbildungen des bronchopulmonalen Bereiches. Archiv fur klinische und experimentelle Ohren-Nasen-und Kehlkopfheilkunde, Band 197, Heft 3, 1970. Springer-Verlag.
18. Bruwer, A., Clagett, O. T., and McDonald, J. R.: Anomalous arteries to the lung associated with congenital pulmonary abnormality. *J. Thorac. Surg.*, 19:6, 1950.
19. Holinger, P. H.: Clinical aspects of congenital anomalies of the larynx, trachea, bronchi and oesophagus (The Semon Lecture, 1960). *J. Laryngol. Otol.*, 75:1, 1961.
20. Hanna, E. A.: Broncho-esophageal fistula with total sequestration of the right lung. *Ann. Surg.*, 159:599, 1964.

Chapter One Hundred Twelve

ESOPHAGOLOGY: ANATOMIC CONSIDERATIONS AND OPERATIVE TECHNIQUES

CHARLES F. FERGUSON, M.D., F.A.C.S.

Diagnostic endoscopic procedures on the esophagus are not as frequently indicated in infants and children as in the adult patient, and are much less commonly performed than bronchoscopic or laryngoscopic investigations. Esophagoscopy, however, carries with it much more danger of complications than a bronchoscopic procedure, mainly because of anatomic differences in the two structures. The esophagus is not simply an open muscular tube, but a potential longitudinal space, with its walls in apposition when at rest. It has two important "pinchcocks"—the cricopharyngeus at its inlet and the esophageal hiatus of the diaphragm at its lower end. The former is a powerful muscle sphincter, which is in a state of tonic contraction most of the time, in order to prevent regurgitation of stomach contents on increased abdominal pressure, and to keep air out of the gastrointestinal tract on inspiration. According to Chevalier Jackson, the cricopharyngeus acts as a veritable gate which, when closed, should never be *crashed,* or it then becomes the "gate of tears" ("Bab el Mandeb").

Although the study of the gross anatomy of the esophagus and its surrounding structures is of great importance, its different appearance and movements in the living patient must be thoroughly appreciated by and entirely familiar to the endoscopist. The esophagus is a most dynamic organ. At rest it has merely a potential lumen, as its thin and elastic walls throughout its extent are in close contact, but it is capable of quickly and extensively expanding this lumen. The esophagus opens during inspiration as the thoracic cavity expands only if air is admitted through the cricopharyngeal inlet. It is not fixed or rigid in location, but is freely movable and follows the cervical and thoracic curves of the spine. It lies behind the trachea and courses downward, backward and somewhat to the left in its lower portion. It passes through an opening in the diaphragm anterior and to the left of the aorta (the diaphragmatic hiatus). There are two "pinchcocks" (the cricopharyngeus above at the sixth cervical vertebra and the diaphragmatic hiatal opening below at the 10th thoracic vertebra) and two areas of otherwise slight compression, that are rarely noted in infants and young children (the aortic crossing at the fourth thoracic vertebra and the left main bronchial compression at the fifth thoracic vertebra.)

The cricopharyngeus is a band of circular muscle fibers from the inferior constrictor muscle, attached laterally to the body of the cricoid cartilage and innervated by the pharyngeal plexus from the vagus nerve. Sensory supply is through the glossopharyngeal into the plexus. Functionally, however, the cricopharyngeus acts independently of the inferior constrictor, relaxing when the constrictor contracts and contracting as the constrictor relaxes. It closes the esophageal inlet by pulling the cricoid cartilage tightly against the posterior pharyngeal wall and the cervical spine. Perforation of the esophagus may occur posteriorly in this region where the circular fibers (cricopharyngeus) and the oblique fibers (inferior constrictors) are thin, sparse and somewhat separated (Fig. 1). Herniation or diverticula also may develop in this region of extreme thinness.

At the lower end there is no true muscle sphincter, as at the inlet, but merely tendons and special bundles of fibers that run from the crura of the diaphragm and wrap around the esophagus, causing a similar "pinchcock" effect. Although not anatomically a true sphincter, the effect is that of a physiological sphincter. Anteriorly and to the left, as the aorta crosses the esophagus, an area of pulsation or even slight compression may be seen or felt as it is transmitted through the esophagoscope. Just below this area, the left main bronchus crosses its anterior wall, running obliquely down toward the left (the trachea lies somewhat to the right).

The musculature of the esophagus consists of an inner circular layer continuous with the inferior constrictor of the pharynx above and the stomach musculature below, and an outer longitudinal layer continuous with the longitudinal muscle layers of the stomach below, merging with the inferior constrictor above, where it is attached to the cricoid cartilage. The muscle in the upper portion of the esophagus is striated and in the lower portion it is the smooth type. The nerve supply is from both parasympathetic and sympathetic nervous systems, the latter from the cervical and thoracic chains. The upper portion of the esopha-

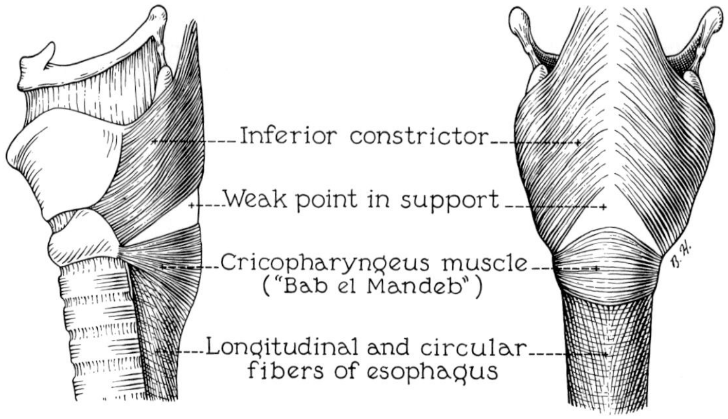

Figure 1. Esophageal musculature, showing weak point in posterior wall. "Bab el Mandeb" is the "gate of tears." (From Jackson, C., and Jackson, C. L.: *Bronchoesophagology.* W. B. Saunders, 1950.)

gus is innervated by the recurrent laryngeal branches of the vagus nerve (parasympathetic).

The slightly pink or yellowish mucosa of the esophagus is smooth and velvety and composed of stratified squamous epithelium. Longitudinal vessels are seen in the mucous membrane, which is thrown up into soft, distinct, longitudinal folds. In the lower portion there are many glands. At the esophagogastric junction the mucosa suddenly changes to a darker pink, almost red color, and these mucosal vessels are less prominent. Here the gastric rugae are noted to be larger and wider as the junction is passed during endoscopic examination and stomach contents become visible.

OPERATIVE TECHNIQUES

In performing esophagoscopy, it must always be borne in mind that the laryngotracheal airway anterior to the pharyngoesophageal food passage may be seriously compressed by the rigid esophagoscope. When general anesthesia is used, as in bronchoscopic procedures (see Chapter 108), a firm endotracheal tube should always be in place before the esophagoscope is passed, to prevent compression of this all-important airway. Since the rigid esophagoscope is introduced by itself, with no assisting laryngoscope, extreme care must constantly be exercised while it is being passed down through the pharynx and esophagus into the stomach.

The position of the head of the patient is all-important in esophagoscopy, and Jackson's "high-low" position must always be strictly observed. (Fig. 2). The head must be kept off the table and behind its edge at all times, so that it may be freely moved at any instant and in any direction. It is raised 15 cm. from the table and held there by a trained assistant, with the face of the patient parallel to the floor (and the head not hyperextended) until the esophagoscope has been passed through the cervical region. The head is then lowered 2 cm. or more below the level of the table, while the esophagoscope goes through the thoracic esophagus, as it follows the curve of the thoracic spine. The esophagoscope should be guided downward very gently, always keeping the lumen ahead in clear view, and never moving the esophagoscope forward until this lumen is straight ahead. If the lumen is not visible, a small, very flexible bougie or lumen finder can be gently passed, and the esophagoscope guided alongside it until the cricopharyngeal area has been navigated successfully.

The esophagoscope is held as a pen or pencil and never grasped by its handle. It

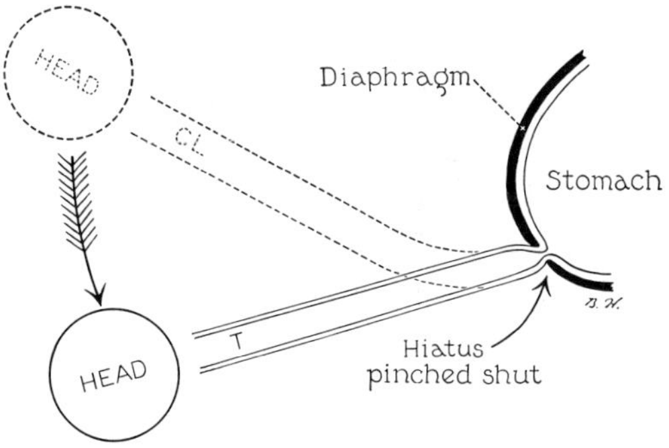

Figure 2. Schema illustrating the "high-low" method of esophagoscopy. Head is dropped from "CL" to "T" position in passing hiatus. (From Jackson, C., and Jackson, C. L.: *Bronchoesophagology,* W. B. Saunders, 1950.)

is always inserted with the handle in a vertical position (pointing upward) so that its bevel lies flat against the posterior wall and its tip does not rough up the very thin muscular wall in this area. It is passed through the right side of the mouth and along the right side of the tongue (not over the dorsum). The tip of the esophagoscope is lifted slightly upward by pressure of the thumb of the left hand, which is holding the mouth open and protecting the lips and teeth. It is moved toward the right pyriform sinus, which is located lateral and just anterior to the right arytenoid cartilage, which is always easily visible (Fig. 3). The cricopharyngeus is then visualized as a tightly closed sphincter, entirely blocking further visibility for the time being. The esophagoscope is then very gently guided ahead, but never forced, with the left thumb still lifting the esophagoscope slightly away from the thin posterior wall, which is a most dangerous area (Fig. 4). In a moment or two this tightly closed sphincter begins to relax, and a tiny lumen appears as a slit anteriorly. The cervical esophagus can then be entered by passing over the posterior bulge of the cricopharyngeus.

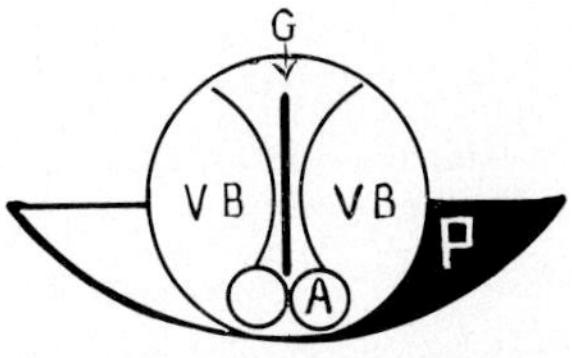

Figure 3. View of right pyriform sinus (top) through which esophagoscope is passed. (G = glottic chink, VB = ventricular bands, A = right arytenoid, P = right pyriform sinus.) (From Jackson, C., and Jackson, C. L.: *Bronchoesophagology,* W. B. Saunders, 1950.)

As the instrument is gently guided along the esophageal pathway, great care must be taken always to have a visible lumen ahead. When the level of heart is reached, where the esophagus turns somewhat forward, the head of the patient is lowered still further. More respiratory movements in the thoracic esophagus are noted than higher up, and these are due to changes in intrathoracic pressure. The head is moved a bit to the right to allow the tip of the esophagoscope to point toward the anterior superior spine of the left ilium, as the esophagus deviates anteriorly and to the left in this region. The rosette at the diaphragmatic hiatus (the closed diaphragmatic "pinchcock") is then entered, and just beyond this constricted area the esophagogastric junction is noted. Fluid then regurgitates from the stomach, and after it is removed by suction, rugae, much larger and redder than those in the esophagus, become visible.

Examination of the esophagus consists of noting the condition of the mucosa, any abnormal movements, dilatation, compressions or pulsations, and any narrowing or stricture. In addition, a tracheoesophageal fistula should be looked for anteriorly, as well as varices, ulcera-

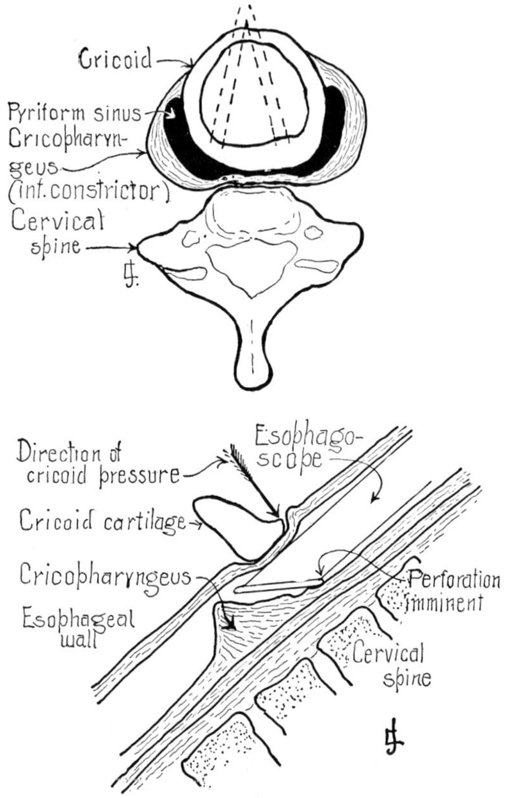

Figure 4. Anatomic basis for introduction of esophagoscope—note the pulling backward of the cricoid cartilage (above) and mounding of the cricopharyngeus posteriorly (below). (From Jackson, C., and Jackson, C. L.: *Bronchoesophagology,* W. B. Saunders, 1950.)

tion, foreign bodies or any abnormal masses. The rugae in the lower esophagus should be inspected for evidence of esophagitis from reflux, competency of the diaphragmatic hiatus, and any retained secretions or food material. The level of the esophagogastric junction is also of importance in a consideration of the so-called "short esophagus."

REFERENCES

Caffey, J.: *Pediatric X-ray Diagnosis.,* 5th Ed. Chicago, Year Book Medical Publishers, 1966.

Jackson, C., and Jackson, C. L.: *Bronchoesophagology.* Philadelphia, W. B. Saunders Co., 1950.

Olsen, A. M.: Recent advances in prognosis of esophageal disease with special reference to studies of esophageal motility. *Ann. Otol. Rhinol. Laryngol.,* 67:1147, 1958.

Chapter One Hundred Thirteen

CONGENITAL MALFORMATIONS OF THE ESOPHAGUS

JOSEPH P. ATKINS, JR., M.D., and JOSEPH P. ATKINS, M.D.

With original drawings by Leon Schlossberg

The esophagus and trachea have a common embryological origin in the foregut. Most esophageal malformations, therefore, also involve the trachea. The development of the foregut is also intimately related to the development of the heart and great vessels anteriorly, to the neural system posteriorly and the diaphragm inferiorly. Therefore, congenital anomalies of these organs frequently produce esophageal aberrations.

Advances in diagnosis and surgery as well as improvements in supportive care have bettered the ultimate prognosis in esophageal malformations. The death rate for these lesions exceeded 70 to 80 per cent only twenty years ago. This figure has been reversed in most malformations and is improving steadily in even severely malformed children.

The purpose of this chapter is to identify and classify (Table 1) the most common anomalies involving the esophagus, to point out their clinical manifestations and to discuss their management. No attempt is made to be exhaustively detailed in this presentation; rather, we wish to present an over-all view of the approach to such patients.

EMBRYOLOGY

At approximately the four weeks' stage of embryonic development, the entodermal layer of the embryo forms a ventral gutter which opens into the yolk sac. This entoderm is projected cephalad and caudad to form a tube. The cephalic end is the foregut, and the caudal end is the hindgut. The cephalad projection, or

TABLE 1. CLASSIFICATION OF CONGENITAL MALFORMATIONS OF THE ESOPHAGUS

A. Congenital absence of the esophagus
B. 1. Congenital atresia (alone) (Type A)
   2. Congenital atresia with tracheo-esophageal fistula
      a. Fistula with upper esophageal segment (Type B)
      b. Fistula with lower esophageal segment (Type C)
      c. Fistula with upper and lower esophageal segment (Type D)
   3. Tracheo-esophageal fistula without atresia
      a. Cleft larynx
      b. Tracheo-esophageal cleft
      c. Broncho-esophageal cleft
      d. Tracheo-esophageal fistula (H fistula) (Type E)
C. Congenital stenosis of the esophagus
   1. Mucosal (webs)
   2. Full thickness (strictures)
D. Duplications
   1. Double esophagus
   2. Enteric duplications
   3. Bronchogenic cysts
E. Diverticula
F. Defects associated with the diaphragm
   1. Patent hiatus (chalasia)
   2. Sliding hiatus hernia
   3. Congenital short esophagus
   4. Paraesophageal defects
      a. Eventration
      b. Hernia of Bochdalek
      c. Hernia of Morgagni
G. Associated vascular anomalies

foregut, is the area from which the pharynx, larynx, trachea and esophagus are ultimately formed.

The separation of the trachea and esophagus occurs by the advancement of folds on each lateral wall of the foregut; these folds join in the midline, splitting the foregut into two tubes. The ventral tube is the respiratory tube which buds, elongates and differentiates to form the larynx, trachea, and lungs. The esophagus is the dorsal tube, and it elongates quickly. During this phase of elongation, the stomach comes to lie intra-abdominally; there is marked proliferation of the epithelial lining and almost complete obliteration of the lumen. At about six to seven weeks of embryonic life, recanalization occurs either by resorption of cells or by a "vacuolization" process in which multiple channels could be present temporarily.

It is theorized that congenital atresias are formed by the lack of vacuolization or recanalization in the esophagus and that fistulas between the esophagus and the trachea are the result of inadequate closure of the laryngotracheoesophageal groove.

The foregut and neural groove are closely associated very early in embryonic life. A dorsal plate of mesenchyme, or entoderm, of the foregut splits to form the primitive vertebral column, or notochord. In cases of persisting connections to the spinal column (i.e., neuro-enteric cysts and duplications) there are often associated vertebral anomalies. This suggests that entodermal "adhesions" may have altered the normal developmental patterns in the separation of the intestinal and nervous systems.

CLINICAL MANIFESTATIONS OF ESOPHAGEAL MALFORMATIONS

The presence of one congenital anomaly increases the chance of a second anomaly; this holds true for esophageal malformations as well. Approximately 50 per cent of patients with atresia of the esophagus have other anomalies (Holder et al., 1964; Waterston et al). This fact should be considered when one anomaly is found. Prematurity is present in about 35 per cent of children with congenital atresia (Rickham). The mere presence of prematurity increases the risk of any anomaly about threefold.

Another consistent association with esophageal defects is the presence of maternal polyhydramnios. Approximately 30 per cent of patients with polyhydramnios have a child with some defect which prevents swallowing (Scott and Wilson). One in fourteen of these mothers has an infant with esophageal atresia. These anomalies prevent the circulation of amniotic fluid through the fetal gut where much of it is resorbed or broken down into meconium. In Waterston's series (Waterston et al.) approximately 85 per cent of mothers of infants with atresia and no fistula had polyhydramnios. Only 32 per cent of mothers of infants with atresias and a fistula had polyhydramnios.

The manifestations of any anomaly involving the esophagus depend upon the severity of the abnormality, the location and whether an abnormal communication with the trachea is present.

The most common symptoms of esophageal malformations are copius salivation, choking, dyspneic attacks, coughing and cyanotic spells. The symptoms may be noted with the first feeding of glucose water in the newborn or may be present before. If esophageal atresia is suspected, studies should be undertaken immediately. If attempts at feeding are continued and esophageal atresia is present, pneumonitis and continued aspiration inevitably occur.

The use of contrast medium as a first step in the diagnosis is to be condemned; it is often unnecessary and will cause pulmonary complications if the contrast medium is aspirated. A water-soluble contrast medium instilled under fluoroscopic control in very small volumes (1 cc.) may be used to outline the proximal pouch and to rule out an upper pouch fistula or multiple fistulas.

Most esophageal malformations, except for the atresia group, produce difficulty in swallowing (particularly solid foods), respiratory distress with or without stridor, and often poor weight gain. When narrowing is present, such as in webs, strictures and vascular compressions, these symptoms are usually present. Regurgitation or vomiting of undigested food is common in diverticula and webs. Vomiting, frequently projectile, or regurgitation of digested food is usually seen in lesions about the hiatus, such as chalasia, hiatus hernia and the "short esophagus" syndrome. The respiratory symptoms are more prominent in the cyst group, i.e., duplications and mediastinal cysts. Stridor is present if the upper airway is compromised.

The onset of symptoms in atresia is usually near birth, but narrowings may present much later in life with any of these symptoms. Holinger (1951) has emphasized that all children who have ingested a foreign body should have complete esophageal studies to rule out a pre-existing congenital lesion in the esophagus after the foreign body has been removed.

CONGENITAL ABSENCE OF THE ESOPHAGUS

To date this anomaly has been 100 per cent fatal. It usually occurs in fetuses with multiple severe abnormalities, and it is not found as an isolated entity. The esophagus may be totally absent, or there may be a fibromuscular cord present in the normal location.

CONGENITAL ATRESIA OF THE ESOPHAGUS

Many authors, beginning with Vogt in 1929, have developed classifications of atresias. Haight (1957) and Waterston (1962 and 1969) have merely used descriptive terminology which seemed more appropriate. For completeness the modified Vogt classification is also listed (Holder et al., 1964) (see Table 1 and Fig. 1).

The various forms of atresia fit into three categories. Pure congenital atresia without any fistula accounts for approximately 10 per cent of the cases in most series (Fig. 1, *A*). The second category refers to congenital atresia with tracheoesophageal fistula. Three types are recognized in this group, depending upon the origin of the fistula in the trachea. The most common category accounts for approximately 85 per cent of all atresias and consists of a blind proximal pouch and the distal esophagus attaching to the trachea (Fig. 1, *C*). The pouch may be high or low. The other variations are fistula of the proximal pouch with the trachea, the distal pouch not having a tracheal connection (Fig. 1, *B*) and, third, a double fistula with proximal and distal pouches attaching to the trachea (Fig. 1, *D*). Each of these accounts for approximately 1 per cent of cases. The third category is not truly an atresia but consists of an isolated tracheoesophageal fistula. Several isolated cases of large bronchial and esophageal connections or failures of fusion of the embryonic laryngotracheo-esophageal groove to close have been described (see Fig. 2) (Terracol and Sweet; Kissane and Smith; Blumberg et al.). However, the most common type is a small fistula between C 7 and T 2, the so-called H fistula; this fistula accounts for approximately 3 per cent of all tracheoesophageal fistulas (see Fig. 1, *E*).

As noted previously, about 50 per cent of the children with atresia have other anomalies. According to Waterston (1962) the prognosis for survival depends upon the birth weight, the severity of associated anomalies and the presence of pneumonia. In healthy infants mortality is now less than 5 per cent, but a grave prognosis (less than 5 per cent survival) exists if birth weight is less than 4 pounds, severe pneumonia has occurred, or another significant anomaly is present.

The prognosis for each type of atresia varies because of differences in the tech-

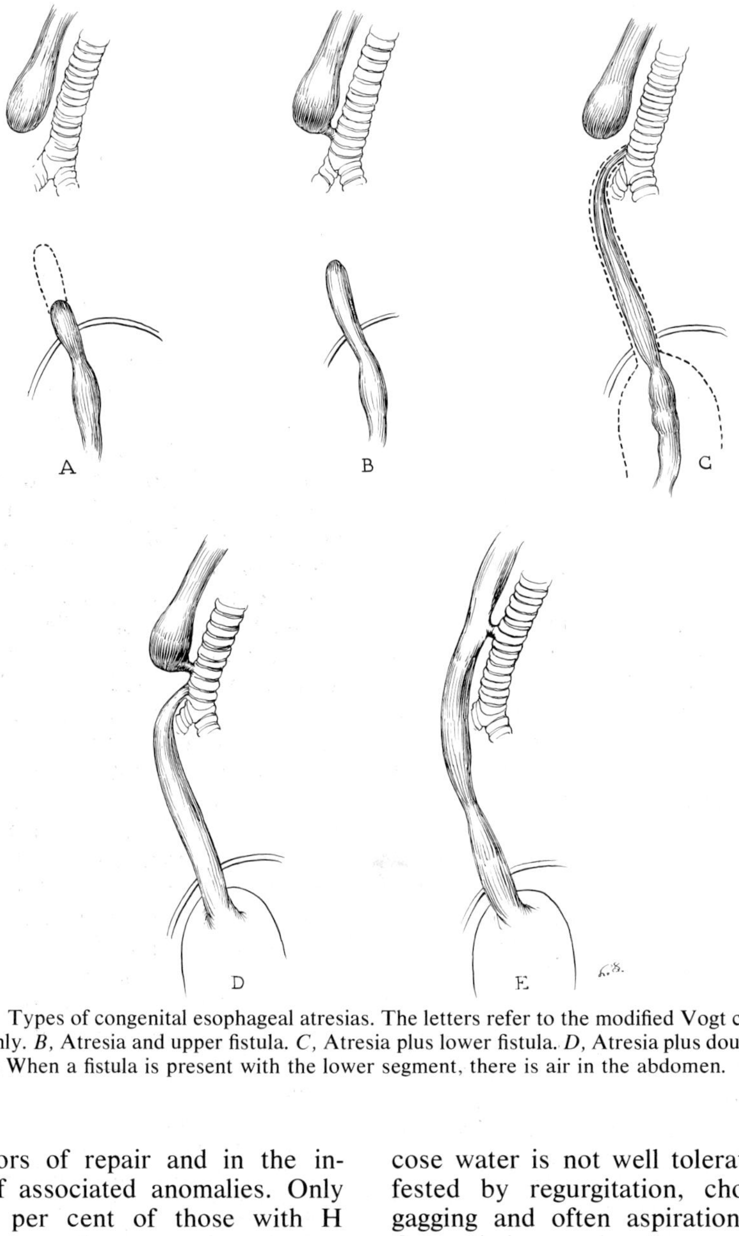

Figure 1. Types of congenital esophageal atresias. The letters refer to the modified Vogt classification. *A*, Atresia only. *B*, Atresia and upper fistula. *C*, Atresia plus lower fistula. *D*, Atresia plus double fistula. *E*, Fistula only. When a fistula is present with the lower segment, there is air in the abdomen.

nical factors of repair and in the incidence of associated anomalies. Only about 27 per cent of those with H fistula have another anomaly, whereas almost 60 per cent of those with pure atresia have a second anomaly. Congenital heart disease and intestinal atresias are the most common accompanying defects (Holder et al., 1964).

Diagnosis

These anomalies are usually first suspected when the initial feeding of glucose water is not well tolerated, manifested by regurgitation, choking and gagging and often aspiration (Fig. 3). Cyanosis is occasionally present. Abundant oral secretions and drooling are common. If no atresia is present, aspiration may be less, and the diagnosis may be delayed. The presence of prematurity and a history of polyhydramnios in the mother should increase the suspicion. Passage of a 10 F. radiopaque nasogastric tube into the stomach will rule out atresia of the esophagus. Position of the nasogastric tube must be checked

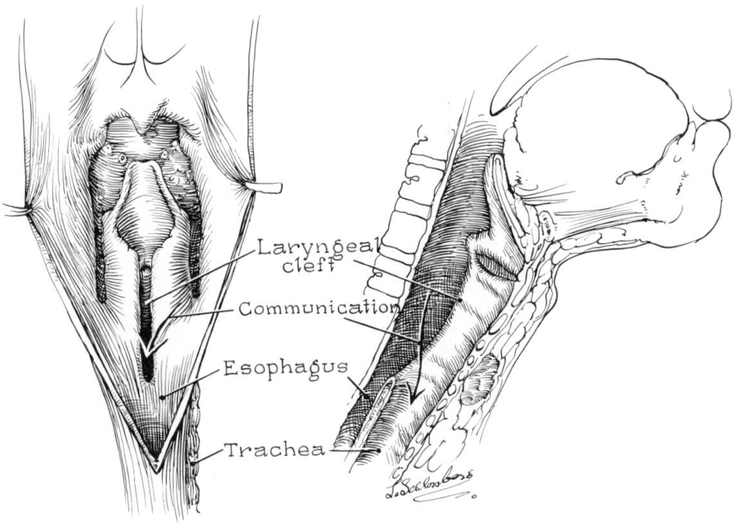

Figure 2. Posterior laryngeal cleft. The most common defect resulting from failure to close the laryngo-tracheo-esophageal groove.

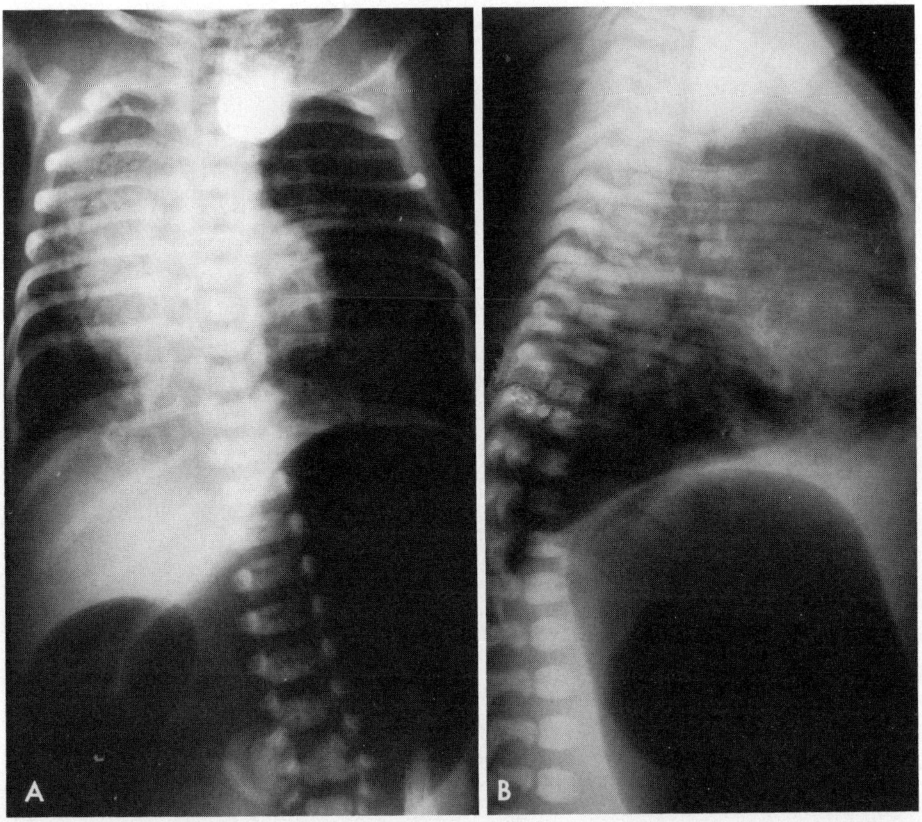

Figure 3. Congenital atresia with esophageal fistula (type C). Posteroanterior (*A*) and lateral (*B*) views showing atresia with a high pouch in a 1-day-old infant with aspiration pneumonia. Air in the stomach indicates a tracheo-esophageal fistula (not seen in these x-rays). There is extensive right-sided pneumonitis.

roentgenographically, by listening over the stomach during air instillation or by aspirating stomach contents.

If the tube meets an obstruction at 8 to 13 cm. or curls up in the esophagus, the diagnosis can be confirmed by air contrast x-ray studies of the upper pouch.

If air has entered the abdomen, a fistula must be present. This is often evident, since distention from swallowed air is usually present. In some cases the air is massive and other atresias (particularly duodenal and anal) must be excluded.

Contrast medium should not be used for routine evaluation of atresia. However, the patient who has coughing episodes and evidence of aspiration pneumonia without atresia (or in whom the diagnosis of atresia is not confirmed by the above studies) should undergo careful fluoroscopic study with a small amount of water-soluble contrast medium to rule out a tracheo-esophageal fistula without atresia. This should be done with cineradiographic techniques while the infant is in the prone position (Fig. 4).

Bronchoscopic examination may help to determine the size and location of the fistula. Dyes, such as methylene blue, may be injected into the esophagus in an attempt to demonstrate the location of the site of fistula.

Esophagoscopic examination need not be carried out in the usual atresia case

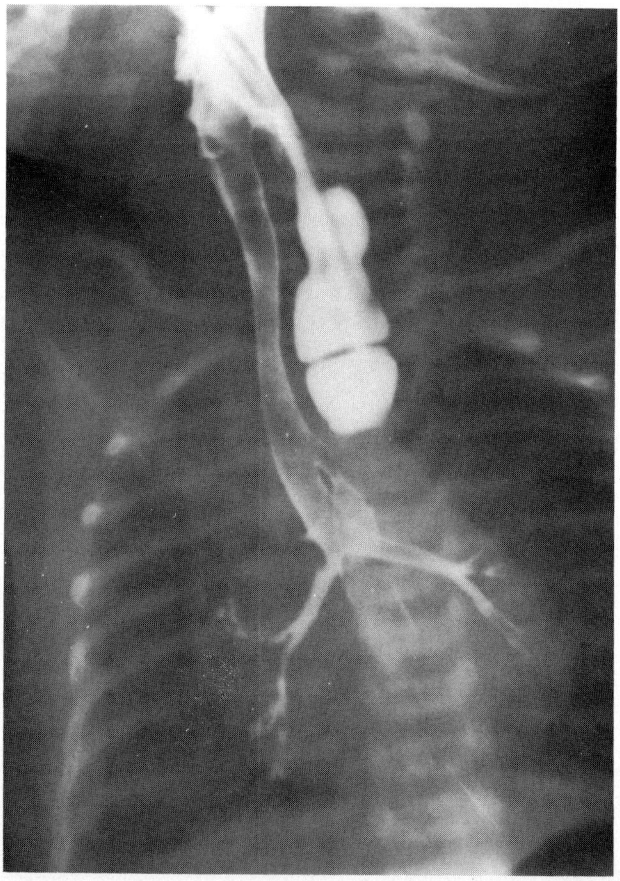

Figure 4. Congenital atresia with tracheo-esophageal fistula (type C). Anteroposterior view with water-soluble contrast medium showing low pouch, spillover into trachea and distal fistula with the esophagus in 1-day-old infant with coughing and difficulty feeding.

and may actually be dangerous. If, on the other hand, the lesion is primarily a stenosis, a membranous web or an H fistula, esophagoscopy is indicated for diagnosis and in some cases for treatment as well.

Treatment

The cornerstone of management in atresia is primary anastomosis of the proximal and distal pouches after ligation of the tracheo-esophageal fistula. This is occasionally not possible in poor-risk patients and in cases in which the proximal and distal pouches are widely separated. Multiple staging procedures have been developed for these cases.

Many factors must be considered before operation. Waterston et al. have produced a series of guidelines to help determine the course of action and have described the mortality rates in these groups (Table 2).

Preoperative hydration, treatment of pneumonia with the use of Replogle tubes (Replogle) and antibiotics, and positioning the patient upright to prevent esophageal reflux through the fistula are important in the preoperative management of these patients. If the patient is in group A or B, primary anastomosis is generally carried out. If the patient is in group C, multiple stage reconstructions are usually done if the infant can be carried over the initial phase of medical management.

The first stage usually consists of cervical esophagostomy, ligation of the fistula, closure of the distal pouch and feeding gastrostomy. Various surgeons use these modalities in different ways. The object is to prevent continued aspiration from the upper esophageal pouch by exteriorizing it. Closure of the distal pouch and ligation of the fistula will prevent retrograde aspiration. The feeding problem may be managed by a feeding gastrostomy or by intravenous hyperalimentation.

Second stage anastomoses with the colon or other intestinal interposition procedures are then done three to twenty-four months later when the infant is in better condition and larger. A retropleural rather than transpleural approach, especially in poor-risk patients, has been recommended to prevent empyema if a complication occurs. The use of local anesthesia has also been recommended (Holder et al., 1964).

TABLE 2. PROGNOSIS IN SURGICAL MANAGEMENT OF ESOPHAGEAL ATRESIA

		Mortality
Group A	Infant over 5½ lbs at birth and well	5 per cent
Group B	1. Birthweight 4 to 5½ lbs. and well 2. Higher birthweight with moderate pneumonia or congenital anomaly	32 per cent
Group C	1. Birthweight less than 4 lbs. 2. Higher birthweight with severe pneumonia and/or severe congenital anomaly	94 per cent

Postoperative care is directed at providing good tracheal toilet, hydration, and treatment of pneumonic and anastomotic complications. Approximately 10 to 20 per cent of the anastomoses develop leaks. The lowest rate appears to be with the Haight anastomosis (Holder et al., 1964; Haight, 1970). However, the postoperative stricture rate appears higher with this method.

Late Complications

Stricture at the anastomosis is the most common late sequela of surgery. The factors influencing formation of these strictures are the technique of anastomosis, tension on the suture line, leaks in the postoperative period, infection and, finally, tissue reaction to suture materials (Rickham).

Esophagoscopic dilatations of the stenosis until an adequate lumen is attained followed by repeated bougienage with mercury bougies (Hurst or Maloney) are often required. If this type of management is unsuccessful, Tucker retrograde bougies may be used through a gastrostomy; they are pulled out of the mouth on a string which was previously passed from the mouth, through the esophagus and out the gastrostomy site. In resistant strictures this is a very safe and successful technique. In general, an adequate lumen is one that does not result in continued dilatation of the proximal pouch.

Many children also have a hoarse cry and respiratory obstruction. This may be due to a form of tracheomalacia or to narrowing of the trachea by closure of the fistula as pointed out by Holinger and Johnson (1963). About 9 per cent (11 of 129) of infants examined postoperatively by Holinger had laryngeal nerve palsies of various etiologies. Some of these patients required tracheotomy to maintain a satisfactory airway.

CONGENITAL STENOSIS OF THE ESOPHAGUS

The esophagus may be stenosed by either mucosal webs or tight strictures. Webs are isolated crescentic diaphragms which may be totally obstructing (i.e., a minor form of atresia) or fenestrated, causing esophageal obstruction. Their presence may be undiscovered for many years. Some of these webs and strictures have not been diagnosed until adulthood or the ingestion of a foreign body, as pointed out by Holinger et al. (1951).

The congenital origin of webs is rarely disputed. They may occur anywhere in the esophagus, although they usually are found in the distal portion near the hiatus. They are only rarely found in the midesophagus.

Strictures or other forms of stenoses are much more complex in etiology than webs. Their congenital origin has been disputed by many (Waterston). However, several cases have been reported to be definitely congenital lesions. These cases are thoroughly discussed by Kissane and Smith. These stenoses may be

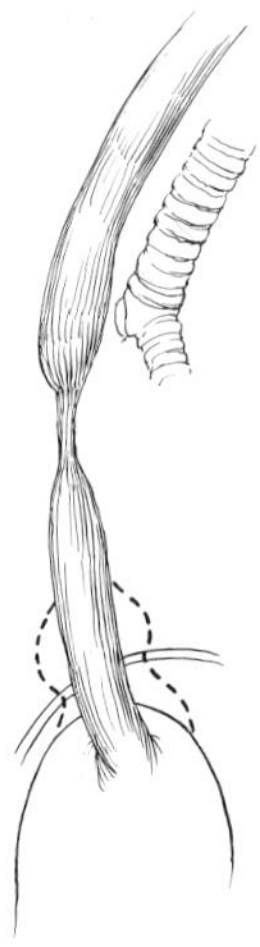

Figure 5. Esophageal stricture. The distal location of this lesion and the often associated hiatus hernia are shown.

either fibromuscular with normal mucosa and represent the same type of pathological process as in pyloric stenosis (Fig. 5), or they may be fully fibrotic strictures. Since most of these occur in the distal esophagus and are associated nearly always with hiatus hernia (Waterston), many authors feel that they are secondary to esophagitis, perhaps even in utero. This would explain the severe fibrosis present in these lesions. However, it seems unlikely that the esophagus should be spared congenital stenoses and minor atresias, since all other areas of the gastrointestinal system have such anomalies.

Diagnosis

Regurgitation, aspiration cyanosis and poor weight gain are the most common symptoms of congenital webs and strictures in infants. The onset of symptoms varies with the severity of the stenosis. In older children, failure to thrive, poor weight gain or difficulty in swallowing solid foods are the usual presenting symptoms. Many are treated for long periods as pure feeding problems until the diagnosis is made.

The diagnosis can be quickly established with a barium swallow or other contrast study of the esophagus. Webs are seen as a diaphragm or plica. Strictures form a longer zone of constriction, often with a threadlike lumen (Fig. 6). Proximal dilatation of the esophagus is usually present.

Webs may be multiple; therefore, the roentgenograms should include the entire esophagus.

Treatment

Dilatation is the treatment of choice in management of both webs and strictures. Esophagoscopy may be required in order to free the weblike stenoses, and frequently endoesophageal bougienage is carried out the initial few times in both forms. Esophagoscopy is required because the lumen is often very narrow, and blind dilatation in such cases may be hazardous. Strictures are much firmer than webs and usually require more procedures in order to maintain an adequate passage. Some strictures have required gastrostomy and subsequent retrograde dilatation by the Tucker method (as described above) or other lumen finding techniques with a string as a guide to the channel.

The success of surgery in the management of congenital stenosis is so poor that it is generally used in only rare instances. The incidence of post-surgical stricture is high (Holinger et al., 1963).

Either longitudinal esophagotomy (Terracol and Sweet) or segmental resection of webs has been recommended (Ravitch et al.). In strictures, resection and primary anastomosis may be performed, or a colon interposition may be done if the stricture is long.

DUPLICATIONS

Three forms of duplications are recognized: the paired organ or double esophagus, the enteric cyst and the bronchogenic cyst. The embryology of enteric cysts has been discussed. The double esophagus syndrome may be due to malformation in the zygote—i.e., a partial twinning phenomenon—or may be a multiple channel created by aberrant recanalization. Most authors feel this does not have a common embryological origin with the cyst. There is usually a distal connection to the esophagus near the hiatus (Fig. 7).

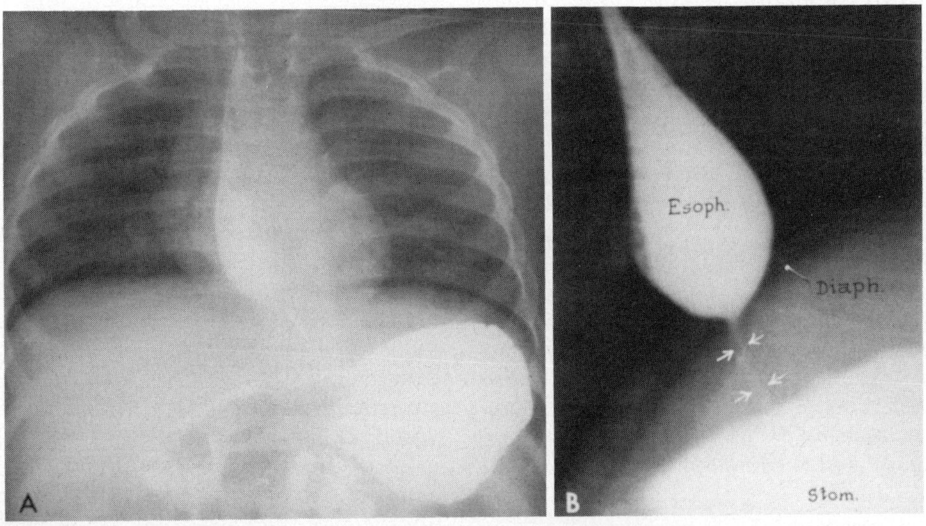

Figure 6. Congenital stenosis of the esophagus (stricture). A 1-year-old female with dysphagia and severe malnutrition since birth is shown. This patient developed severe neurologic deficit secondary to nutritional deficit. The anteroposterior (*A*) and lateral (*B*) views during barium swallow show long stricture in the distal esophagus without hiatus hernia.

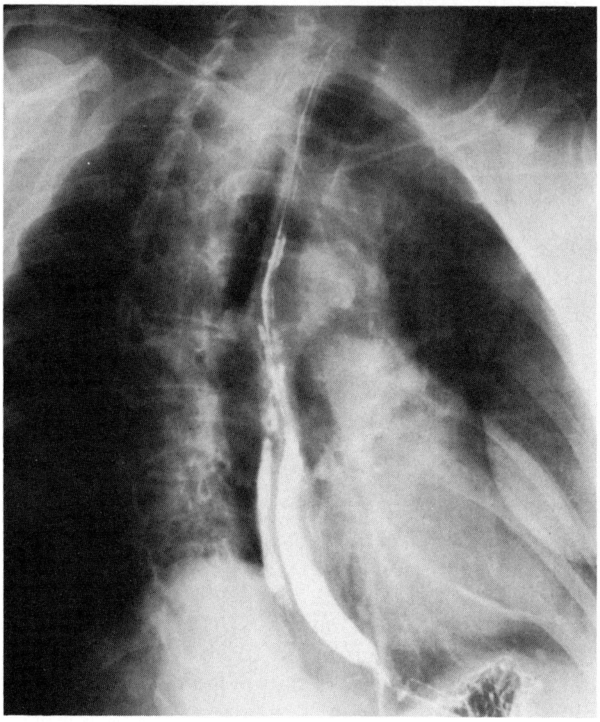

Figure 7. Duplication of the esophagus (double esophagus). This figure shows a 68-year-old white female with a 25-year history of occasional dysphagia which recently has become worse. The oblique view shows an enteric duplication that fills from below.

Bronchogenic and enteric cysts account for about 20 per cent of mediastinal cysts in children (Ravitch and Sabiston) (see Fig. 8). Bronchogenic cysts are true intramural cysts (see Fig. 8) and present as a smooth bulge into the lumen and are incorporated in the muscular wall of the esophagus. They are lined by respiratory mucosa and often contain cartilage within their walls.

Enteric cysts or duplications are not actually connected to the esophageal lumen and do not arise embryologically from the esophagus. They present in this region after rostral migration from their site of origin (probably the stomach) during development. This explains why they have gastric or other intestinal lining rather than squamous epithelium. There may be a fistula to the bowel, but it is usually below the diaphragm.

Diagnosis

Most of the mediastinal cysts are asymptomatic for long periods, especially the intramural (esophageal) type of bronchogenic cyst. This cyst has no secretory mucosa and therefore does not enlarge. There are other forms of bronchogenic cysts that do cause symptoms because of their location particularly near the hilum but are not the subject of discussion here.

Enteric cysts enlarge because of the secretory mucosa and may rupture after causing peptic ulceration of the cyst wall. When this occurs there is primarily a pulmonary presentation. Massive hemoptysis or pneumonitis may occur.

Cineradiographic analysis of the esophagus will usually show displacement by a mass or filling of the lesion from below (Fig. 7). Cervical and thoracic roentgenograms may demonstrate vertebral anomalies (Fig. 9). Two of the most revealing views, however, are the anteroposterior and lateral chest projections which will place the lesion in the posterior mediastinum (Hope and Koop). The only other common lesions in this region are the neuroblastoma

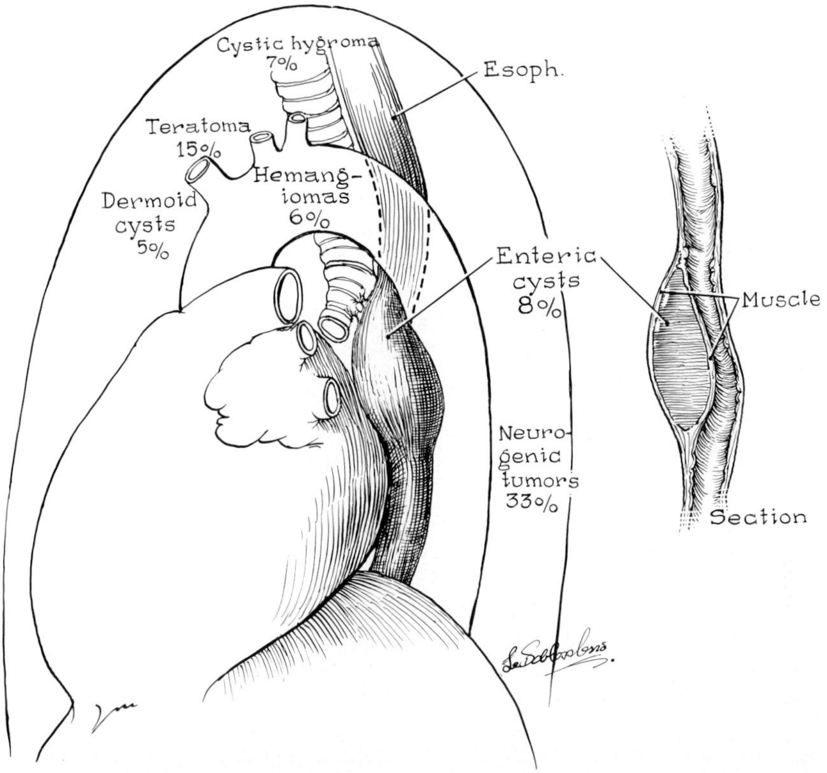

Figure 8. The incidence of mediastinal masses in children. Inset shows a bronchogenic type of enteric cyst within the muscle of the esophagus and with firm adhesions to the trachea (from which they usually arise). (Modified from Ravitch and Sabiston, 1969.)

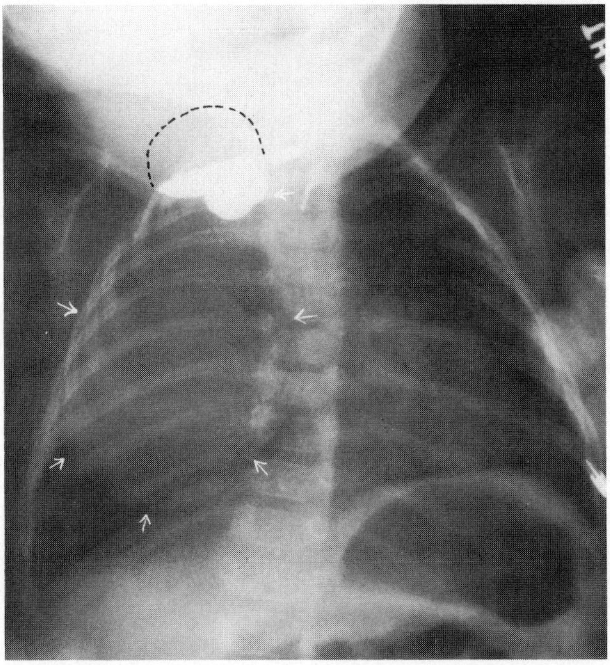

Figure 9. Duplication of the esophagus with cervical myelocele. An infant with a large mediastinal mass and flaccid extremities is shown. The anteroposterior view of the chest during a cervical myelogram shows a mass in the right posterior mediastinum filling the right chest and a large meningomyelocele of the cervical region demonstrating the frequent association of vertebral anomalies and enteric cysts.

group of tumors (Fig. 8). Myelograms may be required to rule out a neuroenteric communication.

Treatment

Exploration after complete evaluation is nearly always required, even in asymptomatic cases (Ravitch and Sabiston). Excision of the lesion is nearly always possible. There is little place for simple marsupialization of the cyst (Cantrell and Herron).

DIVERTICULA

True congenital diverticula probably exist but are quite rare (Grant and Arneil; Nelson). They have been described with other esophageal malformations, particularly tracheo-esophageal fistulas. They are "true" diverticula with complete muscle walls (Fig. 10) unlike Zenker's diverticulum, which usually consists of mucosa and submucosa.

Diagnosis

Cineradiographic studies will differentiate this lesion from the other congenital anomalies of the esophagus.

Treatment

Surgical excision will prevent recurrent aspiration from this abnormality.

DIAPHRAGMATIC HERNIA

Congenital defects about the diaphragm occur in two major forms: (1) the defects at the hiatus, generally including the syndromes of chalasia, sliding hiatus hernias and congenital short esophagus; and (2) the paraesophageal diaphragmatic defects (Fig. 11), which are caused by failure of the septum transversum to fuse, resulting in various herniations into the chest. The most common of these are the hernia of Bochdalek and eventration of the diaphragm. The hernia of Morgagni also occurs but is rarely involved with the esophagus and therefore will not be discussed here.

Chalasia or patent hiatus without hernia is characterized by free reflux in the supine position and vomiting and aspiration. Many authors feel that it is an early form of hiatus hernia without an actual pouch. However, even though it is not demonstrated, a hernia may be present. The important feature is that the treatment is medically oriented by the use of erect position in feeding the infants; the syndrome is completely reversible.

Some authors, particularly Waterston and Rickham, would actually classify all forms of hiatus hernia, stenoses and the short esophagus syndrome as acquired lesions due to reflux, perhaps even in utero. A short esophagus syndrome has been described which developed in only 2 weeks (Atkins). Baffes and Ravitch et al. feel that many are true congenital

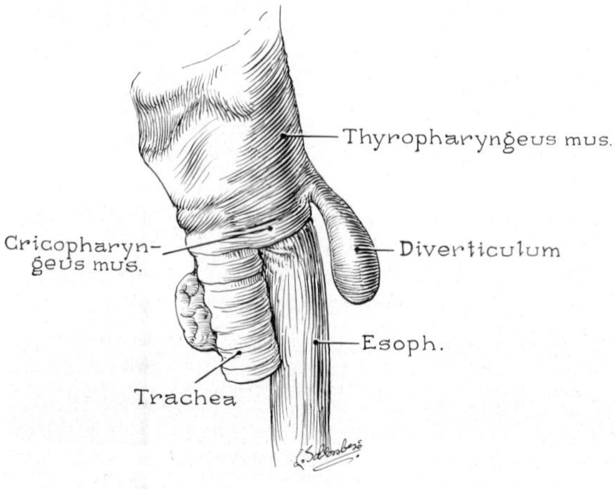

Figure 10. Congenital "true" esophageal diverticulum. The diverticulum has all normal muscular coats. It is often associated with other esophageal anomalies.

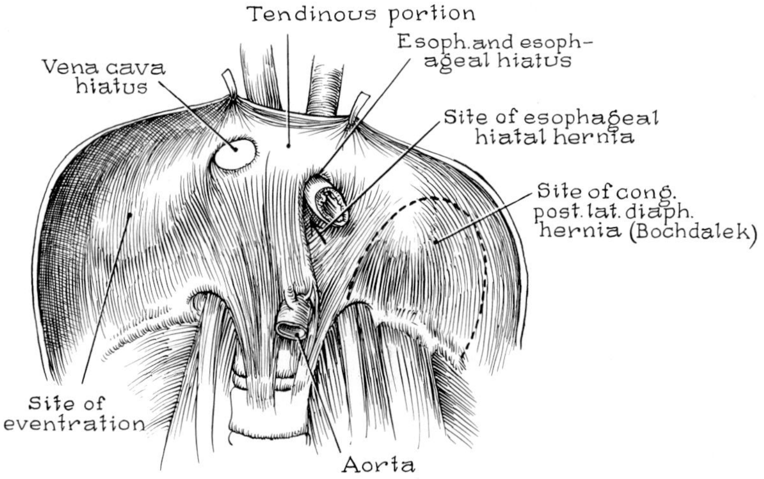

Figure 11. View of diaphragm from below.

lesions). The short esophagus with intrathoracic stomach would then result from a "trapping" of the stomach in the chest by the closure of the diaphragm before elongation of the esophagus (Baffes).

The diagnosis of hiatus hernia is by cineradiographic techniques and may be difficult to demonstrate. Esophagoscopy is needed to establish the diagnosis of esophagitis and to follow the progress of treatment.

Treatment

Management is directed at the prevention of complications, such as vomiting, poor weight gain, anemia, esophagitis, stricture and aspiration, usually through medical therapy unless response is poor. Minor strictures may be treated by dilatation. Plication of the hiatus with the stomach replaced into the abdomen is the usual mode of surgical therapy. Colon interpositions have been recommended if stricture or very short esophagus is present. Esophagogastrectomy in the infant generally results in a chronically poor nutritional status (Waterston).

Congenital paraesophageal defects may occur by a persisting pleuroperitoneal canal (as in the hernia of Bochdalek) or a failure of muscle development between the pleural and peritoneal layers. This results in a thin aponeurotic layer dividing the chest from the abdomen and is called eventration of the diaphragm. The Bochdalek defect is usually a free communication and is a true medical emergency in the newborn. Nearly 75 per cent mortality was reported before surgery was recommended (Hedblom). Butler and Claireaux have emphasized that many die before they can reach the surgeon. Prompt diagnosis and immediate surgery are the keys to improved survival (Ladd and Gross; Gross).

The symptoms of dyspnea and cyanosis are present, and there may be bowel sounds in the chest (the left chest in 80 per cent of cases); displacement of the apex of the heart (especially if a scaphoid abdomen is present) should lead to a chest x-ray. This is usually diagnostic; only pneumatoceles of staphylococcal pneumonia or congenital lung cysts can confuse interpretation (Avery). Bowel markings can be confirmed by contrast studies, but such studies are usually unnecessary and delay therapy.

As the dyspnea increases and the bowel fills with air, more herniation through the defect occurs. Operation at this point is mandatory. By the reduction of the hernia, closure of the defect and water-seal suction on the chest, most of the children will survive. The presence of associated anomalies such as malrota-

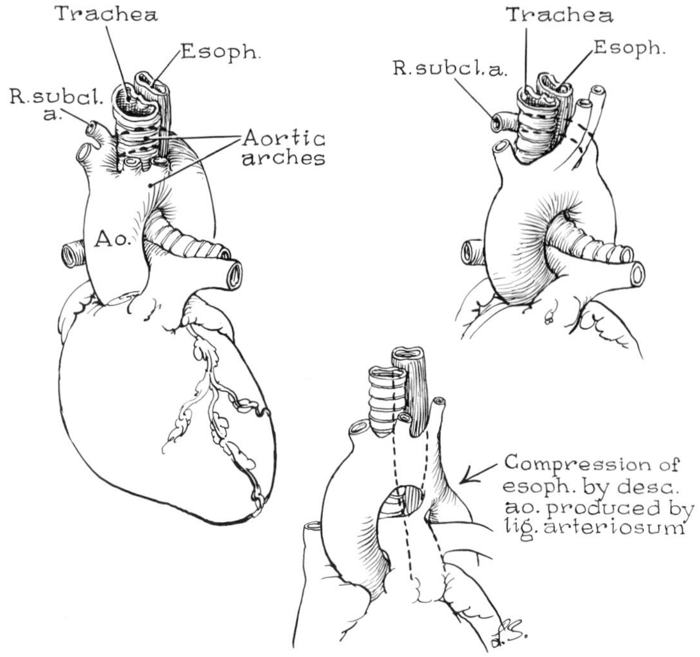

Figure 12. Vascular anomalies causing esophageal symptoms. *Left,* Double aortic arch. *Right,* Anomalous take-off of right subclavian artery. *Center,* Tight ligamentum arteriosum.

tion, hypoplasia of the lung on the ipsilateral side and a very small abdominal cavity contribute to the ultimate success or failure of therapy.

Eventration is far less dangerous than Bochdalek hernias because in eventration there is a peritoneal covering which usually prevents massive intrathoracic herniation. Treatment will depend on the severity of symptoms. If respiratory embarrassment is not too severe, no treatment is required. When necessary, plication of the defect can be done.

ASSOCIATED VASCULAR ANOMALIES

Although they are not strictly esophageal anomalies, malformations of the great vessels may cause symptoms of esophageal obstruction and are in the differential diagnosis of such patients. The most common of these lesions causing esophageal symptoms in children are shown in Figure 12. They are covered in more detail in Chapter 34 in Volume 1.

REFERENCES

Avery, M. E.: The Lung and Its Disorders in the Newborn Infant. Philadelphia, W. B. Saunders Co., 1968.

Baffes, T. G.: Diaphragmatic hernia; in Mustard, W. T., et al. (Eds.): Pediatric Surgery, Vol. I, 2nd ed. Chicago, Ill., Yearbook Medical Publishers, Inc., 1969, Chapter 27, p.342.

Blumberg, J. B., Stevenson, J. K., Lemire, R. J., and Boyden, E. A.: Laryngotracheo-esophageal cleft, the embryologic implications: review of the literature. *Surgery* 57:559, 1965.

Butler, N., and Claireaux, A. E.: Congenital diaphragmatic hernia as a cause of perinatal mortality. *Lancet* 1:659, 1962.

Cantrell, J. R., and Herron, P. W.: Surgery of the Esophagus in Lewis' Practice of Surgery, Vol. 5. Hagerstown, W. F. Prior Co., Inc., 1963, pp. 20–30.

Grant, J. C., and Arneil, G. C.: Congenital diverticulum of the esophagus. *Surgery* 46:966, 1959.

Gross, R. E.: The Surgery of Infancy and Childhood. Philadelphia, W. B. Saunders Co., 1953.

Haight, C.: Some observations on congenital atresia and tracheo-esophageal fistulas of congenital origin. *J. Thorac. Surg.,* 34:141, 1957.

Haight, C.: Congenital esophageal atresia and tracheo-esophageal fistula; in Mustard, W. T., et al. (eds.): Pediatric Surgery, Vol. I. Chicago, Ill.,

Yearbook Medical Publishers, Inc., 1969, pp. 357–382.
Hedblom, C. A.: Diaphragmatic hernia. *J.A.M.A.*, 85:947, 1925.
Holder, T. M., Cloud, D. T., Lewis, J. E., and Pilling, G. P., IV: Esophageal atresia and tracheo-esophageal fistula. *Pediatrics*, 34:542, 1964.
Holder, T. M., and Ashcraft, K. W.: Esophageal Atresia and the Fistula. Chicago, Yearbook Medical Publishers Inc., Current Problems in Surgery, Aug. 1966.
Holinger, P. H., Johnston, K. C., and Potts, W. J.: Congenital anomalies of the esophagus. *Ann. Otol.*, 60:707, 1951.
Holinger, P. H., and Johnston, K. C.: Post-surgical endoscopic problems of congenital esophageal atresia. *Ann. Otol.*, 72:1035, 1963.
Hope, J. W., and Koop, C. E.: Differential diagnosis of mediastinal masses. *Pediat. Clin. North Amer.*, 6:379, 1959.
Kissane, J. M., and Smith, M. C.: Pathology of Infancy and Childhood. St. Louis, The C. V. Mosby Co., 1967, pp. 140–164.
Ladd, W. E., and Gross, R. E.: Congenital diaphragmatic hernia. *New Eng. J. Med.*, 223:917, 1940.
Nelson, A. R.: Congenital true esophageal diverticulum. *Ann. Surg.*, 145:258, 1957.
Potts, W. J.: Congenital deformities of the esophagus. *Surg. Clin. North Amer.*, 31:97, 1951.
Ravitch, M. M., and Sabiston, D. C., Jr.: Mediastinal infections and tumors; in Mustard, W. T., et al. (Eds.): Pediatric Surgery, Vol. I. Chicago, Yearbook Medical Publishers Inc., 1969, pp. 408–428.
Replogle, R. L.: Esophageal atresia. Plastic sump catheter for drainage of the proximal pouch. *Surgery*, 54:296, 1963.
Rickham, P. P., and Johnston, J. H.: Neonatal Surgery. London, Butterworths, 1970. pp. 198–223.
Schaffer, A. J., and Avery, M. E.: Disease of the Newborn, 3rd ed. Philadelphia, W. B. Saunders Co., 1971.
Scott, J. S., and Wilson, J. K.: Hydramnios as an early sign of esophageal atresia. *Lancet*, 2:569, 1957.
Smith, E. I.: The early development of the trachea and esophagus in relation to atresia of the esophagus and tracheo-esophageal fistula. *Contributions to Embryology*, No. 245, 36:41, 1957.
Swenson, O.: Pediatric Surgery, 3rd ed. New York, Appleton Century Crofts, Inc., 1969.
Terracol, J., and Sweet, R. H.: Diseases of the Esophagus. Philadelphia, W. B. Saunders Co., 1958, Chapter 6, pp. 123–152.
Vogt, E. C.: Congenital esophageal atresia. *Amer. J. Roentgen.*, 22:463, 1929.
Waterston, D. J., Bonham-Carter, R. E., and Aberdeen, E.: Esophageal atresia: tracheo-esophageal fistulas. *Lancet*, 2:819, 1962.
Waterston, D. J.: Hiatus hernia and reconstruction of the esophagus; in Mustard, W. T., et al. (Eds.): Pediatric Surgery, Vol. I. Chicago, Yearbook Medical Publishers, Inc., 1969, pp. 392–408.

Chapter One Hundred Fourteen

MECHANICS OF SWALLOWING AND FUNCTIONAL ABNORMALITIES OF THE ESOPHAGUS

ARTHUR M. OLSEN, M.D.

ANATOMY

The anatomy of the mouth and the pharynx has been described in some detail in previous chapters. Structures within the mouth and pharynx do play an important role in the early stages of deglutition, and their role will be recalled in the description of the mechanism of swallowing.

The esophagus itself is a tube with sphincters at the upper and lower ends. It begins at the level of the sixth cervical vertebra and pierces the diaphragm through the esophageal hiatus at the level of the tenth or eleventh thoracic vertebra. The esophagus lies in the posterior mediastinum. Between rather fixed upper and lower points the organ is reasonably mobile. It is essentially a midline structure with some deviation to the right as it enters the thorax. However, in the lower mediastinum the esophagus angulates rather sharply to the left and anteriorly as it approaches the hiatus of the diaphragm.

The muscular layers of the esophagus consist of inner circular and outer longitudinal muscle fibers. Both sets of muscle fibers have a tendency to spiral to some extent (Flavell, 1963). In the upper one-third, striated muscle predominates. In the middle third, the transition to smooth muscle takes place, and in the lower third the walls are composed entirely of smooth muscle. The mucosa is stratified squamous epithelium throughout, with underlying racemose mucous glands. Hayward (1961) has described a columnar junctional mucosa in the terminal esophagus extending 1 or 2 cm. above the esophagogastric junction. The junctional mucosa secretes mucus but no enzymes.

The upper or cricoid sphincter of the esophagus is well defined and consists of the cricopharyngeus muscle, which can be shown to encircle the esophagus and which is attached above to the posterior aspect of the cricoid cartilage (Hollinshead, 1969; Zaino et al., 1970). The cricopharyngeus muscle is actually an extension of the inferior constrictor of the pharynx and in turn blends into the circular fibers of the esophagus.

The lower sphincter has been a debatable anatomic structure. Botha (1962) and Didio and Anderson (1968) described a muscular sphincter but agree that it is not a well-defined structure like the cricoid or pyloric sphincters. Lerche (1950) described a sphincter consisting of the constrictor cardiae muscles. Other authorities such as Lendrum (1937) and Higgs and associates (1965) found no anatomic evidence of a lower sphincter.

As will be brought out later, there is abundant evidence for a physiologic sphincter at the level of the hiatus of the diaphragm (Code et al., 1958; Dornhorst et al., 1954; Fyke et al., 1956), and it would appear to be the principal barrier to reflux (Meiss et al., 1958). Other anatomic entities include the phrenoesophageal ligament described by Harrington (1938) (Fig. 1), by Allison (1951), and by Peters (1955), and considered by these authorities to have considerable importance (Lyons et al., 1956). Although this structure appears to be quite prominent in infants and children (Botha, 1958b), its importance has been minimized by Barrett (1954), who stated that this membrane is so tenuous that ". . . it can be dissected out with the eye of faith. . . ."

Bremner and associates (1970b) found that the membrane played little role in the control of reflux. The encircling fibers of the right crus of the diaphragm form the cardial "sling" (Fig. 2), which helps to maintain the angle of His (Collis

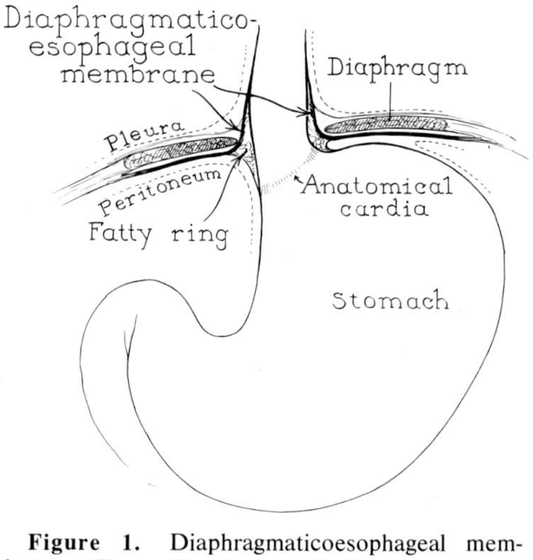

Figure 1. Diaphragmaticoesophageal membrane. (From Harrington, S. W.: Esophageal hiatus diaphragmatic hernia: etiology, diagnosis, and treatment in 123 cases. J. Thorac. Cardiovasc. Surg., *8*:127, 1938. By permission of C. V. Mosby Company.)

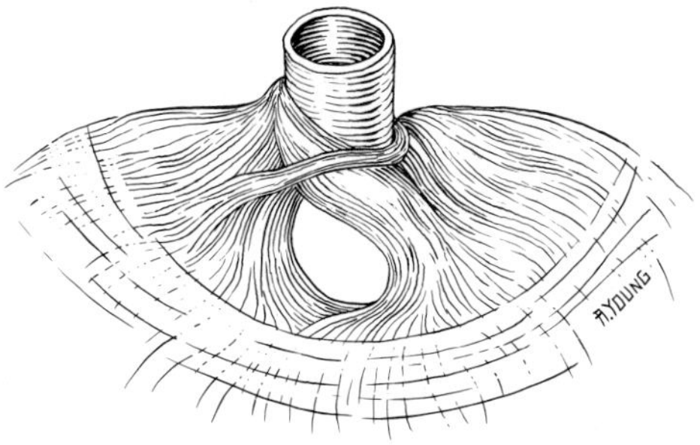

Figure 2. The cardial "sling" formed by the right crus of the diaphragm. (From Carey, J. M., and Hollinshead, W. H.: An anatomic study of the esophageal hiatus. Surg. Gynec. Obstet., *100*:196, 1955. By permission.)

et al., 1954). Botha (1958a, b) and Dornhorst et al. (1954) have emphasized the importance of the mucosal fold at the cardia as a sphincteric mechanism. Finally, the left gastric artery is alleged to play a role in fixing the esophagogastric junction to the hiatus of the diaphragm (Barrett, 1954; Lyons et al., 1956).

The motor nerve supply to the pharynx, the cricopharyngeus muscle, and the esophagus is primarily derived from branches of the vagus nerve (Carlson et al., 1922). The glossopharyngeal nerve is principally sensory to the pharynx (Hollinshead, 1969; Sinclair, 1970), and of course the hypoglossal nerve plays a significant role in the mouth. Branches of the sympathetic nerves are also present in the so-called pharyngeal plexus. In the wall of the esophagus, Meissner's plexus lies in the submucous layer, and Auerbach's plexus can be found between the layers of muscle. The coordination of all of these activities takes place in the "swallowing center" (close to the respiratory center) and is controlled by neurons in the floor of the fourth ventricle (Hightower, 1957).

PHYSIOLOGY

The terms deglutition and swallowing are synonymous. To the endoscopist, the process begins in the mouth and ends in the stomach. However, anatomists (Didio and Anderson, 1968) and certainly the average individual believe that swallowing is over when the bolus reaches the esophagus. In any case, the process of swallowing has traditionally been divided into oral, pharyngeal, and esophageal components (McEwan-Alvarado, 1969).

The oral phase of swallowing is entirely voluntary. Masticated food is carried by the tongue into the pharynx by pressure of the tongue against the hard and soft palate. In the pharynx, the mechanism is more complicated, and is essentially an involuntary process. The glossopharyngeal nerve provides most of the afferent impulses and motor activities are dominated by the vagus (Hollinshead, 1969; Sinclair, 1970). The tongue rises to the hard palate and the soft palate seals off the nasopharynx. The larynx and epiglottis are pulled upward and forward to obstruct the airway. The pharyngeal constrictor muscles propel the bolus toward the esophageal introitus. Simultaneously, the cricopharyngeus relaxes (Fyke and Code, 1955). Food has no place to go but into the esophagus.

Peristalsis in the esophagus has been divided into three types (Templeton, 1944). Primary waves probably begin with the contraction of the pharyngeal constrictors and pass through the esophagus to the cardia. Secondary waves begin in the smooth muscle portion and pass to the stomach. Tertiary waves are not peristaltic and are most readily noted by the radiologist when peristalsis is absent or deficient. Stiennon (1968) states that tertiary waves are caused by simultaneous contraction of longitudinal and circular muscles of the esophagus and are seen when circumstances permit shortening of the organ. These tertiary waves apparently are responsible for the asymptomatic "curling" of the esophagus noted in older people and in many patients with hiatal hernia (Fig. 3).

Relaxation of the lower sphincter does not await the propagation of the peristaltic waves, which take about 10 seconds to reach the cardia. Actually, the lower sphincter relaxes shortly after the peris-

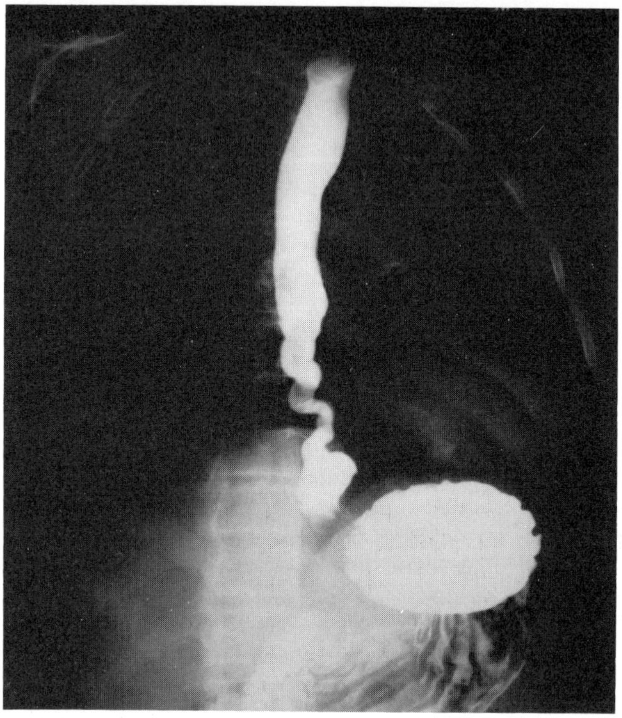

Figure 3. Tertiary waves of the esophagus (the "corkscrew esophagus").

taltic wave is initiated and remains open until the wave rolls through (Fyke et al., 1956). The process of swallowing may be recorded by manometric techniques, which show successively pharyngeal contractions, the relaxation and contraction of the cricoid sphincter (Fig. 4), the peristaltic "profile" in the esophagus (Fig. 5), and the relaxation and contraction of the lower sphincter (Fig. 6).

As has been pointed out, the upper or cricoid sphincter is a well-defined anatomic structure, and maintains a high degree of tone except during its period of relaxation (Fyke and Code, 1955) (Fig. 7 *A*). Resting intraluminal pressures are consistently higher at the level of the upper sphincter (30 cm. of water pressure) than in either the pharynx or the esophagus. The inferior or esophagogastric sphincter provides a weaker (15 cm. of water pressure) but still effective barrier between the esophagus and stomach (Fig. 7 *B*). Because the lower sphincter is difficult to identify anatomically, there has been much discussion regarding the nature of the mechanism that supports the pressure gradient at this level. The presence of an intraluminal resting high-pressure zone is well documented. Anatomic structures that may be important in preventing reflux have already been reviewed.

Despite the possible role of the angle of His (Lyons et al., 1956), the sling produced by the crus of the diaphragm (the diaphragmatic pinchcock) (Collis et al., 1954), the mucosal folds at the cardia (Botha, 1958a), and so forth (Flavell, 1963), it would appear that the sphincter itself is the most important barrier (Belsey, 1966; Bremner et al., 1970b; Meiss et al., 1958; VanTrappen et al., 1960). However, when the sphincter is displaced from its normal location at the hiatus into the thoracic cavity (hiatal hernia), it may lose its effectiveness, and reflux may occur more readily (Atkinson, 1962; Aylwin, 1953; Hiebert, 1970; Kelley, 1965).

To better understand the mechanisms involved, a discussion of pressure rela-

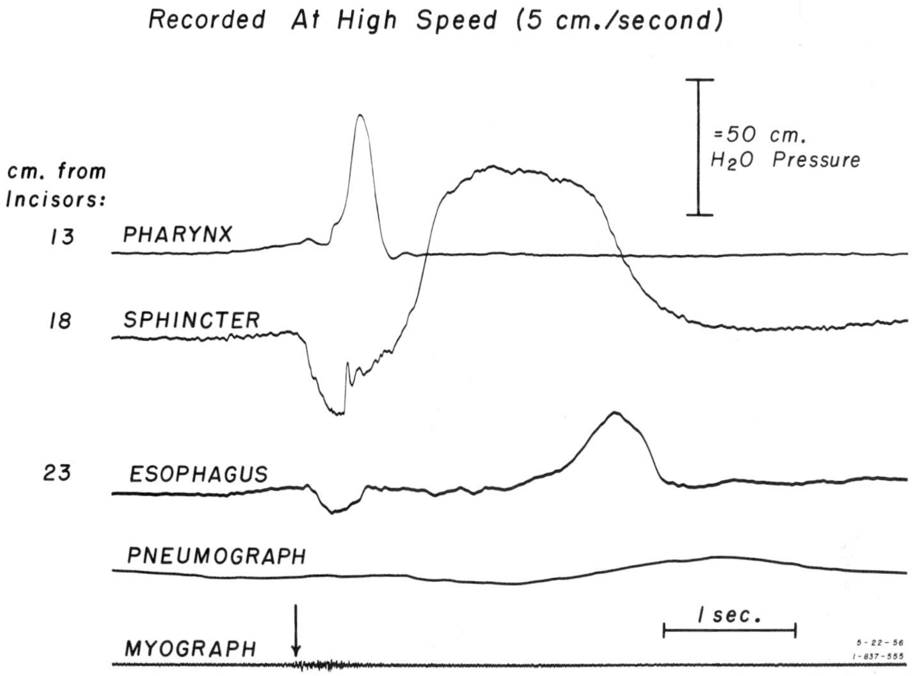

Figure 4. Responses to deglutition in the pharynx at the pharyngoesophageal sphincter. (From Code, C. F., et al.: *An Atlas of Esophageal Motility in Health and Disease.* Charles C Thomas, Publisher, Springfield, Ill., 1958, p. 27. By permission.)

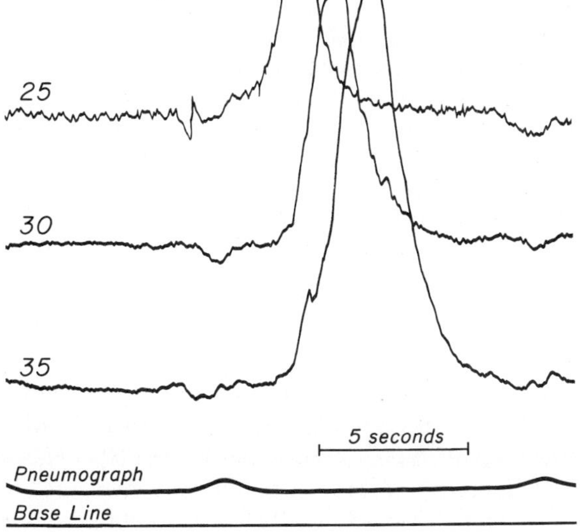

Figure 5. Peristaltic profile of deglutition pressure sequence in esophagus. (From Olsen, A. M.: Study of esophageal motility in health and disease. Ann. Otol., *77*:892, 1968. By permission of Annals Publishing Company.)

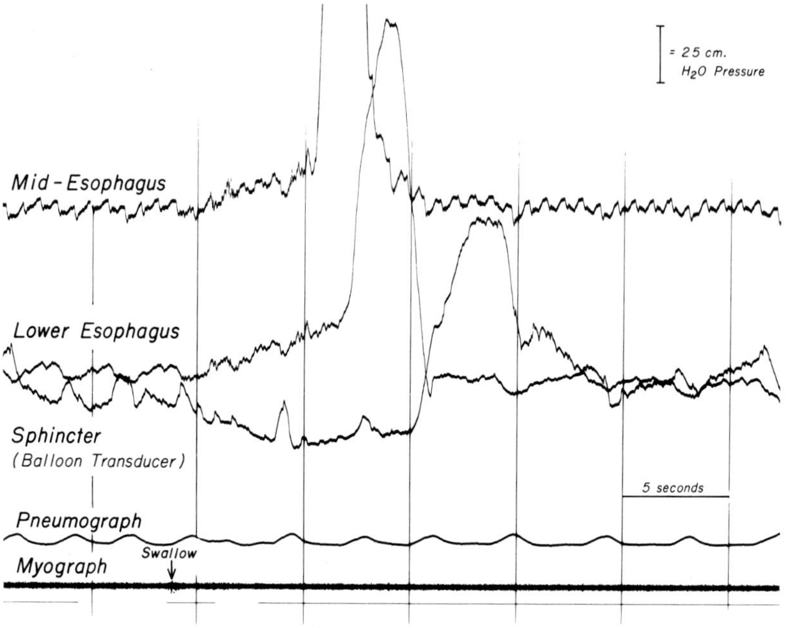

Figure 6. Response to deglutition in lower esophagus and at esophagogastric sphincter. (From Olsen, A. M.: Study of esophageal motility in health and disease. Ann. Otol., *77*:892, 1968. By permission of Annals Publishing Company.)

tionships is necessary. Negative pressures within the thorax (and esophagus) fluctuate with the rise and fall of the diaphragm and are well below intra-abdominal and intragastric pressures (−7 to 10 cm. of water pressure) (Code et al., 1958). Although the difference between intragastric and intraesophageal pressures might appear to provoke regurgitation, it seems likely that the higher intragastric and intra-abdominal pressure may actually strengthen rather than weaken the lower sphincter when it occupies its normal position (Figs. 8, and 9 *A*). However, upward displacement may favor reflux illustrated in Figure 9 *B*. Studies have shown that 28 cm. of intragastric water pressure is required to overcome the lower sphincter in its normal position; however, only 3 cm. of pressure is needed to cause reflux when displaced into the thorax (hiatal hernia) (Flavell, 1963).

Recent studies have suggested that the behavior of the sphincters (especially the lower sphincter) is affected by hormonal and chemical factors (Castell and Levine, 1971; Giles et al., 1969). Hunt and associates (1970) have demonstrated that patients who have reflux esophagitis have a significantly elevated crico-pharyngeal pressure. It would appear that the irritant effect of gastric juice in the esophagus results in increased resting tone of the upper sphincter, thus preventing further reflux into the pharynx and mouth.

The studies of Castell and Harris (1970) suggest that regulation of lower esophageal sphincter pressure may be a physiologic action of gastrin. Subcutaneous injection of pentagastrin results in a marked increase in the resting pressure of the lower sphincter. Although it is known that pentagastrin will elicit a maximal hydrochloric acid response from the gastric mucosa (Berstad and Myren, 1970), the instillation of dilute hydrochloric acid into the stomach results in a fall in esophagogastric sphincter pressure (Castell and Levine, 1971). Conversely, gastric alkalinization stimulates endogenous gastrin release (Posey and Franklin, 1967) and results in increased tone of the lower sphincter (Castell and Levine, 1971). Thus, the

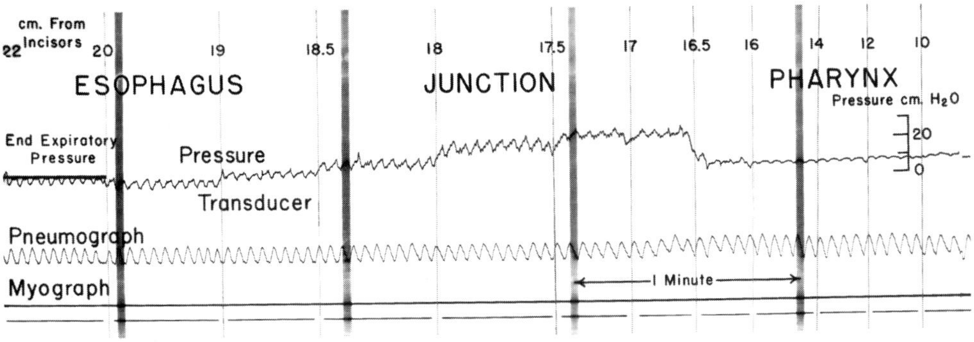

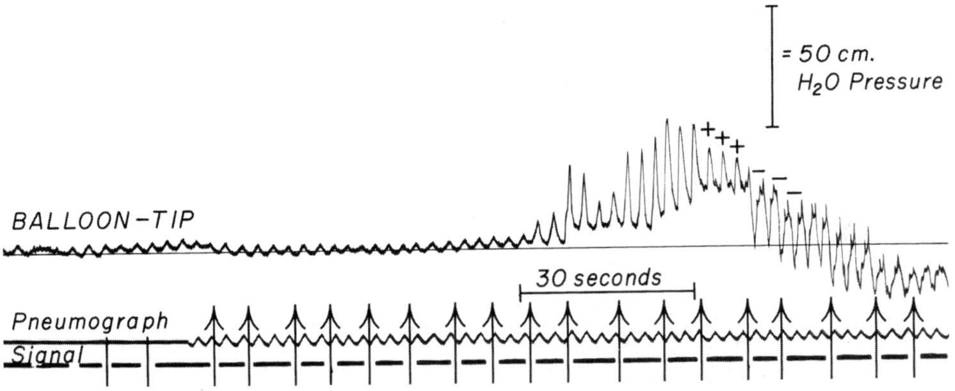

Figure 7. Resting pressures at esophageal sphincters: at the pharyngoesophageal junction (*upper panel*), and at the esophagogastric junction (*lower panel*). (Upper panel from Code, C. F., et al.: *An Atlas of Esophageal Motility in Health and Disease.* Charles C Thomas, Publisher, Springfield, Ill., 1958, p. 22. By permission. Lower panel modified from Olsen, A. M.: Study of esophageal motility in health and disease. Ann. Otol., 77:892, 1968. By permission of Annals Publishing Company.)

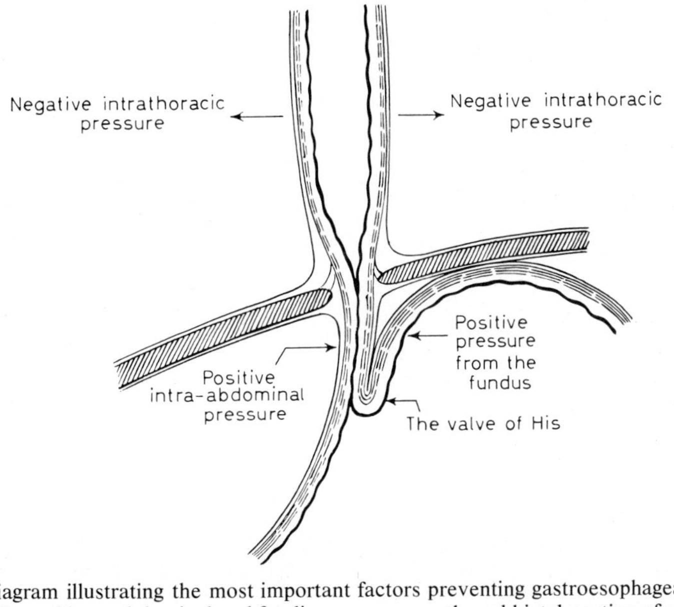

Figure 8. Diagram illustrating the most important factors preventing gastroesophageal reflux. Note in particular the effect of intra-abdominal and fundic pressures on the subhiatal portion of esophagus. (From Flavell, G.: *The Oesophagus.* Butterworth & Co., Ltd., London, 1963, p. 1. By permission.)

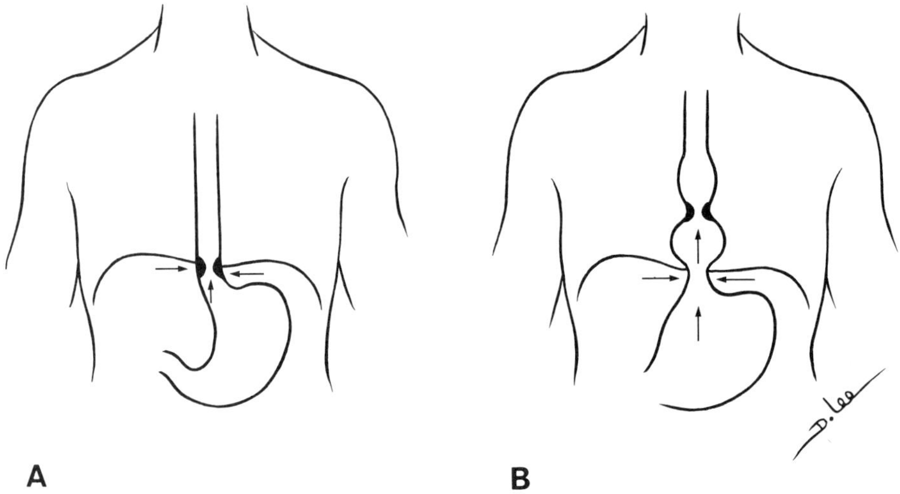

Figure 9. *A*, Diagram showing normal relationships at the hiatus, *B*, Effect of displacement of the lower sphincter into the thorax.

ingestion of antacids in the patient with reflux serves the dual role of neutralizing gastric acid and fortifying the esophagogastric barrier.

Inasmuch as this discussion will be primarily concerned with the problems of the pediatric patient, some discussion of the peculiarities of deglutition in infants is appropriate. The neonate obtains his nourishment by sucking from his mother's nipple or from a bottle (Colley and Creamer, 1958). In the full-term baby, the suckle-swallow reflex is well established (Ardran and Kemp, 1951; Gryboski, 1965). The newborn is an obligatory nose breather for the first three to five weeks of his life. In fact, during sleep the oral passage is closed by elevation of the tongue to the palate.

Sucking movements inhibit respiration, and the pharyngeal mechanism previously described operates very smoothly (Ardran and Kemp, 1970). The tongue sweeps back and upward, the soft palate is elevated, and at the same time the walls of the pharynx constrict. The larynx is elevated and closed and the cricopharyngeus opens. Gryboski (1969) has studied this mechanism in the premature infant manometrically and has found that the suckle-swallow pattern is not as well developed as in the full-term baby. There may be some delay in the opening of the upper esophageal sphincter and esophageal contractions may not be peristaltic. Thus, the premature newborn may have swallowing problems.

Strawczynski and associates (1964) also assessed the mechanism of swallowing with motility studies. They found that although the tone of the esophagogastric sphincter was low in the first two weeks of life, it became normal by the end of one month. Likewise, the fundal-esophageal gradient increases steadily as the child grows and the length of the sphincter also increases. Their studies of normal infants also showed that most of the lower sphincter (up to 80 per cent) is above the hiatus of the diaphragm. Such studies shed some light on the tendency of the infant to regurgitate freely. Blank and Pew (1956), using radiologic techniques, demonstrated reflux in half of the 70 normal infants they studied. Thus, frequent regurgitation is not necessarily an evil omen.

DIAGNOSTIC METHODS

Reference has already been made to some of the techniques that have been used to study the mechanism of swallowing. Ordinary fluoroscopic techniques often leave a good deal to be desired. Cineradiography, however, is helpful in the evaluation of most swallowing problems. It has been employed to study the movements of the tongue and pharynx (Ardran and Kemp, 1951, 1970; Blank and Pew, 1956; Zaino et al., 1970) as well as of the esophagus itself. In evaluating esophagogastric-sphincter competence, the "water siphonage" test may be useful (Crummy, 1966). The radiologist must take advantage of the effects of change of posture in studying the esophageal sphincters, especially in infants and children.

Motility studies are widely used to study swallowing problems (Butin et al., 1953; Code et al., 1958; Fleshler et al., 1958; Harris, 1969; Hightower, 1957). Although such pressure studies are somewhat more difficult to use in infants and children, they can be helpful in the study of both normal (Atkinson et al., 1957b) and abnormal deglutition (Carré and Astley, 1958; Colley and Creamer, 1958; Gryboski, 1965; Gryboski et al., 1963; Kramer et al., 1957; Strawczynski et al., 1964). These manometric techniques are applicable to all stages of swallowing, from sucking to studies of the lower sphincter (Blank and Pew, 1956; Strawczynski et al., 1964).

Esophagoscopy is another useful procedure in studying problems of deglutition, especially those of the lower sphincter (Hiebert, 1970). Milder degrees of esophagitis are best detected by direct vision, especially with the aid of the newer magnifying telescopes or the fiberesophagoscopes. The 5 mm. fiberbronchoscope may be used to examine the infant's esophagus. Usually incompetence of the lower sphincter can be recognized at esophagoscopy. Esophagoscopy is usually indicated in the evaluation of hiatal hernia, achalasia and most esophageal disorders.

The acid diffusion test (Bernstein and Baker, 1958; Siegel and Hendrix, 1963) and studies of esophageal pH (Piccone et al., 1965; Tuttle and Grossman, 1958), have not been used to any extent in children, although they have their usefulness in evaluating heartburn in adults, and may be combined with manometric studies. Correlation of heartburn and other symptoms of reflux with objective measurements of lower sphincter competence and signs of reflux and esophagitis leaves much to be desired in the adult (Kelley, 1965; Maclaurin, 1963; Palmer, 1968; Schuman and Rinaldo, 1966). In the infant and child, we need every available diagnostic aid in the evaluation of swallowing problems, in addition to the most detailed history and the most painstaking examination and observation.

ORAL AND PHARYNGEAL PROBLEMS

Because the three stages of swallowing are intimately related, it is necessary to consider the oral and pharyngeal phases as well as the esophageal phase. Any disturbance of the mouth, tongue or jaws, whether congenital or acquired, will interfere with the propulsion of food from the mouth to the hypopharynx. Usually this is the simplest phase of swallowing and requires little further comment. However, "functional dysphagia" is a problem that may be encountered (Gaarde and Olsen, 1944; Vinson, 1940). After a psychic shock, some individuals have a morbid fear of choking. They masticate with the front teeth ("rabbit-chewers") and they will chew food for long periods of time before attempting to swallow. Functional dysphagia may be responsible for profound malnutrition. Psychiatric therapy is usually the only answer to this problem. Functional dysphagia must be distinguished from "globus hystericus," in which the patient describes a lump in the throat, somewhat akin to the "heart-in-the-mouth" sensation. The patient often feels better after swallowing. The condition is often seen in girls of adolescent age. Globus hystericus is not dysphagia at all. As Harris (1969) has emphasized, dysphagia is a disturbance of the mechanical transport from the mouth to the stomach.

Functional dysphagia must also be separated from "hysterical dysphagia" (Plummer-Vinson or Patterson-Kelly syndrome) (Gaarde and Olsen, 1944), which is perhaps more properly called sideropenic dysphagia. This disorder rarely occurs in children. Characteristically, it is seen in edentulous females past the age of 40, and it may or may not have a functional origin. It is characterized by cheilosis, glossitis, pharyngitis, cracks at the corners of the mouth, achlorhydria, and sometimes splenomegaly. Often there is a "web" at the upper end of the esophagus. Usually the condition can be corrected by dilation of the upper esophagus, reassurance, proper nutrition and administration of iron.

As already indicated, the pharyngeal phase of swallowing is quite complicated. Any disturbance of neuromuscular mechanisms in the throat may produce great difficulty in swallowing, primarily because the opening of the cricoid sphincter is dependent upon a well-coordinated pharyngeal mechanism (Ardran and Kemp, 1951; Utian and Thomas, 1969). Obviously tumors, inflammations such as tonsillitis or retropharyngeal abscess, foreign bodies and diverticula will interfere with swallowing and must always be considered by the physician when swallowing problems occur.

Of great importance are the neurologic disorders that are responsible for hypopharyngeal dysfunction. In the premature infant, the sucking and swallowing reflexes may be deficient. Gryboski 1969) has demonstrated that esophageal contractions may not be peristaltic. Pharyngeal incoordination may occur in the newborn, although in most cases the problem resolves with the growth of the infant (Illingworth, 1969). Dysphagia may occur with a variety of congenital or acquired disturbances in infancy. Logan and Bosma (1967) have reviewed the problems of oral and pharyngeal dysphagia and have listed the various malformations and neurologic and muscular abnormalities that may be responsible (Table 1). If myasthenia is suspected, the administration of edrophonium chloride (Tensilon) may be very helpful, not only for diagnosis but also in the management of the infant's problem (Avery, 1968; Illingworth, 1969).

Other problems to consider in oropharyngeal dysphagia of children and adults include acute bulbar poliomyelitis, botulism, tetanus and any type of cerebrovascular accident. On examination, things to look for include weakness of the palate, regurgitation into the nasopharynx, a nasal voice, pooling of secretions in the hypopharynx and evidence of aspiration into the larynx and trachea. Persistent choking in any child must raise the suspicion of a disturbance in swallowing.

As previously stated, the cricopharyngeus guards the upper end of the esophagus. It remains closed except dur-

TABLE 1. ETIOLOGY OF INFANT ORAL AND PHARYNGEAL DYSPHAGIA*

Malformation

- Ankyloglossia superior
- Choanal atresia
- Cleft lip and palate
- Cysts or tumors
- Laryngeal cleft
- Macroglossia
- Pharyngeal diverticulum
- Pierre Robin syndrome
- Syngnathia

Neurologic or Muscular Abnormality

- Bulbar paralysis
- Cerebral palsy
- Cricopharyngeal achalasia
- DeLange syndrome
- Familial dysautonomia
- Isolated cranial nerve paralysis
- Moebius syndrome
- Myasthenia gravis
- Myotonic dystrophy
- Pharyngeal incoordination
- Suprabulbar paralysis
- Tetanus
- Werdnig-Hoffmann disease

*From Logan, W. J., and Bosma, J. F.: Oral and pharyngeal dysphagia in infancy. *Pediat. Clin. N. Amer.*, 14:47, 1967.

ing the act of swallowing, opening in response to a well-coordinated oropharyngeal mechanism. Failure of this sphincter to open (achalasia of the cricoid) not only results in serious nutritional disturbances but, even more importantly, results in aspiration of food into the trachea and bronchial tree. Thus, aspiration pneumonitis is the most serious consequence, and is often responsible for the early demise of these unfortunate individuals (Olsen, 1970).

Cricopharyngeal spasm (cricospasm) has been described, but it probably is rare in both children and adults. More commonly, the neurologic and functional disturbances already referred to cause the pharyngeal incoordination, which in turn is responsible for the failure of the cricoid sphincter to open. The following case report illustrates the problem of pharyngeal dysfunction associated with central nervous system disease.

This 17-year-old lad entered the hospital in January 1971, after an episode of aspiration pneumonitis. He was a thin, malnourished, markedly underdeveloped boy who appeared many years younger than his age. He had had swallowing difficulties for many years, in addition to all the other problems associated with retarded growth. He had to eat his food very slowly, and frequently he would cough and choke. He had become acutely ill about 10 days before admission and his chest roentgenogram at that time revealed the characteristic appearance of extensive bilateral aspiration pneumonia (Fig. 10). The neurologic examination and the myelograms were consistent with the Arnold-Chiari malformation. Preoperatively it was thought that a bulbar syrinx might be present. At surgery a low-grade astrocytoma was found in the medulla and a decompression was performed. Needless to say, respiratory problems have continued and a gastrostomy was necessary because of persistent difficulties with swallowing and aspiration.

As is well recognized, aspiration pneumonitis is a serious disorder (Olsen, 1970). The arterial blood gases are altered profoundly. The Pa_{O_2} of the boy just mentioned was only 47, even though the chest roentgenogram on admission had shown that marked improvement had taken place by the time he was admitted to the hospital. Not only does recurrent aspiration produce chronic

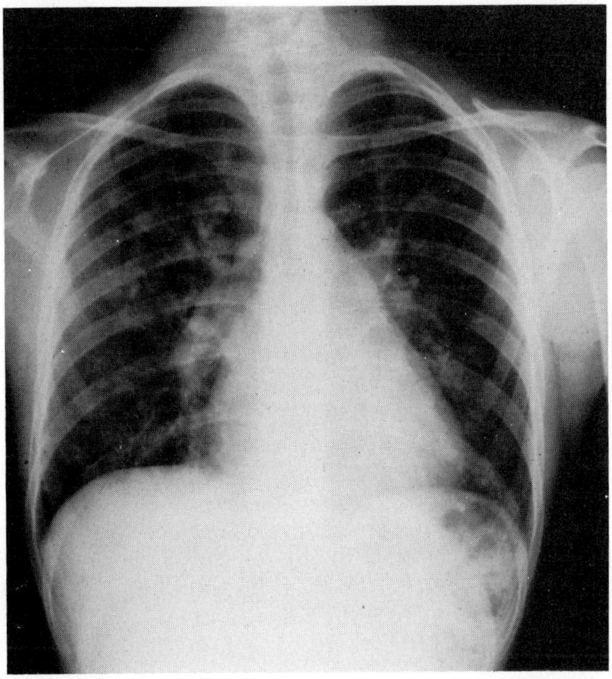

Figure 10. Roentgenogram of the chest of a patient several days prior to admission, showing bilateral aspiration pneumonitis from pharyngeal dysfunction.

tracheobronchitis, but the recurring episodes of pneumonitis lead to pulmonary fibrosis (Davis and Fiuzat, 1967).

Recognition of the dysfunction of the upper sphincter is, of course, most important. A transnasal feeding tube is often necessary for feeding, and tracheal intubation or tracheostomy is frequently required in the acute phases of the patient's illness. Unfortunately, most of the neurologic problems that cause cricopharyngeal achalasia are not amenable to treatment. If true cricopharyngeal spasm is present, a myotomy (Sutherland, 1962) or other sphincter-destroying procedure may be performed on the cricopharyngeal sphincter. The value of cricopharyngeal myotomy in cerebral or brain stem disorders is debatable.

ESOPHAGEAL DISORDERS

ACHALASIA OF THE ESOPHAGUS

Achalasia is not common in children. In a series of 601 patients (Olsen et al., 1953), slightly less than 3 per cent were younger than 15 years of age. However, nearly 10 per cent of all patients could trace their symptoms back to childhood (less than age 15). Hence, it would appear that achalasia often goes unrecognized in children (Ellis and Olsen, 1969).

The principal symptom of achalasia is the sensation of having food stick in the substernal area. Although the individual usually points to the xiphoid as the site of obstruction, it is not uncommon to refer the sense of blockage to the cricoid region. Obstructive symptoms are nearly always intermittent during the first few months of the disease, but become more constant with the passage of time. Although pain (odynophagia) is not a common feature (Olsen et al., 1953, found it in 29 per cent of their patients), it tends to occur most frequently in the early stages of the disorder, and hence may be a prominent part of the disorder in children. The pain is usually substernal and may be radiated to the back, up into the neck and mouth, and occasionally into the shoulders and arms. Usually the pain occurs with the act of swallowing. Salivation occurs commonly, as it does with any other type of esophageal obstruction. Cold foods or fluids are likely to precipitate the obstructive symptoms or pain, and warm foods are usually better tolerated. Solids are more likely to cause trouble than liquids, although the reverse can be true. Regurgitation develops as the disease progresses and is present in the majority of patients.

Certain points in diagnosis of achalasia in children deserve special emphasis. The disorder may appear to develop after injury or psychic shock. The child may be reluctant to eat because of obstructive symptoms or pain on swallowing. Weight loss and malnutrition are common. Too often the problem is thought to be emotional or functional. Painful swallowing must not be ignored. Regurgitation in a child requires careful analysis. If food is returned to the mouth soon after its ingestion, esophageal obstruction should be suspected. Curdled milk comes from the stomach and gastric regurgitation is likely to be delayed after eating. One must remember, however, that delayed regurgitation may occur when the esophagus becomes dilated. Soiling of the child's pillow should always suggest esophageal retention.

Roentgenographic study is the usual method of making the diagnosis (Fig. 11). However, fluoroscopic study is not always easy in children, and cineradiography has some advantages in the diagnosis of esophageal as well as oropharyngeal disorders (Ardran and Kemp, 1970). The characteristic roentgenologic findings (Olsen et al., 1953) are evidence of obstruction at the esophagogastric junction, the conical shape of the terminal esophagus with a beaklike extension into the stenotic zone, and disturbed motility which will vary from nonperistaltic hypermotility in the early (compensated) case to passive "silent" dilatation in the more advanced (decompensated) patients.

Esophagoscopy is especially important in the child to differentiate between

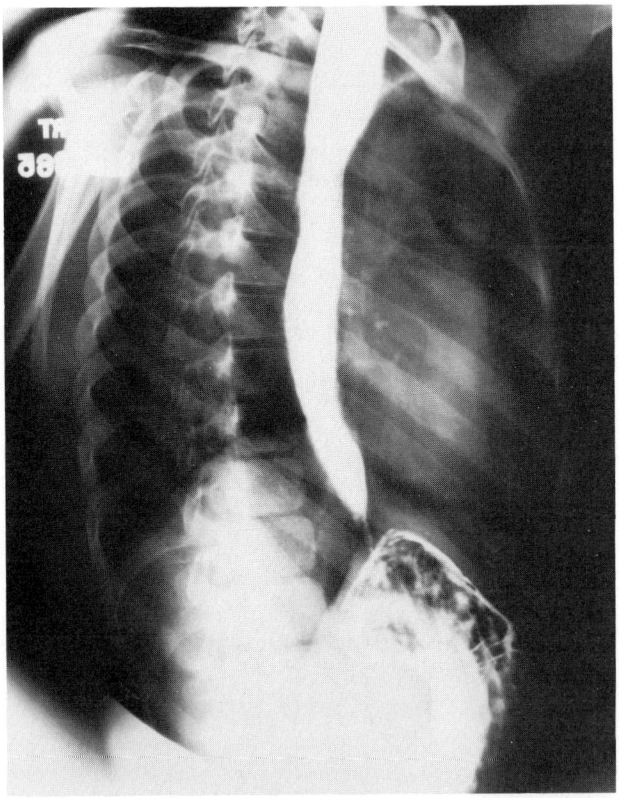

Figure 11. Roentgenogram showing achalasia in a child. (From Olsen, A. M., et al.: The treatment of cardiospasm: Analysis of a twelve-year experience. J. Thorac. Cardiovasc. Surg., *22*:164, 1951. By permission of C. V. Mosby Company.)

achalasia and foreign bodies, strictures or other organic lesions. In the early case, esophagoscopy may be negative, and the scope will pass easily into the stomach even though the roentgenoscopic examination showed a delay in passage of barium into the stomach. At a later stage, retained food and fluid will be found and the cardia will present a "rosette" appearance. Despite a considerable degree of obstruction, the scope will usually pass through the lower sphincter with little or no difficulty. A blunt olive-tipped bougie passed over a previously swallowed thread will encounter a definite but temporary resistance that is quite familiar to the experienced endoscopist (Olsen et al., 1951; Sanderson et al., 1970).

Esophageal motility studies have assisted greatly in diagnosing neuromuscular disorders of the esophagus. The normal resting pressures at the lower sphincter were seen in Figure 5, and the normal responses of the esophagus and the cardia after swallowing were shown in Figure 6. Deglutition patterns in achalasia are contrasted with the normal in Figure 12. Although the resting pressure is normal in achalasia, the disease is characterized by lack of peristalsis and by failure of the lower sphincter to relax in response to the swallowing effort. Motility studies are somewhat more difficult to obtain in children, as they may be unable to cooperate, but they are certainly worth the effort.

Although the cause of achalasia is not known, there is no question that it is an organic disease. Lesions have been described in Auerbach's plexus (Hurst and Rake, 1930: Lendrum, 1937), in the vagus nerve (Cassella et al., 1965), and in the brainstem (Cassella et al., 1964). Obviously, the disease is not amenable to psychiatric therapy and no medications have yet been found that are beneficial. Mecholyl has been shown to be helpful in diagnosis (Kramer and Ingelfinger, 1951) but has no therapeutic

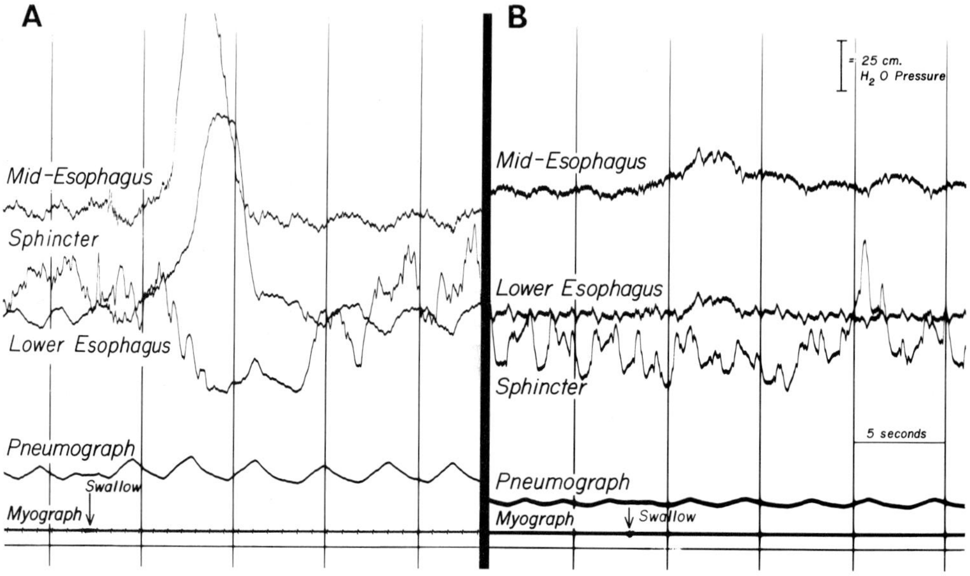

Figure 12. *A,* Normal peristalsis and relaxation of the lower sphincter. *B,* Simultaneous feeble contractions of the esophagus with absence of relaxation in a patient with achalasia. (From Olsen, A. M.: Study of esophageal motility in health and disease. Ann. Otol., *77*:892, 1968. By permission of Annals Publishing Company.)

value. Hence, there is no "physiologic" or curative therapy. The resistance at the esophagogastric sphincter must be lessened by mechanical means, and this may be accomplished by forceful dilatation of the cardia or by surgery. Great care must be taken to weaken the sphincter without producing incompetence.

Forceful dilatation of the cardia may be accomplished with a pneumatic or hydrostatic dilator (Kurlander et al., 1963; Olsen et al., 1951; Sanderson et al., 1970), and good results (for five years or more) can be anticipated in 60 to 80 per cent of adult patients, depending upon the number of dilatations carried out. If permanent relief is not obtained after three properly performed dilatations, it is rarely justified to proceed with further nonsurgical treatment. The author prefers to perform dilatations over a previously swallowed thread (Fig. 13). Some prefer the mercury-weighted tube (Browne and McHardy, 1939); others use a pneumatic dilator passed through an esophagoscope (Thomson et al.,

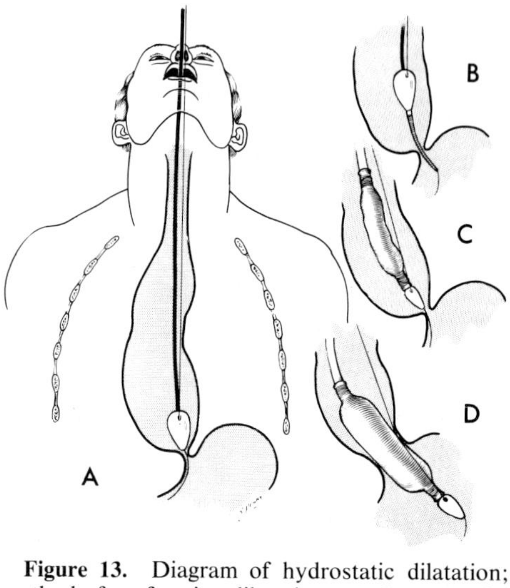

Figure 13. Diagram of hydrostatic dilatation; method of performing dilatations. *A,* Passage of a 41-F olive-tipped bougie into the stomach. *B,* A 50- or 60-F sound is passed into the stomach, guided by a flexible wire spiral. *C,* The hydrostatic dilator is passed to the cardia. *D,* Distention of the hydrostatic dilator across the cardia. (From Olsen, A. M., et al.: The treatment of cardiospasm: Analysis of a twelve-year experience. J. Thorac. Cardiovasc. Surg., *22*:164, 1951. By permission of C. V. Mosby Company.)

1955) or an expanding metal dilator (Starck, 1924) inserted through an esophagoscope.

The most satisfactory surgical procedure is an esophagomyotomy of the Heller type (Ellis, 1962; Polk and Burford, 1964; Tachovsky et al., 1968). Care must be taken to avoid carrying the incision too far onto the stomach, as it is important to preserve the subhiatal portion of the sphincter. Otherwise there is danger of reflux. Satisfactory long-term improvement can be anticipated in over 90 per cent of patients.

The results of forceful dilatation in children have not been good, especially if the child was under 10 years of age (Ellis and Olsen, 1969). Surgical results have been much better (Polk and Burford, 1964; Tachovsky et al., 1968). Hence, in a well-documented case of achalasia in a child, the surgical approach is preferred.

Diffuse Spasm

Symptomatic diffuse spasm is probably quite uncommon in children. However, without manometric studies the diagnosis is difficult (Olsen and Creamer, 1957), and this would be particularly true in children. The roentgen appearance of diffuse spasm varies. Three representative cases are seen in Figure 14. Not infrequently, a roentgen picture similar to that in diffuse spasm may be seen in asymptomatic individuals and has given rise to such terms as curling, corkscrew esophagus, nonsphincteric spasm, and pseudodiverticulosis (see Fig. 3). Reference has been made previously to the tertiary contractions that are seen in older people and in patients with hiatal hernia and that are also seen in patients who have been successfully treated for achalasia.

Symptomatic diffuse spasm usually occurs in emotionally labile young or middle-aged people and is more common in females (Moersch and Camp, 1934). The chief symptom is pain that comes on at intervals and that may be related to eating. The pain is substernal and usually severe, and it radiates to the neck and throat and sometimes to the arms. There may or may not be obstructive symptoms, but the patient rarely regurgitates. At times, diffuse spasm may be associated with disorders of the gastrointestinal tract, such as esophagitis, hiatal hernia, diverticula of the esophagus, peptic ulcer, and gallbladder disease, but often diffuse spasm is seen as an isolated entity. Esophagoscopy (under general anesthesia) is usually negative. When bougies are passed over a thread with the patient awake, a spastic obstruction of the lower two thirds of the esophagus is frequently encountered.

Motility studies are diagnostic in patients with diffuse spasm (Olsen and Creamer, 1957). Resting pressures at both sphincters are normal. However, responses to deglutition are not only simultaneous, but also very powerful in the smooth muscle portion (the lower two-thirds) of the esophagus. In addition, contractions are repetitive and prolonged in most instances. The lower sphincter relaxes normally (Fig. 15).

Treatment of diffuse spasm is not satisfactory. Mechanical dilatation is rarely beneficial. Some patients are treated successfully with "long" myotomy of the Heller type (Ellis et al., 1964).

Other Esophageal Disorders

Occasionally, some patients have clinical and manometric features of both achalasia and diffuse spasm (Sanderson et al., 1967) (Table 2). The term "vigorous achalasia" has been used to describe this group of patients. Contractions are forceful and simultaneous, but not of the magnitude seen in diffuse spasm. Unlike diffuse spasm, the sphincter does not relax with swallowing. Of 72 patients who had this disorder, the youngest was 12 years of age. Pain is a more constant feature in this than in achalasia, but it still does not occur as commonly as it does in diffuse spasm. Obstruction is a constant feature and regurgitation is very common. The roentgen picture and motility findings (Fig. 16) have features of both achalasia and diffuse spasm. Results of treatment with the hydro-

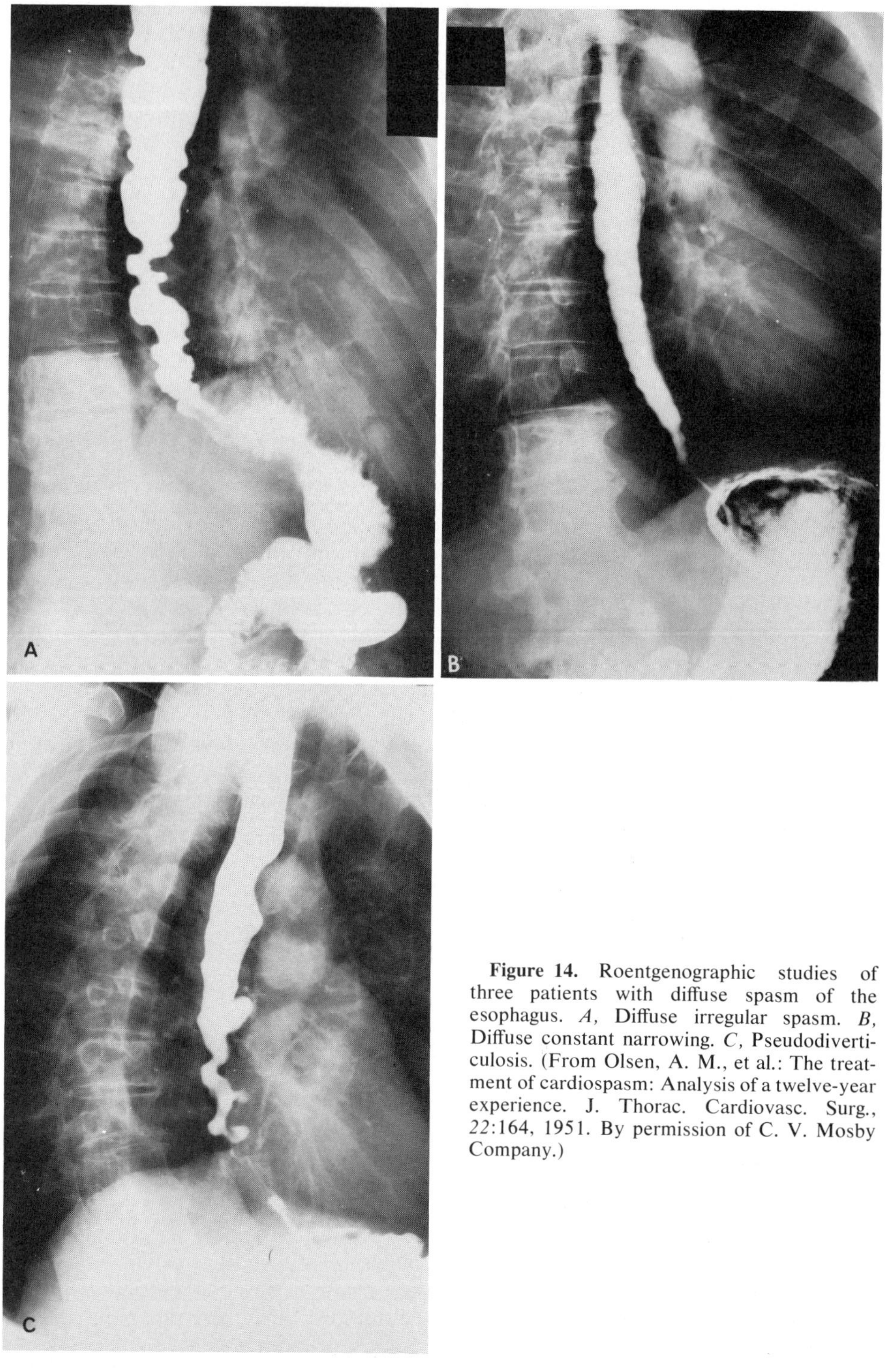

Figure 14. Roentgenographic studies of three patients with diffuse spasm of the esophagus. *A*, Diffuse irregular spasm. *B*, Diffuse constant narrowing. *C*, Pseudodiverticulosis. (From Olsen, A. M., et al.: The treatment of cardiospasm: Analysis of a twelve-year experience. J. Thorac. Cardiovasc. Surg., *22*:164, 1951. By permission of C. V. Mosby Company.)

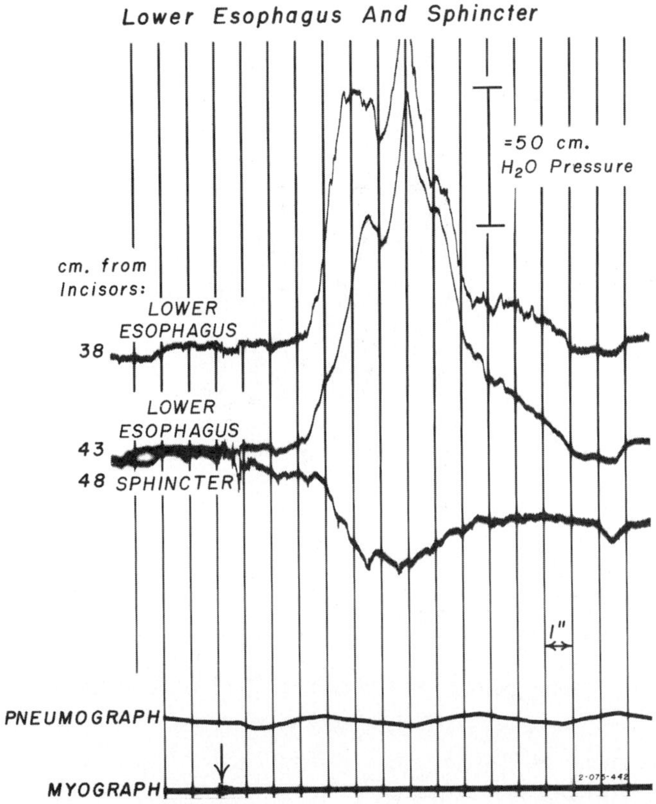

Figure 15. Manometric tracings in diffuse spasm. Contractions are simultaneous, repetitive and of large amplitude. Lower sphincter relaxes normally. (From Code, C. F., et al.: *An Atlas of Esophageal Motility in Health and Disease.* Charles C Thomas, Publisher, Springfield, Ill., 1958, p. 104. By permission.)

TABLE 2. DIFFERENTIAL DIAGNOSIS OF ACHALASIA, DIFFUSE SPASM AND VIGOROUS ACHALASIA*

	Incidence, According to Diagnosis		
Symptom or Sign	Achalasia	Diffuse Spasm	Vigorous Achalasia
Pain	Uncommonly	Almost always	Frequently
Obstruction	Always	Sometimes	Nearly always
Regurgitation	Commonly	Rarely	Frequently
Retention	Frequently	Never	Frequently
Nervousness	Uncommonly	Almost always	Occasionally
Radiologic findings			
Diffuse dilatation	Commonly	Never	Occasionally
Segmental spasm	Uncommonly	Frequently	Commonly

*Modified from Olsen, A. M., Ellis, F. H., Jr., and Creamer, B.: Cardiospasm (achalasia of the cardia). *Amer. J. Surg.*, 93:299, 1957.

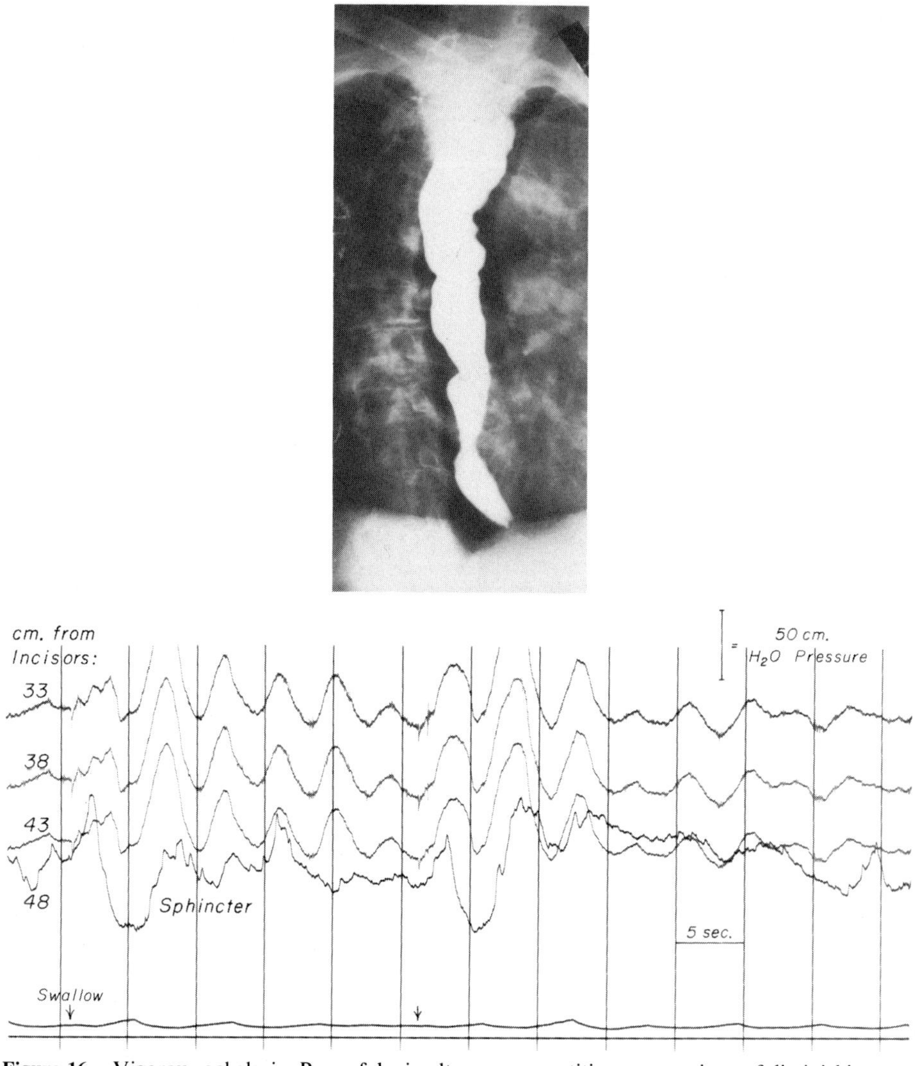

Figure 16. Vigorous achalasia. Powerful, simultaneous, repetitive contractions of diminishing amplitude occur in response to swallow. Relaxation of the lower sphincter does occur, followed by premature contractions. Note barium swallow at left. (From Sanderson, D. R., et al.: Syndrome of vigorous achalasia: Clinical and physiologic observations. Chest, *52*:508, 1967. By permission of the American College of Chest Physicians.)

static dilator are poor, but surgical results are comparable to those with achalasia.

Although scleroderma is not common in children, it should be mentioned because of the frequency of neuromuscular failure of the esophagus in this disorder. This may be demonstrated by manometric studies long before the patient suffers dysphagia. Although the motility pattern varies considerably, the characteristic finding is the absence of peristaltic contractions in all but the uppermost esophagus, where striated muscle is present (Code et al., 1958). The upper sphincter behaves normally. The resting pressures at the lower sphincter may be normal or quite feeble. The sphincter often relaxes poorly after swallowing.

Patients with scleroderma frequently develop varying degrees of esophageal obstruction, often resembling the early phases of achalasia. They are likely to develop reflux esophagitis and go on to have a short esophagus and stricture. The roentgen examination is characterized by lack of peristaltic activity, some dilation, and later the findings of lower esophageal stricture.

Patients with Raynaud's disease may show abnormalities of esophageal motility identical to those seen in scleroderma. Usually these patients have no esophageal symptoms. They may or may not develop the entire picture of scleroderma as time goes on.

Reference has already been made to the swallowing difficulties of patients with dermatomyositis (Donoghue et al., 1960). These can be documented with esophageal motility studies. Changes have also been described in diabetics with neuropathy, in alcoholics with neuropathy and in patients with multiple sclerosis (Daly et al., 1962) and a variety of other neurologic disorders (Fischer et al., 1965; Pierce et al., 1965; Smith et al., 1957).

CHALASIA, HIATAL HERNIA, AND INCOMPETENT CARDIA

The term "chalasia" (Berenberg and Neuhauser, 1950; Neuhauser and Berenberg, 1947) has been used to describe an incompetent sphincter. It is most commonly applied to the sphincter at the esophagogastric junction. By inference, it should be the opposite of "achalasia," and this assumption is not truly valid semantically. Nevertheless, chalasia appears to be a part of our medical nomenclature and refers to the sphincter that permits reflux of gastric content into the esophagus. It need not be synonymous with the "hypotensive" esophagogastric sphincter (Fig. 17), a subject that is currently under study.

The various factors that help to maintain the competence of the lower sphincter were discussed earlier in this chapter. The most important is its location. If the lower sphincter straddles the hiatus of the diaphragm, it is usually quite competent. However, with displacement into the thorax (Atkinson et al., 1957a; Code et al., 1962), reflux is common. Thus, sliding hiatal hernias are the principal cause of incompetence and reflux esophagitis (Allison, 1951; Atkinson et al., 1957a; Schuman and Rinaldo, 1966; Tuttle et al., 1961, Urschel and Paulson, 1967). The size of the hernia does not correlate with the reflux syndrome. In fact, small hernias are more likely to be associated with regurgitation than the larger ones. When the hernia increases in size and the major portion of the stomach has moved into the chest, the competence of the sphincter is often restored. In the adult, the mechanisms involved in the production of sliding hernia and its sequelae are fairly well understood.

In infants and children, the situation is not as clear. Robins and Jankelson described cardioesophageal relaxation in the infant many years ago, and the syndrome of the incompetent cardia is well recognized (Berenberg and Neuhauser, 1950; Neuhauser and Berenberg, 1947). Postural regurgitation is noted in certain infants following any feeding and can be documented by radiology, showing that contrast media pass from esophagus to stomach and vice versa without evidence of any real barrier (Gross, 1953). These infants regurgitate feedings frequently, and the milk is usually curdled and smells sour, thus indicating that it has passed into the stomach before it comes up. The child

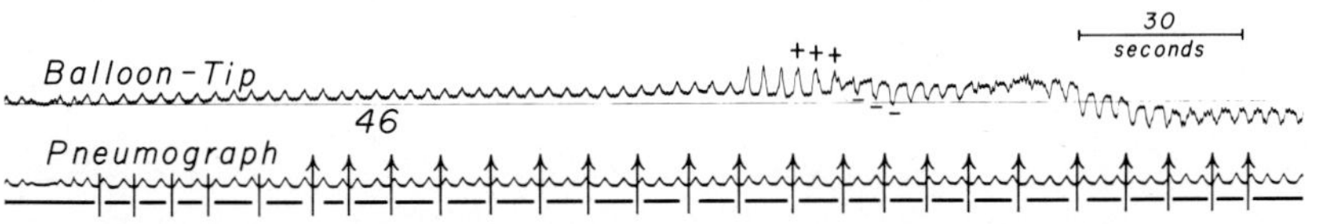

Figure 17. Manometric record of resting hypotensive esophagogastric sphincter. Withdrawal of balloon-covered electromagnetic pressure transducer from the stomach to the esophagus. Resting pressures at esophagogastric junction are low. There is probably an associated small hiatal hernia.

must be held upright after feeding, or the feeding will not be retained. Special chairs or seats have been devised for these children. The prone position for sleeping, with the head elevated 45 degrees, has been suggested. Fortunately, this cardioesophageal relaxation of the newborn usually lasts only a few weeks or a few months (Blank and Pew, 1956; Gross, 1953; Neuhauser and Berenberg, 1947; Polk and Burford, 1964). Finally, the lower sphincter develops normal tone and the problem disappears.

However, chalasia apparently persists in a small percentage of these children (Wyllie and Field, 1946). The frequent episodes of aspiration into the tracheobronchial tree are responsible for repeated attacks of pneumonia and a chronic tracheobronchitis (Davis and Fiuzat, 1967; Husfeldt et al., 1951; Urschel and Paulson, 1967). Pulmonary abscess or bronchiectasis may result and the repeated insults to the lung lead to pulmonary fibrosis and respiratory insufficiency (Olsen, 1970).

The effect upon the esophagus may be equally devastating (Olsen et al., 1960; Olsen and Schlegel, 1965; Wyllie and Field, 1946). Constant reflux of acid gastric content into the esophagus may produce esophagitis and ulceration, healing and cicatrization, and ultimately shortening of the esophagus and stricture. There is experimental evidence to suggest that when peptic ulceration of the esophagus causes a denuding of the squamous mucosa, a columnar type mucosa will grow back in its place, thus producing the "Barrett" esophagus (Bremner et al., 1970a).

There has been much discussion and debate about the short esophagus in children. Is it congenital or acquired (Olsen et al., 1960)? Is there an associated hiatal hernia or is there primary weakness of an otherwise normal esophagogastric sphincter (chalasia)? Husfeldt and as-

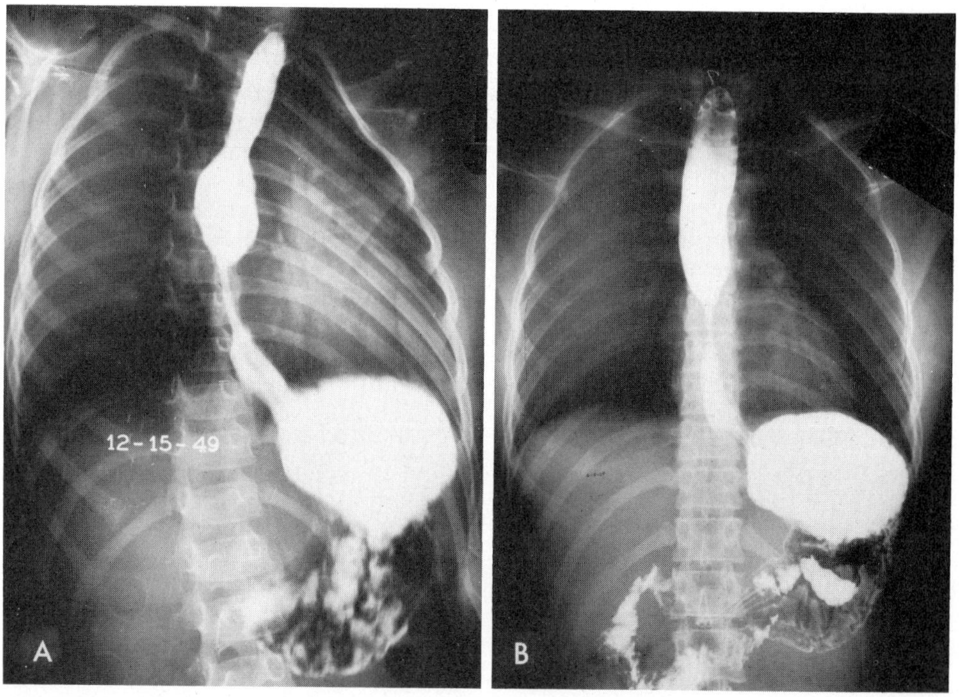

Figure 18. *A*, Short esophagus with stricture in a 5-year-old girl who had had "chalasia syndrome" since early infancy. *B*, The same patient after 20 years of treatment with periodic dilatations.

sociates (1951) felt that hiatal hernia was present in most cases and advocated surgical repair. Others have been unable to demonstrate a hernia.

With or without hiatal hernia, chalasia has been treated surgically by fundoplication procedures of the Belsey (Hiebert and Belsey, 1961) or Nissen (Nissen and Rossetti, 1962) type or modifications thereof. Davis and Fiuzat (1967) recently reported their experience with 18 children who had respiratory problems presumably related to reflux associated with chalasia. Reflux was demonstrated by roentgenologic techniques, including the water siphonage test (Crummy, 1966). The Belsey procedure was performed on nine children, and relief of respiratory symptoms was obtained.

Unfortunately, there are instances in which chalasia persists, esophageal ulceration progresses, and the child is left with a shortened esophagus and a stricture (Olsen et al., 1960) (Fig. 18). In such cases, the management of the stricture is a real problem to the endoscopist. I prefer to treat these children conservatively with periodic dilatations carried out over a previously swallowed thread. However, it may be necessary to resort to surgical management (Ellis, 1956).

Recently our attention has been called to the prevalence of esophageal lesions in individuals who have spastic paralysis (Abrahams and Burkitt, 1970; Holmes, 1971). Most of these patients are children or adolescents. Roentgen studies invariably show evidence of reflux, and in many of the patients a hiatal hernia is demonstrable. Esophagoscopy usually reveals esophagitis, and sometimes the patients are very anemic. Eventually short esophagus with stricture may develop. The reason for the association of reflux with cerebral palsy is not at all clear. Holmes has suggested that these patients may have a primary "chalasia" caused by vagal hyperactivity. Abrahams and Burkitt believe that contributing factors include extensor spasm, incoordination of deglutition accompanied by air swallowing, and the kyphoscoliosis so common in these patients.

SUMMARY

The mechanism of swallowing is complicated, from the time that nourishment enters the mouth until it arrives safely in the stomach. It is indeed remarkable that the healthy newborn child has so little trouble ingesting food. When neuromuscular defects are present, the consequences of imperfect deglutition may be grave. The most serious consequences of incoordination in the act of swallowing tend to occur in the lower respiratory tract. These are usually associated with malfunction of the upper esophageal sphincter, although disorders of the lower sphincter may also result in aspiration and bronchopulmonary disease. Disturbances of function of the esophagus and its lower sphincter may result in organic disease of the esophagus.

REFERENCES

Abrahams, P., and Burkitt, B. F. E.: Hiatus hernia and gastro-oesophageal reflux in children and adolescents with cerebral palsy. *Aust. Paediat. J.*, 6:41, 1970.

Allison, P. R.: Reflux esophagitis, sliding hiatal hernia, and the anatomy of repair. *Surg. Gynec. Obstet.*, 92:419, 1951.

Ardran, G. M., and Kemp, F. H.: The mechanism of swallowing. *Proc. Roy. Soc. Med.*, 44:1038, 1951.

Ardran, G. M., and Kemp, F. H.: Some important factors in the assessment of oropharyngeal function. *Develop. Med. Child. Neurol.*, 12:158, 1970.

Atkinson, M.: Mechanisms protecting against gastro-oesophageal reflux: A review. *Gut*, 3:1, 1962.

Atkinson, M., Edwards, D. A. W., Honour, A. J., and Rowlands, E. N.: The oesophagogastric sphincter in hiatus hernia. *Lancet*, 2:1138, 1957a.

Atkinson, M., Kramer, P., Wyman, S. M., and Ingelfinger, F. J.: The dynamics of swallowing. I. Normal pharyngeal mechanisms. *J. Clin. Invest.*, 36:581, 1957b.

Avery, M. E.: *The Lung and Its Disorders in the Newborn Infant*, 2nd Ed. Philadelphia, W. B. Saunders Company, 1968.

Aylwin, J. A.: The physiological basis of reflux oseophagitis in sliding hiatal diaphragmatic hernia. *Thorax,* 8:38, 1953.

Barrett, N. R.: Hiatus hernia: A review of some controversial points. *Brit. J. Surg.,* 42:231, 1954.

Belsey, R.: Functional disease of the esophagus. *J. Thorac. Cardiovasc. Surg.,* 52:164, 1966.

Berenberg, W., and Neuhauser, E. B. D.: Cardio-esophageal relaxation (chalasia) as a cause of vomiting in infants. *Pediatrics,* 5:414, 1950.

Bernstein, L. M., and Baker, L. A.: A clinical test for esophagitis. *Gastroenterology,* 34:760, 1958.

Berstad, A., and Myren, J.: Effect of graded doses of pentagastrin in patients with and without gastritis. *Gut,*11:299, 1970.

Blank, L., and Pew, W. L.: Cardio-esophageal relaxation (chalasia) studies on the normal infant. *Amer. J. Roentgen.,* 76:540, 1956.

Botha, G. S. M.: Mucosal folds at the cardia as a component of the gastro-oesophageal closing mechanism. *Brit. J. Surg.,* 45:569, 1958a.

Botha, G. S. M.: The gastro-oesophageal region in infants: observations on the anatomy, with special reference to the closing mechanism and partial thoracic stomach. *Arch. Dis. Child,* 33:78, 1958b.

Botha, G. S. M.: *The Gastro-Oseophageal Junction: Clinical Applications to Oesophageal and Gastric Surgery.* Boston, Little, Brown & Company, 1962.

Bremner, C. G., Lynch, V. P., and Ellis, F. H., Jr.: Barrett's esophagus: Congenital or acquired? An experimental study of esophageal mucosal regeneration in the dog. *Surgery,* 68:209, 1970a.

Bremner, C. G., Schlegel, J. F., and Ellis, F. H., Jr.: Studies of the "gastroesophageal sphincter mechanism": The role of the phrenoesophageal membrane. *Surgery,* 67:735, 1970b.

Browne, D. C., and McHardy, G.: A new instrument for use in esophagospasm. *J.A.M.A.,* 113:1963, 1939.

Butin, J. W., Olsen, A. M., Moersch, H. J., and Code, C. F.: A study of esophageal pressures in normal persons and patients with cardiospasm. *Gastroenterology,* 23:278, 1953.

Carlson, A. J., Boyd, T. E., and Pearcy, J. F.: Studies on the visceral sensory nervous system. XIV. The reflex control of the cardia and lower esophagus in mammals. *Arch. Intern. Med.,* 30:409, 1922.

Carré, I. J., and Astley, R.: The gastro-oesophageal junction in infancy: A combined cineradiographic and manometric study. *Thorax,* 13:159, 1958.

Cassella, R. R., Brown, A. L., Jr., Sayre, G.P., and Ellis, F. H., Jr.: Achalasia of the esophagus: Pathologic and etiologic considerations. *Ann. Surg.,* 160:474, 1964.

Cassella, R. R., Ellis, F. H., Jr., and Brown, A. L., Jr.: Fine-structure changes in achalsia of the esophagus. I. Vagus nerves. *Amer. J. Path.,* 46:279, 1965.

Castell, D. O., and Harris, L. D.: Hormonal control of gastroesophageal-sphincter strength. *New Eng. J. Med.,* 282:886, 1970.

Castell, D. O., and Levine, S. M.: Lower esophageal sphincter response to gastric alkalinization: A new mechanism for treatment of heartburn with antacids. *Ann. Intern. Med.,* 74:223, 1971.

Code, C. F., Creamer, B., Schlegel, J. F., Olsen, A. M., Donoghue, F. E., and Andersen, H. A.: *An Atlas of Esophageal Motility in Health and Disease.* Springfield, Ill., Charles C Thomas, Publisher, 1958.

Code, C. F., Kelley, M. L., Jr., Schlegel, J. F., and Olsen, A. M.: Detection of hiatal hernia during esophageal motility tests. *Gastroenterology,* 43:521, 1962.

Colley, J. R. T., and Creamer, B.: Sucking and swallowing in infants. *Brit. Med. J.,* 2:422, 1958.

Collis, J. L., Kelly, T. D., and Wiley, A. M.: Anatomy of the crura of the diaphragm and the surgery of hiatus hernia. *Thorax,* 9:175, 1954.

Crummy, A. B.: The water test in the evaluation of gastroesophageal reflux: Its correlation with pyrosis. *Radiology,* 87:501, 1966.

Daly, D. D., Code, C. F., and Andersen, H. A.: Disturbances of swallowing and esophageal motility in patients with multiple sclerosis. *Neurology,* 12:250, 1962.

Davis, M. V., and Fiuzat, J.: Application of the Belsey hiatal hernia repair to infants and children with recurrent bronchitis, bronchiolitis, and pneumonitis due to regurgitation and aspiration. *Ann. Thorac. Surg.,* 3:99, 1967.

Didio, L. J. A., and Anderson, M. C.: *The "Sphincters" of the Digestive System: Anatomical, Functional and Surgical Considerations.* Baltimore, Williams & Wilkins Company, 1968.

Donoghue, F. E., Winkelmann, R. K., and Moersch, H. J.: Esophageal defects in dermatomyositis. *Ann. Otol.,* 69:1139, 1960.

Dornhorst, A. C., Harrison, K., and Pierce, J. W.: Observations on the normal oesophagus and cardia. *Lancet,* 1:695, 1954.

Ellis, F. G.: The aetiology and treatment of achalasia of the cardia. *Ann. Roy. Coll. Surg. Eng.,* 30:155, 1962.

Ellis, F. H., Jr.: A physiologic operation for ulceration and stricture of the terminal esophagus. *Proc. Staff Meet. Mayo Clin.,* 31: 615, 1956.

Ellis, F. H., Jr., and Olsen, A. M.: *Achalasia of the Esophagus.* Philadelphia, W. B. Saunders Company, 1969.

Ellis, F. H., Jr., Olsen, A. M., Schlegel, J. F., and Code, C. F.: Surgical treatment of esophageal hypermotility disturbances. *J.A.M.A.,* 188:862, 1964.

Fischer, R. A., Ellison, G. W., Thayer, W. R., Spiro, H. M., and Glaser, G. H.: Esophageal motility in neuromuscular disorders. *Ann. Intern. Med.* 63:229, 1965.

Flavell, G.: *The Oesophagus.* London, Butterworth & Company, Ltd., 1963, p. 1.

Fleshler, B., Hendrix, T. R., Kramer, P., and Ingelfinger, F. J.: Resistance and reflex function of the lower esophageal sphincter. *J. Appl. Physiol.,* 12:339, 1958.

Fyke, F. E., Jr., and Code, C. F.: Resting and

deglutition pressures in the pharyngo-esophageal region. *Gastroenterology,* 29:24, 1955.
Fyke, F. E., Jr., Code, C. F., and Schlegel, J. F.: The gastroesophageal sphincter in healthy human beings. *Gastroenterologia,* 86:135, 1956.
Gaarde, F. W., Jr., and Olsen, A. M.: Functional and organic disturbances of the upper part of the esophagus. *Proc. Staff Meet. Mayo Clin.,* 19: 482, 1944.
Giles, G. R., Mason, M. C., Humphries, C., and Clark, C. G.: Action of gastrin on the lower oesophageal sphincter in man. *Gut,* 10:730, 1969.
Gross, R. E.: *The Surgery of Infancy and Childhood: Its Principles and Techniques.* Philadelphia, W. B. Saunders Company, 1953, p. 128.
Gryboski, J. D.: The swallowing mechanism of the neonate. I. Esophageal and gastric motility. *Pediatrics,* 35:445, 1965.
Gryboski, J. D.: Suck and swallow in the premature infant. *Pediatrics,* 43:96, 1969.
Gryboski, J. D., Thayer, W. R., Jr., and Spiro, H. M.: Esophageal motility in infants and children. *Pediatrics,* 31:382, 1963.
Harrington, S. W.: Esophageal hiatus diaphragmatic hernia: Etiology, diagnosis, and treatment in 123 cases. *J. Thorac. Cardiovasc. Surg.,* 8:127, 1938.
Harris, L. D.: Dysphagia. *Adv. Intern. Med.,* 15:203, 1969.
Hayward, J.: The lower end of the oesophagus. *Thorax,* 16:36, 1961.
Hiebert, C. A.: Primary incompetence of the gastric cardia. *Amer. J. Surg.,* 119, 365, 1970.
Hiebert, C. A., and Belsey, R.: Incompetency of the gastric cardia without radiologic evidence of hiatal hernia: The diagnosis and management of 71 cases. *J. Thorac. Cardiovasc. Surg.,* 42:352, 1961.
Higgs, B., Shorter, R. G., and Ellis, F. H. Jr.: A study of the anatomy of the human esophagus with special reference to the gastroesophageal sphincter. *J. Surg. Res.,* 5:503, 1965.
Hightower, N. C., Jr.: Newer concepts of the physiology of deglutition and dysphagia. *Amer. J. Surg.,* 93:154, 1957.
Hollinshead, W. H.: *Anatomy for Surgeons: The Back and Limbs,* Vol. 3, 2nd Ed. New York, Hoeber Medical Division, Harper & Row, Publishers, Inc., 1969, p. 635.
Holmes, T. W., Jr.: Chalasia, peptic esophagitis and hiatal hernia: A common syndrome in patients with central nervous system disease. *Chest,* 60:441, 1971.
Hunt, P. S., Connell, A. M., Smiley, T. B.: The crico-pharyngeal sphincter in gastric reflux. *Gut,* 11:303, 1970.
Hurst, A. F., and Rake, G. W.: Achalasia of the cardia (so-called cardiospasm). *Quart. J. Med.,* 23:491, 1930.
Husfeldt, E., Thomsen, G., and Wamberg, E.: Hiatal hernia and short oesophagus in children. *Thorax,* 6:56, 1951.
Illingworth, R. S.: Sucking and swallowing difficulties in infancy: Diagnostic problem of dysphagia. *Arch. Dis. Child.,* 44:655, 1969.
Kelley, M. L., Jr.: Deglutitive pressure responses in the gastroesophageal sphincters of symptomatic hiatal hernia patients. *Amer. J. Dig. Dis.,* 10:582, 1965.
Kramer, P., Atkinson, M., Wyman, S. M., and Ingelfinger, F. J.: The dynamics of swallowing. II. Neuromuscular dysphagia of pharynx. *J. Clin. Invest.,* 36:589, 1957.
Kramer, P., and Ingelfinger, F. J.: Esophageal sensitivity to Mecholyl in cardiospasm. *Gastroenterology,* 19:242, 1951.
Kurlander, D. J., Raskin, H. F., Kirsner, J. B., and Palmer, W. L.: Therapeutic value of the pneumatic dilator in achalasia of the esophagus: Long-term results in sixty-two living patients. *Gastroenterology,* 45:604, 1963.
Lendrum, F. C.: Anatomic features of the cardiac orifice of the stomach: With special reference to cardiospasm. *Arch. Intern. Med.* 59:474, 1937.
Lerche, W.: *Esophagus and Pharynx in Action: A Study of Structure in Relation to Function,* Springfield, Ill., Charles C Thomas, Publisher, 1950.
Logan, W. J., and Bosma, J. F.: Oral and pharyngeal dysphagia in infancy. *Pediat. Clin. N. Amer.,* 14:47, 1967.
Lyons, W. S., Ellis, F. H., Jr., and Olsen, A. M.: The gastroesophageal "sphincter" mechanism: A review. *Proc. Staff Meet. Mayo Clin,* 31:605, 1956.
Maclaurin, C.: The intrinsic sphincter in the prevention of gastro-oesophageal reflux. *Lancet,* 2:801, 1963.
McEwan-Alvarado, G.: Physiology of deglutition. *Texas Med.,* 65:82, 1969.
Meiss, J. H., Grindlay, J. H., and Ellis, F. H., Jr.: The gastroesophageal sphincter mechanism. II. Further experimental studies in the dog. *J. Thorac. Cardiovasc. Surg.* 36:156, 1958.
Moersch, H. J., and Camp, J. D.: Diffuse spasm of the lower part of the esophagus. *Ann. Otol.,* 43:1165, 1934.
Negus, V. E.: The etiology of pharyngeal diverticula. *Johns Hopkins Med. J.,* 101:209, 1957.
Neuhauser, E. B. D., and Berenberg, W.: Cardio-esophageal relaxation as a cause of vomiting in infants. *Radiology,* 48:480, 1947.
Nissen, R., and Rossetti, M.: Chirurgie de la hernie hiatale et du syndrome de reflux: La fundoplicature et la gastropexie. *J. Chir.,* 83:659, 1962.
Olsen, A. M.: The spectrum of aspiration pneumonitis. *Ann. Otol.,* 79:875, 1970.
Olsen, A. M., and Creamer, B.: Studies of oesophageal motility, with special reference to the differential diagnosis of diffuse spasm and achalasia (cardiospasm). *Thorax,* 12:279, 1957.
Olsen, A. M., Harrington, S. W., Moersch, H. J., and Andersen, H. A.: The treatment of cardiospasm: Analysis of a twelve-year experience. *J. Thorac. Cardiovasc. Surg.,* 22:164, 1951.

Olsen, A. M., Holman, C. B., and Andersen, H. A.: The diagnosis of cardiospasm. *Chest,* 23:477, 1953.

Olsen, A. M., Holman, C. B., and Harris, L. E.: Hiatal hernias in children: Special reference to the short esophagus. *Chest,* 38:495, 1960.

Olsen, A. M., and Schlegel, J.: Motility disturbances caused by esophagitis. *J. Thorac. Cardiovasc. Surg.,* 50:607, 1965.

Palmer, E. D.: The hiatus hernia-esophagitis-esophageal stricture complex: Twenty year prospective study. *Amer. J. Med.,* 44:566, 1968.

Peters, P. M.: Closure mechanisms at the cardia, with special reference to the diaphragmatico-oesophageal elastic ligament. *Thorax,* 10:27, 1955.

Piccone, V. A., Gutelius, J. R., and McCorriston, J. R.: A multiphased esophageal pH test for gastroesophageal reflux. *Surgery,* 57:638, 1965.

Pierce, J. W., Creamer, B., and MacDermot, V.: Pharynx and oesophagus in dystrophia myotonica. *Gut,* 6:392, 1965.

Polk, H. C., Jr., and Burford, T. H.: Disorders of the distal esophagus in infancy and childhood. *Amer. J. Dis. Child.,* 108:243, 1964.

Posey, E. L., Jr., and Franklin, H.: Relation of antral pH to gastrin release and fundal pH in dogs. *Amer. J. Dig. Dis.,* 12:356, 1967.

Robins, S. A., and Jankelson, I. R.: Cardio-esophageal relaxation. *J.A.M.A.,* 87:1961, 1926.

Sanderson, D. R., Ellis, F. H., Jr., and Olsen, A. M.: Achalasia of the esophagus: Results of therapy by dilation, 1950-1967. *Chest,* 58:116, 1970.

Sanderson, D. R., Ellis, F. H., Jr., Schlegel, J. F., and Olsen, A. M.: Syndrome of vigorous achalasia: Clinical and physiologic observations. *Chest,* 52:508, 1967.

Schuman, B. M., and Rinaldo, J. A.: Relative frequency of esophagitis and gastritis in patients with symptomatic hiatus hernia. *Gastroint. Endosc.,* 12:14, 1966.

Siegel, C. I., and Hendrix, T. R.: Esophageal motor abnormalities induced by acid perfusion in patients with heartburn. *J. Clin. Invest.,* 42:686, 1963.

Sinclair, W. J.: Initiation of reflex swallowing from the naso- and oropharynx. *Amer. J. Physiol.,* 218:956, 1970.

Smith, A. W. M., Mulder, D. W., and Code, C. F.: Esophageal motility in amyotrophic lateral sclerosis. *Proc. Staff Meet. Mayo Clin.,* 32:438, 1957.

Starck, H.: Die Behandlung der spasmogenen Speiseröhrenerweiterung. *Munchen. Med. Wschr.,* 71:334, 1924.

Stiennon, O. A.: On the cause of tertiary contractions and related disturbances of the esophagus. *Amer. J. Roentgen.,* 104:617, 1968.

Strawczynski, H., Beck, I. T., McKenna, R. D., and Nickerson, G. H.: The behavior of the lower esophageal sphincter in infants and its relationship to gastroesophageal regurgitation. *J. Pediat.,* 64:17, 1964.

Sutherland, H. D.: Cricopharyngeal achalasia. *J. Thorac. Cardiovasc. Surg.,* 43:114, 1962.

Tachovsky, T. J., Lynn, H. B., and Ellis, F. H., Jr.: The surgical approach to esophageal achalasia in children. *J. Pediat. Surg.,* 3:226, 1968.

Templeton, F. E.: *X-ray Examination of the Stomach: A Description of the Roentgenologic Anatomy, Physiology, and Pathology of the Esophagus, Stomach, and Duodenum.* Chicago, University of Chicago Press, 1944, p. 104.

Thomson, S., Negus, V. E., and Bateman, G. H.: *Diseases of the Nose and Throat: A Textbook for Students and Practitioners,* 6th Ed. London, Cassell & Company, Ltd., 1955, p. 776.

Tuttle, S. F., Rufin, F., and Bettarello, A.: The physiology of heartburn. *Ann. Intern. Med.,* 55:292, 1961.

Tuttle, S. G., and Grossman, M. I.: Detection of gastroesophageal reflux by simultaneous measurement of intraluminal pressure and pH. *Proc. Soc. Exp. Biol. Med.,* 98:225, 1958.

Urschel, H. C., Jr., and Paulson, D. L.: Gastroesophageal reflux and hiatal hernia: Complications and therapy. *J. Thorac. Cardiovasc. Surg.,* 53:21, 1967.

Utian, H. L., and Thomas, R. G.: Cricopharyngeal incoordination in infancy. *Pediatrics,* 43:402, 1969.

VanTrappen, G., Texter, E. C., Jr., Barborka, C. J., and Vandenbroucke, J.: The closing mechanism at the gastroesophageal junction. *Amer. J. Med.,* 28:564, 1960.

Vinson, P. P.: *The Diseases and Treatment of Diseases of the Esophagus.* Springfield, Ill., Charles C Thomas, Publisher, 1940.

Wyllie, W. G., and Field, C. E.: The etiology of intermittent oesophageal regurgitation and haematemesis in infants. *Arch. Dis. Child.,* 21:218, 1946.

Zaino, C., Jacobson, H. G., Lepow, H., and Ozturk, C. H.: *The Pharyngoesophageal Sphincter.* Springfield, Ill. Charles C Thomas, Publisher, 1970.

Chapter One Hundred Fifteen

STRICTURES AND BURNS OF THE ESOPHAGUS

JOHN F. DALY, M.D.

INTRODUCTION

Strictures of the esophagus in infants and children are of either the acquired or the congenital type. The acquired stricture is more common and is the result of fibrosis following trauma, infection, chemical injury or surgical procedure. The congenital stricture is the result of failure of the normal development of the esophagus and is considered to be a variant of the important group of atresias that occur in the esophagus. Congenital strictures and webs may involve any of the several layers that make up the esophageal wall; they may be membranous, muscular or fibromuscular. It may be impossible in some instances to determine whether the stricture is congenital or acquired, since an inflammation of the esophagus may have gone undetected until the stricture produced obstruction and dysphagia.

CONGENITAL STRICTURES

Congenital strictures may occur at any level, but most frequently they are found in the middle and lower third of the esophagus. They may be single and involve short segments of the esophagus and appear as shelves, webs or rings, or they may be multiple or involve long segments, up to 10 cm. of the esophagus.

Clinical Picture

Regurgitation and difficulty in swallowing in infants are common problems that respond to simple measures such as change in the formula and regulating the feeding schedule. However, when the symptoms persist or become progressive and the infant fails to gain weight, or the dysphagia is associated with cough and difficulty in breathing, the cause is to be sought in the upper gastrointestinal tract. Strictures may exist without producing symptoms. The stricture may not be detected until strained baby food or solid food is added to the diet or a foreign body obstructs the lumen. Many children with strictures have a history of being poor or slow eaters.

Diagnosis

The three methods for detecting the presence of a stricture are taking roentgenograms of the esophagus with contrast media, passing a flexible catheter or bougie, and esophagoscopy.

The esophagogram gives the essential information about the stricture—its location and extent, the amount of dilatation above it, and the presence of other anomalies of the esophagus, such as short esophagus, incompetence of the esophagogastric junction or a hiatus hernia. By passing a catheter or flexible bougie, a fixed point of obstruction can be detected. The size of the catheter or bougie that just passes through the obstruction is a simple method of calibrating the degree of stenosis.

Esophagoscopy not only confirms the presence of the stricture, but gives additional information about its character. By esophagoscopy, the stricture may appear as a crescentic shelf or a symmetrical narrowing; the mucosa may be normal or congested and velvety; the stricture may be soft and yielding to the pressure of the tip of the esophagoscope, or it may be firm. These characteristics are important in determining the prognosis for successful management.

Treatment

Thus, the single soft stricture may yield to one or two dilatations and gastrostomy will be unnecessary. The firm, unyielding, fibrous strictures and those involving a long segment of the esophagus will require a program of dilatations over several months. When the stricture is narrow and unyielding and the nourishment of the infant cannot be maintained by oral feedings, a gastrostomy is indicated. Retrograde dilatations are started after the gastrostomy has healed, i.e., at the end of two to three weeks.

The majority of congenital strictures respond to dilatation. Persistence in dilatations over a period of several months will be rewarded with good esophageal function. When dilatations fail to maintain an adequate lumen (28 F. for an infant; 40 F. for a child), or when the program of dilatations is not feasible, surgical resection of the stricture and reanastomosis of the esophagus should be done. However, an adequate trial of dilatations should be tried first, since stricturing at the site of anastomosis may occur following surgery and may require dilatations.

ACQUIRED STRICTURES

Acquired strictures are the result of contraction of fibrous tissue in the healing phase of an inflammatory reaction in the esophagus. There are three groups of acquired strictures: (1) strictures formed as a result of incompetence of the esophagogastric junction with reflux esophagitis, (2) strictures at the anastomotic sites following esophageal surgery, and (3) strictures due to burns of the esophagus.

STRICTURES DUE TO PEPTIC ESOPHAGITIS ASSOCIATED WITH HIATUS HERNIA AND SHORT ESOPHAGUS

Incompetence of the esophagogastric junction may be present at birth. The reflux of gastric contents into the lower esophagus produces an esophagitis. Strictures may form rapidly and, with edema, lead to complete obstruction of the esophagus. Usually there is a very definite but brief period of normal feeding that precedes the development of regurgitation and vomiting. The obstruction may progress rapidly to complete inability to swallow in a period of a week. The aspiration of secretions and the inability to swallow feedings creates an emergency situation. Feedings by mouth must be discontinued; a feeding gastrostomy should be done and the secretions removed from the hypopharynx by continuous suction. On this regimen, with the child placed in a semi-upright position in the crib, the edema around the stenosis subsides by the end of a week. The lumen opens and the child is able to swallow secretions.

At this point, the suction can be discontinued and a thread suspended from the head of the crib is gradually introduced into the mouth. With the infant swallowing it, it finds its way through the esophagus into the stomach. It is then retrieved through the gastrostomy opening by using a suction tip. The thread is used to pull a heavier string through the esophagus and out the gastrostomy opening. The upper end is brought out through the nose and the ends are tied, making a continuous loop. Retrograde dilatations are started as soon as the gastrostomy is healed. The dilatations are carried out daily at first and then every two to three days. As soon as the esophagus is dilated to 28 F., oral feedings are started. Dilatations with flexible weighted bougies can be continued at home. When there is no further tendency for the stenosis to contract, the gastrostomy is allowed to close. These measures will succeed in restoring the lumen so that at the end of a year the child has no further difficulty.

Maintaining the infant in the upright position in a specially constructed crib controls the reflux esophagitis in most infants. The esophagus heals and the strictures, when they present, can be easily dilated. However, when the esophagitis persists and the strictures re-form, in spite of adequate dilatations and other measures to correct reflux esophagitis, surgical correction of the incompetent esophagogastric junction will be necessary.

The repair of hiatus hernia is successful in infants and children under the age of 2 years. In older children, where the esophagitis has been well established, stricture formation is more fibrous, and hiatus hernia and shortening of the esophagus are present, it may be necessary to resect the esophageal stenosis and protect it by interposing a segment of colon between the upper resected esophagus and the stomach. The colon interposition operation has been successful in 70 to 80 per cent of the children with this clinical picture.

ANASTOMOTIC STRICTURE FOLLOWING SURGICAL PROCEDURES ON THE ESOPHAGUS

As surgical procedures have been used with greater frequency to correct congenital and acquired defects of the esophagus, strictures following surgical procedures have become more common. The factors that influence the formation of a surgical stricture are: (1) the type of anastomosis, (2) the tension on the suture line, (3) the occurrence of a leak, (4) how extensive the mobilization of the esophagus was, (5) the tissue reaction to the suture material, and (6) the presence of infection. Of these factors, tension seems most important, according to Schultz and Clatworthy. They found that when the anastomosis was made with marked tension, 60 per cent developed strictures, whereas when adequate and good tissue was available for the anastomosis, only 10 per cent developed strictures. Leaks and inflammation around the anastomosis will produce a dense fibrous stricture and will be much more difficult to manage.

Since stricturing following esophageal surgery is common, roentgenograms are done on the tenth to the fourteenth postoperative day, particularly if the feeding problems persist. In over half of the patients, some narrowing at the site of anastomosis will still be present at this time because of edema. The swelling subsides in ten days to two weeks. If the nutrition of the infant can be maintained, no treatment is required. However, if there is an increase in difficulty in swallowing, or if the child fails to gain weight, then a catheter should be passed through the site of anastomosis and its lumen calibrated. If the lumen is less than 28 F., dilatations with catheters or tapered bougies should be instituted. If the stenosis is soft, the lumen will rapidly respond to the dilatations. However, if there is a tendency for the lumen to diminish and the stricture does not respond to dilatations with weighted bougies, then a string should be introduced, as described previously, and retrograde dilatations using the Tucker type of retrograde dilators should be started. Retrograde dilatation is more effective and safer than prograde dilatation. This is particularly true in surgical anastomotic strictures because of the angulation at the site of anastomosis.

Most strictures will respond to dilatations over a period of three to four months, and only about 20 per cent require dilatations beyond that point (up to 12 months). In the late and hard strictures that usually result from infection and fistula formation, an adequate lumen cannot be maintained, and revision of the anastomotic site will be necessary.

Less common are the strictures resulting from foreign bodies that have remained in the esophagus and caused ulceration, and the trauma attendant on difficult removal of the foreign bodies. Strictures may follow the removal of a diverticulum, or they may occur at the site of islands of gastric mucosa in the esophageal wall—the "Barrett" lesions of the esophagus. Stricture may also occur in achalasia due to chronic inflammation of the esophageal wall and secondary fibrosis. Systemic infection may also produce an esophagitis that heals with stricturing. Typhoid and scarlet fever are the two systemic diseases that produce ulceration and stricture formation.

STRICTURES RESULTING FROM BURNS OF THE ESOPHAGUS

Burns of the esophagus and their complications are the cause of a great deal of suffering. They require prolonged treatment and repeated hospitalizations, often extending over many years. The treatment required is a financial burden to the community and to the parents. Since it is an entirely preventable disease, its primary treatment should be aimed at prevention. Although state and federal legislation requires that caustic agents be marked as poisonous, these measures have had only limited success in eliminating the hazard for children.

The National Clearinghouse for Poison Control Centers reported 76,155 accidental ingestions by children under the age of 5 in the year 1969; 1322 ingested acid or alkali agents; 523 ingested some form of lye. Since only about 10 per cent of the ingestions are reported to the poison centers, it has been estimated that about 5000 ingestions of lye by children occur each year.

Other preventive measures could be instituted, such as requiring the agent to be packaged in containers with caps that are difficult for children to remove. However, it would not eliminate the hazard of the concentrated liquid form of lye. Even the residue in the empty bottle or cap is sufficient to cause severe burns of the mouth, pharynx and esophagus. An educational program should be directed to parents, warning them of the hazards of caustic agents left within the reach of children and recommending the elimination of such agents from the household. However, Sobel has investigated the psychiatric implications of accidental poisoning of children and suggests that it is an expression of hostility between the child and parent. The exploratory instincts of children account for some of the ingestions, but in many it is an expression of insecurity or rebellion against parental authority. The health problem is important enough to ban the marketing of caustic liquid drain cleaners from the home.

Pathology

The clinical picture and the subsequent course of the burn of the esophagus can best be understood by a review of the pathology. Belinoff, Krey, Rosenberg, Leape and others have contributed significantly to an understanding of the pathology of this lesion. The severity of the lesion depends upon the corrosive agent swallowed, its nature, its concentration, the quantity ingested and the duration of contact with the tissue.

Corrosive Agents

Cleaning agents containing sodium hydroxide are the most frequent cause of severe burns of the esophagus. There are many common household agents that produce burns of the esophagus. Sulfuric acid, nitric acid, acetic acid and other agents are also responsible for burns of the esophagus, but are less common.

Chemical Nature of the Agent

Acids and alkalis are destructive to tissue. Sodium and potassium hydroxide and ammonia produce severe burns and account for more than half of all corrosive strictures occurring in the esophagus. Alkalis have the ability to penetrate to the deeper layers of the esophagus because they produce a liquefying necrosis. All layers become involved in an intense inflammatory reaction. Acid solutions produce coagulative necrosis, which prevents deeper penetration into the tissues. Lysol is a common agent for household cleaning; however, it rarely produces an esophagitis severe enough to cause stricturing.

Concentration of the Agent

Small quantities of a concentrated caustic taken into the mouth and then expectorated may produce lesions in the esophagus as the agent mixes with the saliva and is swallowed. The more concentrated the agent swallowed, the more severe will be the injury, in both depth and extent. Holger Krey has shown that there is a definite quantitative relationship between the depth of penetration of the lye and its concentration, as follows: a 10-second contact of normal (3.8 per cent) solution of sodium hydroxide with esophageal mucosa produced a necrosis of the mucosa and submucosa and involved some fibers in the inner longitudinal layer in rabbits. A solution of 3 N. (10.7 per cent) of sodium hydroxide produced necrosis extending to the circular muscle. A solution of 5 N. (16.4 per cent) sodium hydroxide produced necrosis extending through the whole esophageal wall and affecting the periesophageal tissue to some extent.

The significance of these figures is obvious when one realizes that cleaning agents and washing powders have anywhere from 8 to 50 per cent caustic soda as the chief ingredient. Liquid-plumer, which has a concentration of 30 per cent sodium hydroxide, produces the severest form of burns of the esophagus. Leape and his associates have shown that even a 3-second exposure to Liquid-plumer produced marked necrosis and swelling of the epithelium, which progressed to ulceration of the esophageal mucosa and an intense inflammatory reaction. There was extensive necrosis of the esophageal wall, in addition to mucosal ulceration and widespread thrombosis of the submucosal arterioles and venules.

Quantity and Duration of Contact

The greater the quantity of the agent swallowed, the more extensive the lesion and the likelihood of involvement of the stomach and duodenum. However, even a small amount of concentrated 30 per cent solution of sodium hydroxide found on the cap of a container is sufficient to produce extensive necrosis of the esophagus.

Histologic Changes

Belinoff, in a study of burned esophagi of dogs, divided the course of corrosive lesions into four stages: (1) necrosis, (2) ulceration, (3) granulation, and (4) scar formation.

In the acute phase, lasting two to three days, cell death takes place by coagulation of the intercellular proteins. A zone of intense inflammatory reaction develops in the surrounding area and thrombosis of the arterioles and veins takes place. The necrotic tissue sloughs, leaving an ulcerated surface with an acutely inflamed base. Ulceration occurs in severe burns of the esophagus within 48 hours. All the layers of the esophagus are usually involved in the inflammatory reaction. Grossly, areas of ulceration and slough are found in the oropharynx, the epiglottis, the posterior surface of the arytenoids, at the cricopharyngeus and at the crossing of the left main bronchus and cardia. The severest burns occur in the lower and middle third of the esophagus.

The inflammatory reaction and the repair begin with a proliferation of fibroblasts and the formation of new vessels. By the end of the second week, granulation tissue has started filling in the defects and fibroblasts are laying down collagen. The swelling and edema of the tissue, plus the contraction of the collagen fibers, produce narrowing of the esophagus, and adhesions begin to form between the granulating surfaces; pockets and bands thus develop. The inflammatory reaction involves the muscle coats and also the myenteric plexus of Meissner and of Auerbach, producing degenerative changes that prevent normal muscular activity and peristalsis. The esophageal lumen becomes narrowed and is made up of multiple channels and pockets that finally become completely occluded.

Injury to the esophagus and the stomach is most severe in ingestion of the concentrated liquid form of sodium hydroxide. The entire esophagus may slough and the stomach disintegrate.

Clinical Picture

The clinical course varies according to the severity of the esophagitis and may be divided into three types: (1) mild esophagitis, (2) moderate to severe esophagitis, and (3) severe esophagitis with complications.

Mild Esophagitis

Mild cases of esophagitis are those produced by weak acids or alkalis. Soreness of the mouth and slight dysphagia are present. The child is in no acute distress and there are no indications either locally or systemically of a burn. Often the history of ingestion is not definite or ingestion is only suspected by the parents. In suspected cases of ingestion, diagnostic esophagoscopy is necessary to establish or eliminate the presence of a burn.

Severe Uncomplicated Esophagitis

This form is produced by strong acids and alkalis and is almost invariably present with the ingestion of lye. Soreness of the mouth and severe dysphagia, nausea and vomiting and a rise in temperature are common symptoms. These account for the greatest number of cases and the clinical picture is due to the injury to the esophagus. The clinical course of uncomplicated severely burned esophagus may be divided into three phases, the acute phase, the intermediate or latent phase and the chronic or obstructive phase. The *acute phase* lasts for about three days and is characterized by dysphagia and a slight rise in temperature. The *intermediate or latent phase* lasts two to three weeks and is characterized by gradual improvement and disappearance in symptoms. This apparently favorable clinical course frequently leads one to believe that all is going well in the esophagus.

The *chronic or obstructive phase* begins about the third week and its onset is marked by the return of dysphagia, which may progress rapidly to complete obstruction in a few days. This corresponds to the time of the greatest contraction of collagen fibers of the inflamed esophagus. Even after the third or fourth week, when obstruction has become complete, a lumen may be present, so that a string can be introduced into the esophagus and the lumen preserved for future dilatations.

Severe Esophagitis with Complications

In severe esophagitis with complications, the injury to the esophagus is severe and extends to the periesophageal structures, or it is extensive and involves the gastrointestinal tract, particularly the stomach and the duodenum. The clinical picture is more grave and presenting signs and symptoms are those of the complications. Mediastinitis, esophageal perforation, pericarditis, chemical gastritis and peritonitis, pulmonary edema and laryngeal obstruction are some of the clinical complications. The prognosis in this group is poor and the mortality rate is high. This type of severe esophagitis with complications is seen particularly with the ingestion of liquid lye.

Diagnosis

The infant or child who presents with a history of having swallowed a corrosive agent requires a diagnostic workup to determine whether or not the agent has produced damage to the mucosal surfaces of the esophagus. The absence of burns of the mouth and pharynx does not eliminate the possibility of burns of the esophagus. For this reason, a diagnostic workup should include x-ray studies of the esophagus and an esophagoscopy.

X-ray studies in the early phases of burns of the esophagus are of little value in determining the extent and severity of the injury; only in the severely burned patient is complete atony present. The most important diagnostic procedure is esophagoscopy. It has proved to be accurate and informative. It permits direct examination of the extent and severity of the burn and it provides a means of following the progress of healing. The procedure is potentially dangerous but if it is carried out with care by a skilled endoscopist, injury to the organ can be avoided. Esophagoscopy should be done on all patients who give a history of swallowing a corrosive agent. It is done under general anesthesia. *The esophagoscope is passed to the first burned area in the esophagus and no further!* By following this policy, the danger of perforation is avoided. Passage of a scope and manipulation of the esophagus that is severely burned may cause perforation. The danger is at its greatest at about the third week, when the esophagus becomes very friable and is easily penetrated by bougies.

Treatment of Burns of the Esophagus

The object of treatment of burns of the esophagus is to prevent stricture formation, to treat the complications, to treat the strictures that develop and to reconstruct a substitute esophagus where the function of the esophagus cannot be maintained.

Neutralization of the agent is of questionable value. Dilute acetic acid, half-strength vinegar or citric acid has been used to neutralize alkalis and sodium bicarbonate for acids. However, it has been proved that unless these agents are taken immediately after the ingestion, they are of no value. Kiviranta could find no evidence that attempts to neutralize substances after one minute had any effect on the clinical course of the patient. This has been confirmed by the work of Leape.

Vigorous attempts at washing out the stomach have little value and run the risk of perforation of the esophagus or stomach. Maloney recommends having the patients drink large quantities of water.

Prevention of Stricture

The treatment directed at the prevention of strictures is based upon three factors: (1) the control of infection with the use of antibiotics, (2) the control of fibrous tissue production by steroid therapy, and (3) the prevention of adhesions by dilatations. Basically, these form the essential features of the various regimens that have been used in various clinics in dealing with corrosive esophagitis.

The earliest efforts directed toward preventing stricturing of the esophagus were made by Belinoff in 1920 and by Bokay in 1924. They reported success in preventing stricture formation in the patients with severe burns of the esophagus by the passage of weighted bougies. The weighted bougies were passed each day in increasing sizes to the largest size tolerated by the patient. Dilatations were continued until the esophagus healed. Frequency of the dilatations was decreased as the esophagus showed less tendency to contract. The bougienage was continued for months if necessary. Often the patient was given bougies to pass at home.

The effectiveness of the bougienage was due to the separation of the ulcerated areas and breaking up of adhesions before strictures could form. The esophagus thus healed as a smooth tube rather than one distorted by pockets and by blind channels and strictures. The method also accurately calibrated the lumen from day to day. Thus, if in the second or third week the esophagus admitted progressively smaller bougies, it indicated that the method would not succeed and that gastrostomy would be necessary, and that the patient should swallow a string to preserve the lumen for retrograde dilatation. The weighted bougies are not effective dilators of contracting scar tissue. The method was safe and was successful in maintaining normal swallowing function in 80 to 85 per cent of the patients. It was generally accepted and forms part of many therapeutic regimens.

The next advance in prevention of strictures was the use of corticosteroids, as reported by Rosenberg in 1951 and by Weisskopf in 1952. They demonstrated in both experimental animals and humans that corticosteroids controlled the production of granulation tissue and thus stricture formation, and that corticosteroids could be used safely if the infection were controlled by antibiotic therapy. Normal swallowing function was preserved in 80 to 90 per cent of the patients. Strictures that formed on this regimen were soft and yielded to a few dilatations. Most clinics use this method or the preceding one, or a combination of both.

Another factor that stimulates the production of granulation tissue is the entrapment of food in the granulating surface. Krey has demonstrated that burns did not heal when rabbits were fed by mouth. Food particles stimulated foreign body reaction. Daly and Cardona preferred to introduce a soft, small-caliber feeding tube and eliminate all oral feedings. Others have recommended a gastrostomy for feeding, thus putting the esophagus at rest.

Cardona has eliminated bougienage, feeling that it is traumatic, delays healing and does not significantly improve results. Holinger and others point to the dangers of an indwelling nasogastric tube. Some physicians permit oral feedings after the third day or as tolerated by the patient.

Although authors from clinics reporting an extensive experience with the treatment of the burned esophagus recommend regimens differing in detail, all agree on two points: that early treatment should be instituted to prevent strictures and to maintain the lumen of the esophagus, and that dilatations with weighted bougies and therapy with corticosteroids and antibiotics are both effective measures in preventing strictures. Thus, it is necessary for the physician to use his judgment in the selection of the preventive methods to be applied to the individual patient with an uncomplicated burn of the esophagus.

Regimen for Early Treatment of Burns of the Esophagus

When ingestion of an alkali or acid occurs or is suspected, the infant or child should be admitted to a hospital to establish the diagnosis and to start therapy. Oral feeding is discontinued. A small polyethylene nasogastric tube is passed and left in place until healing is complete. The feeding tube also serves to maintain the lumen of the esophagus. The nasogastric tube has not caused complications in the author's experience at Bellevue Hospital.

Corticosteroid Therapy

Corticosteroid therapy is prescribed according to the weight of the child, starting with 40 mg. of prednisolone per day for one week and gradually reducing it to a maintenance dose until healing is complete. Also, penicillin is given throughout the period of healing.

Esophagoscopy is done during the first three days and before the fourth day. If burns are not found or if they are of a mild degree, without ulceration, the regimen is discontinued and the child is discharged from the hospital. Follow-up esophagoscopy is repeated at two-week intervals to check the progress of healing.

The danger of perforation by the esophagoscope is an ever-present risk and is greater in the child with an inflamed esophagus. Great care and expertise are needed to avoid perforation.

TREATMENT OF STRICTURES RESULTING FROM BURNS OF THE ESOPHAGUS

If the burned esophagus does not respond to preventive measures, and strictures do form, it is essential to introduce a string into the esophagus to maintain the lumen. If a gastrostomy has been done, the end of the string is retrieved from the stomach through the gastrostomy opening. The upper end of the string is brought out through the nose. The ends are tied, forming a continuous loop. Retrograde dilatations with Tucker-type bougies are started on a daily schedule and continued until a satisfactory lumen has been established and the tendency of the strictures to contract has diminished. The patient can then continue the dilatations by introducing the weighted bougies himself, either the Hurst bougies or tapered Maloney-type bougies.

If a gastrostomy has not been done, strictures may be dilated from above with the Jackson-Plummer dilators over a previously swallowed string. Several yards of heavy black silk string should be swallowed, so that the string becomes well anchored in the small intestine. Dilatations can be accomplished also by passing esophagoscopes of gradually increasing caliber, using the string as a guide. Prograde dilatation is suitable for uncomplicated strictures. The danger of perforating the esophagus is always greater in the prograde dilatation than in the retrograde method. Dilatations are performed twice a week. A lumen of 26 to 28 F. is adequate for an infant, one of 40 F. for a child and one of 45 F. for an adult.

When the lumen is 30 F. or less, only liquids can be swallowed. The frequency of the dilatations is diminished as the tendency for the strictures to contract diminishes. Mendelsohn and Maloney have reported improved results with dilatation by the submucosal injection of corticosteroids at the site of stricture.

Complications Resulting from Too Forceful Dilatation

It is axiomatic to stop if blood is noticed on the bougie. Bleeding indicates that the mucosa has been broken, and further dilatation may result in a tear and perforation. Occasionally a periesophageal reaction will occur following dilatation. Treatment with antibiotics for a period of two weeks is usually adequate to control the reaction. Dilatation may be resumed at the end of two weeks, dropping back to smaller bougies.

REPLACEMENT OF A NON-FUNCTIONING ESOPHAGUS

When injury to the esophagus is so extensive that adequate swallowing function cannot be maintained, the esophagus should be replaced with a colon transplant or a gastroesophageal tube fashioned from the greater curvature of the stomach. Resection of the esophagus and stomach and replacement with a colon transplant is indicated as an emergency procedure when the burn is severe and perforation of the organ is imminent.

In children who have ingested liquid agents containing 30 per cent sodium hydroxide, immediate resection of the esophagus and stomach and replacement with a segment of colon is a life-saving procedure. Ritter et al. have treated two patients with early esophagogastrectomy followed by a colon interposition at a later date. The primary esophagogastrectomy lessened morbidity, the hospital convalescence and complications from severe burns produced by liquid caustics.

REFERENCES

Bartlett, M. D., Faxon, H. H., and Waddell, W. R.: Treatment of reflux esophagitis with stricture. *New Eng. J. Med.,* 262:551, 1960.

Belinoff, S.: Treatment of corrosive esophagitis. In

Terracol, J., et al.: Les Maladies de l'Oesophage. Paris, Masson et Cie, 1958.

Bokay, J.: Salzer's treatment of lye poisoning. *Wien. Klin. Wschr.*, 37:282, 1925.

Cardona, J. C., and Daly, J. F.: Current management of corrosive esophagitis: An evaluation of results in 239 cases. *Ann. Otol. Rhinol. Laryng.*, 80:521, 1971.

Daly, J. F.: The early management of corrosive burns of the esophagus. *Surg. Clin. N. Amer.*, 34:343, 1954.

Daly, J. F.: Corrosive esophagitis. *Otolaryng. Clin. N. Amer.*, 119:131, 1968.

Daly, J. F., and Cardona, J. C.: Corrosive esophagitis. *Amer. J. Surg.*, 93:242, 1957.

Daly, J. F., and Cardona, J. C.: Acute corrosive esophagitis. *Arch. Otol.*, 74:629, 1961.

Fearon, B.: The endoscopic management of congenital atresia of the esophagus with or without tracheo-esophageal fistulas and of congenital tracheo-esophageal fistula without atresia of the esophagus. *Ann. Otol.*, 68:1047, 1959.

Flood, C. A.: Clinical features in the management of esophageal hiatal hernia. *J.A.M.A.*, 100:314, 1960.

Gross, R. E.: *Surgery of Infancy and Childhood.* Philadelphia, W. B. Saunders Co., 1953.

Haight, C.: The management of congenital esophageal atresia and tracheal-esophageal fistula. *Surg. Clin. N. Amer.*, 41:1281, 1961.

Haight, C.: The esophagus. In Benson, C. D., et al. (Eds.): *Pediatric Surgery.* Chicago, Year Book Medical Publishers, Inc., 1962, Chap. 23.

Haight, C.: Discussion of Schultz and Clatworthy's paper. *Arch. Surg.*, 87:124, 1963.

Hanson, E. L., Daly, J. F., and Davis, D. A.: Ulceration associated with an islet of columnar epithelium in the mid-esophagus: New evidence for an acquired etiology of Barrett's syndrome. *J. Ped. Surg.*, 5:370, 1970.

Hays, D. M., and Synder, W. H.: Results of conventional operative procedures for esophageal atresia in premature infants. *Amer. J. Surg.*, 106:19, 1963.

Hohf, R. P., Kimball, E. R., and Ballenger, J. J.: Rupture of the esophagus in the neonate. *J.A.M.A.*, 181:939, 1962.

Holder, T., and Ashcraft, K.: *Current Problems in Surgery: Esophageal Atresia and Tracheo-Esophageal Fistula.* Chicago, Year Book Medical Publishers, 1966.

Holinger, P.: Endoscopic aspects of esophagitis and esophageal hiatal hernia. *J.A.M.A.*, 98:312, 1960.

Holinger, P. H., and Johnston, K. C.: Postsurgical endoscopic problems of congenital esophageal atresia. *Ann. Otol.*, 72:1035, 1963.

Jacobziner, H.: Accidental chemical poisonings: Fatalities due to ingestion of corrosives. *N.Y. State J. Med.*, July, 1963, p. 1969.

Kiviranta, U.: Korrosion des oesophagus und des ventrikels. *Acta Otolaryng.* (Stockholm), Suppl. 81:1, 1949.

Krey, H.: On the treatment of corrosive lesions in the oesophagus. *Acta Otolaryng.* (Stockholm), Suppl. 102:1, 1952.

Leape, L. L., Ashcraft, K. W., Scarpelli, D. G., and Holder, T. M.: Hazard to health—liquid lye. *New Eng. J. Med.*, 284:578, 1971.

Longino, L. A., Woolley, M. M., and Gross, R. E.: Esophageal replacement in infants and children with use of a segment of colon. *J.A.M.A.*, 90: 1187, 1959.

Mendelsohn, H. J., and Maloney, W. H.: The treatment of benign strictures of the esophagus with cortisone injection. *Ann. Otol.*, 79:900, 1970.

Miller, C. L., and Warren, R. O. Y.: Steroid treatment of lye burns of the esophagus. *J.A.M.A.*, 170:1525, 1959.

Morrison, L. E.: Experience with dilatation of the esophagus following surgery for esophageal atresia. *Ann. Otol.*, 68:580, 1959.

Olsen, A. M., Code, C. F., and Clagett, O. T.: Role of motility patterns in the diagnosis of esophageal disease. *J.A.M.A.*, 172:319, 1960.

Reynolds, R. P., and Morrison, W. W.: Congenital malformation of the esophagus. *Amer. J. Dis. Child.*, 21:339, 1921.

Ritter, F. N., Gago, O., Kirsh, M. M., Korman, R. M., and Orvald, T. O.: The rationale of emergency esophagogastrectomy in the treatment of liquid caustic burns of the esophagus and stomach. *Ann. Otol.*, 80:513, 1971.

Rosenberg, N., Kunderman, P. J., and Moolten, S. E.: Prevention of experimental strictures of esophagus by cortisone. *Arch. Surg.*, 63:147, 1951.

Rosenberg, N., Kunderman, P. J., Vroman, L., and Moolten, S.: Prevention of experimental esophageal stricture by cortisone. *Arch. Surg.*, 66:593, 1953.

Salzer, H.: Early treatment of corrosive esophagitis. *Wien. Klin. Wschr.*, 33:307, 1920.

Schultz, L. R., and Clatworthy, H. W., Jr.: Esophageal strictures after anastomoses in esophageal atresia. *Arch. Surg.*, 87:120, 1963.

Sobel, R.: The psychiatric implications of accidental poisoning in childhood. *Pediat. Clin. N. Amer.*, 17:653, 1970.

Strawczynski, H., et al.: The behavior of the lower eosphageal sphincter in infants and its relationship to gastroesophageal regurgitation. *J. Pediat.*, 64:17, 1964.

United States Department of Health, Education and Welfare, Public Health Service: Food and Drug Administration: Tabulation of 1969 reports. Bullentin, National Clearinghouse for Poison Control Centers, Sept.-Oct., 1970.

Waterson, D. J., Bonham-Carter, R. E., and Aberdeen, E.: Oesophageal atresia: Tracheo-oesophageal fistula. A study of survival in 218 infants. *Lancet*, 1:819, 1962.

Weisskopf, A.: Effects of cortisone on experimental lye burn of the esophagus. *Ann. Otol.*, 61: 681, 1952.

Chapter One Hundred Sixteen

THE RADIOLOGIC ASPECTS OF THE AIR AND FOOD PASSAGES

MARIE A. CAPITANIO, M.D., and JOHN A. KIRKPATRICK, M.D.

The radiologic examination plays an important role in the diagnosis of obstructing lesions of the respiratory tract and the esophagus. It is possible in most instances to delineate the site of obstruction and to define the pathophysiology produced by the obstructing lesion. A radiologic diagnosis, therefore, depends on a knowledge of normal anatomy and physiology of the neck and chest, and on a knowledge of those lesions that are most apt to occur in the various age groups and in each of the sexes.

THE AIRWAY

Technique

There are several radiographic techniques that can be utilized to define an obstructing lesion of the airway. Initially, there must be a "basic" examination that reveals the *entire* airway in all instances of suspected airway obstruction. The initial x-ray study should include the neck exposed in the lateral position during inspiration and expiration, and frontal and lateral examinations of the chest. The exposure of frontal films of the thorax during inspiration and expiration is often a part of the initial examination. After a careful review of the initial examination, additional radiographs and fluoroscopy can be added when necessary.

Because infants and young children are unable to cooperate as well as older children, it may be difficult to obtain satisfactory radiographs of the neck and chest during both inspiration and expiration. This problem can be easily resolved by a fluoroscopic examination of the neck and chest and the exposure of appropriate spot films during the different phases of respiration. In addition to, or in place of, a frontal film of the chest during expiration, lateral decubitus films may be obtained to determine the presence of air trapping in the lungs. A film of the chest in the frontal projection is exposed while the patient is lying on one side and then repeated with the patient lying on his other side. The lung on the dependent side is expected to be underaerated. If all or part of the lung traps air, the involved area will remain expanded and be hyperlucent (Fig. 1).

After review of the initial roentgen studies, an abnormality may be better defined by the addition of oblique views of the chest, tomography, a barium swallow, bronchography or angiography.

Roentgen Signs of Airway Obstruction

Direct Signs. Significant roentgen signs of airway obstruction are mass, overaeration, underaeration and deformity.

Mass lesions in the airway or mediastinum are readily visible on radiographs, since they are of water density and stand out in sharp relief by virtue of the air in the respiratory tract that surrounds them

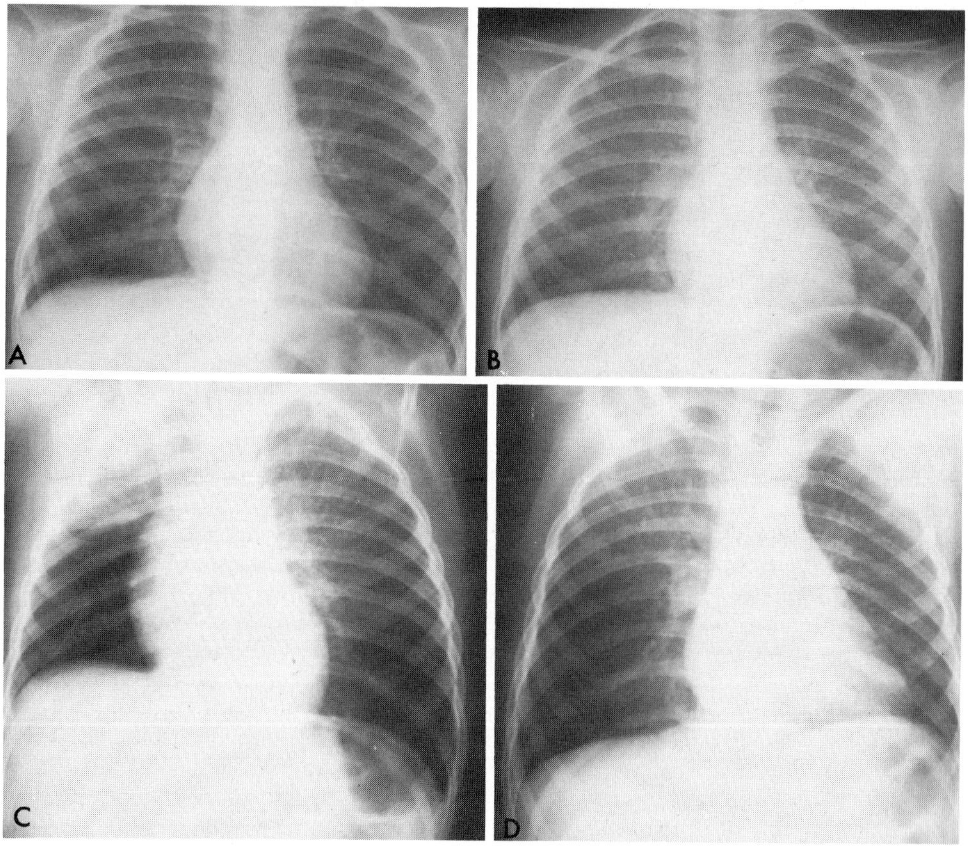

Figure 1. Peanut in the right lower lobe bronchus. Air trapping in the right lower lobe is most apparent on a right lateral decubitus film (*C*) as compared to erect frontal (*A*) and lateral (*B*) chest x-rays. *D*, Normal left lateral decubitus.

(Fig. 2). Though the exact nature of the mass cannot be ascertained on the basis of its roentgen appearance, it is possible to arrive at an appropriate differential diagnosis, depending on the location of the mass, the age and sex of the patient, the effect of the mass on surrounding structures, and the characteristics of calcifications within the mass if they are present. Radiopaque foreign bodies present no problem in diagnosis; on the other hand, nonradiopaque foreign bodies will be visible radiographically only as a mass of water density if they are of sufficient density and size. Nonradiopaque foreign bodies or masses that are not large or dense enough to be visible may still cause varying degrees of obstruction, and their presence is suspected by virtue of other radiographic signs of airway obstruction.

Overaeration and *underaeration* are most valuable roentgen signs of airway obstruction. In general, obstructing lesions in the upper respiratory tract will result in overaeration or distention of the airway proximal to the site of obstruction during inspiration, and, depending on the severity of the obstruction, the airway below the obstruction will be normally aerated or underaerated.

Obstructing lesions in the lower respiratory tract may present in one of two ways: as obstructive emphysema or as atelectasis. Obstructive emphysema occurs as the result of a "ball-valve" mechanism produced by the obstructing lesion, which permits air to flow past the

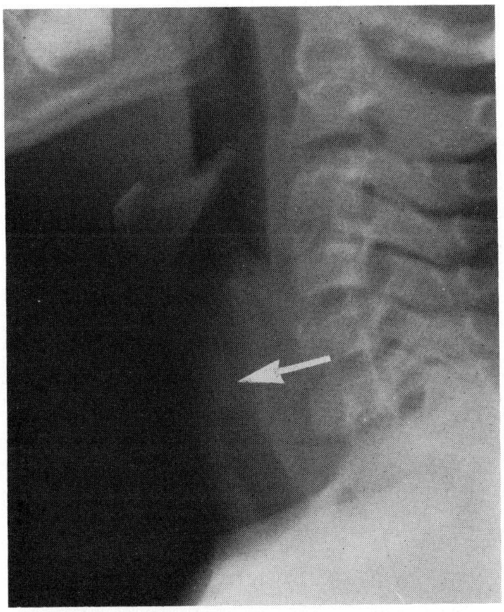

Figure 2. Subglottic granuloma presents as a soft tissue mass (arrow).

site of obstruction in a bronchus into the lung during inspiration but will not permit air to be evacuated from the lung during expiration. Air enters the lung because the bronchus dilates during inspiration, permitting sufficient patency of the lumen of the bronchus at the site of the obstructing lesion, but on expiration the bronchus narrows, and this normal reduction in caliber, added to the compromise afforded by the obstructing lesion, occludes the lumen and prevents air from leaving the lung. As a result, the involved lung, lobe or segment appears hyperlucent. Atelectasis results when the obstruction completely occludes the bronchus during both phases of respiration (Fig. 3).

When a large segment or a number of segments of one lung are involved, by either obstructive emphysema or atelectasis, there will be a shift of the heart and mediastinum during expiration. In instances of obstructive emphysema, the shift is away from the involved side, and when atelectasis is present the shift is toward the involved side (Fig. 4).

Deformity of the trachea is highly significant in the diagnosis of airway obstruction in infants and children. Normally, the trachea is in the mid-mediastinum in front of and slightly to the right of the esophagus. It is seen as a relatively uniform, sharply delineated column of air in both the frontal and lateral projections. Buckling of the trachea at the level of the thoracic inlet is seen frequently in the infant, because the trachea is not yet firmly fixed in the mediastinum, but this does not compromise the airway. Lesions that compromise the caliber of the airway are, as a rule, readily detected on roentgenographic examination because of the contrast afforded by the distorted pattern of air within its lumen. Alterations in the caliber and configuration of the trachea are most significant in the diagnosis of certain entities, such as esophageal atresia, vascular ring and croup.

INDIRECT SIGNS. Obstructing lesions of the upper airway may be suspected when a paradoxical change in the size of the heart between inspiration and expiration is noted; that is, the transverse diameter of the heart is smaller during expiration than during inspiration. (Normally, the heart appears larger during the expiratory phase of respiration than during the inspiratory phase of respiration.) This phenomenon is readily explained by the Valsalva and the Mueller maneuvers. The Valsalva maneuver involves breathing *out* against a closed glottis or an obstruction in the upper airway, and during it, the intrathoracic pressure tends to be less negative, which results in a decrease in the volume of venous blood returning to the heart; thus the heart appears small. During the Mueller maneuver, which is breathing *in* against a closed glottis or an obstruction in the upper airway, the intrathoracic pressure is more negative, facilitating the return of venous blood to the heart; thus the heart appears large (Fig. 5).

The presence of interstitial pulmonary emphysema, pneumomediastinum or pneumothorax implies that there is a peripheral air block beyond the major bronchi (Fig. 6). An obstruction of a small bronchus may result in rupture of a respiratory bronchiole or alveolus, allowing air to escape into the interstitial tissues

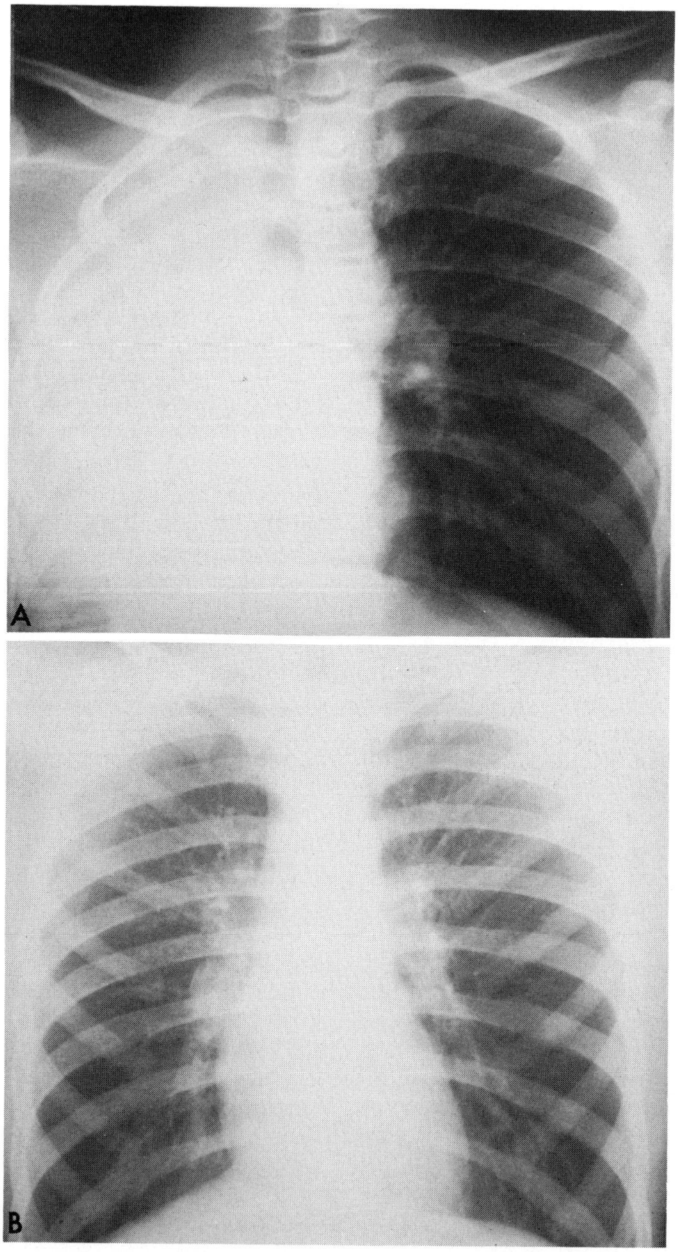

Figure 3. *A*, Atelectasis of right lung in a patient with asthma *(B)* cleared readily after mucus plug was coughed up.

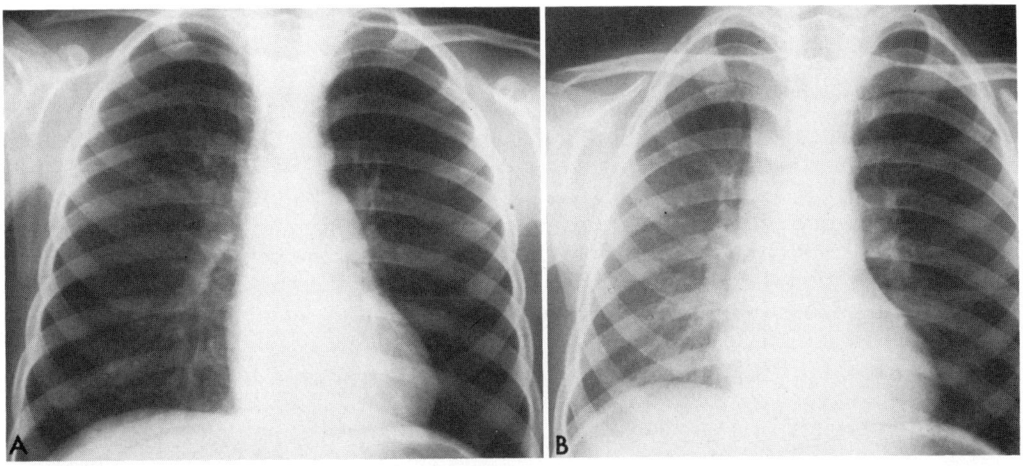

Figure 4. *A*, Obstructive emphysema of left lung produced by peanut in main bronchus. *B*, Note shift of the heart and mediastinum away from the abnormal side during expiration.

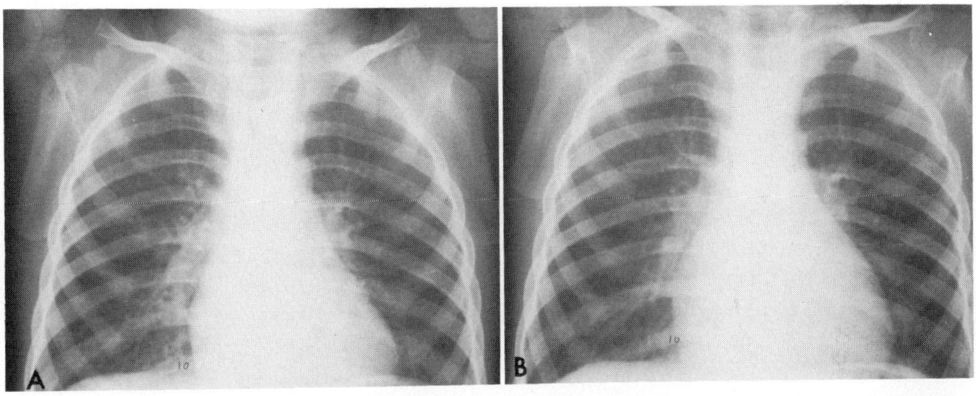

Figure 5. Mueller-Valsalva maneuver. The heart is larger during inspiration (*B*) than during expiration (*A*) in this 2-year-old child, who has the subglottic granuloma illustrated in Figure 2.

Figure 6. Interstitial air in newborn infant with hyaline membrane disease. Note the streak of air in the right upper lobe.

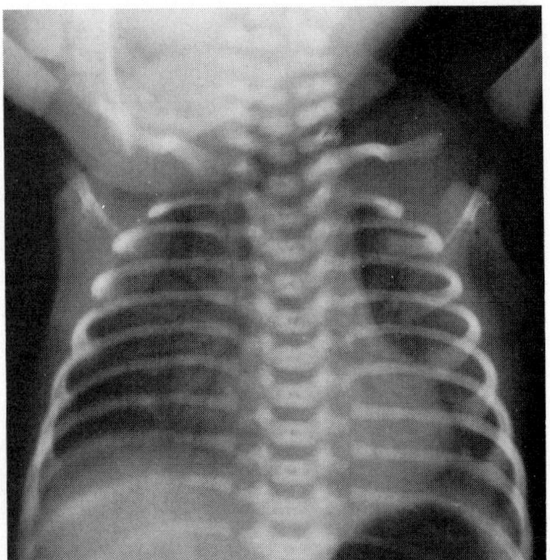

of the lung. This appears radiographically as a streak of air or cystic collection of air surrounded by compressed lung that is dense but that varies in thickness. At times, the interstitial air will pass along the vascular sheaths to the hilum and into the mediastinum, producing a pneumomediastinum. Characteristically, a pneumothorax results when the air breaks out of the mediastinum into the pleural space. It is exceedingly rare in children to have a pneumothorax develop from rupture of a subpleural bleb (Fig. 7) (Campbell, 1970).

A persistent localized pneumonia that does not clear in the expected time with treatment should be suspected of being related to an obstructing lesion, and in most instances this will be a foreign body. The lower and middle lobes are most commonly affected in instances of foreign bodies. Diffuse chronic pulmonary infections may be manifestations of a tracheoesophageal fistula or chronic aspiration.

AIRWAY OBSTRUCTION

The Trachea and Bronchi

There are a number of developmental anomalies that may cause respiratory distress by producing varying degrees of obstruction at the tracheal or bronchial level. Notable among these are the developmental anomalies of the great vessels, the so-called "vascular rings." The double aortic arch and the right aortic arch with an aberrant left subclavian artery and left ligamentum arteriosum produce a similar deformity of the trachea and esophagus that is visible on barium swallow. In the frontal projection, the trachea may appear normal, but not infrequently the trachea well above the carina may be displaced slightly to the left by the right aortic arch, and the distal trachea and carina displaced slightly to the right by the left aortic arch. The deformity of the trachea is best appreciated on the lateral film study of the chest in

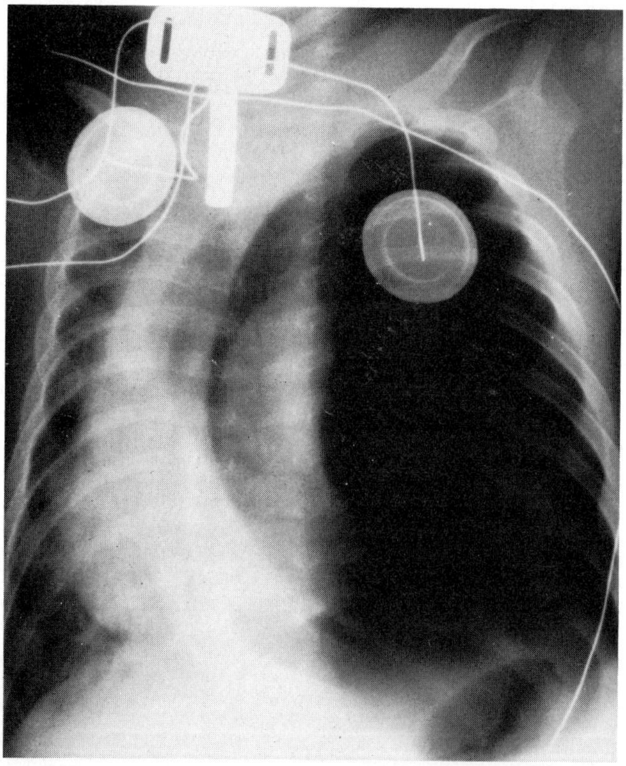

Figure 7. Tension pneumothorax.

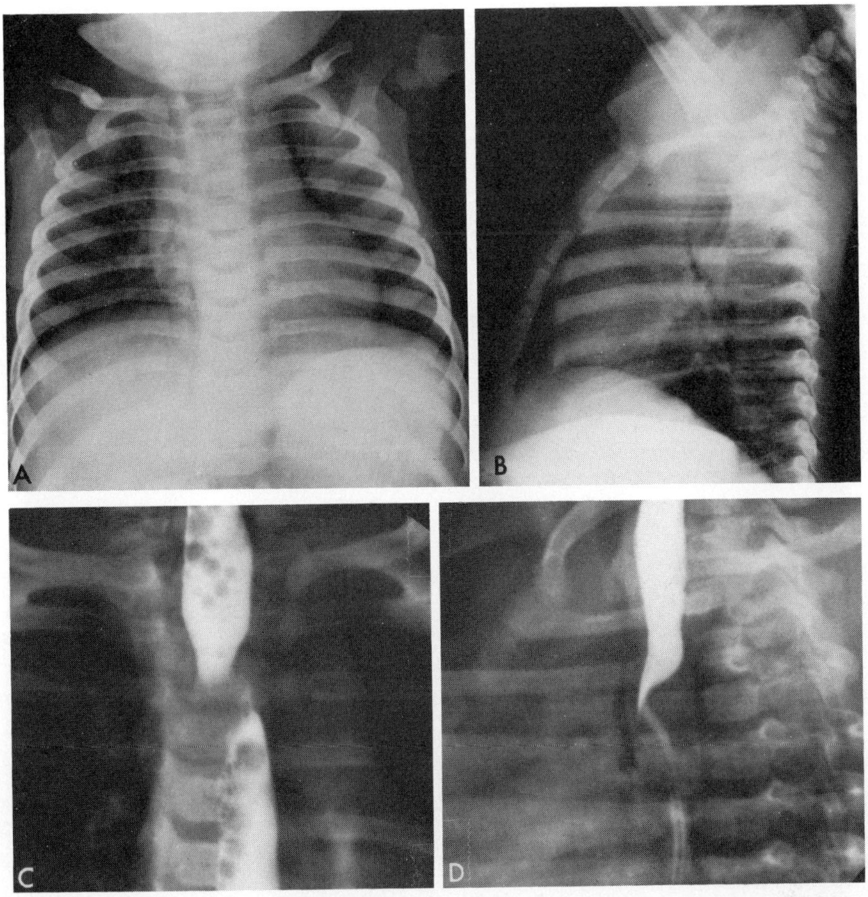

Figure 8. Double aortic arch. In the frontal view *(A)* the trachea appears normal; in the lateral view *(B)* the trachea is S-shaped in contour, reflecting the presence of an anterior and posterior arch. There are bilateral *(C)* and posterior *(D)* indentations on the esophagus.

which the trachea appears S-shaped in contour, reflecting the presence of an anterior and a posterior arch. In the presence of such a vascular ring, there will be bilateral and posterior indentations on the barium-filled esophagus (Fig. 8). A constant local compression of the trachea anteriorly, below the thoracic inlet at the level of the manubrium, suggests an "anomalous" innominate artery (Fig. 9). The "pulmonary sling" or aberrant left pulmonary artery may result in varying degrees of atelectasis or obstructive emphysema of the right lung. The diagnosis of a pulmonary sling is suggested when roentgenograms of the chest reveal an alteration in aeration of the lungs, particularly the right lung, anterior bowing of the right bronchus (Fig. 10) and a low left hilum (Fig. 11). At times there may be an anterior indentation on the barium-filled esophagus, which is produced by the left pulmonary artery as it courses from the right pulmonary artery between the trachea and esophagus to the hilum of the left lung (Fig. 12). The definitive diagnosis is made by pulmonary arteriography (Fig. 13). Common to all the vascular anomalies is a high incidence of associated anomalies of the trachea and bronchi, notably stenosis of these structures (Fig. 14). Thus, surgical correction of such vascular anomalies may not relieve the patient's respiratory distress. It is advised that a tracheogram and a bronchogram be performed prior to surgery, to define any associated anomalies of the airway that may be corrected if possible

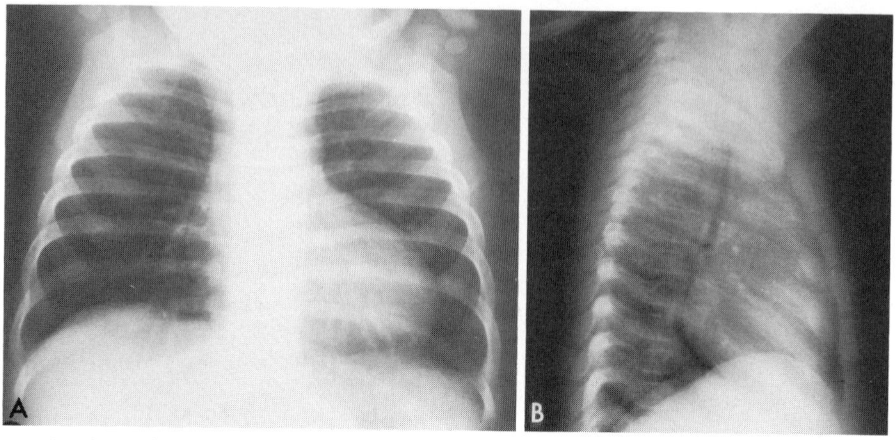

Figure 9. Anomalous innominate artery. The trachea appears normal in the frontal view *(A)*, but in the lateral view *(B)* there is an anterior impression on the trachea at the level of the manubrium.

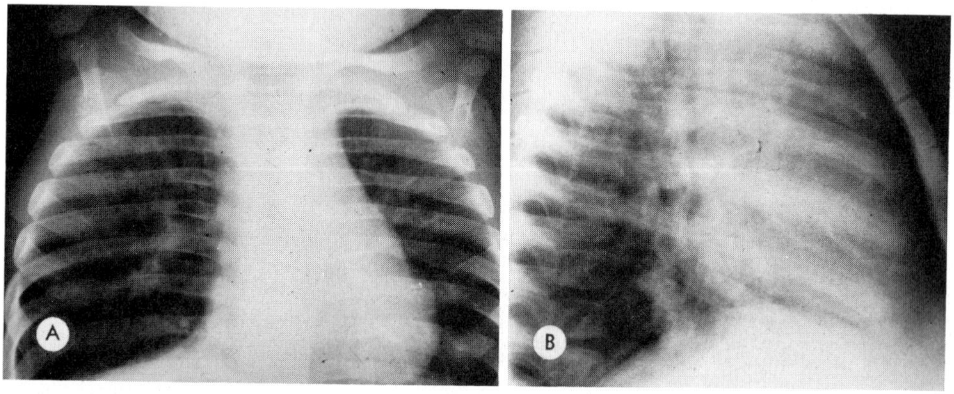

Figure 10. Pulmonary sling. *A*, The right middle and lower lobes are atelectatic. *B*, The right bronchus is bowed anteriorly.

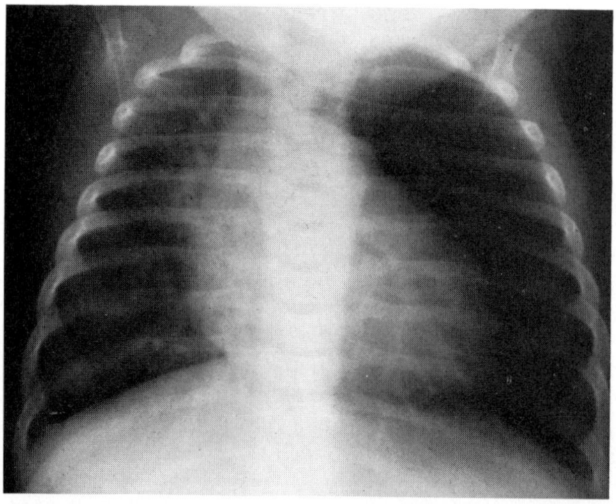

Figure 11. Pulmonary sling. The left hilum is low and the lungs are overaerated.

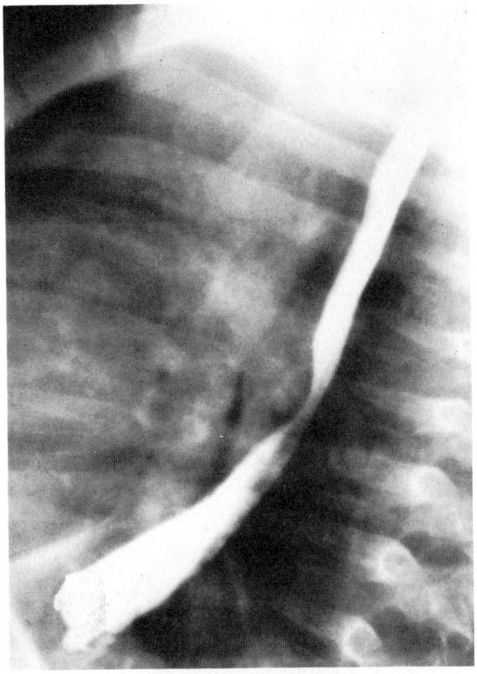

Figure 12. Pulmonary sling. There is an anterior indentation of the esophagus just below the carina.

at time of surgery (Capitanio et al., 1971).

Esophageal atresia commonly produces respiratory distress when the distended esophageal pouch impinges on the trachea posteriorly, narrowing its lumen.

Congenital stenoses of the trachea as isolated phenomena are exceedingly rare. These may be generalized, involving the entire trachea; funnel-like, with the trachea becoming progressively narrower to the level of the carina; or segmental, which may be a single localized area of narrowing or multiple localized areas of narrowing (Fig. 15).

A child with atresia or severe stenosis of a bronchus frequently presents with recurrent pneumonia and varying degrees of respiratory distress. The chest roentgenogram of such a patient often reveals an area of overaeration in which may be seen a nodular density representing a plug of mucus that dilates the bronchus just distal to the site of obstruction (Fig. 16).

Respiratory infections in infants and young children tend to be diffuse in nature and viral in origin. The inflammatory process results in edema of the mucosa of the trachea, bronchi and bronchioles. The generalized narrowing of the airway results in overaeration of the lungs. With treatment, the inflammatory reaction readily subsides and the lungs become normally aerated. There are, however, inflammatory processes that may lead to permanent obstruction of the bronchioles or bronchi, with resultant overaeration of the lungs. *Bronchiolitis fibrosa obliterans* or *obliterating bronchiolitis* results from organization of fi-

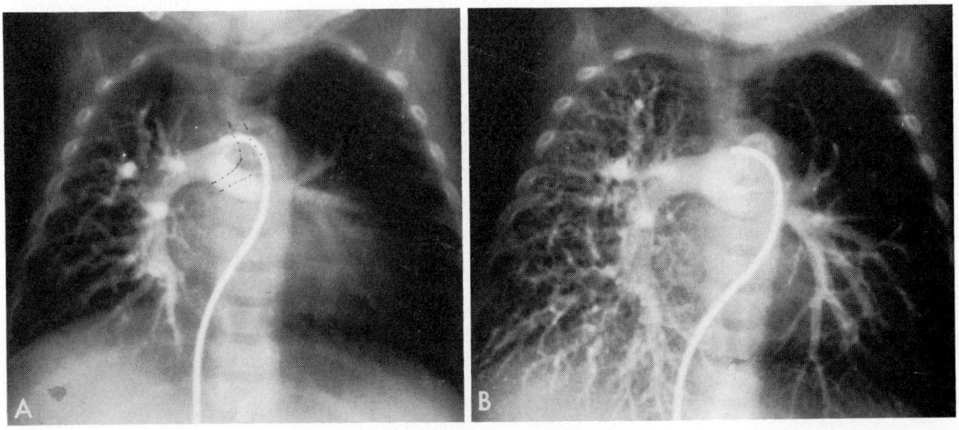

Figure 13. Pulmonary sling. The left pulmonary artery arises from the right pulmonary artery; note the low left hilum.

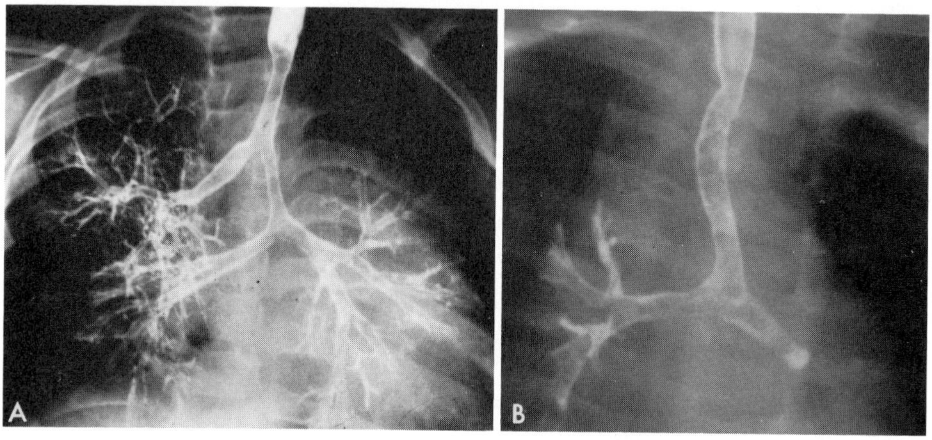

Figure 14. Pulmonary sling. (*A*), A tracheal bronchus to the right upper lobe is evident, as well as stenosis of the lower trachea. (*B*), In addition to mild compromise of the right main bronchus there is associated stenosis of the left bronchus.

brinous exudate in the bronchiole in response to local injury. It has been reported as a complication of measles, adenoviral infections, influenza, or scarlet fever, or following the inhalation of irritant substances such as nitric or sulfuric acid fumes. The involved bronchioles and bronchi are destroyed and replaced by fibrous tissue and the bronchi proximal to the obstruction dilate, resulting in bronchiectasis (Fig. 17).

Foreign bodies are by far the most common causes of obstruction in the airway in the pediatric age group. Obstructive emphysema, atelectasis and persistent pneumonia are the most common roentgen manifestations of foreign bodies in the lower respiratory tract (Fig. 18). Most often, aspiration of a foreign body produces symptoms of respiratory distress immediately. Not infrequently, however, it is only in retrospect that a history of a foreign body is obtained, and then only when the offending agent has been removed at bronchoscopy or surgery are the details remembered by the patient or his parents. It is worth reiterating that a child with a persistent atelectasis or pneumonia may well have aspirated a foreign body.

The *papilloma* is the most common tumor of the airway in the pediatric age group and may involve the trachea and bronchi as well as the upper airway. Depending on the location of the lesions, they may produce varying deformities of the trachea, atelectasis, obstructive emphysema or recurrent pneumonia.

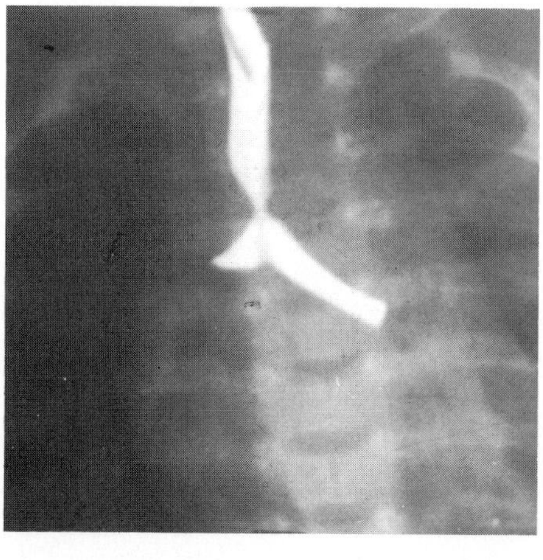

Figure 15. Tracheal stenosis. A local area of stenosis of the trachea is seen just above the carina.

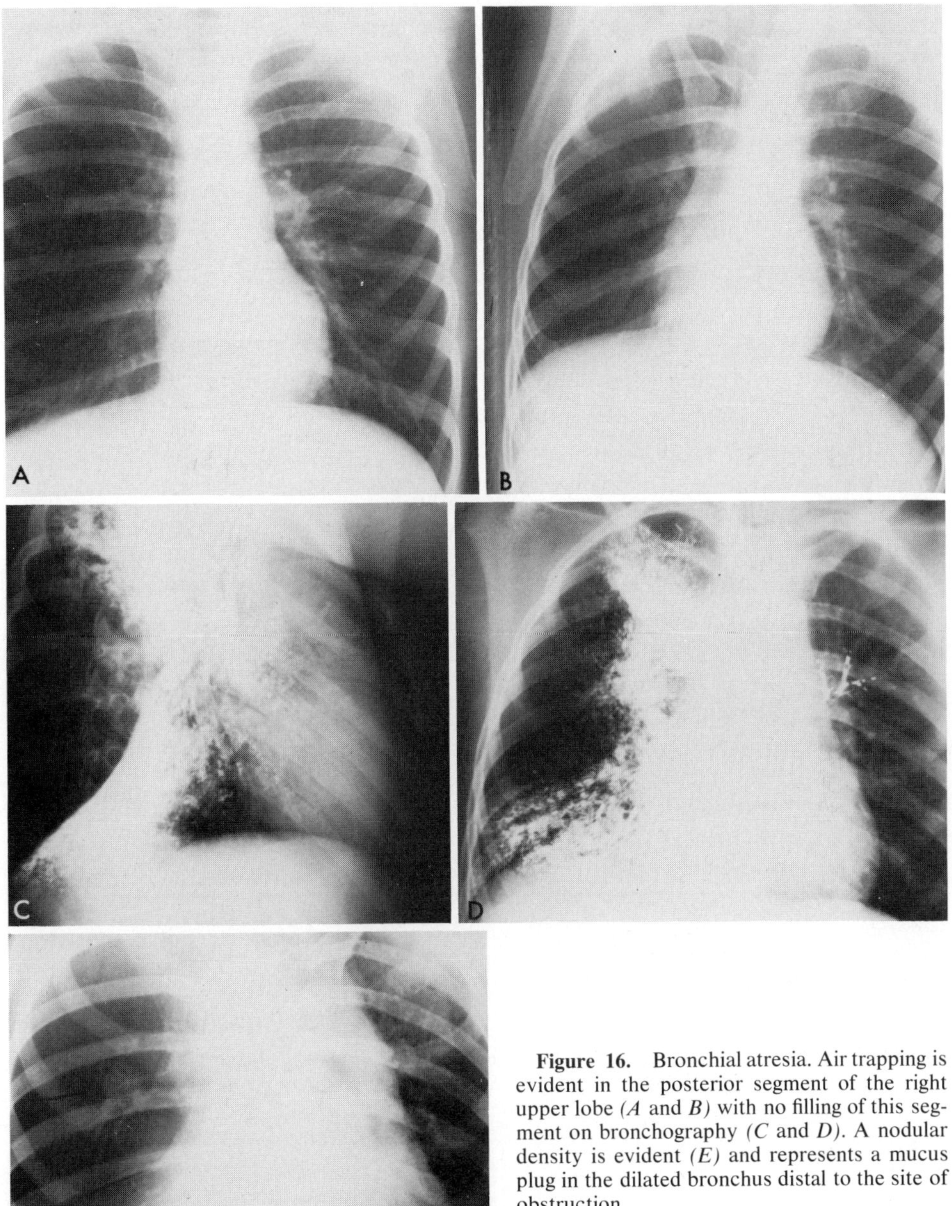

Figure 16. Bronchial atresia. Air trapping is evident in the posterior segment of the right upper lobe *(A* and *B)* with no filling of this segment on bronchography *(C* and *D)*. A nodular density is evident *(E)* and represents a mucus plug in the dilated bronchus distal to the site of obstruction.

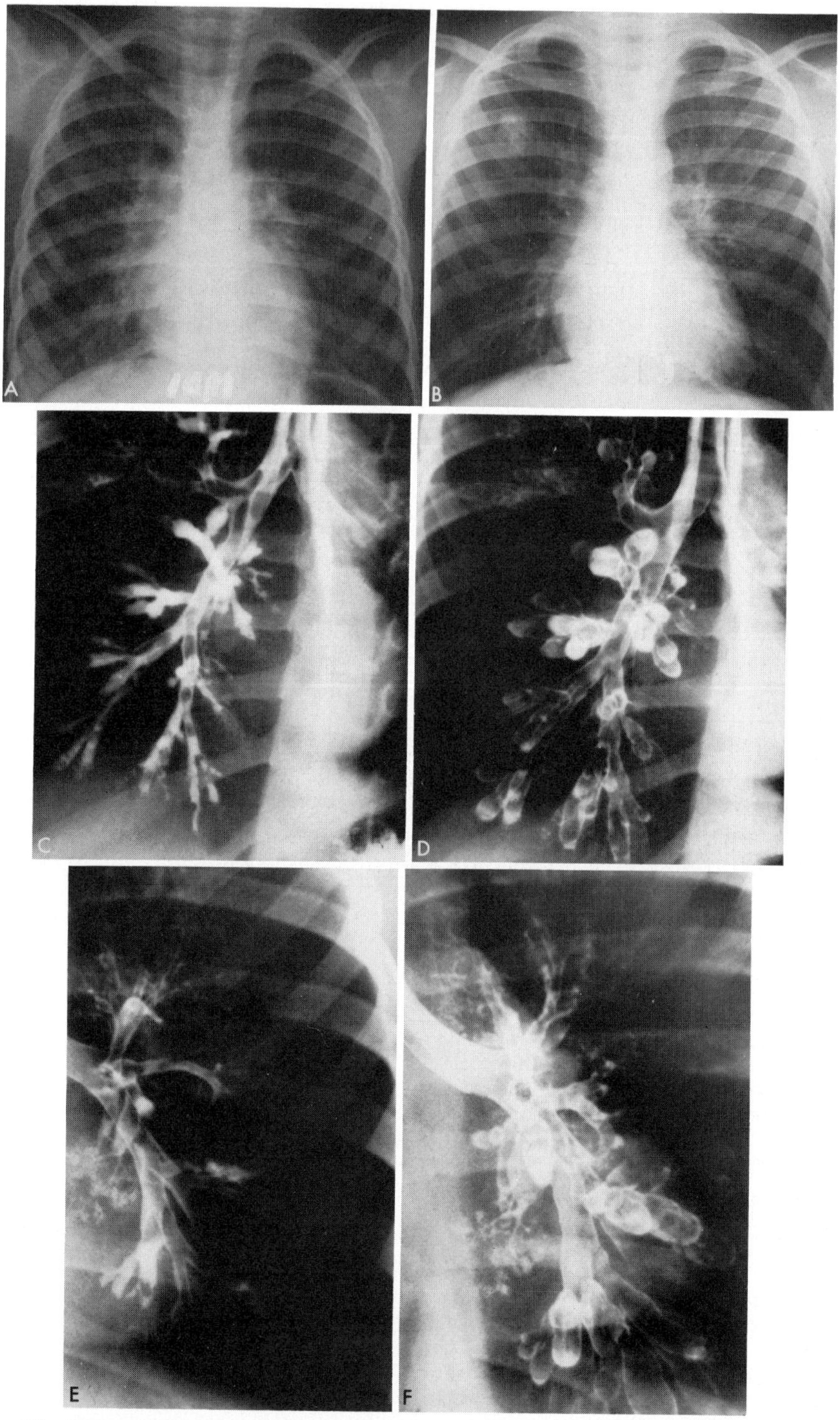

Figure 17. Obliterating bronchiolitis. *A*, Measles pneumonia. *B*, Bilateral obstructive emphysema developed following the pneumonia. *C* to *F*, Bronchography demonstrates bilateral obstructive bronchiectasis with the bronchi dilating during inspiration and narrowing during expiration.

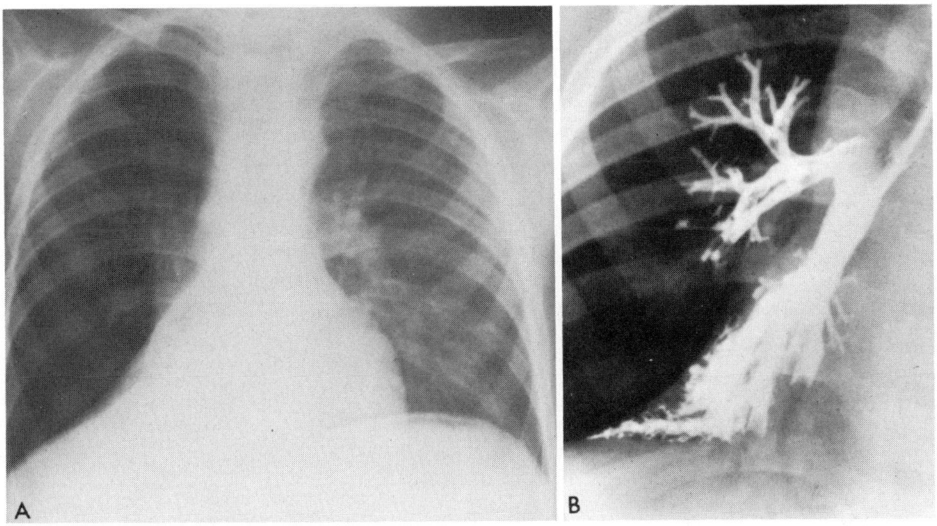

Figure 18. Foreign body. *A*, Persistent atelectasis of the right lower lobe was caused by aspiration of timothy grass. *B*, Bronchogram.

THE ESOPHAGUS

Technique

The manner in which the esophagus of a child is examined radiographically depends upon the nature of the abnormality that is suspected. Thus, the approach will differ considerably when utilized to define esophageal atresia as opposed to the defining of an esophageal stenosis or defining abnormalities of deglutition. In most instances, the roentgen examination of the esophagus is carried out by the administration of a radiopaque contrast material, either by the oral route or via a catheter positioned in the esophagus. A barium-water mixture is an appropriate and safe contrast material. It is not desirable to use water-soluble iodine-containing contrast materials, since these are irritating to the mucosa if aspirated into the airway. Before doing a contrast examination of the esophagus, film studies of the neck in the lateral projection and of the chest in frontal and lateral projections are obtained. The initial examinations of the neck and chest are first carefully reviewed, as these may reveal findings that could negate the contrast study of the esophagus or alter the approach to the esophagram.

An esophageal atresia can be defined in several ways radiographically. On the lateral film study of the thorax, it may be seen as a fluid- or air-filled pouch impinging on the trachea posteriorly (Fig. 19); a radiopaque catheter may be placed in the esophageal pouch and film studies of the chest in frontal and lateral projections will reveal the tube coiled in the pouch or its tip at the blind end of the pouch. Via a tube in the esophagus, the atretic pouch may be distended with air and recorded on appropriate roentgenograms. Finally, under fluoroscopic observation, approximately 0.25 ml. of radiopaque material may be instilled into the esophageal pouch via an *end hole* catheter, and then appropriate spot films made with the infant in the erect position (Fig. 20). When this last approach is utilized, the contrast material is immediately aspirated following exposure of the films. An end hole catheter must be utilized rather than a catheter with side holes in order to prevent the contrast material from spilling over into the trachea via a hole in the side of the catheter that may lie above the cricopharyngeus.

The posterior pharyngeal wall is apparently relatively easy to perforate with a catheter, and a catheter may be passed into the soft tissues of the mediastinum,

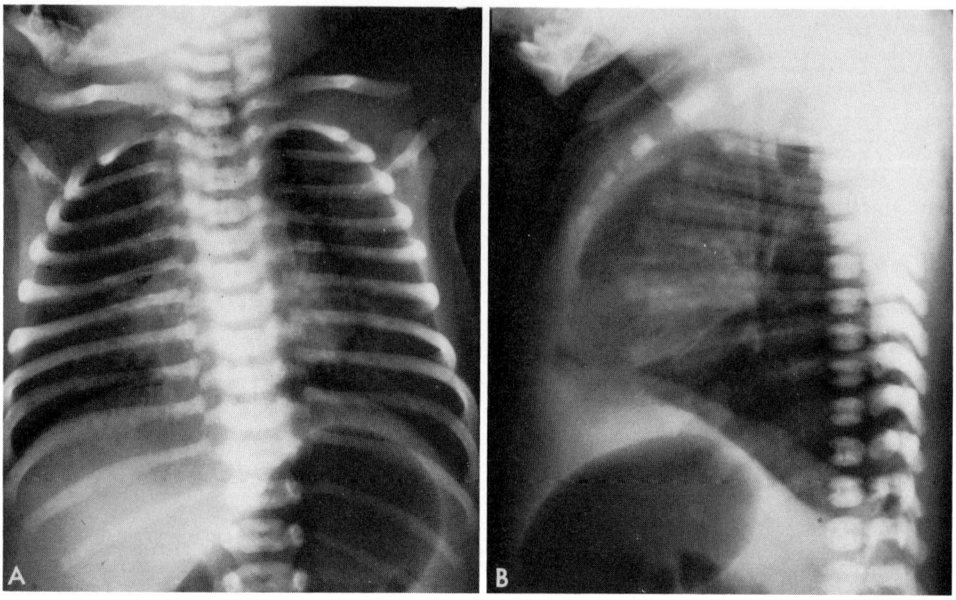

Figure 19. Esophageal atresia with tracheoesophageal fistula. The atretic esophageal pouch is distended with air, and in the lateral view it can be seen compressing the posterior wall of the trachea *(B)*. Air in the gastrointestinal tract below the diaphragm indicates the presence of an associated tracheoesophageal fistula.

where obstruction is finally encountered, giving rise to suspicion of esophageal atresia. The instillation of a small amount of contrast material through the tube will readily demonstrate the presence of an irregular cavity posterior to the esophagus. The irregularity of the contrast bolus at the site of obstruction will readily differentiate it from a smooth, rounded atretic esophageal pouch.

Infants who have an H-type tracheoesophageal fistula or pharyngeal incoordination will frequently present with difficulty in swallowing and recurrent or chronic pneumonia. The esophagram is extremely helpful in differentiating these two conditions. Under fluoroscopic observation, with a feeding tube positioned in the distal esophagus and the child placed with the right side down in the lateral or prone oblique position, the esophagus is distended with contrast material that is introduced via the nasoesophageal catheter. In this instance, it is preferable to use a thin barium-water mixture, as oily contrast materials may be too thick to pass through a tracheoesophageal fistula. The catheter is slowly withdrawn and the proximal esophagus distended with barium, taking great care that the contrast material never goes above the level of the cricopharyngeus muscle. The diagnosis of an H-type fistula is made when contrast material appears in the trachea (Fig. 21). If contrast material appears in the trachea at a time when barium has gone above the cricopharyngeus, it is impossible to know if this entered the trachea through a fistula or spilled over from above and was aspirated.

If no fistula is present, the baby is then given a barium-water mixture by bottle. The swallowing act is observed fluoroscopically with the infant in the lateral position. Note is made as to the motility of the palate. The child who has poor palatal function will be unable to attain velo-palatine closure, and contrast material will reflux into the nasopharynx and at times out the nares. A discoordination of pharyngeal function results in spill-over into the trachea (Fig. 22). In such instances, spasm of the cricopharyngeus may be observed as a persistent filling defect posteriorly on the barium-filled cervical esophagus. Poor palatal function and discoordinate pharyngeal function may be observed in immature infants and in children with a disorder of the central nervous system (Singleton et al., 1971).

The presenting complaints in instances of esophageal stenosis are difficulty in swallowing, especially swallowing solid foods, and frequent regurgitation of undigested food. At times a bolus of food may become lodged at the site of a stenosis and obstruct the esophagus. In the latter instances, roentgenograms of the chest may reveal a dilated, fluid-filled esophagus that displaces the trachea forward. An air-fluid level may be seen on a radiograph exposed with the patient in the erect position. To define an esophageal stenosis, the esophagus must be maximally distended with the contrast agent. The examination is first carried out using a relatively thin barium-water mixture, to be certain that there is no abnormality in the swallowing act. If the swallowing act is normal and no area of stenosis is identified, the patient is then given a thick barium paste. The esophagus can be more adequately distended by the use of paste, and thus a stenosis that was not evident initially may become apparent (Fig. 23).

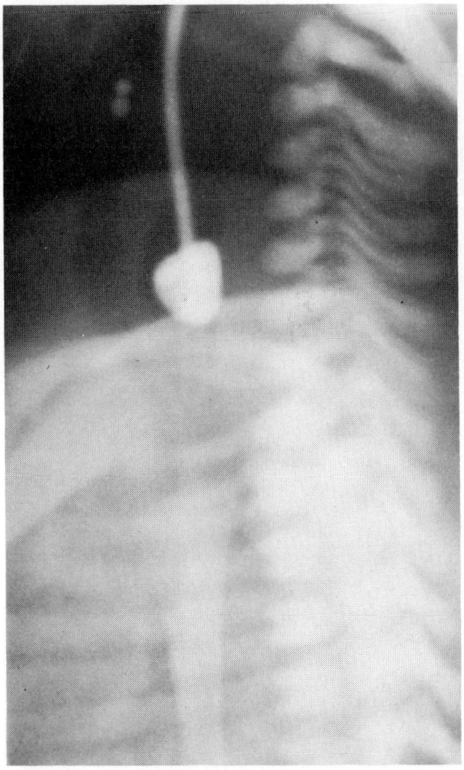

Figure 20. Esophageal atresia with tracheoesophageal fistula. A small amount of opaque material is utilized to determine the level of the esophageal atresia.

Esophageal Abnormalities

In 70 per cent of instances of *esophageal atresia,* there is an associated communication between the trachea and the esophagus, and most often this is a fistula between the trachea and the distal esophagus. The second most common type is an isolated atresia of the proximal esophagus. Whenever there is a communication between the trachea and the esophagus below the level of the atresia, the intestinal tract will be distended by air, which readily enters the gastrointestinal tract through the fistula as the child breathes. Conversely, the child who has an isolated esophageal atresia will have a gasless abdomen. In both instances, varying degrees of inflammatory disease in the lungs may be evident either because of spill-over into the trachea from the esophageal pouch or because of reflux of gastric contents into the esophagus and through the fistula and into the trachea.

The diagnosis is suspected shortly after birth, as the child may exhibit excessive oral secretions, and an obstruction is encountered in an attempt to pass a catheter into the esophagus. Even if no obstruction is encountered in such an infant, the possibility of esophageal atresia should not be excluded. It is possible, in instances of esophageal atresia with tracheoesophageal fistula, to unknowingly pass a catheter into the trachea, then through the fistula into the distal esophagus and subsequently into the stomach.

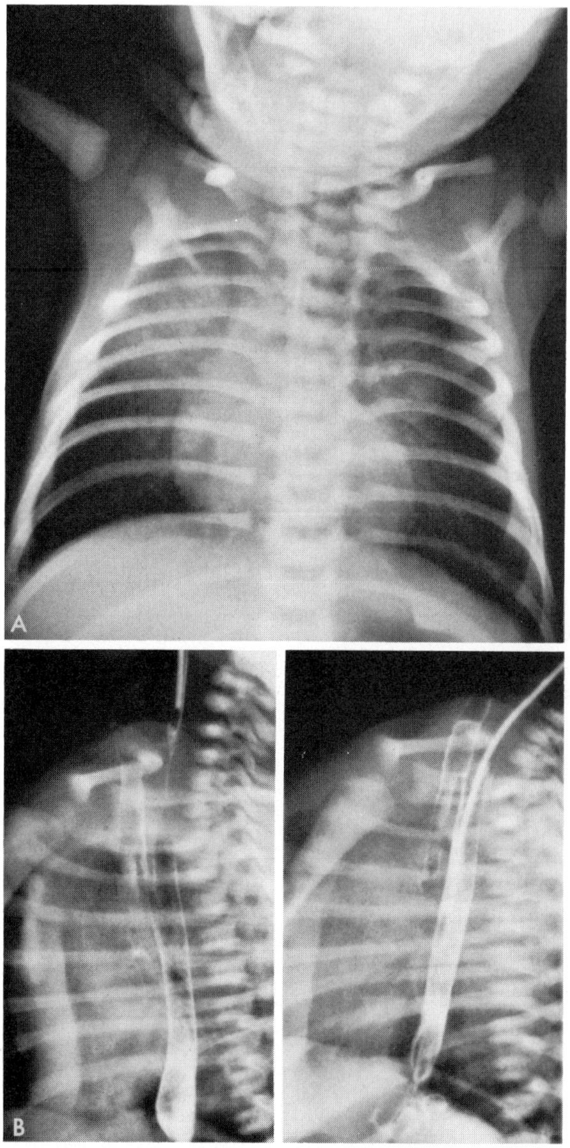

Figure 21. H-type tracheoesophageal fistula. *A*, Persistent bilateral pneumonia resulting from the tracheoesophageal fistula (*B*).

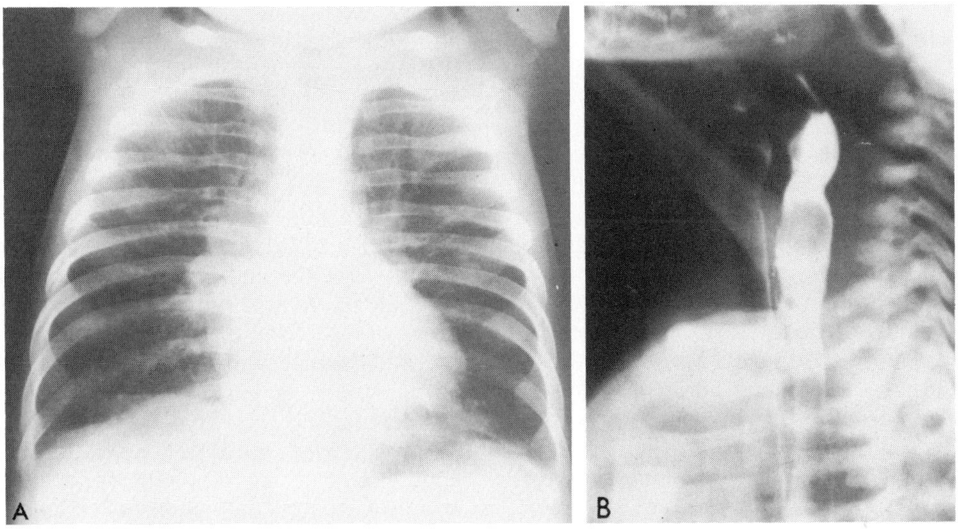

Figure 22. Aspiration. Bilateral pneumonia persisted *(A)* because of chronic aspiration *(B)*.

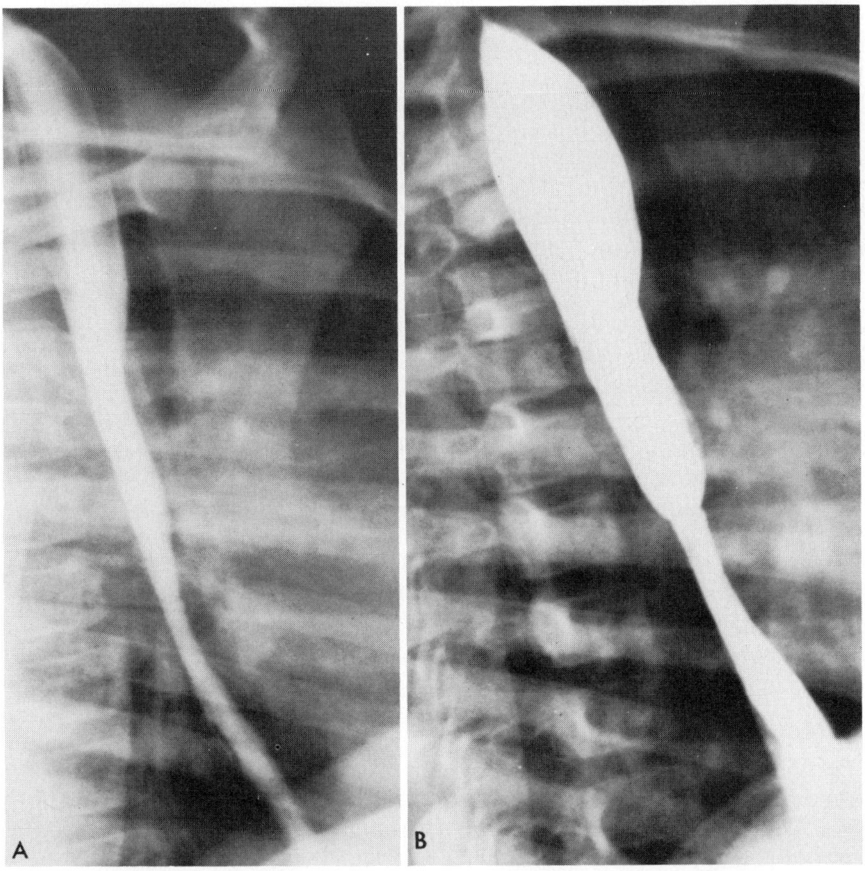

Figure 23. Esophageal stenosis. The esophagus appears normal when it is distended with a barium-water mixture *(A)*, but the web stenosis in the distal esophagus is obvious when the esophagus is distended with a barium paste *(B)*.

Only a lateral film study of the chest will correctly identify the course and location of the catheter.

Esophageal atresias with or without tracheoesophageal *fistulae* are surgically correctable lesions, and the diagnosis should be made as early as possible, as results are best when the child is clinically well at time of surgery. In addition to the anatomic abnormality, which is readily corrected surgically, there is a physiologic abnormality that persists throughout the life of the patient. In all instances of esophageal atresia, there is an abnormality of the motility of the proximal esophagus such that no effective primary peristaltic wave forms. It is this abnormal motility of the esophagus, rather than the relative narrowing at the site of the anastomosis, that is most often responsible for large boluses of food becoming lodged and obstructing the esophagus at the line of anastomosis. Most patients adjust to this physiologic disability in time.

Most *congenital stenoses* of the esophagus occur in the distal third of the esophagus. The commonest type is a local weblike area of narrowing; the less common type is a long, tubular segment of narrowing. The latter is frequently more difficult to identify on an esophagram unless the entire esophagus is well distended.

The *ingestion of caustic substances* is a common and serious problem encountered in the pediatric age group. Such ingestions may lead to burns of the lips, oral cavity, pharynx, esophagus, larynx and trachea. Depending on the severity of the burns, extensive fibrosis and obstruction of the esophagus and airway may develop. The roentgen examination plays an important part in the evaluation of such a patient. The roentgen examination of the neck aids in determining the extent and severity of the burns in the pharynx, larynx and trachea, as manifested by the degree of edema and obstruction of the airway that is present (Fig. 24). The roentgen examination of the chest will aid in determining whether mediastinitis or aspiration pneumonia has occurred.

The esophagus is examined radiographically by means of the esophagram. Because such patients may have difficulty in swallowing, a thin barium-water mixture is used initially. Burns of the esophagus will be manifested radiographically as edema of the mucosa, and in such instances the mucosal folds will not be sharply defined and may appear slightly irregular and thicker than normal (Fig. 24 *B*). In severe burns, ulcerations and even perforations may be evident. During the acute phase of esophageal burns, there is no narrowing of the esophagus; this usually occurs about 10 to 14 days after the insult, when fibrosis develops (Fig. 24 *C*). The upper and middle thirds of the esophagus are most commonly affected in instances of alkali burns.

When acid-containing caustic substances are ingested, burns are most likely to be found in the distal esophagus and stomach and may later result in gastric obstruction if fibrosis develops. Contrary to common belief, chlorine bleach in sufficient amounts will produce burns of the esophagus in the same manner as other alkaline agents (Biklazi et al., 1969).

One of the most frequent requests for a roentgen examination of a child is to locate a *foreign body* that has been ingested. There are several anatomic points where foreign bodies frequently will be lodged in the esophagus—at the level of the cricopharyngeus, at the level of the aorta or carina of the trachea, and at the esophagogastric junction. Whenever a foreign body is lodged in the esophagus at a point other than those mentioned, an underlying abnormality of the esophagus, such as an area of stenosis, must be suspected (Fig. 25). If the foreign body is radiopaque, no other roentgen study is done until the foreign body has been removed, and then an esophagram is performed to exclude the presence of an esophageal stenosis and to determine if the esophagus has been traumatized by the foreign body. If a foreign body has been lodged in the esophagus for any length of time, there may be ulceration and perforation of the

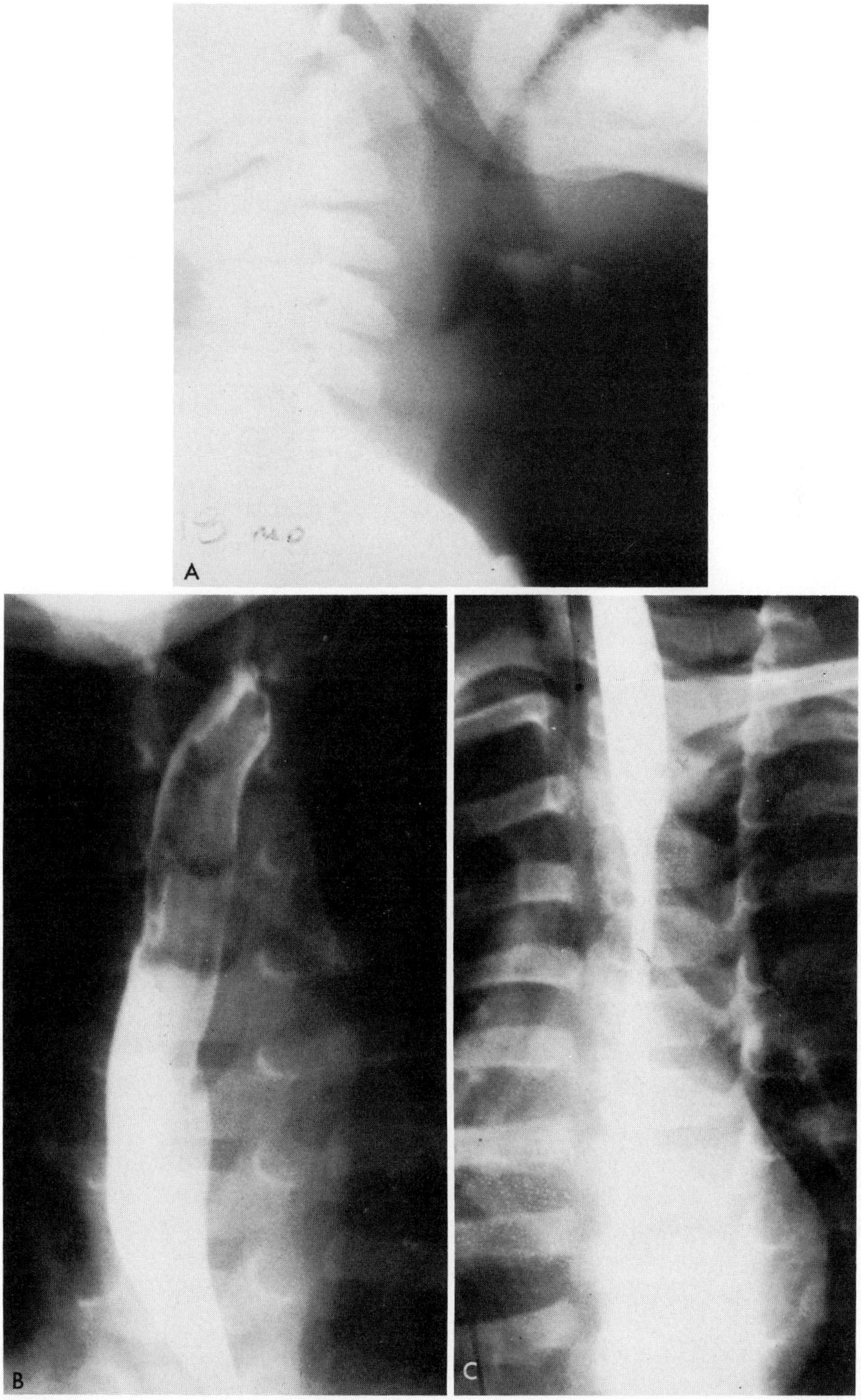

Figure 24. Caustic ingestion. *A*, Marked edema of the epiglottis and aryepiglottic folds indicates the presence of burns. *B*, The esophageal folds are thickened, reflecting edema due to esophageal burns. *C*, Approximately one month later, marked narrowing of the esophagus is evident.

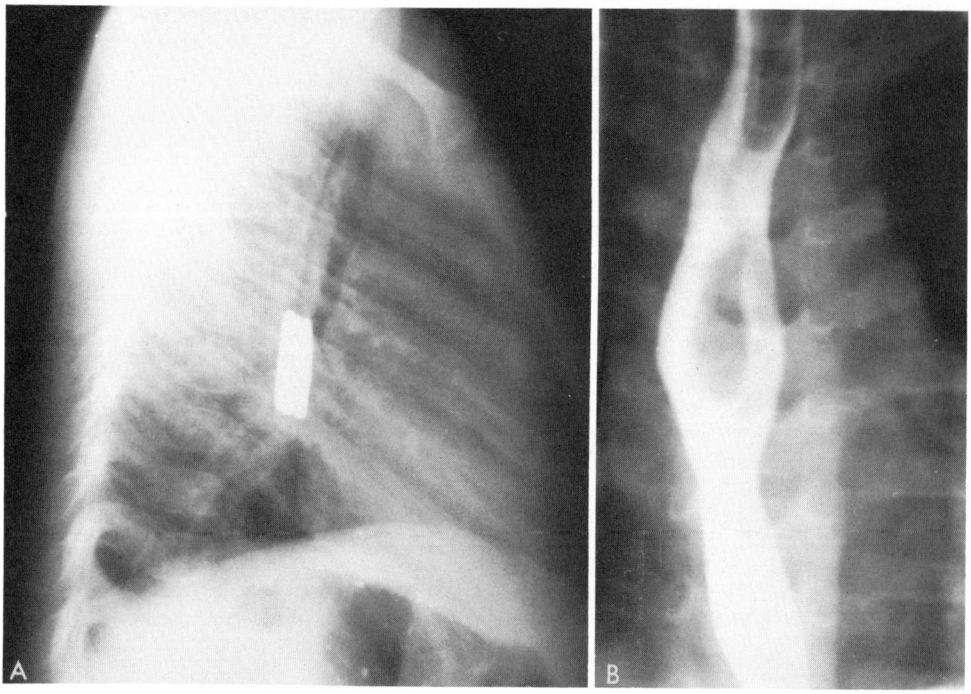

Figure 25. Esophageal foreign bodies. *A,* Three coins are seen on the lateral view. *B,* There is a tubular area of stenosis of the esophagus.

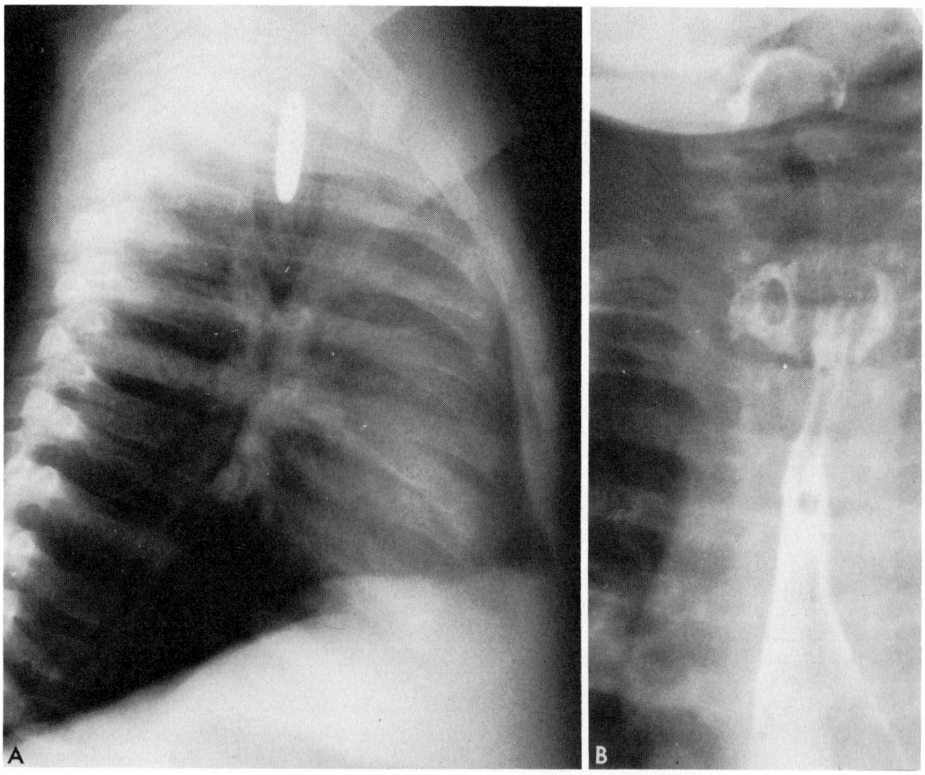

Figure 26. Esophageal foreign body. *A,* A coin is lodged in the esophagus at the level of the aortic arch. *B,* An area of erosion of the esophagus is seen where the coin had been lodged.

esophagus, even if the foreign body is a smooth object, such as a coin (Fig. 26). Coins are among the most common objects ingested. When coins are lodged in the esophagus, they will always appear as a round disc on frontal films of the chest, whereas coins lodged in the larynx or trachea will always be seen on end. In addition to a frontal film of the chest, a lateral film should also be exposed, as a number of coins may be lodged in the esophagus at the same level and appear as one on the frontal film. Not until the lateral film of the chest is reviewed will the exact number of coins actually present become apparent.

SUMMARY

There are a variety of radiologic techniques readily available for the diagnosis of obstruction of the respiratory tract and the esophagus. Any special study must be preceded by a basic examination that includes as a minimum the neck in the lateral position and frontal and lateral exposures of the chest. After these are studied, then the techniques just discussed are utilized to define the underlying abnormality. It must be kept in mind that the lesion may be congenital, acquired, traumatic or neoplastic, and that the nature of the abnormality may often be suspected on the basis of associated or indirect effects on the involved or adjacent structures as well as by its direct visualization.

REFERENCES

Berdon, W. E., Baker, D. H., Borduik, J., and Mellins, R.: Innominate artery compression of the trachea in infants with stridor and apnea. *Radiology,* 92:272, 1969.

Biklazi, H. B., Thompson, E. R., and Shumrick, D. A.: Caustic ingestion: Current status. *Arch. Otolaryng.,* 89:770, 1969.

Campbell, R. E.: Intrapulmonary interstitial emphysema: A complication of hyaline membrane disease. *Amer. J. Roentgen.,* 110:449, 1970.

Cantrell, J. R., and Guild, H. G.: Congenital stenosis of the trachea. *Amer. J. Surg.,* 108:297, 1964.

Capitanio, M. A., and Kirkpatrick, J. A.: Upper respiratory tract obstruction in infants and children. *Radiol. Clin. N. Amer.,* 6:265, 1968.

Capitanio, M. A., and Kirkpatrick, J. A.: Roentgen examination in the evaluation of the newborn infant with respiratory distress. *J. Pediat.,* 75:896, 1969.

Capitanio, M. A., and Kirkpatrick, J. A.: Roentgenographic evaluation of intestinal obstruction in the newborn infant. *Pediat. Clin. N. Amer.,* 17:983, 1970.

Capitanio, M. A., Ramos, R., and Kirkpatrick, J. A.: Pulmonary sling. *Amer. J. Roentgen.,* 112:28, 1971.

Culiner, M. M.: Obliterative bronchitis and bronchiolitis with bronchiectasis. *Dis. Chest,* 44:351, 1963.

Greenfield, H., and Herman, P. G.: Papillomatosis of the trachea and bronchi. *Amer. J. Roentgen.,* 89:45, 1963.

Greenough, W. G.: Congenital esophageal strictures. *Amer. J. Roentgen.,* 92:994, 1964.

Griscom, N. T.: Persistent esophagotrachea. *Amer. J. Roentgen.,* 97:211, 1966.

Gross, R. E., and Neuhauser, E. B. D.: Compression of the trachea or esophagus by vascular anomalies; surgical therapy in 40 cases. *Pediatrics,* 7:69, 1951.

Kirkpatrick, J. A., Cresson, S. L., and Pilling, G. P.: The motor activity of the esophagus in association with esophageal atresia and tracheoesophageal fistula. *Amer. J. Roentgen.,* 86:884, 1961.

LaDue, J. S.: Bronchiolitis fibrosa obliterans. *Arch. Int. Med.,* 68:663, 1941.

Rosenblum, H. D., Alavi, S. M., and Bryant, L. R.: Pulmonary parenchymal spread of juvenile laryngeal papillomatosis. *Radiology,* 90:654, 1968.

Singleton, E. B., and Wagner, M. L.: *Radiologic Atlas of Pulmonary Abnormalities in Children.* Philadelphia, W. B. Saunders Co., 1971.

Steele, R. W., Metz, J. R., Bass, J. W., and Dubois, J. J.: Pneumothorax and pneumomediastinum in the newborn. *Radiology,* 98:629, 1971.

Swischuk, L. E.: Anterior tracheal indentation in infancy and early childhood: Normal or abnormal? *Amer. J. Roentgen.,* 112:12, 1971.

Tsai, S. H., and Jenne, J. W.: Mucoid impaction of the bronchi. *Amer. J. Roentgen.,* 96:953, 1966.

Willis, R. A.: *The Pathology of the Tumors of Children.* Springfield, Ill., Charles C Thomas, 1962.

Wittenborg, M. H., Gyepes, M. T., and Crocker, D.: Tracheal dynamics in infants with respiratory distress, stridor, and collapsing trachea. *Radiology,* 88:653, 1967.

Wittenborg, M. H., Tantiwongese, T., and Rosenberg, B. F.: Anomalous course of left pulmonary artery with respiratory obstruction. *Radiology,* 67:339, 1956.

INDEX